Ophthalmic Plastic Surgery

OPHTHALMIC
PLASTIC SURGERY

FOURTH EDITION

Sidney A. Fox, M.S. (OPHTH.), M.D., F.A.C.S.

*Clinical Professor of Ophthalmology, New York University School of
Medicine; Visiting Ophthalmologist, Bellevue Hospital; Consultant
Ophthalmologist, Bronx, V. A. Hospital, Goldwater Memorial Hospital
and Hospital for Joint Diseases and Medical Center*

Grune & Stratton   New York and London

GRUNE & STRATTON, INC.
757 Third Avenue
New York, New York 10017

Library of Congress Catalog Card Number 75-100073

International Standard Book Number 0-8089-0646-1

Printed in the United States of America (G-B)

To My Wife—Again

Preface to the Fourth Edition

Every edition of a book has a way of battening on its progenitor. This fourth edition is no exception. It is bigger and fatter and longer than its predecessor. It contains more text and more illustrations.

In extenuation it must be said that the size of the book is due neither to unplanned nor uncontrolled elephantiasis but to the fact that the past ten or fifteen years have seen a steady evolution—almost revolution—in methods of lid repair. No single step in this change has been particularly startling but the cumulative result is dramatic indeed. One has but to compare this volume with the textbooks of thirty and twenty years ago (even Fox's Third Edition), to realize how the specialty has advanced. As a result, while some material has been retained, much was discarded and much more added. All the chapters have been revised; most of them have been completely rewritten, three are new. The book is as up-to-date as publishing time will allow and hence, I believe, more valuable than its predecessor.

Happy the author whose book is popular enough to go into multiple editions. It gives him the opportunity to change previously unalterable opinions which time has proven false. It also permits him to add new technics and to discard outmoded operations. But there is an obverse to the coin. Frequent editions require a constant state of alertness for new procedures and new technics which seem to have lasting merit. Decisions are not always easy and infallibility is not one of man's commoner assets. Hence, constant revision and rewriting is necessary no matter how burdensome. With all the labor, I am thankful to have had the opportunity for revision again so soon.

The perspicacious reader will note that the organization of the book has been drastically changed and the classifications simplified. The presentation of cases now proceeds in orderly fashion from the simple extramarginal lesions to the most complicated reconstructions. As always, the book is directed to the practicing ophthalmologist, not the surgical specialist. Bibliographies have been expanded and brought up to date. They are not encyclopedic but any interested reader can get a good start here for thorough investigation of any subject in ophthalmic plastic surgery.

I have been accused of wasting too much space on historical facts in my books. The headlong advance of scientific medicine—and this includes ophthalmology—is now so rapid that little time is left for contemplation and study of its various affects on the human being. Even less important apparently is the historic early origin of many of our modern scientific principles and technics. Many "new" revelations and operations are offered whose provenance, with little change, existed scores of years ago.

I do not apologize for my interest in the historical. Here, as in previous volumes, I have permitted myself a few reflective looks backward and behind the scenes. There are not many as versatile as Iri, court physician to a pharaoh about 2500 B.C. who, history tells us, was "an oculist of both eyes, shepherd of the rectum, magician and scholar." But I find it interesting that Dieffenbach, who contributed so much to ophthalmic plastic surgery, was not an ophthalmologist; that Syzmanowski was a Russian military surgeon; that the immortal Bowman started out as a professor of anatomy and Thomas Wharton Jones as a professor of physiology. There are countless such recondite historical facts, too many for inclusion. This is my way of trying to humanize and quicken dead eponyms into something more than cold faceless abstractions. The fact that Argyll Robertson's full name was Douglas Moray Cooper Lamb Argyll Robertson is not of the slightest scientific significance. However, it is interesting that he achieved greatness despite the onus of such nomenclature and it somehow brings him closer to us.

As for illustrations: The book contains 308 figures. This is approximately one-third more than the previous edition. Many old ones were discarded, many redrawn and even more new ones added. I do not know how many more hundred single drawings and photographs this represents but I would guess that at least half of all these figures are new. No attempt has been made to create a complete set of pretty matched illustrations. Old favorites have been kept because I could find no better ones. Thus, the illustrations are a somewhat heterogeneous collection but they have one quality in common: clarity. If they showed what was done clearly, they were used—old or new, halftone or pen and ink. A plain black and white line drawing is often more enlightening than the elaborate halftone with its many shadings—as shown here.

This volume has two new contributors: Dr. Joseph Newall, who wrote the chapter on radiotherapy; and Dr. Perry Robins, who contributed the section on chemosurgery. I am grateful to both these men, specialists in their respective fields, who have been kind enough to give of their time and skill to help round out this book. Both contributions are completely unedited. While, as indicated elsewhere, I may not agree wholeheartedly with everything they say, their right to say it was unchallenged.

This is the sixth book for which Mr. Lou Barlow has done the illustrations and Mr. Walter S. Lentschner the photographs. They have my sincere thanks. This is also the sixth book for which Miss Helen Holoviak has given unstintingly of her patient, skillful and unflagging assistance with all the stenography and editing involved in this undertaking. Without this team of dedicated collaborators this book would have been a poorer thing.

SIDNEY A. FOX

Contents

CHAPTER 1

Anatomy: Brow and Lids, Orbit, Lacrimal Apparatus

BROW AND LIDS

BETTER THAN any other organ in the body, the eye is guarded by its own protective and sanitary mechanisms which serve it through all the ordinary wear and tear of daily seeing as well as in most of the unusual vicissitudes that life throws on it and at it.

Most of the eye lies buried in the orbit but even its exposed anterior surface is shielded by the overhanging brow above, the lids in front, and the nose and cheekbones to the sides and below. However, it is the eyebrow and lids which are the important protective elements of the eye. In their exposed position, they are the first bulwarks against the irritations and injuries to which the eye is constantly subjected. The jutting overhang of the brow is a stationary defense. The reflexly acting lids, constantly in motion, constitute a mobile guard against the dust, smoke, glare, heat, cold, foreign bodies and the thousand and one insults of man and nature. It is not remarkable that the brow and lids suffer many injuries. What is a matter for wonder is that this occurs so often leaving the eye intact.

Surface Anatomy of the Eyebrow

The eyebrow is a horizontal eminence separating the upper lid from the forehead. It is covered with an arching growth of hair which is thickest medially and tapers off to a thin line laterally. The supply of brow hair is not standard and varies with the individual. In some, the hairs are abundant and thick; in others, they are thin and sparse. In general, they partake of the character of the scalp hair and, since they are important cosmetically, the similarity becomes significant in plastic surgery when one is forced to restore the eyebrow. Medially, where thickest, the hairs of the brow tend to grow somewhat below the orbital margin. Temporally they form a thin line a little above the lateral orbital border. In general, the hairs of each brow are directed outward toward the temple except those closest to the glabella, which run straight upward. The glabella is usually clean of hair. Occasionally it contains a few short hairs; more rarely, it is so thickly covered that there is no separation at all between the eyebrows. In ancient Greece this was considered a mark of beauty.

Surface Anatomy of the Lids

Below the protective hirsute prominence of the brow lie the apposed upper and lower lids. When closed they protect the cavelike opening which is the orbit. Together they extend from the brow above to the cheek below and from the frontomaxillary orbital margin medially to the frontozygomatic orbital margin laterally. When closed they offer a

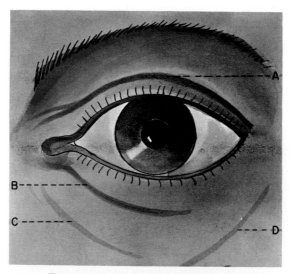

FIG. 1.   The Palpebral Furrows.
A. Superior.   C. Nasojugal.
B. Inferior.   D. Malar.

waterproof, hermetically sealed shutter which is difficult to pry open against resistance.

Lid Furrows

The skin of the lids shows several furrows which are important surgical landmarks (fig. 1). The most important is the upper palpebral furrow in the upper lid (usually absent in the Mongolian races) which marks the attached upper border of the tarsus and establishes the limit between smooth and folded parts of the conjunctiva. Most of the levator attachment to the skin is below this line. Hence, above the superior palpebral furrow, where the skin has no attachment to the levator, the skin is loose and tends to overhang the furrow as the lid moves up. In the lower lid the homologous inferior palpebral furrow is rarely defined as clearly and, indeed, is often absent except in infancy. Also in the lower lid two other faint furrows can sometimes be made out in older individuals: the malar and nasojugal. The former is seen more often. The latter marks the position of the facial artery and vein extending to the medial canthus. These furrows mark the site of attachment of the skin to the lower temporal and nasal periosteum of the orbital margin respectively. Surgically these landmarks are important because they indicate fascial barriers which limit the passage of hemorrhage and inflammation to and from the orbit.

Palpebral Fissure

When the eyelids are closed normally, as in sleep, the line of juncture between the two lids is not a perfectly straight line but one which rises slightly at its medial end and drops perceptibly at the lateral end. The reverse is true when the eye is open, for then the lateral canthus is higher than the medial. When open naturally, the lids uncover an irregular ellipse, the palpebral fissure, in which most of the cornea and a little of the sclera is framed. In infants under one year the palpebral fissure measures 18 to 22 mm. in length; in adults this opening usually measures from 25 to 28 mm. horizontally and 7 to 11 mm. vertically; the average width is 9 mm.

In proptosis and high myopia more of the globe is visible. In infants the palpebral fissure is relatively much wider with the upper lid border usually lying at the upper limbus and the whole cornea exposed. Since the fissure is also shorter horizontally it tends to assume more of a circular shape than oval.

In upward and downward movement of the eye, the palpebral fissure changes not only in size but also in shape when it moves away from the straight-ahead position. This is due to two factors: (1) the action of the ocular muscles, and (2) the orbital fat. Thus, in upward movement the upper lid is pulled not only upward but somewhat backward. (In other words, the upper lid movement is not entirely analogous to a "window blind" as has been erroneously stated.) This backward movement causes downward and somewhat forward displacement of the semisolid orbital fat and is aided by the concomitant relaxation and forward movement of the lower lid muscle fibers. On downward movement of the lids, the reverse takes place with the superior rectus and levator relaxing and moving forward and the fascial expansions of the inferior rectus contracting with backward movement of the lower lid thus displacing orbital fat upward and backward.

As a result of all this, the plane of the palpebral fissure moves not only upward and downward but rotates on a frontal axis and remains constantly parallel with the cornea no matter what the position of the globe.

An analogous situation is noted on lateral and medial gaze. Thus when the eye is moved temporally, the lateral commissure moves somewhat backward also and the plica and caruncle are pushed slightly forward. Conversely, on looking medially, the caruncle and plica are somewhat retracted and the lateral commissure protrudes. In addition, there is often a slight narrowing of the palpebral fissure probably due to slight attendant orbicularis contraction.

The curve of the upper lid is greatest at the juncture of its inner and middle thirds, that of the lower lid at the juncture of the middle and outer thirds. With the eyes open, the lateral canthus is somewhat higher than the medial in all eyes. In the white races this difference in height is only 2 or 3 mm. In the Mongolian races it is greater and a distinct slant upward and outward is to be noted. Also the shape of the Mongolian fissure tends to be different than that of the Caucasian. It is usually somewhat longer relatively, with the medial half being somewhat wider (fig. 2).

As has been stated, the palpebral fissure is not a perfect ellipse.

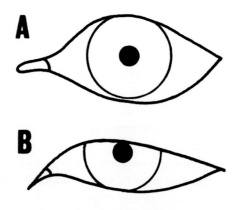

FIG. 2.   The Palpebral Fissure Outlines.
A.   Caucasian.   B.   Oriental.

Laterally the lids meeting at the outer commissure form a sharp, acute angle, the lateral canthus, and lie flush against the eyeball. At the medial canthus the fusion of the two lids is more rounded, and the medial commissure is 5 to 7 mm. away from the globe, being separated by the lacus lacrimalis (the lake of tears), which contains the plica semilunaris and, more medially, the caruncle. The plica semilunaris is a fold of conjunctiva which in humans is a vestigial remnant of the nictitating membrane or third eyelid of the lower species.

The caruncle is a reddish, irregular, fleshy little eminence measuring about 4 or 5 mm. vertically and 3 mm. across, lying between the plica and medial canthus. It is actually a modified form of skin and contains sebaceous glands and a few hairs. The caruncle is not a particularly handsome structure, taken by itself, but it is an important cosmetic adjunct in the over-all picture of the eye. Its absence or malposition is readily noticeable. Hence, it is important to know that it is attached not only to the plica semilunaris but also to the sheath of the medial rectus muscle. When displaced by an improper dissection of this muscle the eye acquires a "stary" or "glassy" look. This was frequently seen in earlier days when tenotomies of the medial rectus were more common.

Most of the opening and shutting of the eye is done by the upper lid. Opening is accomplished by a unique muscle, the levator palpebrae superioris, which pulls the lid up from in front of the cornea when the eye opens. The lower border of the upper lid then overrides the upper limbus and is normally situated approximately halfway between the pupillary border and the limbus in average illumination (when the pupil is 3 to 4 mm. in size). However, this may vary as much as 2 or 3 mm.

The border of the lower lid is usually just at the lower limbus but may be a trifle lower. The lower lid takes but little part in the process of opening and shutting of the eye. Its only movement is a slight rise when the eye is shut and a slight lowering when the orbicularis and inferior rectus relax and the eye is opened. However, due to its attachment to the globe via the fascial expansion of the inferior rectus, the lower lid moves 4 to 7 mm. between upward and downward gaze.

Lid Margins

The margin of the lids is almost 2 mm. in width and covered with modified skin. The anterior edge of the margin, from which the cilia project in several rows, is rounded. The cilia are arranged in two or three irregular rows being longer, more numerous and coarser in the upper lid than in the lower. It has been estimated that there are normally about 100 cilia in the upper lid and approximately 50 in the lower. They are usually about 2 mm. long but show much variation in different individuals. They curl upward in the upper lid and downward in the lower. The cilia thus serve to protect the eye against flying particles from both above and below. When lost they usually grow back in 8 to 10 weeks. They rarely change color and do not ordinarily grow lighter with age.

The posterior edge of the lid border is sharp and fits closely against the globe. When examined carefully, the openings of the meibomian glands may be noted just in front of the posterior edge of the lid border.

Also to be noted on the lid margin is the intermarginal groove, a faint grayish line just anterior to the openings of the meibomian glands, which marks the natural anatomic division of the lid between the tarsus and orbicularis. This "gray line" is a ready-made cleavage plane supplied by nature for the surgeon, always available and usually identifiable, unless much trauma, pathology or scarring have preceded operative procedure. An incision here splits the lid easily into skin-muscle and tarsoconjunctival laminae, and the surgeon has two clean tissue surfaces with the best possible conditions for normal postoperative healing.

The portions of the lid which bound the plica semilunaris lose the above characteristics. Here they are completely rounded both anteriorly and posteriorly and are bare of cilia. At a point opposite the plica, a small pinhead mound of tissue, the papilla lacrimalis, rises slightly above the surface of the border, and in both lids it is pierced in the center by the punctum lacrimale, which is the opening into the canaliculi. (See below.)

In working on the closed lids which cover the orbital opening, the orbit may be divided into quadrants which contain the following important structures: upper temporal—the lacrimal gland; upper medial—the pulley of the superior oblique; lower medial—the origin of the inferior oblique. The lower temporal quadrant, with no important structure, is the least vulnerable. Most of the eye and its muscles are located behind the upper lid when closed, and the line of lid closure marks the lower corneal limbus.

Surgical Anatomy of the Eyebrow

The brow is akin to the scalp in structure. Its layers from without inward are skin, subcutaneous tissue, muscles (note the plural), submuscular areolar tissue and pericranium. The skin is firmly attached to the fibrous subcutaneous fascia and though thick is exceedingly mobile, because the fascia, in turn, is connected to the multiple muscle layer beneath it, and all three layers move as one.

The muscle layer consists of three muscles whose fibers are so intermingled that it is difficult to identify them in this region (fig. 3): (1) The orbicularis oculi is the most superficial, and its horizontal fibers just reach the brow at its highest point. It is the sphincter of the eye and

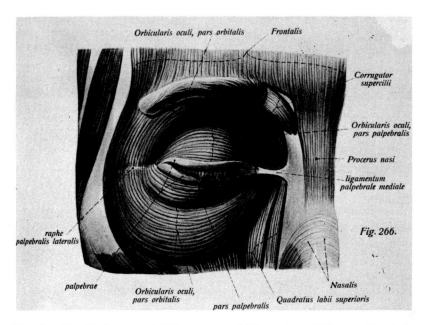

FIG. 3. The Eyebrow and Lids: Frontal Dissection. (Sobotta, J.: Atlas der deskriptiven Anatomie des Menschen. Courtesy J. F. Lehmans Verlag, München.)

is discussed more fully below. (2) The vertical frontalis raises the eyebrow and lid and creases the forehead. (3) The oblique corrugator supercilii draws the eyebrow medially and creates the vertical folds above the nose in midforehead.

The frontalis, the anterior half of the long, flat occipitofrontalis, takes its origin from the epicranial aponeurosis anterior to the coronal suture. It is inserted into the skin and subcutaneous layer of the eyebrow, mingling here with the fibers of the other two muscles, the orbicularis and corrugator. By its action it draws the scalp forward, creases the forehead and raises the eyebrow, which in turn raises the upper lid, thus opening the eye widely: the expression of astonishment is the result. This ability to raise the lid makes it important in the repair of certain types of ptosis.

The corrugator supercilii muscle lies deep to the orbicularis and frontalis under the medial half of the eyebrow. It is a narrow band of muscle which takes its origin from the medial end of the superciliary ridge. From here it passes temporally and somewhat upward to about the center of the eyebrow where it sends fibers through the two other overlying muscles to insert into the skin and subcutaneous fibrous layer. The two corrugators acting as a team pull the eyebrows together and wrinkle the skin above the nose vertically: thus the frown is expressed.

The submuscular tissue layer is thinner than the subcutaneous layer and is areolar in structure. Its attachment to the brow is a rather loose one and, since the frontalis is not attached here at all, the products of hemorrhage and infection find their way easily from above the brow into the upper lid between the orbicularis and the septum orbitale.

The vascular supply of the eyebrow is by way of the supraorbital and temporal arteries and veins. The sensory nerve supply is from the fifth cranial nerve.

Surgical Anatomy of the Lids

The lids are multilaminated structures made up of layer upon layer of tissue, each distinctive and each serving a purposeful function. The following tissues in anteroposterior arrangement go to make up the lids: (1) skin, (2) subcutaneous areolar tissue, (3) orbicularis, (4) submuscular tissue layer, (5) septum orbitale with the tarsal plates, (6) the levator (upper lid), (7) Müller's muscles, and (8) the conjunctiva.

Skin of the Lids

The skin of the lids, as has been pointed out so frequently, is probably the thinnest in the body. In the aged, it becomes even finer and almost as diaphanous as tissue paper. Furthermore, it stretches easily, and the superior palpebral furrow is marked by a fold of skin, wider temporally, which hangs down to the lid margin. The other palpebral furrows also become more prominent in older individuals. The skin is attached loosely over the eyelids (except at the tarsi) but firmly at the brow, cheek, lid margins and canthi.

Subcutaneous Layer

The subcutaneous layer is areolar tissue, thin and loose, which has little attachment to the subjacent orbicularis muscle and is easily infiltrated by edema, fluid or hemorrhage.

Orbicularis Muscle

The orbicularis oculi (fig. 4) is the muscle which brings the lids together and closes the eye. It is a flat, sheetlike muscle whose fibers, originating from the medial palpebral ligament, run in elliptical pattern around the palpebral fissure and spread outward in ever widening concentric arcs of fibers. These fibers cover the lids, overlap the adjacent eyebrow, temple and cheek and fuse into the lateral raphé in front of the lateral palpebral ligament. For ophthalmologic purposes the muscle is conveniently divided into orbital and palpebral portions.

The orbital portion of the orbicularis is the peripheral part of the muscle which rises from the medial margin of the upper and lower orbital rim. In the upper lid it sweeps upward to cover the corrugator

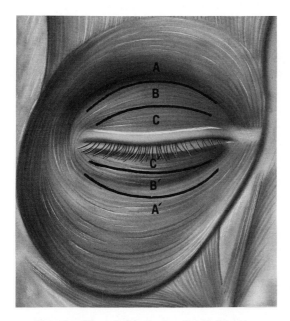

FIG. 4. The Orbicularis Oculi Muscle.
A.A' Orbital portions.   B.B' Preseptal muscles.
BC and B'C' Palpebral portions.   C.C' Pretarsal muscles.

supercilii, fuse with frontalis and overlap the adjacent temporal muscle laterally. Below, it spreads downward behind the skin of the cheek to cover part of the malar bone. This orbital portion of the orbicularis is the part used to squeeze the lids together firmly in spasm. "Crow's feet" beyond the lateral canthus of the eye mark the lines of tension left in the skin by its contraction. It is normally used in sneezing, laughing, crying, etc.

The palpebral portion, confined to the lids, runs from the medial canthal ligament to the lateral palpebral raphé. Medially it is also attached to the superior maxilla. Anatomically it may be further subdivided into two parts as suggested by Jones and Boyden. The pretarsal portion or muscle lies on the anterior surface of the tarsus being separated from it only by the fibers of the levator which pass through to attach to the skin. Beyond the tarsus is the preseptal portion of the palpebral muscle which covers the orbital septum. The palpebral portion of the orbicularis is thinnest at the attached border of the tarsus and is firmly joined to it; it is less firmly attached to the septum. It is covered by layers of loose areolar tissue which separate it from the skin anteriorly and which permits easy infiltration of the lid by edema and hemorrhage. There is no fat between these layers. It is this part of the orbicularis muscle which acts reflexly to close the eye in sleep, against danger and to blink away offending substances. Ravetta and his co-workers have pointed out that these subdivisions of the orbicularis have poorly defined limits and are anatomic rather than actual.

Two localized bundles of orbicularis fibers have special names:

1. The tensor tarsi, or Horner's muscle, is a scant bundle of orbicularis fibers whose origin is behind the lacrimal sac. As it passes forward and temporally, it divides into two narrow slips which surround both canaliculi and merge with the fibers of the orbicularis covering the tarsi. It helps the canaliculi to siphon away the tears, and it is this bundle of fibers, along with the lacrimal fascia and the posterior attachment of the medial palpebral ligament, which keep the lower lid in place after section of the anterior fibers of the medial canthal ligament as in dacryocystectomy.

2. The muscle of Riolan is a narrow band of striated muscle fibers which lies subconjunctivally in the dense tissue of the posterior portion of the lid margin in the neighborhood of the openings of the meibomian glands. It is separated from the palpebral portion of the orbicularis and the roots of the cilia by the glands of Moll (fig. 6). Medially it merges with Horner's muscle. The muscle of Riolan helps to bring the lid margins together and is the muscle which is thought by some to cause senile entropion by contracting sharply as a result of conjunctival inflammation and irritation, thus inverting the lid. This is impossible for two reasons: First, its position on the lid margin precludes this. Secondly, it is too negligible and scrawny a muscle to be capable of this.

The orbicularis is also supplied by the facial nerve.

Submuscular Layer

The submuscular layer of areolar tissue is important surgically for two reasons: (1) Because of its connection with the submuscular layer of the brow, it is the plane along which infection from the brow may spread. (2) Most of the main blood vessels and nerves supplying the lids lie in this area. Hence to anesthetize the lids fully and most easily by infiltration one should inject beneath the orbicularis fibers.

Fascia Orbitalis (Septum Orbitale; Palpebral Fascia)

The septum orbitale and the tarsal plates form a continuous layer of fibrous tissue which constitutes the only firm framework of the lids.

The septum orbitale is attached to the periosteum of the orbital rim along its whole periphery and is a continuation of the dura mater. In the upper lid it blends with the fibers of the adjacent levator aponeurosis at varying distances above the attached tarsal border and thus does not insert into the tarsus as a separate entity. In the lower lid it proceeds from the lower orbital rim upward to blend with the fascial expansion of the inferior rectus without inserting into the tarsus. Medially the upper and lower extensions blend with the posterior crus of the canthal liga-

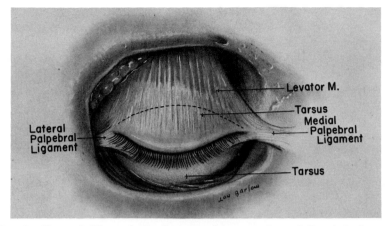

FIG. 5.   Frontal View of the Levator Aponeurosis and Its Attachments.

ment to insert into the posterior lacrimal crest. Laterally they fuse to form the posterior layer of the palpebral raphé, the anterior layer of which is formed by the fusion of the upper and lower orbicularis fibers.

The septum orbitale is not of uniform thickness but has weak areas, especially medially, in the upper lid and below the tarsus in the lower lid. In the aged and not so aged this permits the herniation of orbital fat and helps cause the "baggy" lids. It is not a rigid membrane and moves easily with the lids in all directions. It is important surgically because, in general, the septum orbitale tends to prevent hemorrhage and infection which arise on either side of it from invading the other side.

The Levator Muscle

The levator palpebrae superioris, which raises the upper lid and thus opens the eye, takes its origin above the optic foramen under the lesser wing of the sphenoid. Its fibers are grouped together into a flat little band not unlike the other extraocular muscles. It advances forward just below the orbital roof and above the superior rectus muscle. Near the front of the orbit close to the equator of the globe it loses its fleshy appearance abruptly and becomes a wide triangular fibrous aponeurosis which at first is separated from the septum by a layer of oribital fat. More anteriorly it becomes firmly connected with the septum orbitale and spreads out medially and laterally to occupy the whole width of the orbit (fig. 5).

Its main and most important attachment is to the skin of the upper lid in front and above the tarsus. Its fibers penetrate the orbicularis in small multiple bundles to reach the skin (fig. 6). It is also attached firmly to the upper anterior two-thirds of the tarsus. It sends off two projections medially and laterally, the "horns." The lateral horn attaches to the orbital tubercle by way of the canthal ligament; the medial joins

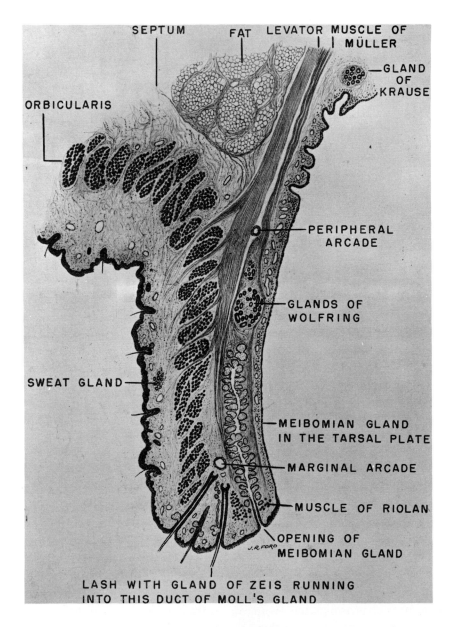

FIG. 6. Sagittal Section Through the Upper Lid. (Wolff, Eugene: The Anatomy of the Eye and Orbit. Courtesy W. B. Saunders Co., Philadelphia and Toronto.)

the medial canthal ligament. On its way, the lateral horn, much the stronger and thicker of the two, indents the lacrimal gland into two lobes, forming orbital and palpebral portions which remain fused posteriorly. (See anatomy of the lacrimal gland below.) This should be remembered in all operations on the lacrimal gland. Another posterior attachment is via its sheath to the superior rectus muscle and the superior conjunctival fornix.

Along with some of the other extraocular muscles the levator derives its nerve supply from the third cranial nerve. By its action it raises the upper lid and draws it under the brow.

Palpebral Muscles (of Müller)

The superior palpebral muscle (of Müller) is a thin sheath of unstriped muscle fibers lying just behind the aponeurosis of the levator. Above the tarsal plate the two muscles are loosely connected by fine fibrils of connective tissue. Müller's muscle attaches to the upper border of the tarsus (fig. 6).

The inferior palpebral muscle in the lower lid is a weaker counterpart of the superior muscle. It originates from the sheath of the inferior rectus muscle and inserts into the lower border of the inferior tarsus. A fascial expansion from the inferior rectus muscle and Lockwood's ligament runs upward to insert on the anterior surface of the inferior tarsus. Some fibers from the expansion of the inferior rectus also penetrate the orbicularis to attach to the skin of the lower lid thus forming an analogue—albeit a poorly developed one—of the levator aponeurosis. Both muscles are supplied by sympathetic nerve filaments and their action is to assist in widening the palpebral fissure. (It is likely that some of the very mild forms of ptosis can be explained by weakness of the superior palpebral muscle.)

Tarsi

The tarsi are firm, semielliptical, flat little structures of thickened fibrous tissue in which lie the meibomian glands of which there are about 25 in the upper lid and 20 in the lower. Much the larger is the upper tarsus which is usually 11 to 12 mm. wide in the center. The lower tarsus is somewhat thinner and is only about 5 mm. at its widest. Both tarsi are slightly convex outward and loosely attached to the overlying orbicularis muscle. Posteriorly, on the other hand, they are so firmly attached to the conjunctiva that it is difficult to separate the two. The tarsi are thickest at the straight free border and thinnest at the attached curved border where they merge into septum orbitale. At their medial and lateral extremities they are attached by thick fibrous bands to the bones of the skull (fig. 5).

The lateral palpebral ligament is attached to the lateral orbital wall at the tubercle of the zygomatic bone 3 mm. behind the orbital rim, posterior to the lateral raphé of the orbicularis and the attachment of the levator. This attachment which is posterior to the anterior plane of the globe keeps the lateral commissure close against the eyeball.

The medial palpebral ligament is a wider band of connective tissue (fig. 5). Its main attachment, a broad one, is on the frontal process of the superior maxilla, well in front of the anterior lacrimal crest after crossing the lacrimal fossa and the dome of the lacrimal sac. It also sends a small slip to attach to the posterior lacrimal crest. The prominence of the medial palpebral ligament is easily noted on the frontal process of the maxilla and is a landmark in lacrimal sac surgery. The lateral palpebral ligament, on a more posterior plane, cannot be seen and can only be palpated when the lids are pulled medially and the ligament pulled forward. Thus the medial palpebral ligament is attached outside the orbit, while the lateral palpebral ligament has its attachment more posteriorly inside the orbit.

This position of the medial ligament may explain the frequency of avulsion of the lower lid at the medial canthus after trauma and also why the punctal area is the first to evert in cases of senile ectropion.

Conjunctiva

The conjunctiva is the posterior or internal layer of the lids. It is a membrane common to both the lids and eyeball. From the posterior surface of the lids it passes on to the eyeball and at the limbus it changes its character to form the epithelium of the cornea. Hence it lies interposed between the eye and lids in double thickness and forms a closed chamber whose entrance is through the palpebral fissure. For anatomic purposes it may be divided into three distinct areas: palpebral, fornical and bulbar.

The palpebral conjunctiva is a transparent, highly vascular layer of mucous membrane which is so strongly attached to the tarsi of the upper and lower lids as to be practically inseparable from them surgically. Between the tarsi and the upper and lower fornices, however, it is but loosely attached to the adjacent thin layer of Müller's muscle.

The conjunctiva of the fornices runs almost continuously around the inside of the lids forming a cul-de-sac whose greatest depth (8 to 10 mm.) is under the upper lid, the superior fornix, which reaches the superior orbital rim. The inferior fornix, somewhat shallower, almost reaches the lower orbital rim. Temporally the lateral fornix extends behind the equator of the eyeball. Nasally the lacus lacrimalis with its contents breaks the continuity of this conjunctival pocket.

The fornix conjunctivae bears several important relationships to contiguous structures. It is adherent to the fascial expansions of the recti and levator muscles. Though this attachment is a loose one, it is sufficient to deepen the fornices when the muscles contract. This relationship is additionally important when incisions of the upper and lower fornices are made. Thus a knife passed vertically up through the conjunctiva of the superior fornix will split the fibrous connection between the levator and superior rectus muscles. Inferiorly it will pass through the aponeu-

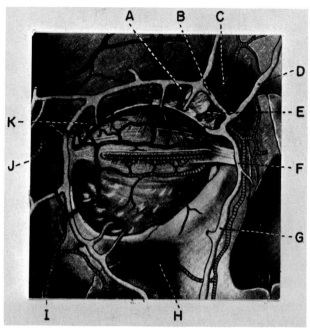

FIG. 7.   The Vascular Supply of the Lids.

A.   Supraorbital artery.
B.   Supraorbital vein.
C. and E.   Frontal artery.
D.   Frontal vein.
F.   Angular vein and artery.

G.   Facial vein and artery.
H.   Infraorbital artery.
I.   Transverse facial artery.
J.   Superficial temporal artery.
K.   Lacrimal artery.

(Wolff, Eugene: The Anatomy of the Eye and Orbit. Courtesy H. K. Lewis & Co. Ltd., London; Blakiston Co., Philadelphia.)

rotic layer between the inferior rectus and inferior oblique muscles.

Where not in contact with the muscle sheaths, the fornix conjunctivae is in close relation to the orbital fat. Hence fractures or infections at the base of the skull will allow blood and inflammatory processes to find their way under the bulbar conjunctiva.

The bulbar conjunctiva is quite loosely adherent to Tenon's capsule beneath it. This, together with the slackness furnished by the fornices, permits easy movement of the eyeball in all directions. Close to the cornea, however, it unites firmly with Tenon's capsule and the subjacent sclera and makes this the ideal location for fixation of the globe in surgical procedures.

Vascular Supply of the Lids

The vascular supply and drainage of the lids is fortunately a rich one (fig. 7). Hence the lids can stand a good deal of traumatic and surgical insult with an excellent chance of retaining their integrity. In fact, the ophthalmic surgeon has learned to take this for granted

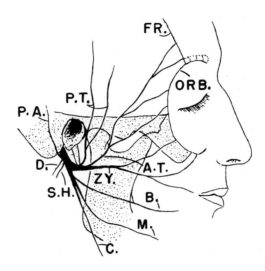

Fig. 8.   Distribution of the Terminal Facial Nerve Fibers.

FR. Edge of frontalis.	S.H. Stylohyoid.
ORB. Edge of orbicularis.	ZY. Zygomatic.
P.T. Posterior temporal.	B. Buccal.
A.T. Anterior temporal.	M. Mandibular.
P.A. Posterior auricular.	C. Cervical.
D. Digastric.	

(Wolff, Eugene: The Anatomy of the Eye and Orbit. Courtesy H. K. Lewis & Co. Ltd., London; Blakiston Co., Philadelphia.)

to such an extent that little thought is usually given to blood supply preliminary to surgery. And unless there has been a tremendous amount of injury and scar formation, this attitude is probably justified. However, knowledge of the approximate position of the main vessels of drainage and supply sometimes becomes important, because it is as valuable to know how to avoid bleeding as it is to know where to obtain vascular supply. For the requirements of the ophthalmic plastic surgeon the following résumé is adequate. Greater detail is available to any one desiring it in the many textbooks on this subject.

The arterial supply of the lids is derived mainly from the ophthalmic artery. Nasally the superior and inferior medial palpebral arteries penetrate the orbital septum above and below the medial palpebral ligament respectively. They run temporally to anastomose with the homologous lateral superior and inferior palpebral arteries derived from the lacrimal artery to form three tarsal arcades or arches. The two main tarsal arcades run close to each lid margin between the tarsus and the orbicularis muscle. The third tarsal arch, the arcus superioris tarsalis, lies anterior to the upper border of the upper lid tarsus. Occasionally what amounts to a fourth tarsal arcade may be made out at the attached border of the inferior tarsus. From these arcades, branches run forward and backward to supply all the lid tissues and to anastomose with each other.

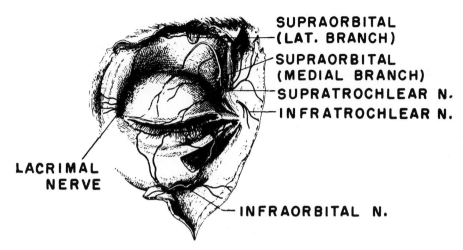

SUPRAORBITAL
(LAT. BRANCH)

SUPRAORBITAL
(MEDIAL BRANCH)

SUPRATROCHLEAR N.

INFRATROCHLEAR N.

LACRIMAL
NERVE

INFRAORBITAL N.

FIG. 9. The Sensory Nerve Supply of the Lids. (Wolff, Eugene: The Anatomy of the Eye and Orbit. Courtesy H. K. Lewis & Co. Ltd., London; Blakiston Co., Philadelphia.)

The venous supply to the lids is more ample and complex than the arterial and is especially rich in the upper and lower fornices and anterior and posterior to the tarsi. One group, pretarsal, empties into the angular and superficial temporal veins. A deeper retrotarsal group empties into the muscular tributaries of the ophthalmic vein.

Lymph Supply of the Lids

The lymph vessels of the lateral two-thirds of the upper lid and lateral third of the lower lid enter the parotid lymph nodes. The medial third of the upper lid and medial two-thirds of the lower lid drain into the submaxillary lymph nodes at the angle of the mandible. More centrally, both lymph pathways drain into the deep cervical nodes.

Nerve Supply of the Lids

As has already been indicated, the motor nerve supply to the lids is from the seventh cranial nerve to the orbicularis (fig. 8), from the third cranial nerve to the levator and by way of the sympathetic to Müller's muscle.

The sensory supply is from the fifth cranial nerve as follows (fig. 9): The upper lid is supplied mainly by the supraorbital and supratrochlear branches of the frontal nerve with the help of filaments from the infratrochlear (from the nasociliary) medially and from the lacrimal nerve laterally. The latter also supplies the lateral surface of the lower lid. The main sensory nerve supply to the lower lid is from the infraorbital branches of the maxillary nerve with the infratrochlear helping out medially. These sensory nerves form a plexus close to the margin between the orbicularis muscle and tarsus.

THE ORBIT

The orbit has been variously described as a quadrilateral pyramid, an irregular cone, and a pear-shaped figure of which the optic nerve is the stalk. These are all rather rough descriptions of the bony cavity which houses the eye (fig. 10).

Anteriorly its opening is somewhat quadrilateral in shape but with rounded corners. The opening is directed slightly laterally and tilted so that the upper and lower margins slope downward mediolaterally. The depth of the orbit is about 40 mm. and its volume has been estimated at about 30 cc. The roof, floor and lateral wall are roughly triangular in shape, the medial wall is somewhat quadrangular.

The roof is made up mostly of the frontal bone with the lesser wing of the sphenoid contributing a small part at the posterior apex. The anterolateral angle contains the fossa which lodges the orbital lobe of the lacrimal gland. About 4 mm. from the orbital margin is the trochlear fossa, a small depression which holds the pulley of the superior oblique muscle. The roof is rather thin and fragile especially in old age when bone absorption may cause bony dehiscences with the periorbita coming in direct contact with the dura.

The medial wall of the orbit is made up from before backward of the angular process of the frontal bone (above), the lacrimal bone (below), the lamina papyracea of the ethmoid and the lateral part of the sphenoid. This is by far the thinnest and most fragile wall of the orbit. The lacrimal sac lies anteriorly in this wall in a fossa surrounded by the lacrimal fascia. The ethmoid air cells are, of course, in close relation to the lamina papyracea and also to the lacrimal bone.

The floor of the orbit is made up of the zygomatic bone anterolaterally, the orbital plate of the maxilla centrally and the orbital process of the palatine bone posteriorly. It contains the infraorbital canal with its vessels and nerves. The floor slopes slightly downwards mediolaterally and is the shortest of the orbital boundaries. It lies above the maxillary sinus—a very important anatomic and pathologic relationship. The inferior oblique muscle originates just lateral to the opening of the nasolacrimal canal and passes, close to the floor, backward, outward and upward to its lateral attachment.

The outer wall is made up of the orbital portion of the zygomatic bone anteriorly and the orbital surface of the great wing of the sphenoid posteriorly. As required by its exposed position, it is the thickest of the orbital walls. The orbital tubercle lies just behind the orbital rim and gives attachment to the lateral palpebral ligament, the lateral horn of the levator and the suspensory ligament of the eyeball.

The margin of the orbit is made up of three bones. The frontal above, the zygomatic inferolaterally and the maxilla inferomedially. The

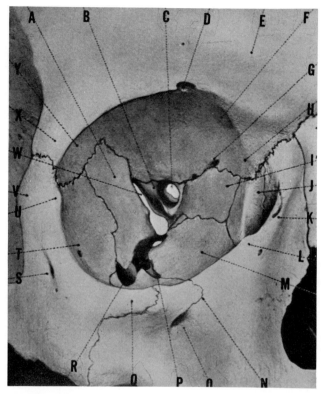

FIG. 10.   The Orbit.

A. Orbital plate of great wing of sphenoid.
B. Lesser wing of sphenoid.
C. Optic foramen.
D. Supraorbital notch.
E. Superciliary ridge.
F. Trochlear fossa.
G. Anterior ethmoidal foramen.
H. Medial angular process.
I. Ethmoid bone.
J. Lacrimal bone and fossa.
K. Sutura Notha.
L. Lacrimal tubercle.
M. Orbital plate of maxilla.
N. Infraorbital suture.
O. Infraorbital foramen.
P. Infraorbital groove.
Q. Marginal process.
R. Inferior orbital fissure.
S. Zygomaticofacial foramen.
T. Zygomatic foramen.
U. Lateral orbital tubercle.
V. Zygomatic tubercle.
W. Superior orbital fissure.
X. Lateral angular pocess.
Y. Fossa of lacrimal gland.

(Wolff, Eugene: The Anatomy of the Eye and Orbit. Courtesy H. K. Lewis & Co. Ltd., London; Blakiston Co., Philadelphia.)

height of the orbital opening is about 35 mm. and the width about 40 mm. The lateral orbital margin is the strongest and does not reach quite as far forward as the medial. The inferior orbital margin is slightly raised above the orbital floor. The medial margin contains the anterior lacrimal crest, the anterior boundary of the lacrimal fossa above and is continued below by the internal angular process of the frontal bone.

The pia and arachnoid continue into the orbit as coverings for the optic nerve. The dura forms the outer dural sheath of the optic nerve and then splits off to form the periorbita, the inner lining of the whole orbit to the orbital margin where it continues as the fascia orbitalis and also as the periosteum of the bones of the face.

The periorbita is tightly adherent along the sutures, at the fissures and foramina and at the trochlear fossa. Elsewhere it strips away readily.

THE LACRIMAL SYSTEM

The Lacrimal Gland

The lacrimal gland is a small flattened lobulated organ, yellowish pink and somewhat darker in color than the orbital fat. It consists of two lobes formed by the temporal edge of the levator aponeurosis which cuts into it so deeply that the lobes are connected only by a thin bridge of glandular tissue posteriorly (fig. 11).

The orbital (superior) lobe of the lacrimal gland is somewhat oval shaped. It lies well hidden in the lacrimal fossa of the frontal bone behind the upper lateral rim of the orbit. It is composed of tightly packed lobules and measures approximately 20 by 12 by 5 mm. It is covered in front by the skin, orbicularis muscle, fascia orbitalis and a thin layer of orbital fat. Posteriorly it lies on the levator aponeurosis medially and more laterally on the fascial expansion which passes from the sheath of the superior rectus to the lateral rectus muscle. While the upper pole of the lobe is usually free, the lower pole is fixed to the orbital fascia and the expansion sheath of the lateral rectus. Hence dissection here should be done carefully in order not to injure the muscle sheath.

The anterior edge of the orbital lobe is thin and is the only part that extends beyond the orbital rim. The posterior edge is thick and merges into the mass of orbital fat lying between the superior and lateral rectus muscles as well as into the glandular tissue connecting it to the palpebral lobe. The lacrimal nerve, artery and vein, all branches of the parent ophthalmic nerves and vessels, enter the gland about the center of its posterior edge.

The palpebral (inferior) lobe of the lacrimal gland is about one-third to one-half the size of the orbital lobe. It is thinner, less compact, diffuse in outline and composed of a number of small discrete lobules. Posteriorly it is confluent with the orbital lobe and presents the same relations. Anteriorly it extends well beyond the orbital margin beneath the aponeurosis of the levator medially. Laterally it lies partly on Müller's muscle but mostly on the lateral palpebral conjunctiva above the tarsus of the upper lid. It is firmly attached to the conjunctiva.

The lacrimal ductules are 10 to 12 in number with about two-thirds coming from the palpebral lobe. All open into the conjunctival sac about

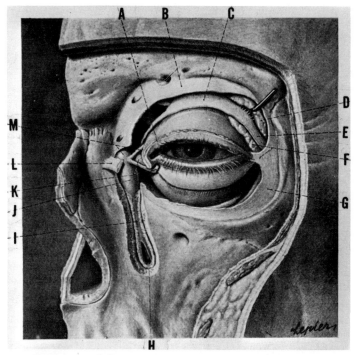

FIG. 11. The Lacrimal System.

A. Inferior lacrimal punctum.
B. and G. Orbital septum.
C. and E. Levator aponeurosis.
D. Orbital portion of lacrimal gland.
F. Palpebral portion of lacrimal gland; lateral canthal ligament.
H. and I. Nasolacrimal duct.

J. Lacrimal sac.
K. Lower canaliculus; posterior layer of medial canthal ligament.
L. Anterior portion of medial canthal ligament.
M. Superior canaliculus; dome of lacrimal sac.

(Pernkopf, Eduard: Anatomie des Menchen. Courtesy Urban & Schwarzenberg, Munich.)

5 mm. above the upper border of the tarsus just in front of the *outer* part of the superior fornix. However, one or two of the larger ones frequently open into the outer part of the *lower fornix*.

Accessory Lacrimal Glands

The glands of Krause are accessory lacrimal glands similar in structure to the main lacrimal gland. They are situated under the conjunctiva from the fornices to the convex border of the tarsi. As many as twenty have been described in the upper lid and eight in the lower. Similar glands have been described by Wolfring (1872).

The conjunctiva also contains goblet cells, more numerous in the bulbar area, which secrete a mucus to help lubricate the conjunctiva. When these are destroyed, as in xerosis conjunctivae, ocular dessication takes place even in the presence of a normally functioning tear gland.

Hence they are of extreme importance to the lubrication and well-being of the eye.

The Lacrimal Passages

On each lid margin, at the junction of its ciliary and lacrimal portions, lies the lacrimal papilla, a slight elevation situated on the posterior edge of the margin.

The punctum is a minute round or oval opening 0.2 to 0.3 mm. in diameter which lies at the summit of the papilla and is the opening into the canaliculus. The area is relatively avascular and hence the papillae are paler in color than the surrounding tissue. Both puncta are about 6 mm. from the medial canthus with the lower about 0.5 mm. more lateral than the upper.

Both puncta normally lie against the globe. Because of the position of the caruncle the upper punctum lies between the caruncle and semilunar fold; the lower between the globe and semilunar fold.

The canaliculi are about 10 mm. long the first 2 mm. run vertically from the punctum. The tube then makes a right angle bend at a slight dilation, the ampulla, and runs horizontally for about 8 mm. to join the lacrimal sac. The direction of the upper canaliculus is slightly downward and of the lower slightly upward. The canaliculi, about 0.5 mm. in diameter, first run along the lid margin on the conjunctival side then dip deeper under the canthal ligament to pierce the lacrimal fascia usually separately. They then unite just above the center of the lacrimal sac at a point of diverticulum called the sinus of Maier.

The vertical part of the canaliculus is surrounded by the lacrimal fibers of the orbicularis muscle which form a sort of sphincter for the punctum. Fibers from the same muscle surround the horizontal tube and serve to drain the tears away. The muscle fibers continue in the superior and inferior portions of the medial palpebral ligament to insert in the anterior and posterior lacrimal crests. This is the lacrimal division of the orbicularis muscle and the fibers inserting into the posterior lacrimal crest are called Horner's muscle (see description of orbicularis muscle above).

The lacrimal sac lies in the fossa lacrimalis which is in the lower part of the medial orbital margin and is an excavation in the bone formed by the frontal process of the maxilla and the lacrimal bone. The fossa is bounded anteriorly by the anterior lacrimal crest of the maxilla which merges inferiorly with the lower orbital margin. Posteriorly the fossa is bounded by the posterior lacrimal crest, a part of the lacrimal bone which is continuous above with the medial orbital margin. The sac is completely surrounded by periorbita which splits at the posterior lacrimal crest, one layer following the bone and lining the fossa, the other passing over the sac to the anterior lacrimal crest. This layer of periorbita is termed the lacrimal fascia.

Embryologically, histologically, and anatomically the sac and naso-lacrimal duct are identical and form one tube, the upper part of which dilates to form the sac (fig. 11). The lacrimal sac is a membranous tube about 12 mm. long and 4 to 8 mm. wide with a capacity of about 2 cc. although it can dilate to hold a great deal more. The upper part of the sac, the fundus, is a closed end lying some 3 to 5 mm. above the medial canthus. Inferiorly the sac merges into the nasolacrimal duct. The point of union being marked by a slight constriction inside the bony canal.

The course of the sac is downward, slightly backward (15° to 25°) and also slightly lateral. Its direction is usually given as a line joining the medial canthus with the homolateral first upper molar tooth.

Medially the relations of the lacrimal sac correspond to the medial fossa wall in which it lies. Laterally it is covered by the lacrimal fascia anterior to which lies the anterior limb of the medial palpebral ligament over the upper half of the sac. This blends with the lacrimal fascia above the ampulla.

Anterior to the ligament are the fibers of the orbicularis, the angular vessels and the skin. The angular vein lies 6 to 8 mm. nasal to the medial canthus under the skin. Occasionally a smaller tributary vein crosses the canthal ligament even more medially. In order to avoid cutting these it is safest to make skin incisions 2 to 3 mm. from the medial canthus.

The lower half of the lacrimal sac lies below the canthal ligament and is covered in front only by skin, orbicularis fibers, and the anterior layers of the septum orbitale and lacrimal fascia. Since it is not confined here by the medial canthal ligament, there is no resistance to infectious swelling. Hence acute dacryocystitis always manifests itself *below* the medial canthal ligament and it is here that swellings occur and abscesses open.

Lateral to the sac the inferior oblique muscle usually takes origin from the floor of the orbit and the fascia covering the sac. The inferior palpebral and infraorbital vessels also lie in this region.

The nasolacrimal duct is a direct continuation of the lacrimal sac and opens into the inferior meatus of the nose. It is something less than three-quarters of an inch in total length. The upper half inch, the intra-osseous portion, runs in the bony canal. The lower one-quarter inch, the meatal portion, extends below the bony canal and lies in the mucous membrane of the lateral wall of the nose. The position of this opening into the nose varies: While it is usually found at some point in the lateral wall it may emerge high up near the roof of the inferior meatus. The shape of the opening may be oval, round or a mere slit. It is quite difficult to find. To add to this difficulty a flat fold of mucous membrane termed the valve of Hasner may cover the opening, although it is normally patulous.

The tear-conducting mechanism works beautifully—in normal circumstances. The tears produced by the lacrimal gland are swept over the eyeball lateromedially to the medial canthus by the normal blinking process. Oily tarsal secretion keeps the tears from spilling over the lid margin.

Since only about 0.5 to 0.65 of a cc. of tears are normally produced in twenty-four hours and since most of these are disposed of by evaporation, the tear conducting mechanism has little difficulty. But it does not take much to upset it because there is little leeway (see Chapter 23). The main factors in tear conduction are the action of various parts of the orbicularis muscle. To this must be added the active help of the puncta and canaliculi; the former by their capillarity and the latter by drawing the tear fluid into their lumen aided by the pars lacrimalis muscle. There is still some controversy about the relative importance of these various elements and the possible more refined physiologic actions of the lacrimal sac and nasolacrimal duct. These refinements and quodlibets are left to the anatomists and physiologists for settlement.

The lacrimal passages get their blood supply from the superior and inferior palpebral branches of the ophthalmic artery, the angular branch of the facial artery and from the infraorbital and nasal branches of the maxillary artery. The veins drain into the angular, the infraorbital and nasal veins. The nerve supply comes from the trigeminal nerve. The infratrochlear nerve supplies the sac and upper part of the duct. The anterior superior alveolar nerve supplies the lower part of the duct.

The foregoing discussion of the surgical anatomy of the brow, lids, orbit and lacrimal system is obviously not exhaustive. It is a short résumé of the important anatomic highlights of these structures which should be, and no doubt are, familiar to every ophthalmic surgeon. For more detailed studies of the subject the reader is referred to the many excellent works which are available.

REFERENCES

ADLER, F. H.: Physiology of the Eye. St. Louis, C. V. Mosby, 1950.
CUNNINGHAM, D. J.: Textbook of Anatomy. New York, William Wood & Co., 1921.
DUKE-ELDER, S., and WYBAR, K. C.: The Anatomy of the Visual System. St. Louis, C. V. Mosby, 1961.
EISSLER, R., and LANGENECKER, L. P.: The common eye findings in Mongolism. Am. J. Ophth. 54:398, 1962.
FINK, W. H.: Anatomical study of the orbital fascia. Suppl. Am. Acad. Oph. Oto. Sept.-Oct., 1959.
GRAY, H.: Anatomy of the Human Body, ed. 24. Philadelphia, Lea & Febiger, 1946.

HILDRETH, H. R.: Insertion of the levator palpebrae muscle. Am. J. Ophth. *24*:749, 1941.

JONES, L. T., and BOYDEN, G. L.: The lacrimal apparatus. *In* Coates, Schenk, and Miller (Eds.): Otolaryngology. Hagerstown, Md. W. F. Prior Co. 1955, Chap. 29.

KESTENBAUM, A.: Applied Anatomy of the Eye. New York, Grune & Stratton, 1963.

PERKOPF, E.: Topographische Anatomie des Menschen. München, Urban & Schwarzenberg, 1960.

RAVETTA, C. A., RAVETTA, A. M., WEIL, B. A., CREMONA, E. G., *and* SORANO, J. E.: Revision Anatomica del Augulo Interno de la Orbita. Arch Oftal. B. Air. *42*:246, 1967.

SOBOTTA, J.: Atlas der deskriptiven Anatomie des Menschen. München, J. F. Lehmann's Verlag, 1920.

SPALTEHOLZ, W.: Hand Atlas der Anatomie des Menschen, Leipzig, Verlag von S. Hirzel, 1929.

WEEKS, W. W.: Surgery of the Eye. New York, privately published, 1937.

WHITNALL, W. E.: The Anatomy of the Human Orbit. London, Oxford Press, 1932.

WOLFF, E.: Anatomy of the Eye and Orbit, ed. 6. Philadelphia, W. B. Saunders Co., 1968.

CHAPTER 2

Technical Details

A CHAPTER ON THIS SUBJECT is usually written to be ignored, hence it is not proposed to dwell too long on the technical details surrounding plastic surgery. Anesthesia, instruments, pre- and postoperative care, asepsis, etc. do not differ markedly here from any other branch of general or ophthalmic surgery. No dogmatic details concerning instruments and their sterilization, operating room technics, etc. will be given. Each surgeon has his own methods and routines and who shall say which is the best?

The author's preferences will be indicated. No doubt these will often be quite different from the preferences of others. This does not matter. In surgery there are many ways of doing the same thing and many of them are good. The routines and methods touched on here have worked well for the author. Other technics have undoubtedly also worked well and will continue to do so.

ASEPSIS

The ophthalmic surgeon does not have to be told of the importance of asepsis. Surrounded as the eye is by brows, lashes, lacrimal and nasal orifices—all incapable of surgical sterilization—the risk of infection is constantly present.

While the complications of infection in lid surgery are not as catastrophic as those of intraocular surgery, they can be sufficiently severe to interfere with or totally nullify operative results. Not only that, but their destructive effects may hamper further reparative surgery. Hence strict asepsis is a sine qua non of all eye surgery including plastic surgery. The most carefully planned and beautifully executed procedure can be completely nullified by a moment of carelessness or forgetfulness resulting in a break of sterile technic.

The preoperative preparation of the patient can be accomplished in

26

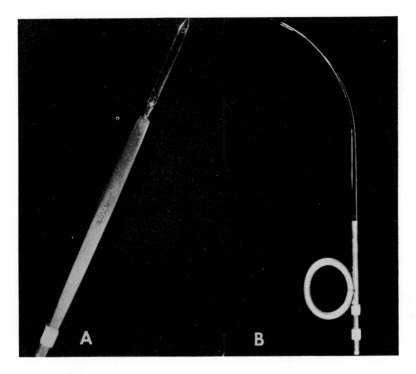

FIG. 12.
A. Reese ptosis knife.   B. Wright ptosis needle.

many ways. The author prefers washing the whole upper half of the patient's face (brow to tip of nose) with green soap and water, then painting the whole area with Merthiolate 1:1000. Half strength iodine, Metaphen, Zephiran (1:1000) are all good. The eyes are thoroughly irrigated preoperatively.

INSTRUMENTS

It is useless to suggest the instruments and materials to be used. Each surgeon has his favorites and will continue to use those familiar to him. Furthermore, in the average case it will matter little what size knife or scissors is used, whether the blade is a millimeter or two longer or shorter, or whether the handle is round or square. What is important is that incisions be made cleanly and with as little trauma and crushing of surrounding tissue as possible. Sharp instruments help. Also the surgeon will be wise to employ the hand the Almighty taught him to use best. Ambidexterity is pretty but is not of much use in plastic surgery.

Of special instruments the author has few to suggest. He has found the Reese ptosis knife, Wright needle (fig. 12) and the Ehrhardt and ptosis clamps (fig. 13) of great value. The fascia stripper (fig. 14), of course, is handy for taking fascia. As for the rest, both straight and

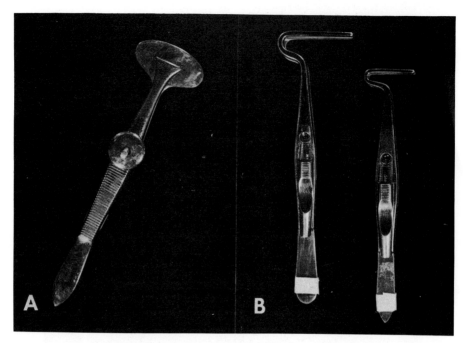

FIG. 13.
A. Ehrhardt clamp.   *B.* Ptosis clamps.

curved blunt pointed scissors are important. Obviously it is more difficult to cut a straight line with curved scissors than with straight scissors. Instrument nurses seem to find this hard to understand sometimes.

The author has fairly well abandoned the use of the Graefe knife in plastic surgery. The well sharpened detachable surgical blades now available for general surgery have been found quite adequate since the instrumental requirements of plastic surgery are much less exacting than those of cataract and corneal surgery. Thus a sharp new blade is available at a moment's notice for each operation and can be discarded after use. The two shapes which have been found particularly useful are the small round-bellied blades for skin incisions (No. 15) and the sharp-pointed, somewhat triangular blades especially useful for splitting the lid margin (No. 11).

The regulation Stevens or Lester forceps and the Stevens scissors are adequate for most cases except where grafts are to be taken from other parts of the body. In taking skin from the thigh, abdomen or supraclavicular region and in removing fascia from the thigh, a heavier surgical scissors and rat-toothed surgical forceps are necessary.

Newer electric dermatomes, large and small, are now available in every well-equipped operating room. They make the life of the ophthalmic surgeon a good deal easier and he should familiarize himself with their use. Blades should be renewed constantly so that they are razor sharp;

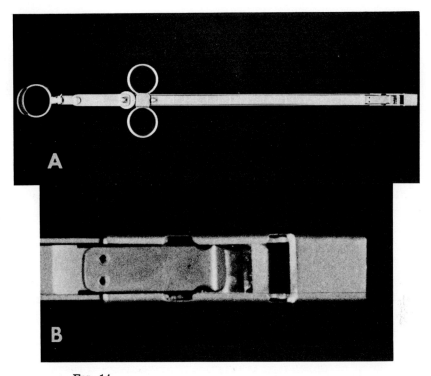

FIG. 14.
A. Fascia stripper.   B. Close-up of cutting head.

a dull blade can macerate a graft and make it useless. Description of the use of dermatomes is inadequate. One must see them, handle them and use them to become their master. They are discussed more fully in Chapter 3.

As for the rest, a review of the operating technic will provide a list of all the possible additional instruments such as clamps, millimeter rule, compasses, etc. which are the tools of the plastic surgeon's trade.

The sharp instruments are sterilized in Post's solution or Zephiran 1:1000. If Post's solution is used they should be thoroughly washed afterward in sterile water and dried. All other instruments are autoclaved as are all solutions to be used at the operating table.

ANESTHESIA

At one time or another all types of anesthesia are useful in ophthalmic plastic surgery. However, the author confesses a preference for local anesthesia wherever possible. The advantages of local over general anesthesia may be listed as follows:

1. The greater safety of local anesthesia is obvious especially in the older age group. This is especially true among cardiacs, nephritics, arteriosclerotics, etc.: also there is less incidence of pulmonary and embolic complications and there is less bleeding.

2. Local anesthesia assures the surgeon the cooperation of the patient when necessary.

3. A field obstructed by the masks, tubes, inhalators, etc. of general anesthesia makes the operation more difficult.

4. These paraphernalia and the hands of the anesthetist increase the danger of contaminating the operative field. And there is no danger of explosion when local anesthesia is used.

5. Postoperative nausea is avoided.

6. Time may not always be important, but this author has wasted many a weary half hour waiting for a patient to succumb to the wiles of the general anesthetist. It is a pleasure not to have to go through this. And here a quotable quote from the Lancet of March 18, 1967 may not be amiss:

> As a mere journeyman surgeon, I am grateful to the anesthetists who kindly allow me to operate during their anesthetics. They are so full of charm and science that, as the endpoint of a half-hour induction approaches, I am allowed to feel that I also serve by standing and waiting—a pawn in the advancement of knowledge. The most pedestrian pieces in my surgical repertoire now attain the dignity of an appendage to original pharmacological research. I am forgiven when gentle traction on the pedicle of a pile spoils the oscillograph recording; and if my thumb on the aorta fails to agree with the monitoring console, it is only indirectly and politely implied that my thumb should be sent for servicing and recalibration. . . .

This is a bit far removed from the field of ophthalmology but not so far that it cannot be apropos.

Local Anesthesia

Local anesthesia may be obtained by (1) instillation, (2) infiltration or (3) nerve block.

1. Instillation anesthesia is of value only in minor repairs of the conjunctiva and as a preliminary to infiltration anesthesia. For this purpose any of the local anesthetics in general use are quite adequate. The author prefers proparacaine HCl. 0.5 per cent.

2. For infiltration anesthesia, the solutions most frequently used are lidocaine or procaine hydrochloride 1 to 2 per cent. Using a stronger solution does not enhance the depth of the anesthesia. As a matter of fact, the 1 per cent solution is just as effective as the 2 per cent in duration and depth of anesthesia. Unless otherwise contraindicated by age or disease, the anesthesia is always given in a solution of 1:50,000 epinephrine. This not only cuts down capillary and small vessel bleeding but slows absorption by vasoconstriction and hence reduces the possibility of

toxic effects. Epinephrine 1:1000 may also be used as a surface hemo-static unless contraindicated.

For inflamed and scarred tissues and for those which have been previously worked over many times, hyaluronidase, 6 turbidity reducing units added to each cubic centimeter of anesthetic solution, is excellent. It facilitates infiltration, helps the spread of the anesthetic solution and the duration of the anesthetic is not shortened materially. Epinephrine may be contraindicated in vascular disease and where general anesthesia is also used.

Infiltration anesthesia is adequate in most operative procedures on the lids, socket and surrounding areas. It is preferred in working on the thin atrophic tissues of the aged where it helps to swell the bulk of the tissues. However, it can be a liability where landmarks such as lid furrows are to be preserved (as in the correction of dermachalasis, in ptosis work, etc.).

A good habit to acquire is the marking out of the areas to be incised with alcoholic gentian violet, brilliant green or some other antiseptic dye, before the injection of anesthetic. This permits the proper placement of incision lines before the skin has been ballooned out and the surface anatomy distorted.

3. For nerve block, 1 per cent lidocaine or procaine in 1:50,000 epinephrine solution is used. Nerve block is of value in the extensive operations around the orbit where infiltration is not desired. It is also valuable in the presence of an inflammatory process and in ptosis surgery. Nerve block is useful in those cases where it is required that the tissues not be ballooned out or distorted in any way, and is often used in combination with light general anesthesia. The free border of the lid is easily anesthetized by nerve block. For this, knowledge of nerve distri-bution is important (fig. 9).

For anesthesia of the upper lid, the supraorbital nerve may be found by palpating the superior notch and the nerve lying approximately at the junction of the inner and middle thirds of the superior orbital rim (fig. 15A). A skin wheal is raised and the needle pushed backward and slightly downward close to the orbital roof with the solution injected as the needle is advanced behind the orbital fascia. One and one-half or two cc. suffices. It is then redirected medially and more solution injected to catch both the more medial of the supraorbital and supra- and infra-trochlear branches of the frontal nerve. Injection of the lacrimal nerve (fig. 15C) completes akinesia of the upper lid.

Hildreth and Silver recommend a single injection for block of the upper lid. A 4 cm. needle is inserted exactly in the midline of the orbit following the roof all the way. Then exactly 0.5 cc. of anesthetic solution is injected. This gives anesthesia of the whole upper lid except for the extreme nasal and temporal ends. This injection blocks both the frontal

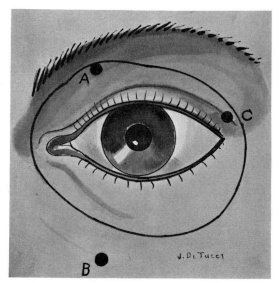

FIG. 15.   Sites of Injection for Nerve Block.
A.   Supraorbital nerve.   C.   Lacrimal nerve.
B.   Infraorbital nerve.

and lacrimal nerves and is ideal for ptosis work because muscle motility is retained.

The infraorbital foramen lies 4–5 mm. below the lower orbital margin in the same vertical plane as the supraorbital notch (fig. 15 at B). For block of the infraorbital nerve, the needle is introduced at this point and directed laterally and posteriorly. About 2 cc. of solution is injected. All patients receiving local anesthesia are given oxygen intranasally.

General Anesthesia

General anesthesia is used in operative procedures on the very young or on those adults who are too apprehensive, senile or mentally incapable of cooperation. It is also sometimes the better choice in major procedures where there has been a good deal of cicatrization or where inflamed tissues are hard to anesthetize. The introduction of hyaluronidase has simplified this latter problem a great deal. However, if general anesthesia is to be used, the type of anesthesia and method of administration must be left to the judgment of the anesthetist.

It is well to acquaint the anesthetist with the general character and approximate duration of the contemplated procedure so he will know how best to cooperate. If oral mucous membrane is to be taken, intubation will have to be done through the nose. The duration of the operation may influence the choice of anesthetic. The anesthetist should be placed on the side opposite the eye to be operated on. This gives both him and the surgeon more freedom of movement.

If general anesthesia cannot be avoided, it is even possible to do the long lacrimal procedures with considerable diminution in bleeding by using hypotensive general anesthesia.

It will be found in general that most cases can be done under local anesthesia with comfort and less preoperative and postoperative inconvenience to both patient and surgeon.

AKINESIA

It is sometimes advantageous to get paresis or paralysis of the lids. For akinesia of the orbicularis muscle the method of O'Brien is excellent: A solution of 1 or 2 per cent lidocaine or procaine in 1:50,000 epinephrine is injected over the condyloid process, anterior to the tragus and just below the posterior portion of the zygomatic process. The patient opens and closes his mouth a few times and the condyloid process is located. The needle is inserted to a depth of almost a centimeter when the bone is encountered, care being taken not to injure the periosteum. About 1 cc. of solution is injected. The needle is withdrawn slightly, pushed upward more superficially toward the eye and more solution injected as the needle is pushed forward. It is withdrawn again, pointed downward slightly and still more solution injected. Thus all the branches of the nerve are anesthetized. Hyaluronidase may be used to advantage here too.

The method of Atkinson is as effective and may be preferred by some. The needle is inserted at the point in line with the lateral margin of the orbit at the inferior edge of the zygomatic bone. It is directed upward about 30° lateral from the vertical close to the bone. Atkinson advises that 3 to 4 cc. of solution be injected as the needle advances upward. The landmarks for the injection are easily located and one rarely fails to obtain a complete akinesia of the orbicularis.

An injection for complete facial nerve block is recommended by Nordath and Rehman. They inject 3 cc. of 1 per cent mepivacaine just below the pinna of the ear.

SUTURES

Vague references to the use of horsehair, leather and cotton sutures go back to the first millenium B. C. However, the use of sutures was attended by so much infection, understandably, that little use was made of them until Lister in 1865 showed that a suture was safe if sterilized. Improvement in suture material and needles then followed rapidly and they have now attained their indispensable role in surgery.

Braided silk is preferred throughout as the best all-purpose suture for both skin and conjunctival closure. The 5–0 can be used for most purposes except lash grafts where 6–0 is perhaps better. The 4–0 braided silk suture is used for tarsorrhaphies and wherever greater tensile strength is required. In other words, the suture gauge is adjusted to the tissue under repair and to the tension placed upon it.

Normal lid skin is so thin that subcuticular sutures are rarely indicated. Once beyond the movable lid skin, however, buried sutures are useful. The skin of the brow especially, and the zygomatic area are excellently adapted to subcuticular closure, and the final cosmetic result is enhanced by them as they help to avoid suture marks. Relaxation sutures in ophthalmic plastic surgery are relatively simple and are best used as buried sutures. In most cases 3–0 or 4–0 plain catgut is preferred. The simple interrupted subcuticular suture usually suffices for most purposes.

Horsehair, linen, nylon, dermal, cotton, steel wire, etc., all have their champions as suture materials for particular purposes and technics. There can be no objection to any of these, providing the surgeon has used them before and knows what to expect of them. The author has seen no repair, however complex, which could not be fully consummated with good result with adequate supplies of silk and catgut sutures of the proper fineness.

Wire sutures are not used routinely by the author. (The only possible exception is when bone fragments are to be held together.) The object of suturing is to bring two tissue surfaces together for a sufficiently long time to allow nature to do the healing. This means that there must be *no tension on the tissues*. If tissues are pulled together by main force and held together by sutures of greater tensile strength than the tissues themselves, the latter will pull away. On the other hand, if tissue surfaces are sufficiently relaxed to come together easily, chromic catgut or silk of adequate guage will be more than ample. They are also easier to handle.

Sutures swaged on needles are preferred for their convenience. The needles should be firm, of adequate gauge, tensile strength and size for skin work. One attempt at poking a fine corneoscleral needle through brow skin will be worth more than a couple of hundred words here. Only cutting needles should be used.

Sutures should not be tied too loosely as they tend to loosen still further with the subsidence of operative edema. On the other hand, tissues should not be strangulated by sutures that are too tight. Firm apposition of the wound edges without dimpling of the skin will give the best healing and will leave no suture marks. In grafting, the knot lies on the host skin side to reduce irritation of the grafted tissue to a minimum.

At postoperative dressings, when the area around the suture appears red and puffy, the suture should be removed immediately. The same holds true in cases where the suture appears to be too tight and the tissue is strangulated.

Ordinarily, sutures are removed on the fourth to sixth day. Stitch marks in the skin are rarely seen if sutures are removed by the sixth day unless they have been tied too tightly. On the other hand, if removed much earlier, before the initial lag phase of the healing process is over, there is danger that the wound will open and the healing scar will stretch. It is far better to leave sutures in five or six days to get a good firm union than to remove them in two or three days and have a wound reopen. The healing then takes longer and scarring is a certain result.

SURGICAL PEGS

Those who have done any amount of plastic surgery have been bedeviled at one time or another by the rubber pegs used to prevent sutures from cutting through tissues. Often the pegs dig into the tissues and macerate the skin. Moreover, passing sutures through a tiny square of rubber is a nuisance, time consuming and requires the help of an assistant. The following easily made peg has been found excellent for use in plastic surgery:

A rectangle of oiled silk, measuring 4 by 4 inches, is folded into four thicknesses along one length, giving a quadruple fold of oiled silk measuring 1 by 4 inches. It is then stiched along the border which does not have the free edge. This stitching is placed one-fourth inch from the edge.

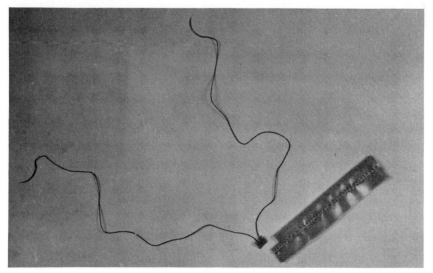

FIG. 16.   Surgical Pegs of Oiled Silk.   (Fox, S. A.: Courtesy American Journal of Ophthalmology.)

When needed, the needles are passed through the stitched edge easily and rapidly and a peg of any desired size is cut from the whole piece (fig. 16). One such piece of oiled silk suffices for 12 to 16 pegs, depending on the size desired. These pegs are soft enough so that they do not macerate the skin and sufficiently firm to prevent the sutures from cutting through the tissues. They have the additional virtue of not requiring an assistant to hold one end of a tiny rectangle barely allowing room for a needle to come through.

PLASTIC CONFORMERS, LENSES AND MOLDS

The use of plastic conformers for many purposes in ophthalmic plastic surgery has proved a welcome and beneficial innovation. These conformers are made of methyl methacrylate, the same material that is used in the manufacture of plastic eye prostheses. In the author's experience, they have never caused sufficient irritation or tissue reaction to prevent their use. Such reactions have, however, been reported.

Conformers are of primary importance in filling the empty socket when lid reconstruction is done because they provide counter-pressure to the pressure bandage. They must never be so large that force is necessary to close the lids over them. On the other hand, if they are too small they fail to fulfill their function. Hence various sizes and shapes should be on hand in a 1:1000 Zephiran solution, ready for instant use (fig. 17). Another use of the conformer is to fill out the socket after enucleations and secondary implants into Tenon's capsule to prevent edema and consequent extrusion of the implant and conjunctiva. Scleral conformers and contact lenses are also used as protective lenses over the bulb in lid surgery and are a good precaution.

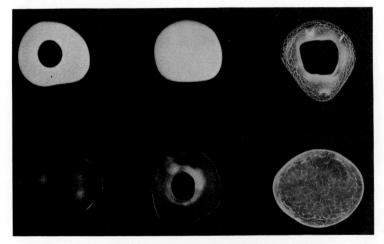

FIG. 17. Plastic Conformers.

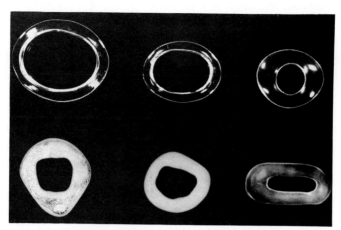

FIG. 18.   Plastic Skeleton Conformers.

A second type, the skeleton or open conformer (fig. 18), is useful to keep a socket on stretch after reconstruction or grafting and thus prevent it from shrinking. The opening keeps secretions from damming up behind it and allows for the toilet of the socket without removal of the conformer.

Plastic plates are also used to elevate the ptosed globe and for the repair of supratarsal depressions (see Chapter 21).

PREPARATION OF THE PATIENT

Plastic surgery of the traumatized lids and socket—especially those injuries resulting from warfare and severe industrial injury—may vary from the plastic surgery required after the excision of neoplasms. The battered lids seen in army hospitals months and years after injury are severely scarred and often have poor blood supply and a low vitality. Occasionally sutures pull out of tissue as if it were butter and pedicle flaps may have to be delayed several times before viability can be assured. On occasion, tubed pedicles have to be brought up because local tissues do not have sufficient blood supply to support either pedicle or free grafts. Also the skin of the younger individual does not have the distensibility—the "stretchability" one might say—of the older man whose subcutaneous tissues are beginning to absorb and whose skin is beginning to sag.

Neoplasms play at least as important a part as trauma in lid surgery. Modern medicine is extending the life span so that more individuals than ever before are enabled to enjoy the fruits of old age including some of its diseases and neoplasms. As a consequence, members of the older age group, vessels of old age diseases, form an appreciable part of the patients treated.

One learns from sad experience that preoperative preparation can occasionally be as important to the success of a plastic procedure as the actual technic of operation. In some cases a high caloric, high vitamin diet and general physical build-up may be necessary.

The general condition of the patient is important in any operative procedure and should be investigated. All possible foci of infection should be checked: A special search should rule out chronic dacryocystitis, blepharitis, meibomitis, conjunctivitis, etc. In addition to the routine examination of blood, urine and serology, blood clotting time, a/g ratio and sedimentation rate may be important to forestall later trouble.

Ophthalmic plastic surgery is not commonly surgery of emergency. Hence preoperative preparation need not be hurried. Also, it is limited surgery, usually localized to a small area and hence there is rarely the danger of general shock.

Nor does plastic surgery carry with it the faint but constant threat of disaster as does intraocular surgery. However, it does help to have the patient comfortable and cooperative as much as circumstances will permit. Preoperative sedation is therefore important. If the patient is admitted to the hospital the night before operation, a good night's sleep is important. The type of sedation used should be that with which the surgeon is familiar and has used so that he will know what to expect.

Some prefer 100 to 200 mg. of pentobarbital sodium (Nembutal) or an equivalent barbiturate such as secobarbital (Seconal), others prefer nonbarbiturates of which there are a number of good ones on the market. For the elderly and infirm 0.5 to 1.0 Gm. of chloral hydrate is still a tried and true medicament.

Patients to be operated on in the morning are given a repeat dose of the sedative plus 50 to 100 mg. of meperidine Hcl (Demerol). Chlorpromazine HCl (Thorazine) 25 mg., prochlorperazine (Compazine) 10 mg. or equivalent tranquilizing and antiemetic medication helps prevent preoperative and postoperative nausea and enhances the action of the other drugs.

The object in local anesthesia is not to "knock the patient out." (If this is desired then general anesthesia should be used.) In fact it may even be dangerous since such deep sedation is neither controllable nor trustworthy. But the patient should be sedated enough to take the edge off his fear and reduce his preoperative tension—most patients have these whether they admit it or not.

Prophylactic chemotherapy or antibiotics are a moot point with surgeons and a highly personal matter. There is little use in ordering such medication unless it is prolonged at least over a three or four day period. On the other hand, there would seem to be little indication for a full course of antibiotics in a healthy individual on whom a minor plastic procedure is to be done, and there is always the question of allergy and building of tolerance in the patient unnecessarily. In the case of the old, the infirm and the multioperated, on whom long and complicated procedures are to be done the surgeon must decide in each case whether the exhibition of prophylactic therapy against infection is warranted. Certainly where it is definitely indicated as in septic cases, pre- and postoperative antibiotics and chemotherapeutics are a must and a Godsend. Infection is a dreaded complication in plastic surgery. With the modern methods and tools at the surgeon's disposal and reasonable care, it need be a rare complication.

There is little or no good evidence to show at this time that steroids delay healing. As a matter of fact, some authorities believe that a patient who has been on steroids for some time preoperatively should receive even larger doses while in the hospital. The patient's personal physician should be consulted in this matter.

Postoperative Treatment

The type and method of postoperative dressing can be important to the comfort of the patient, the ease of subsequent handling of the wound and the ultimate healing.

It need not be reemphasized that all bleeding should be stopped before the wound is closed. In grafting it could easily mean death of a graft unless this is done. Over suture lines material such as perforated rubber dam, plastic sheets like Telfa, Adaptic or the coarser Parrisin mesh or some equivalent may be used to prevent adhesion of sutures to dressings and thus make subsequent removal easy. The perforations permit drainage if any is present. Petrolated dressings macerate skin and are not as useful except possibly when used on raw surfaces such as donor areas from which split skin grafts have been taken.

Pressure bandages are often used. They can be made simply by fluffing up a number of 4 by 4 gauze sponges which are held in proper position with a few strips of adhesive. An excellent alternative is the tie sutures described in figure 26, Chapter 3. These sutures should not be used to exert pressure but simply to hold the fluffs in place. Over this a good firm pressure dressing or head roll is placed. With this procedure it is almost impossible to exert too much pressure on the graft. The patient, however, may have cause to complain: Knots should be tied so that they do not lie over bare skin. Also tight bandages, while not lethal to the graft, may be uncomfortable to the patient and may even cause edema and suggillation of the opposite eye due to fascial communication over the nose. In such cases one or two vertical cuts are made in the lower margin of the head roll to ease the tension.

Pain is controlled according to the custom and experience of the surgeon with whatever medicaments he prefers. After plastic surgery, unless hemorrhage has been severe and more is feared, the patient may be allowed up early and given more freedom than after intraocular surgery.

Postoperative disorientation may be induced by too much sedation in some cases. Bilateral eye patching is another predisposing factor to be kept in mind.

Proteolytic enzymes have been suggested to reduce postoperative hemorrhage, edema and swelling. Their use by the author has not convinced him completely of their efficacy. However, this may be due to the relatively short experience with them; some reports are quite favorable. There is one caution: Allergic reactions may be encountered.

The tendency now is to get patients out of bed—especially the elderly—as soon as possible. Unless hemorrhage is expected or is to be contained, there is no contraindication to bathroom privileges almost immediately after operation even after extensive lid surgery. In most cases the patient is freely allowed out of bed the next day.

REFERENCES

ATKINSON, W. S.: Local anesthesia in ophthalmology. Tr. Am. Ophth. Soc. 32:399, 1934.
———: Use of hyaluronidase with local anesthesia in ophthalmology. Arch. Ophth. 42:628, 1949..
———: Akinesia of the orbicularis. Am. J. Ophth. 36:1255, 1953.
———: The development of ophthalmic anesthesia. Am. J. Ophth. 5:1, 1961.
FOX, S. A.: A new type of surgical peg. Am. J. Ophth. 29:586, 1946.
GARTNER, S., and BILLET, E.: Mortality during general anesthesia. Am. J. Ophth. 45:847, 1958.
HAVENER, W. H.: Ocular Pharmacology. St. Louis, C. V. Mosby, 1966.
HILDRETH, H. R., and SILVER, B.: Sensory block of the upper eyelid. Arch. Ophth. 77:230, 1967.
KIMURA, S. J., and GOODNER, E. K.: Ocular Pharmacology and Therapeutics. Philadelphia, F. A. Davis, 1963.
NORDATH, R. P., and REHMAN, I.: Facial nerve block. Am. J. Ophth. 55:143, 1963.
O'BRIEN, C. S.: Local anesthesia. Arch. Ophth. 12:240, 1934.
PADGETT, E. C.: Skin grafting. Springfield, Ill., Charles C Thomas, 1942.
POST, M. H.: Prevention of infection in eye surgery. Am. J. Ophth. 32:679, 1949.
POST, M. H., JR.: Prevention of infection in ophthalmic surgery; further studies. Trans. Am. Ophth. Soc. 50:295, 1952.
SCHEIE, H. G.: Long-lasting local anesthetic agents in ophthalmic surgery. Arch. Ophth. 53:177, 1955.
TASSMAN, I. S.: Hyaluronidase in ophthalmology Am. J. Ophth. 35:683, 1952.
VAN LINT, A.: Paralysie palpébrale temporaire provoquée l'opération de la cataracte. Ann. d'ocul. 151:420, 1914.

CHAPTER 3

Grafts

BY DEFINITION a graft is a portion of tissue used to replace a defect in a similar tissue. Technically, therefore, whenever a scar is excised and the edges of the resultant wound undermined and brought together, grafting is being done, although it is not thought of as such. Yet tissue has been moved to cover a defect. Sliding or advancing grafts (French or Celsus flaps) are little more than this except that the flap may be cut from its surroundings to allow for easier movement.

The terminology of grafting is large and many descriptive terms of the various types of grafts exist. Only those of paramount interest to ophthalmologists will be mentioned here.

An *autograft* is a graft taken from the patient's own body.

A *homograft* (isograft) is a tissue graft taken from another individual.

A *heterograft* is tissue taken from a different species or a graft derived from synthetic or nonorganic material.

A *zoögraft* is a heterograft taken from an animal.

A *free* graft is a segment of tissue removed entirely from its location and planted in a new bed.

A *flap* or pedicle is a graft a portion of which still retains its original attachment. There are many types of pedicle grafts:

A sliding or advancement flap is one whose pedicle is slid or advanced forward from its bed without change of direction (fig. 59).

A rotated pedicle, as its name implies, is one which is twisted away from its original position in another direction (fig. 80).

A transposed flap is one used to assume the position of another flap. The Z plasty is a good example of this (fig. 54).

A hammock flap is one left attached at both ends for better blood supply (fig. 205).

A delayed flap is one which is dissected up then resutured to its original position for a while in order to assure its blood supply before being moved to a new position (fig. 137B).

A tubed flap is a combined hammock and delayed flap. The strip of tissue is dissected up but left attached at both ends. The raw edges are sutured together to form a tube with the raw surface on the inside. After blood supply has been assured one attachment is cut free and advanced. When a "take" has been assured the other end is advanced similarly. This may be repeated several times caterpillar fashion until the area to be grafted is reached, the tube opened and grafted into position.

A physiologic flap is one which contains the main blood vessels supplying the part.

The last three named flaps are rarely used in ophthalmology. There are in addition bridge, twisted, tunneled and composite flaps (fig. 130) which are also of rare concern here.

Grafting requirements in ophthalmic surgery are, in general, simple. Judged by the lesions and involvements seen in general plastic surgery, ophthalmic lesions of the lid and brow are relatively small in area hence grafting requirements are usually comparatively minor. But this does not always make the repairs simple. The lids are complex in anatomy and physiology. The eye, when present, is a constant challenge to the care and watchfulness of the surgeon lest its integrity be impaired and permanent damage be done. Hence, though the areas involved are small, the repair of lid deformities is a highly specialized and sometimes formidable procedure.

HISTORICAL SUMMARY

The history of skin grafting is a fascinating one and records of surgical interest in eyelid deformities go back to ancient days. Thus the Hindu literature contains descriptions of plastic procedures by Susruta in the seventh century B.C. During the time of Hippocrates, technics for the correction of such conditions as entropion, ectropion and trichiasis are said to have been devised and Aetius has given us the first such account in his Tetrabiblion. Celsus in the first century A.D. is credited with having devised the first sliding flaps, although these must have been known before his time. In the Middle Ages interest in plastic surgery quickened and the records of plastic repairs during these days are relatively more numerous.

In general there were three methods of grafting. The French method amounted to little more than excision and closure with or without undermining. The Italian method initiated by Togliacozzi was the property of a few Italian surgeons who kept their secrets in the family by passing them along from father to son. This was primarily a nasal plastic procedure in which the arm was fastened to the face until a skin "take" was accomplished. This, in turn, had been borrowed from the old Indian method.

Early in the nineteenth century the rotation of pedicles from adjacent areas, became popular and was generally adopted. The names of von Graefe, Dzondi, Fricke, Dieffenbach and Arlt, to mention but a few, are important in these early developments. Von Graefe reported the first successful blepharoplasty by means of a sliding flap in 1818. But for a long time skin grafting remained a hit and miss proposition— mostly miss. It was based on the universally accepted belief that a graft must never be separated from its source of blood supply until it had "taken."

Then, beginning with Reverdin in 1869, the whole concept of skin grafting was revolutionized. Too little is known about the important role that ophthalmologists and ophthalmic pathology played in this development. Reverdin showed that pinch grafts removed from their donor area would grow on granulating surfaces. From here on developments came thick and fast. In 1870 Lawson, an ophthalmologist, reported using Reverdin's method for the repair of an upper lid ectropion and in 1871 Driver used a free graft from the upper lid, with tarsorrhaphy, to repair the opposing lower lid.

In 1872 Le Fort reported the successful repair of ectropion with a free full thickness graft. In the same year Ollier showed that larger split skin grafts would survive on granulating surfaces and De Wecker urged all ophthalmologists to use this method. In 1874 Thiersch reported successful "takes" with even larger and thinner free split skin grafts and Everbusch became such an enthusiastic disciple of this type of grafting that it became known in Europe as the Thiersch-Everbusch method. In 1873 Sichel reported on the use of small multiple free full thickness grafts with tarsorrhaphy for the repair of ectropion and in 1875 Wolfe, a Scotch ophthalmologist, used one large free full thickness graft for the repair of ectropion. This method was immediately taken up in this country by such ophthalmologists as Wadsworth (1876), Aub (1879), Noyes (1880), Weeks (1889) and many others.

It makes no difference that no great distinction was made in those early days between autografts, homografts or even heterografts; or that infection was ever present and made "takes" uncertain. The free skin graft had been born and was here to stay once it had outlived its precarious early days.

Despite all these epoch-making developments, of which only a few are reported, free grafting was slow in catching on. The most important obstacle was probably infection which was a familiar and persistent companion of all surgery not so many years ago. And then again, old concepts die hard; especially wrong ones, it would seem. Thus, in 1904, Czermak was still advising against the use of free grafts and as late as 1936 Wheeler found it necessary to chide ophthalmologists with the fact that they were still dominated by the idea of the necessity of pedicles for grafts and "in doing so, they accept a serious handicap."

The past 35 years, however, have supplied experience, understanding and refinement. The homograft and heterograft were discarded (although the homograft is now the center of much research) ; infection has become less and less a danger. The present day ophthalmic surgeon now uses free lid skin grafts without hesitation. In addition he makes use of free whole skin grafts and split skin grafts from the temporal and cephaloauricular region as well as from the upper arm, abdomen and thigh.

The conjunctiva also was a source of much investigation and Teale in 1860, reported cure of a symblepharon by using a conjunctival pedicle. In 1884 Bock used mucous membrane for the repair and replacement of conjunctival surfaces and Stellwag repaired symblepharon with it. Stellwag also reported the use of vaginal mucosa to replace conjunctiva. About the same time rabbit conjunctiva was a popular tissue in the replacement of human conjunctiva. This, however, soon went the way of all zoögrafts and was perforce discarded.

Early attempts at cilia grafting in the nineteenth century were initiated by Dieffenbach and preceded, as always, by experiments in zoögrafting on lower animals and even birds. Human cilia were first painstakingly transplanted singly. All these attempts were unsuccessful. Finally "takes" in hair-bearing grafting were attained by the inclusion of several rows of hair on the edge of a skin pedicle swung down from the forehead for an upper lid reconstruction. The next and final step was the free graft transplant of narrow strips of hair-bearing brow skin to form the ciliary border of a reconstructed lid. This was first reported by Paul Knapp in 1908. Others since then have improved this method to its present status.

SKIN GRAFTING

As stated above, skin grafting requirements in ophthalmic plastic surgery are relatively simple as compared to those of general plastic surgery. These requirements are met most often by free skin grafts either full thickness or epidermic. Dermal and intermediate skin grafts are more rarely used. Free skin grafts are hardy and failures with them are not common.

If grafted skin is to be used after resection of a neoplasm, the amount needed should be measured before resection, otherwise skin retraction may seem to make the graft requirement larger than it actually is. However, when cicatrized areas are to be grafted, they should be incised, undermined and the wound edges allowed to retract ad maximum before measurement in order not to underestimate the amount of needed skin.

When faced with a skin grafting problem the surgeon must immediately make a number of definite decisions:

What kind of graft shall be used—free or pedicle?

What is the best source if a free graft is to be used?

What skin will furnish the best color match?

If free, shall the graft be full thickness or split skin?

Free Whole Skin Grafts

In working on the lids there is one perfect answer to all the above questions: Use lid skin to replace lid skin if at all possible. Nothing works more easily nor gives a better result with less scarring and it is an exact match in texture and color. Another important factor is that it is so loosely attached that there is practically no shrinkage when removed from its bed. This means that the skin can be cut as an inlay almost exactly to pattern.

In cutting free skin grafts from the upper lid the lower incision should be in the lid furrow parallel with the lid margin. The upper incision completes the spindle (fig. 19), the length and width of which depend on the size of graft needed. When incisions are so placed the normal lid fold is least disturbed and the scar lies in the normal furrow where it is least noticeable.

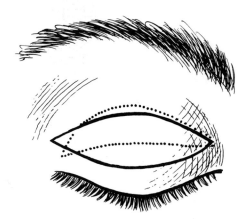

FIG. 19. Outline of Free Full Thickness Skin Graft from Upper Lid (dotted lines). The lower incision can usually be placed in the lid furrow to minimize scarring. Note that with the lid pulled down the furrow assumes a convex curve parallel with the lid margin (solid lines).

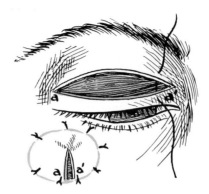

FIG. 20. Shaping of Skin Spindle to Fit a Round Defect (see text).

A spindle of skin approximately 1.5 cm. wide and 4 cm. long can be taken from many lids without fear of causing lagophthalmos. (In the young the spindle should be somewhat narrower.) Even where slight difficulty in closing the lid is experienced, this soon passes away as the skin stretches. Furthermore, sometimes more can be taken later if necessary.

Where a lower lid is involved, skin from an ipsilateral upper lid may be used and thus only one eye need be bandaged. For an upper lid graft the contralateral upper lid may be used as the donor. Lower lids can rarely be used as donors for upper lid grafting in young individuals. Even in the aged, where there has been atrophy and stretching of the skin with pronounced "bagginess" of the lower lids, care should be taken in resecting skin; ectropion is too easily caused here. In general, then, where only one lid or both lower lids are involved, free whole skin grafts preferably from the upper intact lids should be the choice if available.

The best way to take lid skin is in spindle shape. However, since not all defects are spindle shaped, the graft, which is elastic, can sometimes be pulled out of shape somewhat to fit the bed. At other times the graft may be taken a little larger and shaped to the dimensions of the defect. In the case of an almost circular defect the skin spindle may be shaped into the defect (fig. 73) as illustrated in figure 20 with the central slit opening left open for drainage.

If somewhat heavier grafts are needed as in cases where tissue loss is deep, or if lid skin is not available and epidermis (see below) is not desirable, then free whole skin grafts may be obtained from other sources. These are the cephaloauricular angle (fig. 21), the temple (fig. 22), the supraclavicular area if not hair bearing (fig. 23), the inside of the arm, the thigh and the lower abdomen.

Not one of these sources furnishes an exact match in texture or color, all these skins being thicker and of varying shades. However, the first three named (cephaloauricular, temple, and supraclavicular) are the best of the lot and with the passage of time blend in fairly well with the

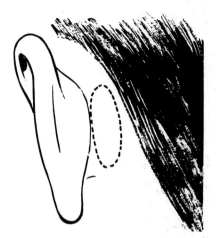

Fig. 21.   Skin Graft from Cephaloauricular Area.

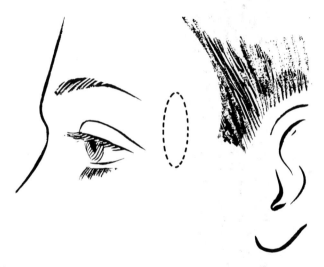

Fig. 22.   Donor Area of Skin Graft from the Temple Region.

host skin. Hence, though less desirable, these sources are adequate. In cases of severe face burns, the match is better because the skin is usually paler after such injuries. One may even use more than one source in order not to make too large a scar in one area. Thus one may use one graft from the cephaloauricular angle and another from the temple, etc. However, it should be remembered that in all cases other than lid skin, the graft must be cut one-quarter to one-third larger than the bed to allow for shrinkage. Also tension lines should be studied so that they are not cut across as this makes for more shrinkage.

Free whole skin grafts have sometimes been used to advantage as filling material for depressions in the bony wall around the socket and for supratarsal depression of the upper lid after long-standing enucleations

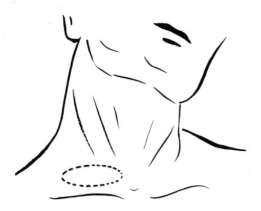

FIG. 23.   Donor Area of Skin Graft from the Supraclavicular Region.

and fractures of the orbital floor. They are best taken from the thigh, abdomen or inner arm where an adequate supply is always available. After excision the surface of the skin should be painted with 30 per cent trichloracetic acid and the epithelium scraped off. Enough should be taken so that it can be doubled over and implanted as a sort of sausage, raw surface outward. Overcorrection should be aimed for since the skin may shrink 50 per cent or more.

Epidermal Grafts

If whole skin is not available another type of free skin graft, the epidermal or split skin graft, may be used to advantage. The best source for this tissue is the inner aspect of the arm, the lower abdominal wall or the upper thigh in that order. In battle casualties from World War II it was not unusual to see ectropion of two, three or all four lids as the result of tank and plane gasoline explosions. Industrial accidents furnish similar injuries (fig. 185). This type of graft is ideal for such cases as enough tissue can usually be obtained to supply all four lids at once if necessary.

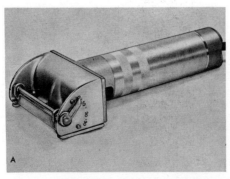
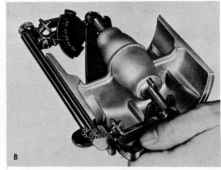

FIG. 24.

A.   Padgett Electric Dermatome.   *B.*   The Hand Dermatome.

With the aid of the modern electric dermatome (fig. 24A) split skin grafts of any desired size and thickness may be taken quickly and simply and require no great skill if the surgeon remembers that reasonable counterpressure is necessary. Hence the firm thigh is better as a source than the soft abdominal wall which caves in on pressure. In this one respect the older machines, such as the Padgett (fig. 24B) which use cement, are better because the skin is lifted up and no counterpressure is required.

Epidermis is also especially useful after burns because it furnishes a good color match for skin that has been blanched by fire. It will grow on flat granulating surfaces, cartilage and bone and is useful for socket lining after exenterations and in socket reconstructions. It is much surer of a "take" on granulation tissue than free whole skin on pedicle flaps.

Taking Epidermis

With a little experience the newer Padgett dermatome is a good instrument for obtaining split skin grafts of any size and shape up to 4 inches by 8 inches. The operator is advised to put in a preliminary period of assembling and adjusting the instrument. It is not at all difficult to learn how to use it successfully. The underlying principle is an adhesion by means of cement between the skin and the dermatome drum of the instrument which enables the operator to cut a graft of any desired thickness. The procedure is as follows:

The dermatome is locked into its stand (fig. 25A). The thickness of graft desired is set in the scale. The cement is now applied to the drum of the dermatome in a thin, even coating according to the size of graft desired. The donor skin area is prepared in the usual fashion and then wiped off with ether. The skin should be dry and free of blood or oil. A smooth, thin, uniform coat of cement is then brushed on over an area of skin somewhat larger than the size of the graft desired. When the cement has dried and the skin no longer shows glistening highlights—a matter of less than five minutes—the skin is ready for the taking of the graft. There is no hurry as the cement remains sticky for a long time after drying.

The edge of the cement-coated drum is placed on the cement-coated skin surface. After a few seconds the drum edge is tilted upward slightly to raise the skin and put it on slight stretch (fig. 25B). The surgeon moves the knife handle horizontally in a sawing motion while rotating the drum slowly and carefully (fig. 25C). When the end of the cement-coated skin is reached a knife stroke or two cuts the skin graft loose from the patient.

The drum is next locked into position on the stand again and the graft picked up by grasping it with hemostats at the four corners (fig. 25D). Handling of the graft may be further facilitated by a tape which

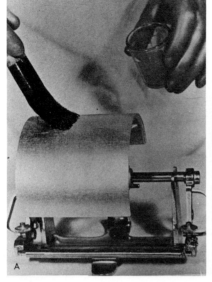
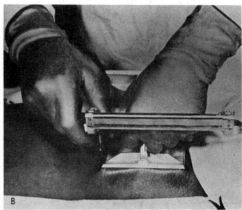
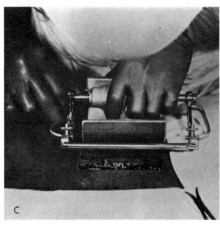
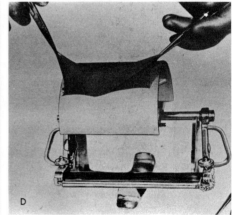

FIG. 25.   Use of Padgett Dermatome.

A. Coating the drum with a thin   C. Cutting the graft.
     layer of cement.   D. The graft is picked up with
B. The drum is placed on the donor area.   hemostats.

is cemented to the drum before the graft is taken. After taking, the
tape is pulled off and the graft and tape applied to the recipient area.
The donor skin area is coated with cement according to the size and
shape of graft desired; thus, only the required amount of skin and no
more is taken.

    Although the usual limits of thickness for the various types of
graft are indicated on the dermatome scale, it is well to know that thickness is indicated in thousandths of an inch. The usual thickness for
grafting a granulating surface is .010 to .014 of an inch. This is about

the thickness necessary to reline a socket. There will be some contracture with this thickness. Hence the socket should be dissected generously.

In cases of cicatricial ectropion where appearance and minimal contracture is important, the graft should be somewhat thicker—up to .020 to .024 of an inch. In the adult this still leaves sufficient subepithelial elements in the skin base for early regeneration. However, in taking abdominal skin from a woman who has been pregnant several times, the thickness should be less due to a thinning out of the abdominal skin. In a young child of 12 or 14 the thickness should be .016 inch or less, in a baby .010 or .012 of an inch—no more.

Pedicle Flaps

The discussion so far has been limited to free skin grafts which are the author's preference wherever possible. However, situations will present themselves where one cannot use free grafts and where pedicle grafts are preferable. In ophthalmic surgery the two most common types of pedicles are the sliding or advancing pedicle and the rotated pedicle. Tubed pedicles are rarely used although the occasion for them may arise. The use of a biologic flap is practically never called for. The advantage of pedicles is that they carry their blood supply with them. The disadvantage is that they cause more scarring. They are valuable:

(1) Where the area involved contains much scar tissue which cannot be completely removed and the requirements for a good "take" of a free graft are lacking because blood supply will be inadequate and too much shrinkage will occur. Here a pedicle with its own blood supply will be preferable.

(2) When after resection of all fibrous tissue one has a deep bed which an ordinary free skin graft will not fill, a pedicle flap with its subcuticular tissue to fill in the depression must be considered. This can be used where the blood supply is poor and the shrinkage is less than that of any free skin graft except lid skin.

(3) Where a whole lid is to be reconstructed, especially the upper lid, a pedicle graft is practically inevitable (fig. 137).

(4) In repairs around the brow, temple and nasolabial angle, where the skin is thick, pedicle grafts may have to be used, especially if previous surgery has already been carried out and blood supply is impaired. Sometimes one or two sliding flaps may be resorted to instead. The resultant scarring is no less, and the choice is between Scylla and Charybdis. However, under these conditions little other choice exists.

The foregoing discussion has dealt entirely with autogenous skin grafts. This is the only type of graft which can survive permanently anywhere on the host. Intensive research is now being carried out in many quarters on homografts. At this writing homografts of kidneys, hearts and even arms and legs of varying longevity are being reported.

With the help of whole body irradiation followed by bone marrow transplantation to restore hematopoietic function, remarkable advances have been made. In skin grafting, however, the exact reason and mechanism of homograft rejection by immunologic response is not yet known. The importance of the gamma globulin factor in antibody production is obviously great as proved by the survival of homologous skin grafts in cases of agammaglobulinemia. The use of fetal transplants also seems to be making some headway against the immunologic antibody response. But at present skin homografts are limited clinically to temporary use in severe burns and permanently only in identical twins. Otherwise skin autografts and homografts look alike only during the first six days then the latter begin to disintegrate and are usually sloughed off completely in three or four weeks.

Elements of Successful Skin Grafting

One of the main elements in successful skin grafting is infinite attention to detail. Full understanding of these details is perhaps better obtained by the trial and error of experience than by formal exposition. However, broad essential principles can be outlined. Some are obvious. Others are learned only through failure. All are important.

Asepsis is the underlying requirement in plastic surgery. Infections, however slight, prevent "takes" and ruin chances for primary union. In cosmetic surgery this is disastrous. These days, when strict asepsis can be buffered by the use of antibiotics and chemotherapy, infections can be reduced to a minimum if ordinary care is taken in the preoperative preparation of patient and instruments. This requires no elaborate technics and was discussed in the previous chapter.

Surgical preparation of the graft bed includes several simultaneous chores: First and foremost is the removal of scar tissue. This cannot be overemphasized. The extent to which a graft can shrink almost to nothing as the surgeon stands by helplessly in horrified amazement is something hard to describe. After one such experience, however, one will never again fail to resect all scar tissue from the recipient bed.

While granulation tissue may not prevent a take, too much of it will cause shrinkage, hence it should be scraped as thin as possible and smoothed out. The smoother the graft bed in all cases the smoother and surer the healing. This applies only to epidermic grafts. Whole skin grafts should not be planted on granulation tissue.

Adequate blood supply should be available. If this is questionable, as previously mentioned, a pedicle graft will have to be considered. All bleeding must be stopped before the graft is laid. A slight ooze, however, will be stopped by the pressure bandage.

Preparation of the graft is important. If lid skin is used, the graft is cut just a trifle larger than the recipient bed. Grafts from other areas should be taken at least one-quarter and preferably one-third larger. Grafts in general should not be larger than two inches square, preferably somewhat less. If more skin is needed, it is better to take two pieces. The graft should be handled by sutures passed through the corners so that the edges are not crushed by instrumentation. In general the thinner the graft the surer the take, especially where the blood supply is uncertain.

It is better to avoid hair-bearing donor sites if possible. Hair has a startling faculty of appearing even when only epidermis (with the hair follicles presumably left behind) has been taken. Conversely, it frequently fails to appear when carefully grafted. It is probably better not to shave these donor sites so that if hair is present on any part it may be seen and avoided.

Grafts are kept alive the first few days by lymph absorption until a new blood supply is acquired. The first three days the graft survives only by diffusion of nutrition and metabolites from plasma. It seems fairly well estblished now that free skin grafts survive by blood flow through the same capillary network that existed before they were excised. In other words, the graft's original capillary network remains unchanged. This does not depend on the nature of the host bed, whether freshly prepared or a week-old bed with established granulations is used. It takes about a week for a recognizable circulatory flow to develop. Before that, although the vessels are filled by imbibition, there is no flow. Within 48 or 72 hours the color of the graft begins to change from a dead white to a blotchy blue and then, slowly, to a healthy pink.

Circulation at the edges of the graft is attained as early as the fourth day by peripheral capillary buds which grow from the surrounding host into the graft and again the color begins to change from bluish to a more healthy pink. Once vascularization has been achieved the cellular union of host and graft occurs. In other words, the fate of the graft is decided on the fourth or fifth day.

Obviously if the graft is too thick it will die if vascular supply is acquired too slowly. Hence the raw surface should be carefully cleaned of all subcutaneous tissue including fat. This also prevents contracture.

Getting the graft into its bed should be accomplished without stretching. It must fit snugly into place and it is better to have it slightly oversize than too small. When suturing into place, bites should be taken close to the edge with knots tied on the host side. Five–0 braided silk is adequate in most cases. It is a good idea to make a small (about 5 mm.) central incision with a sharp knife as an avenue for the escape of accumulated blood beneath the graft but only if necessary. This will sometimes mean the difference between failure and success if a bleeder has been overlooked or if bleeding should recur and lift the graft from its bed.

In split skin grafting the graft edges should overlap the bed amply to assure complete coverage (fig. 185). While seroma is not common in split skin grafting, it may occur due to epithelialization of its dermal surface by proliferation of cells of the divided hair follicles. In such cases the epithelium must be curetted off the dermal surface before the graft can be made to adhere to its bed.

In pedicle grafting the ratio of pedicle width to length should be no less than 1 to 3 and preferably 1 to 2½. Here too the graft should be cut somewhat larger than the bed to overcome expected shrinkage although there is less here than in most free grafting except lid skin. It should fit into the recipient bed without too much tension and twisting so that the blood supply is not interfered with. Also, the less instrumentation the better.

Ligatures to tie off bleeders are to be avoided if possible as they may act as a foreign body under the graft and cause necrosis. Antiseptic and styptic powders will clump and act similarly and should also be eschewed.

Dressing of the grafted area should be done carefully with a layer of Cilkloid, Telfa or some similar material over which a thick layer of cotton is arranged to fill in and smooth out all depressions. This is held in place by tie sutures (fig. 26), strips of adhesive or scotch tape. Over this a firm pressure dressing is applied by any method which the surgeon prefers. Obviously tie sutures are not used to exert pressure but simply to hold fluffed cotton or gauze in place. The pressure is exerted by the headroll or bandage applied over it. The thin split skin grafts should be covered by tinfoil or a conformer, if availble, to keep them in place before the layer of cotton and pressure bandage is applied. The object is to assure immobility, thus avoiding rupture of early forming lymph and blood channels, and to cause close adherence of the graft to the bed to prevent the pooling of serum and blood under the graft.

Pressure is important to assure a "take." Too much pressure will obviously be detrimental. Too little is as bad since the fibroblastic layer between bed and graft must be kept at a minimum; otherwise too much scar tissue will result during the healing process and the graft will shrink. In free grafts, if a good layer of cotton or gauze fluffs is applied freely, and over this a pressure bandage, it is almost impossible to apply too much pressure and if all other rules are followed a good "take" should result. In pedicle grafts a firm dressing is necessary but not so much pressure as in free grafting because a good blood supply is presumably assured from the base of the graft.

Denuded donor areas from which split skin has been taken do not bleed much but there is always a slow ooze. This should be dried up as much as possible, covered with nonadherent gauze and securely bandaged. The dressing is left in place for 10 days at which time the whole area is

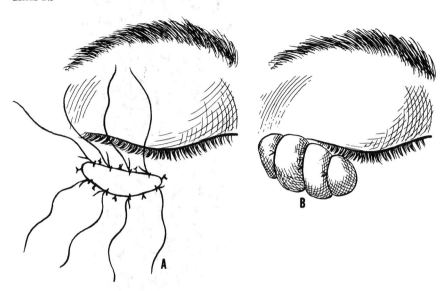

FIG. 26. Tie Sutures.
A. As the graft is sutured into place some sutures are left long for ties.
B. Sutures are tied over dressing to hold it in place.

usually reepithelialized, and no further dressing is necessary. If a full thickness skin graft has been taken, the wound edges are undermined if necessary, sutured and dressed in the usual manner.

All dressings are left in place 5 or 6 days without disturbance, i.e., until blood supply is assured. Patients are kept in bed the first 24 hours and then are allowed bathroom privileges only, for the next 48 hours. If the graft is large and a "take" precarious, activity is limited as much as possible until the first dressing.

On the sixth day dressings are removed, the grafted areas are carefully cleansed and sloughed sutures picked off. The pressure dressing is reapplied for 3 or 4 more days. At the next dressing the graft will be a healthy pink in color and fine new blood vessels will be seen coursing into it. All the sutures are removed and the wound is dressed every other day (no pressure) until complete healing has taken place.

AUTOGENOUS FREE FULL THICKNESS LID GRAFTS

Full thickness lid grafts, i.e., transference of sections of one whole lid to another lid, is the most recent of the important breakthroughs in ophthalmic plastic surgery. This technic has been used by the author with satisfaction (see Chapter 11) and offers a welcome new method of handling lid reconstructions requiring replacement of more than half a lid.

We have come far from the days of Wheeler's dictum that lid wounds must be closed by halving to avoid notching. We know now that closure can be made directly without notching if the wound is carefully sutured anteriorly and posteriorly and at the margin. Such surgery would be impossible if a lid had no inherent "give" and if it were not possible for a lid to lose a considerable amount of tissue without requiring tissue replacement. However, where the elasticity of the lid is not enough, the rest can be made up by a full thickness autogenous free lid graft in cases of large lid defects.

The technic of full thickness lid grafting is not difficult. The graft is best taken at the lateral canthus where, if necessary, canthotomy, cantholysis and an advancement graft can be made to assist closure of the donor site. This is not always necessary if the lid is lax enough or the graft small enough. Once taken, the graft should be seated immediately because of its tendency to shrink; hence all other surgery should have been completed in the recipient lid.

Since there is no vascular bed, as in the case of a flat skin graft, healing takes place by vascularization from the edges of the wound and no pressure is required. But the graft must be firmly sewed into position with numerous closely placed sutures on the skin and conjunctival surfaces. Despite the paucity of vascular source, healing is rapid and the graft appears normally pink and healthy on the fifth day. In fact, healing seems better and more rapid here than with a free lid skin graft.

Grafts are seated where possible in the medial portion of the coloboma, thus enabling closure by a previously advanced lateral graft. Hence full thickness grafting is particularly suitable for central and medial lid lesions. It is quite probable that as this technic becomes more widely accepted it will be used more and more for the smaller and medial colobomata which do not require tissue from the lateral canthus.

Mucous Membrane Grafts

The conjunctiva itself and buccal mucosa, in the order named, are the best sources of mucous membrane for grafting purposes in ophthalmic plastic surgery. Small segments of conjunctiva from the upper and lower fornices are available (fig. 27) for defects in either bulbar or palpebral conjunctiva of the same or contralateral eye. They may be used as pedicle grafts or free grafts and are useful in the repair of symblepharon and recurrent pterygium. (See Chapter 12 for full discussion.)

Buccal mucosa is best for the larger grafts required in socket and cul-de-sac reconstruction. It should be noted that buccal mucous membrane tends to retain its pinkish color and hence should be used in the palpebral fissure only if a thin layer is taken with a mucotome (fig. 28A) as it would otherwise be a conspicuous cosmetic blemish. If taken thin enough, the pinkish color is practically unnoticeable (fig. 28B).

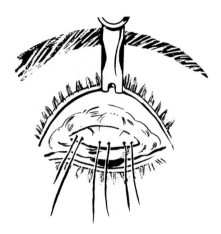

FIG. 27.   Donor Area of Conjunctival Graft from the Upper Fornix.

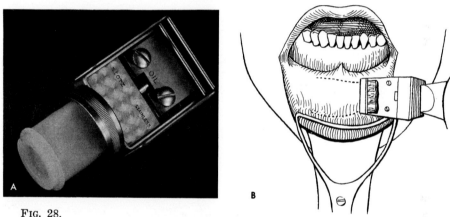

FIG. 28.

A. Head of Castroviejo electro-mucotome. *B.* Taking buccal mucosa with mucotome.

The best source of buccal mucosa is the lower lip in the area between the vermilion border and the frenulum (fig. 29). The cheek furnishes a somewhat thicker mucosa and this is a bit more difficult to get as the cheek must be turned out sufficiently to give adequate exposure and this is not always easy (fig. 30). Exposure of malar mucosa is best obtained by pressure on the cheek from without while it is everted by a pair of clamps or sutures held by an assistant. The opening of the parotid gland should first be located lest it be inadvertently injured.

After the patient has rinsed his mouth several times with a solution of potassium perborate, the area is infiltrated with a 1 per cent solution of procaine to which a few drops of epinephrine 1:1000 have been added. This injection should be made quite superficially to assist in taking as thin a graft as possible. The mucosa to be resected should be outlined with a knife and it should be remembered that it has been stretched by the anesthesia.

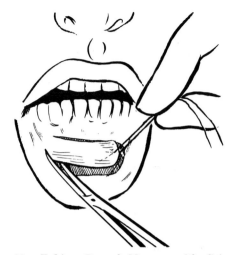

FIG. 29.   Taking Buccal Mucosa with Scissors.

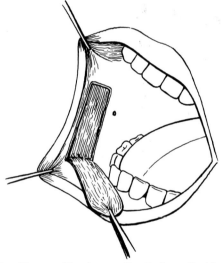

FIG. 30.   Mucous Membrane Graft from Inside of Cheek.

Dissection is carried out with a long narrow knife blade or a small blunt pointed scissors, whichever is preferred by the surgeon. It is much better to spend a little more time doing this than to attempt to trim off the excess later. The mucosa tends to curl up and contract making subsequent trimming a laborious task and requiring that it be pinned out on a flat surface if it is to be done at all adequately. Time and trouble will be saved if the submucous tissue and fat are left behind at the outset.

In the taking of buccal mucous membrane bleeding, which is usually profuse, must be controlled. Suction and sponging is done frequently to prevent the swallowing or inhalation of blood. Cotton spindles can be inserted on both sides of the jaw, i.e., between cheek and jaw and tongue and jaw to aid in absorption.

The denuded bed needs no suturing and will granulate in nicely. The patient has little discomfort after 24 hours but should have a bland mouthwash t.i.d. and a soft diet. On the fifth day after operation the donor bed will be filled in with grayish-white membrane through which a fine network of new blood vessels may be seen (fig. 31A). By the tenth day the membrane is pinkish and much more vascular. At this time the patient may have a regular diet but the lip should be washed after each meal. Within two weeks (unless the graft has been unusually large) the dehiscence is practically healed (fig. 31B).

A spindle measuring 1 cm. by 2 cm. of unstretched buccal mucous membrane can easily be taken, and more can be taken if necessary at a later date. However, too many incisions of the area will result in fibrosis. Enough is available from the mouth for complete reconstruction of a cul-de-sac. Both cheeks in addition will be necessary for a whole socket. In the latter case the surgeon should consider epidermis which makes an adequate socket lining (see Chapter 20).

Castroviejo's electro-mucotome has eased the problem of taking thin mucous membrane grafts (fig. 28A). A graft 0.3 to 0.4 mm. thick is adequate for a bulbar conjunctival repair: The one disadvantage of this useful little instrument is that not quite as large a piece of mucous membrane is obtainable as when taken by hand. However, the ease with which a graft can be obtained makes up for this defect in selected cases and two narrow strips may be taken from the same lip, if necessary (fig. 28B). In using the mucotome good counterpressure is required. This may be obtained by injecting sufficient anesthesia superficially so that the mucous membrane is tense. Also an assistant should support the injected lip from below or draw it out with a pair of forceps to supply sufficient tension.

Mucous membrane will shrink. The bed as in all grafts must therefore be cleaned of fibrous tissue before the graft is sutured into place. The graft must be kept on stretch by sutures or a conformer for at least three

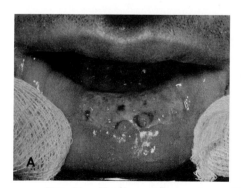
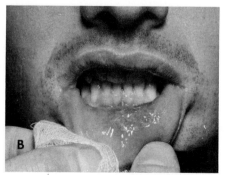

FIG. 31.   Healing of Donor Area after Resection of Mucous Membrane.
A.   Five days later.   B.   Fourteen days later.

weeks and preferably longer. If the socket is empty, as large a conformer as can be conveniently gotten into the socket without forcing should be used. All these technics will be discussed subsequently in greater detail in their respective places.

Peritoneal grafts to replace conjunctiva have not proved successful in the author's hands. The use of prepucial skin and vaginal mucosa to replace conjunctiva has been reported. They have not been used by the author. Buccal mucosa is more readily accessible than nasal mucosa.

HAIR-BEARING GRAFTS

Of all grafts, hair-bearing grafts are probably the least gratifying cosmetically, the results frequently being considerably less than an unqualified success. In the case of lash grafts especially, the result is often an irregular array of sparse cilia growing in all directions. Attempts at making these grow in one direction by "training" and collodion, so glibly mentioned in the literature, rarely succeed in making them look natural. However, the attempt is always worthwhile and should be made, for occasionally one is agreeably surprised by a luxuriant growth which is almost normal in appearance. Usually this happens inexplicably when least expected. Absence of lashes is a noticeable cosmetic blemish which is more serious in the upper than the lower lid. In the lower lid they are usually shorter and somewhat lighter and hence their absence is less noticeable (see Chapter 13 for fuller discussion).

Lash Grafts

The best source of hair for lid lashes is the medial end of the eyebrow where the hairs are numerous. If these are unavailable for some reason, scalp hair from the occipital or temporal region may be used.

The normal lashes curl up in the upper lid and down in the lower lid; hence the eyebrow chosen for the source of the graft is important for the hairs of the eyebrow also sweep up and out on each side. If both eyebrows are intact, the choice is simply made. The ipsilateral brow will supply lashes growing in the proper direction for the upper lid, i.e., upward and outward. And a graft from the contralateral brow, turned upside down, will supply lashes for the lower lid which grow downward and somewhat outward (fig. 160). If the brow hair on the same or opposite side is missing, one must perforce use the same procedure with hairs from the one brow and attempt to train them to grow properly.

Failing both eyebrows, a hair-bearing skin graft is taken from the hair line of the temporal region behind the ear (fig. 32) or from the occipital region (fig. 33). These are less preferable because of the greater thickness of scalp skin. Only dire necessity will drive one to this expedient. Here also the direction of hair growth must be watched.

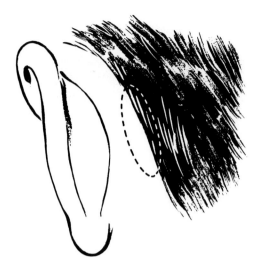

FIG. 32. Hair-Bearing Graft from Temporal Region.

When the eyeball is present, the choice of proper lash direction has more than cosmetic importance, for trichiasis with all its connotations is a constant danger. Even with proper choice, the danger of trichiasis is always present, for the hair follicles have a perverse way of becoming displaced and disorganized even when most carefully handled.

This operation is always simpler when perfomed in the presence of an anophthalmic socket, for then the choice of hair direction—although for cosmetic reasons it should be the same as with an eyeball present—may be subject to more compromise since the fear of damage to the globe from trichiasis is absent.

It might be pointed out that modern cosmetic specialists have produced artificial eyelashes which are excellent. These are primarily for the upper lid. However, it is unlikely that a male patient would avail himself of this artifice. Dyes are also available which, when tattooed on carefully at the lid edge, give some appearance of verisimilitude (fig. 166).

Further details of lash grafting procedures are given in Chapter 13.

Eyebrow Grafts

If the hairs of one brow have been lost and the other brow is intact, with plentiful hair, the simplest procedure is to rotate a hair-bearing pedicle consisting of half the intact brow to take the place of the one destroyed. For complete details of the technic see figure 164. It suffices to say here that, while this type of graft may be a cosmetic necessity and should be tried, it is not one of the most successful of grafts. (Figure 164E shows one of the better results.) When the opposite brow is not available as a source of hair, the occipital and temporal regions of the scalp can supply free hair-bearing tissue.

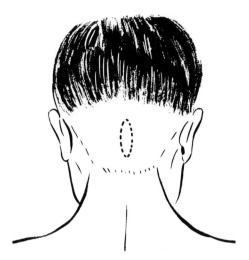

FIG. 33.   Hair-Bearing Graft from Occipital Region. (Hair need not be shaved but
should be clipped short.)

In all these grafts it is important to make sure that they are so placed that the hair will grow in the proper direction. The hair of the brow usually grow toward each temple. The hair of the scalp, whether from the temporal region behind the ear or from the occipital region, grow downward. Hence the graft is cut lengthwise in the direction of hair growth and set in the recipient bed so that the upper part is the most medial. Thus the direction of the grafted eyebrow will be outward. Before it is taken the hair should be clipped short but not shaven to help identification. Inserting a white suture into the upper tip and a black suture into the lower will also help avoid reversal.

The graft should be cut at least 33 per cent larger than the bed to allow for shrinkage and for loss of the hair follicles along the cut edges. If too wide after the take it can always be narrowed by dissecting away the excess (see Chapter 13 for further details of eyebrow grafting).

CARTILAGE GRAFTS

In former days cartilage auto- and homografts were used quite frequently in the repair of fractures of the orbital floor and for the filling in of depressions around the bony foramen of the socket (fig. 34).

Free autografts of ear and rib cartilage are available for these purposes, ear cartilage being used in those rare instances where lid grafting is necessary and rib cartilage for orbital and periorbital defects. Ear cartilage is obtained from the pinna by careful dissection on the back surface of the ear (fig. 35). There is never enough taken to cause concern. Rib cartilage is obtainable from the right sixth and

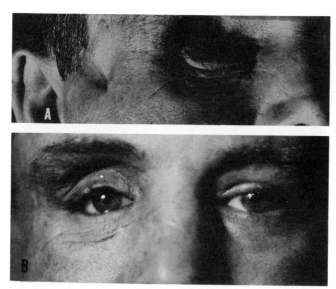

Fig. 34. Reconstruction of Bony Dehiscence of the Temple with Preserved
Cartilage.
A. Depression in right temporal region.
B. Three weeks after repair.
(Fox, S. A.: Courtesy Archives of Ophthalmology.)

seventh ribs under local anesthesia. A curved skin incision is made over
the junction of the sixth and seventh costal cartilages and the fascia and
muscles are exposed. These are separated by blunt dissection, the rib
fascia cut and rib cartilage exposed. A piece of cartilage with perichondrium cut to thickness and size is excised, the bleeding stopped and the
wound closed in layers. Fresh cartilage shrinks somewhat and should
be taken about 25 per cent larger than the defect. It is easily cut to
pattern with a sharp scalpel and should be fastened into its bed in a
bony defect or in the floor of the orbit with 20 day chromic catgut
sutures to assure its remaining in place during the healing process. The
tissues over the cartilage graft are closed in layers and a firm dressing
is applied for 6 or 7 days. At this time the sutures are removed, the
wound carefully cleaned and the dressing reapplied for 5 more days.

Preservation of the material is not difficult. When obtained at
autopsy the cartilage is cleaned of all attached tissue, including perichondrium. It is placed in a solution composed of 2 parts of aqueous
merthiolate 1:1000 and 2 parts of isotonic solution of sodium chloride
for 48 hours. It is then transferred to a similar fresh solution daily for
3 days, being cultured before each transferral and cleaned of all adherent
strands of perichondrium which might have been overlooked originally.
These strands have a tendency to separate after cartilage has soaked for
several days. Rarely do cultures show any growth after the first 48
hours. After 3 successive sterile cultures, the material is stored perma-

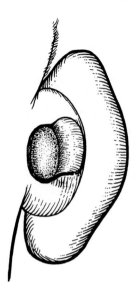

FIG. 35.   Donor Area for Ear Cartilage Graft.

nently at icebox temperatures in a solution of 1 part of aqueous merthiolate 1:1000 and 3 parts of isotonic solution of sodium chloride. Two successive daily cultures are obtained before the graft is used. The material has been stored for several months by the author and found excellent for use. Successful use of cartilage stored as long as two years has been reported. Seventy per cent alcohol may also be used as a storage medium.

Preserved cartilage has been used in the past by the plastic surgeon in reconstructions of the nose, ear, forehead, chin and other facial structures. This will probably always remain its greatest sphere of usefulness. But it can also be used effectively by the ophthalmic surgeon in reconstructions in and about the orbit (fig. 34).

Since preserved cartilage is "dead" tissue, the question of what happens to it after grafting is pertinent. In the case of preserved human rib cartilage buried in human hosts, experimental studies showed microscopic invasion by the surrounding host tissues and areas of absorption. There were also areas of calcification and early formation of bone. This process, however, was very slow and the bulk of the graft was still present two years after transplantation.

In recent years inert plastic materials of various composition, density and elasticity have begun to replace the various organic tissues described here. These have proved quite successful and few side effects or contraindications have been noted. This tends to make the replacement problems in plastic surgery a good deal easier. Hence the use of cartilage and bone autografts has recently tended to become less and less in ophthalmic plastic surgery.

BONE GRAFTS

Bone autografts may also be used for the repair of fractures of the orbital floor and for filling in other bony defects. Bone is available from the crest of the ilium above the anterior superior spine which can supply all the cancellous bone which an ophthalmic surgeon needs. It is easily obtained and also easily shaped at the operating table. Taking the graft is something of a chore, but no more so than obtaining a cartilage autograft. The procedure is as follows:

A 10 cm. incision is made over the iliac crest above the anterior' superior spine down to periosteum. The latter is also incised and raised with an elevator. As much of the exposed bone as required is removed and the periosteum resutured with heavy chromic catgut. The skin is closed with interrupted silk sutures.

The patient should be allowed up early. There is some pain over the donor site for the first 2 or 3 days but this rapidly disappears as healing takes place.

Bone banks have been established which permit the use of bone homografts. What has been stated previously about the advantages of using cartilage homografts also applies to bone. If available, a bone homograft is excellent for socket repair. It has to be shaped to pattern at the operating table and this is somewhat more time-consuming. But histologic evidence seems to show that the graft acquires a blood supply and is replaced by living bone from the host if placed in contact with bone which has been stripped of its periosteum and then covered with host periosteum. This makes it a desirable modality which the author has used with satisfaction. Here also the use of methyl methacrylate, silastic and supramid plates is gradually replacing the necessity for autogenous or homologous bone in the repair of orbital fractures.

TARSAL GRAFTS

Since the object of plastic surgery is to restore the injured part as nearly as possible to its previous state, the problem of replacing the tarsus keeps coming up in reconstructive surgery. In the author's experience, however, this problem has been more academic than real, and the necessity for tarsal reconstruction has not arisen too often except after large tumor excisions.

The usual difficulty in reconstructing a lid is not to make it thick enough but to keep it reasonably thin. The tissues become so thickened by inevitable scarring during the process of surgery that the transplantation of cartilage or tarsus to replace tarsus frequently becomes a work of supererogation which would have been best left undone in the majority of cases.

Where the defect is small, the absence of tarsus from part of a lid is of little consequence. In large reconstructions after tumor excision, where sufficient lid skin and conjunctiva is available, the problem of lid stiffening does arise and here cartilage or tarsus may be required. Also, in rare instances, where the tarsus has previously been resected for some reason, need for its restoration may arise. However, where skin other than lid skin is used, it is usually so much heavier that no further thickening of the lid may be necessary.

The tarsus is still valuable for use as a sliding graft though not as much as formerly. The best example is the Hughes procedure for lower lid reconstruction in which a sliding graft from the ipsilateral upper lid is used to reconstruct the lower lid. Similar use may be made of the tarsus for repair of lid notches, congenital colobomata, etc. According to Hughes its use is indicated not only because tarsus is needed per se but even more because it makes an excellent bed on which to graft skin and cilia for lashes.

It may also be used as a free graft and transferred from one lid to another. A free tarsal graft from an upper lid may be used in a lower lid or in the opposite upper lid. It may also be shifted to another position in the same lid. However, what has been said previously concerning the use, or abuse, of cartilage grafts also applies here. In small lid defects there seems little purpose in using free tarsal grafts. As a matter of fact, if a small loss of tarsus is to be replaced by a segment of tarsus from another lid, it seems legitimate to ask why the injured lid cannot get along without it if the donor lid can. Indeed, the remarkable thing is how much tarsus a lid can spare and still function normally. Many a trachomatous lid has been deprived of most of its tarsus with the lid better off for it.

Fascia, Muscle, Fat, Dura and Sclera Grafts

At various times autogenous fascia, fat and muscle tissue have been used for filling in depressions due to trauma in and around the socket. Fascia is an ideal tissue for this purpose because of its low metabolism. Transplanted, it will thrive almost anywhere provided it is well covered. While there is shrinkage, this diminution in volume is not as great as that of fat or skin. Years ago—it seems prehistoric now—fat was a favorite tissue for implantation into Tenon's capsule after enucleation. This has now been abandoned because of its propensity to vanish almost completely.

Both fascia and muscle are available from the outer aspect of the thigh or from the tensor fascia lata just below the anterior superior spine of the ilium. This can be taken without hesitation since the amount usually needed is small and can easily be spared. Fat, if desired, is also available from this site or from the abdominal wall.

The tissue over the depression to be filled in should be prepared as for other grafting procedures. It is incised and the depression fully exposed. All bleeding is stopped. The graft, whether skin, muscle or fascia, is set in place with sutures if necessary. The covering of the graft is then done in layers and a pressure dressing applied.

Fascia and de-epithelialized skin are useful to fill out the supra-orbital depressions of the upper lid in cases of old anophthalmic sockets. The technic of this procedure will be discussed later (Chapter 21). It is a useful tissue to have at one's disposal.

Obtaining Autogenous Fascia for Ptosis Surgery

Fascia is obtained as follows: After the usual presurgical preparation of the area a vertical 3 inch incision is made in the lower lateral aspect of the thigh. The incision is carried through skin and subcutaneous fat down to fascia lata. Bleeding is contained with pressure and catgut ties. The upper and lower ends of the wound are undermined by blunt dissection so that an extra half or three-quarter inch of fascia is exposed at each end. The lips of the wound are drawn well apart so as to give good exposure and two vertical incisions are made in the fascia 4 to 5 mm. apart. If a bilateral operation is planned the strip of fascia is cut about 10 mm. wide and then split into thinner vertical ribbons. The resultant strip of fascia about 4 inches long, is freed from the subjacent muscle by blunt dissection or by a muscle hook placed behind it to separate it from the muscle. When the strip of fascia is freed along its whole length its upper and lower attached ends are cut and the fascia wrapped in warm moist gauze until ready for use (fig. 36).

The wound in the leg is closed with deep 3–0 chromic interrupted sutures and stout interrupted silk skin sutures. A firm dressing is applied.

An alternative method is the use of a fascia stripper which simplifies the procedure somewhat. The fascia is exposed through a 1.5 inch vertical incision. Some prefer to use a short horizontal incision although this gives less exposure. The fascia is freed anteriorly and posteriorly by a blunt, long-bladed scissors in order to allow free passage to the fascia stripper (fig. 37A). A tongue of fascia is threaded into the stripper at the lower end of the wound. This is grasped with a clamp, held taut and the stripper is moved upward cutting a 10 cm. (about 4 inches) strip of fascia (fig. 37B). Closure is then made as above. Obviously not all of the fascial wound can be reached for closure. The patient is kept in bed for 24 hours and ambulation is then begun slowly. The donor site is quite painful for several days.

Fascia is a slippery tissue which does not hold sutures well. When using it, sutures should be tied tightly and insured with over-ties, i.e., additional sutures tied over the knot.

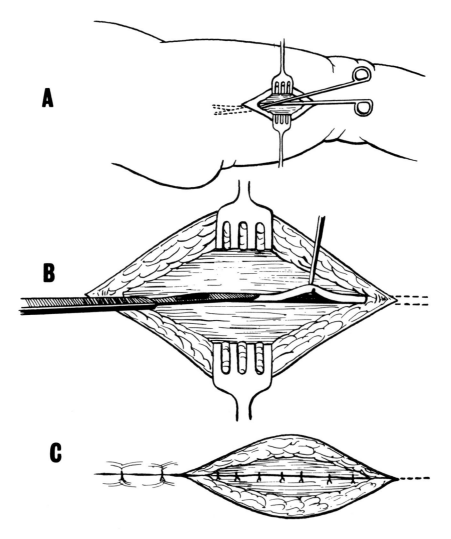

Fig. 36. Taking Fascia by the Open Method.

A. A vertical 3 inch incision is made through skin and subcutaneous fat in the lower lateral aspect of the thigh. The lips of the wound are undermined as are the upper and lower ends.

B. The lips of the wound are retracted and two longitudinal incisions are made outlining the fascial strip.

C. The ends are cut off and the wound is closed in layers (see text).

Homologous Grafts

The use of homologous grafts of fascia, dura and sclera has been reported. The method of obtaining, sterilizing and storing these tissues is described in detail by Reeh and Mason. These, like all homografts, act as a framework into which host fibroblasts migrate and form new layers of collagen as the homologous graft degenerates and is absorbed.

Homologous dura is useful in filling out supratarsal and other

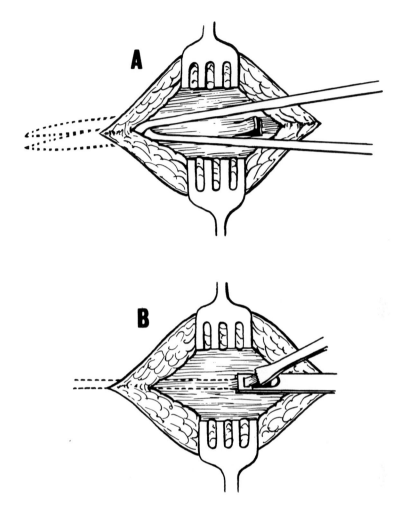

FIG. 37.   Taking Fascia with the Fascia Stripper.
A.   A 1.5 inch vertical incision is made through skin and fat in the lower lateral aspect of the thigh and the fascia is cleanly exposed. (Some prefer a short horizontal incision.) By means of a long, blunt tonsil scissors passed upward, the fascia is freed from the overlying skin and fat for about 5 inches. A strip of fascia is dissected up and the scissors is passed upward behind the fascia to free it from the underlying muscle.
B.   The end of the fascial strip is passed through the open end of the fascia stripper and the fascial end is grasped with forceps. The stripper is passed up and the fascial strip is cut off (see text). Closure is as described in Procedure 36.

depressions around the eye as well as in the repair of mild enophthalmos. Homologous and heterologous fascia absorbs too rapidly to be of any value in frontalis ptosis surgery. Preserved sclera may be used to repair scleral defects such as staphylomata and to replace tarsus when the patient's own tissue is not available. Bodian has reported the use of homologous sclera in frontalis suspension.

REFERENCES

VON ARLT, C. F.: Cited by Beard, C. H., Opthalmic Surgery, ed. 2. Philadelphia, P. Blakiston's Son & Co., 1914, p. 222.

AUB, J.: Ectropion treated by transplantation of flaps without pedicle. Arch. Ophth. 8:95, 1879.

VON BLASKOVICS, L., and KREIKER, A.: Eingriffe am Auge. Stuttgart, Ferdinand Enke, 1938.

BOCK, E.: Die Propfung von Haut und Schleimhaut auf oculistischen Gebiete. Vienna, W. Braumuller, 1884.

BONOLA, A.: The methods of obtaining skin grafts for palpebral reconstruction. Ann. ottal. e clin. ocul. 81:105, 1955.

BROWN, J. B.: Cited by Peer, L. A., Cartilage transplanted beneath the skin of the chest in man. Arch. Oto. 27:42, 1938.

————, and CANNON, B.: Full thickness skin grafts from the neck for function and color in eyelid and face repair. Ann. Surg. 121:639, 1945.

CELSUS: Cited by Zeis, E., Handbuch der plastischen Chirurgie. Berlin, G. Reimer, 1818, p. 13.

CLAY, G. E., and BAIRD, J. M.: Restoration of orbit and repair of conjunctival defects with grafts from perpuce and labia minora. J.A.M.A. 107:1122, 1936.

CONWAY, H., STARK, R. D., and JOSLIN, D.: Observations on the development of circulation in skin grafts. Plast. Reconstr. Surg., 8:312, 1951.

CRAWFORD, H.: Dura replacement: An experimental study of derma autografts and preserved dura homografts. Plast. Reconstr. Surg. 19:299, 1957.

CZERMAK, W.: Die augenärtzlichen Operationen. Vienna, Karl Gerolds Sohn, 1893–1904, p. 213–215.

DE WECKER, L.: La greffe dermique en chirurgie oculaire. Ann. d'ocul. 68:62, 1872.

DIEFFENBACH, J. F.: Uberpflanzung Vollig gettrennter Hautstücke bei einer Frau und Wiedranheilung einer grossenteils der abgehauenen Wange. J. d. Chir. u. Augenh. 6:482, 1824.

DZONDI, C. H.: Bildung eines neuen untern Augenlides aus der Wange J. d. pract. Heilk. 47:99, 1818.

————: Zweiter Jahresbericht von den merkwürdigsten Krankenheitsfallen und Operationen in dem Institute des Professors Dzondi zu Halle. Mag. f. d. ges. Heilk. 6:1, 1819.

EDGERTON, M. T., PETERSON, H. A., and EDGERTON, P. J.: The homograft rejection mechanism. Arch. Surg. 74:238, 1957.

EVERBUSCH, O.: Uber die Verwendung von Epidermistransplantationen bei den plastischen Operationen an den Lidern und der Conjunctiva. München. med. Wchnschr. 34:1, 19, 1887.

FILATOV, V. P.: Tissue therapy in ophthalmology. Am. Rev. Soviet Med. 2:53, 1944.

FOX, S. A.: Use of preserved cartilage in plastic surgery of the eye. Arch. Ophth. 38:182, 1947.

————: Basic techniques of lid surgery: Their origins and their apocrypha. Am. J. Ophth. 50:384 (Sept.), 1960.

FRICKE, J.: Die Bildung neurer Augenlider nach Zerstorungen, etc. Hamburg, Perthus & Besser, 1829.

GRADENIGO, P.: Scritti oftalmologici del conte Pietro Gradenigo. Padua, Stabilimento della Società Cooperativa Tipografica. 1904, pp. 155, 157.

GREEAR, J. M.: The use of buccal mucosa in restoration of the orbital socket. Am. J. Ophth. 31:445, 1948.

HARTMAN, E.: Eye surgery in wartime. Am. J. Ophth. 25:1448, 1942.

HIPPOCRATES: Cited by Beard, C. H., op. cit.

HUGHES, W. L.: Reconstructive Surgery of the Eyelids. St. Louis, C. V. Mosby, 1954, p. 138.

KNAPP, H.: Methoden der blepharoplastik. Klin. Monatsbl. Augenh. *9*:424, 1871. (Discussion by Driver.)

KNAPP, P.: Zwei Fälle von Lidplastik nach Budinger. Klin. Monatsbl. Augenh. *46* (II):317-322, 1908.

KRUSIUS, F. F.: Uber die Einpflanzung lebende Haare zur Wimpernbildung. Deutsche Med. Wchnschr. *40*:958, 1914.

LAGRANGE, F. Fractures of the Orbit. London, University of London Press, 1914.

LAWSON, G.: On the successful transplantation of portions of skin for the closure of large granulating surfaces. Lancet, *2*:708, 1870.

LE FORT, L. C.: Blepharoplastie par un lambeau complètement détaché du bras et reporté a la face. Bull. et mém. Soc. de Chir. *1*:39, 1872.

LE GROUS, R.: The technique of using free full-thickness palpebral skin grafts. Arch. Ophth. *10*:367, 1950.

LEWIS, G. K.: Skin flaps in reconstruction of head and neck following excision of malignant lesions. Trans. Am. Acad. Ophth. & Oto. *64*:660, 1960.

LITTLEWOOD, A. H. A.; Seroma: An unrecognized cause of failure of split-thickness skin grafts. Brit. J. Plast. Surg., April, 1960.

MOWLEM, R.: Bone and cartilage transplants. Brit. J. Surg. *29*:182, 1941.

NOYES, H. D.: Formation of an eyelid by transfer of large piece of skin without pedicle. Med. Rec. *17*:344, 1880.

O'CONNOR, G. B.: Merthiolate—a tissue preservative and antiseptic. Am. J. Surg. *45*:563, 1939.

OLLIER, L.: Sur les greffes cutanées de l'autoplastique. Bull. et mém. Acad. de Chir. *1*:243, 1872.

PADGETT, E. C.: Skin Grafting from a Personal and Experimental Viewpoint. Springfield, Ill., Charles C Thomas, 1942.

PAULUS AEGINITA: Cited by Zeis, E., op cit.

PEER, L. A.: The fate of autogenous human bone grafts. Brit. J. Plast. Surg. *3*:233, 1950.

————: Transplantation of Tissues. Baltimore, Williams and Wilkins Co., 1959.

PIERCE, G. W., and O'CONNOR, G. B.: Reconstructive surgery of the nose. Ann. Otol. Rhin. & Laryn. *45*:563, 1939.

PRESSMAN, J. J., BERMAN, W., and SIMON, M. B.: Primary repair of defects following the surgical removal of tumors of the face. Arch. Surg. *79*:921, 1959.

REEH, M. J., and MASON, N. S.: Use of homologous dura mater, fascia and sclera in ophthalmic plastic surgery. Highlights of Ophthalmology. *4*:242, 1961.

REESE, J. D., and STARK, R. B.: Principles of free skin grafting. Bull. N. Y. Acad. of Med. *37*:213, 1961.

REVERDIN, J. L.: Greffe epidermique—experience faite dans le service de M. le Docteur Guyon a l'hopital Necker. Gaz. d. hop. *43*:15, 16, 1870.

ROBERTSON, D. M.C.L.A.: Notes on some points of procedure in the operation of direct transplantation of skin grafts for the cure of ectropion. Pract. *57*:160, 1896.

ROMANES, G. J.: Treatment of established symblepharon with split skin homograft. Brit. J. Ophth. *37*:236, 1953.

ROSEN, E.:Heterogeneous conjunctival transplantation. Am. J. Ophth. *29*:193, 1946.

ROSONOFF, H. L.: Ethylene oxide sterilized, freeze-dried dura mater for the repair of pachymeningeal defects. J. Neurosurg. *16*:197, 1959.

SINGER, M.: Some basic causes for failure in grafting skin and mucous membrane to the lids and socket. Trans. Am. Acad. Ophth. & Oto. *60*:679, 1956.

SICHEL, A.: Blepharoplastie par greffe dermique. Bull. Acad. de méd. *4*:574, 1875.

STELLWAG, VON CARION K.: Ruckblicke auf den augeartzlichen Propfungsversuche und ein neuer Fall von Schleimhauttubertragung. Alg. Wien. med. Ztg. *34*:341, 1889.

STERN, W. E.: The surgical application of freeze-dried homologous dura mater. Surg. Gynec. & Obst. *106*:159, 1958.

TAGLIACOZZI, G.: De curtorum chirurgia per insitionen libri duo. Venice, G. Bindonus, 1597.

TEALE, T. P. JR.: On relief of symblepharon by transplantation of conjunctiva. Royal Oph. Hosp. Reports, 1860–1861, pp. 3 and 253–258.

THIERSCH C.: Uber die feineren anatomischer Veranderungen bei Augenheilung von der Haut auf Granulationen. Arch. klin. Chir. *17*:318, 1874.

VANNAS, M.: On the use of rib cartilage for the correction of cosmetic defects caused by enucleation. Acta. Ophth. *24*:225, 1946.

WADSWORTH, O. F.: Case of ectropion cured by transplantation of a large piece of skin from the forearm. Trans. Int. Ophth. Cong. New York, D. Appleton & Co., 1876, p. 237.

WEEKS, J. E.: A case of restoration of the tegument of the upper lid by transplanting a flap without pedicle. Arch. Ophth. *8*:92, 1889.

WHEELER, J. M.: Collected Papers. New York, Columbia University Press. 1939, pp. 124; 356; 423.

WOLFE, J. R.: A new method for performing plastic operations. Med. Times & Gaz. *1*:608, 1876.

CHAPTER 4

Basic Technics

GENERAL CONSIDERATIONS

THIS MAY WELL BE the most important chapter of all because it outlines in detail the fundamental technics on which most of the procedures described in the rest of the book are based.

The historic roots of ophthalmic surgery are buried deep in antiquity. This is as true of adnexal surgery as it is of the globe. It is only something less than 150 years since we have had a formalized, regular and trustworthy literature for the recording of scientific proceedings and the publication of scientific papers. Hence prior to this time most of our scientific "facts," with a few exceptions, have come down to us second, third or fourth hand, taken on faith, based on hearsay or founded in rumor.

With all this we have gradually evolved over the years from sources known and unknown a body of fundamental technics in lid surgery which we use over and over again and which are in many respects apart and different from those of tectonic surgery elsewhere in the body. This had to follow because the lids are unique in many ways:

First, the upper and lower lids together form a sphincter muscle which acts voluntarily and reflexly to protect the eye and the opening into the orbit.

Second, one set of lids is part of a team which includes the opposite set. These four lids work together reflexly, and very often to our chagrin this happens whether one eye is patched or not. Hence after cataract surgery or skin grafting we often have to patch both eyes to assure immobility of the operated eye.

Third, the unique anatomy of the lids enables us to manipulate them in ways which are not always possible elsewhere. Lid skin is so thin and has so few contractile elements that it can be grafted without allowing for contraction. Again, the structure of the lid in layers which are easily split into two laminae and which heal with practically no scarring is something of which we take advantage constantly.

It goes without saying that a surgeon should know the anatomy of his surgical field. It is not impossible to cause a ptosis where one did not exist before. And the author has seen hypotropia and diplopia as the result of too free a dissection for dermachalasis of the lower lid. This could have been avoided, it would seem, by a rudimentary knowledge of the course of the inferior oblique muscle. Knowledge of adnexal anatomy not only obviates errors but helps the surgeon to take advantage of the specialized structure of the lids.

The presence of the eye and the necessity for its protection both during operation and immediately thereafter must guide the surgeon's work at all times. It colors his thinking and guides his planning. It is an ever present hazard which the surgeon trained in eye work has learned to accept almost automatically. Others will ignore it to their sorrow. Corneal injury and irreversible eye muscle damage can be the result. The necessity for protecting the eye by secure closure with patch, suture or tarsorrhapy cannot be stressed too much.

Nature has been bountiful in supplying the lids with nerves and blood vessels so that they can withstand a good deal of surgical insult. This is a useful state of affairs for the ophthalmic surgeon, for it is comforting to know that however severe the trauma and no matter how complicated the repair, there is an excellent chance that healing will take place normally and without incident.

The more common basic technics used in ophthalmic plastic surgery are listed below.

INCISION AND CLOSURE

A glance at figures 1 and 4 will show that the normal course of the lid furrows and of the orbicularis fibers is roughly parallel with the lid margins. Hence, wherever possible, lid incisions should lie in the normal furrow or should parallel the direction of the orbicularis fibers (fig. 38). Such incisions are less conspicuous and heal better because there is no tendency to gaping from vertically cut muscle fibers. Obviously, vertical incisions cannot be avoided and frequently have to be made. Sometimes, however, they may be minimized to some extent by beveling or staggering to obviate a long vertical scar and a tendency to ectropion.

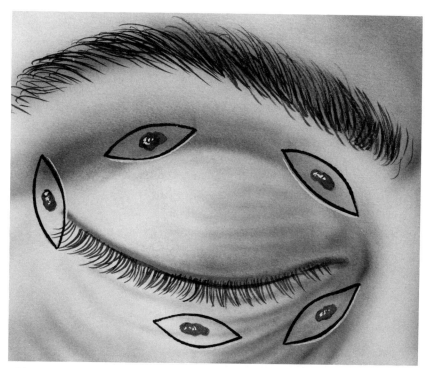

FIG. 38.   Preferred Placement of Incisions for Resection of Lid Lesions.

In making incisions one should proceed boldly yet carefully. They should be long enough to expose fully the area to be worked on. They should be made cleanly and accurately, taking care not to injure important structures. A cleanly incised wound will heal more rapidly and with less deformity than a ragged one. If the skin and subcutaneous tissues are yielding, as they frequently are in the aged, they should be held on stretch; hence the importance of marking out areas to be incised with alcoholic gentian violet or some other antiseptic dye, before they are distorted by pull and distended by infiltrative anesthesia.

Closure should be made by careful approximation with slight eversion of the skin lips to forestall depression when reorganization and healing take place. When closed the lips of the wound should lie together snugly without puckering. This implies sufficient relaxation of the wound edges either by undercutting or by subcuticular relaxation sutures or both if necessary. All incisions leave scars. Hence while sufficient incision to give adequate exposure must be made unhesitatingly, unnecessary incisions should be avoided.

SCARS

Scars are the result of trauma or surgery and the need for their excision and repair is sometimes encountered. The surgeon cannot prevent the traumatic scars which are brought to him; he can do a great deal to minimize his own surgical scars. These may be due to retained blood clots and wounds sutured too tightly or too loosely. Infection is a constant menace and keloids are a dreaded though fortunately uncommon complication in scar formation. In trauma early closure and clean healing makes for less scar; secondary closure increases it.

When scars are resected incisions should be made on each side close to the scar which is then cleanly excised. If the scar is deep, especially if close to bone, only the superficial portion is removed, one of the wound edges is amply undermined and drawn over the scarred area so that it is covered by healthy skin and the wound is sutured. However, over the area of the movable lids, the scar must be excised in toto no matter how deep. Over bony areas soft subcutaneous tissue should be interposed, if possible, between bone and skin to prevent adhesion of skin to bone and consequent sinking and distortion of the scar (fig. 39).

TEMPORARY PARACENTRAL (MEDIAN) TARSORRHAPHIES

Tarsorrhaphy (blepharorrhaphy) is the surgical fusion of the upper and lower lid margins. It may be classified in many ways: It is total or partial depending on whether all or only a portion of the palpebral fissure is occluded. It is called lateral, medial or paracentral (median) depending on its position in the palpebral fissure. Also, it may be temporary or permanent depending on the use to which it is put. The construction of a temporary tarsorrhaphy is simple. The technic of the permanent tarsorrhaphy is of necessity somewhat more elaborate. For a discussion of the construction and uses of the permanent tarsorrhaphy see Chapter 10.

Bowman is given credit for introducing the temporary paracentral tarsorrhaphy as we know it. This was modified and improved by Argyll Robertson and then by Panas. However, there are earlier precedents. Back in 1836 Lisfranc did the first recorded total tarsorrhaphy for an anterior staphyloma and Mirault in 1851 used two such tarsorrhaphies in a repair of cicatricial ectropion to prevent pull on the lid.

The temporary tarsorrhaphy is a fundamental procedure in plastic surgery. It is almost always central or paracentral, i.e., somewhere between the center of the lid and the canthi. It serves not only to protect the globe when pressure must be applied to the area, it also helps to splint the lids and reduce their movement to a minimum, thus aiding the healing process after grafting and similar procedures. The technic as originally described by Bowman and perfected by Panas is simple and usually leaves practically no scar on the lid margin. The surgeon should have no hesitancy about using it. It is much better to create an unnecessary tarsorrhaphy than to jeopardize a cornea or lose a graft. An example of its use is shown in figure 40 as an adjunct to the correction of cicatricial ectropion. Note that the tarsorrhaphies may be so placed as

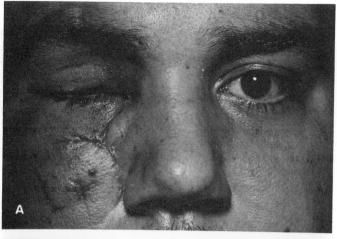

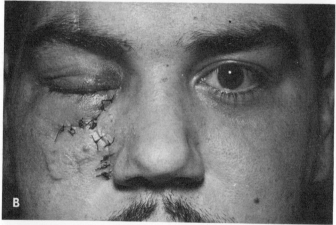

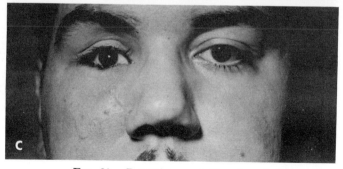

FIG. 39. Resection and Repair of Scar.
A. Old irregular scar of right cheek.
B. Appearance before removal of sutures.
C. Appearance four weeks later.

to leave the patient's vision unobstructed. The uses of the temporary paracentral tarsorrhaphy may be summarized as follows:

1. To protect the cornea in operative procedures about the lids, after orbital surgery and when pressure must be applied.

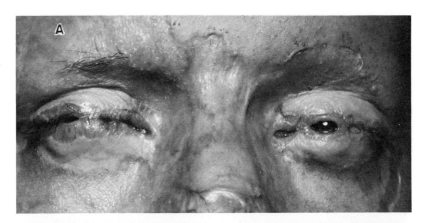

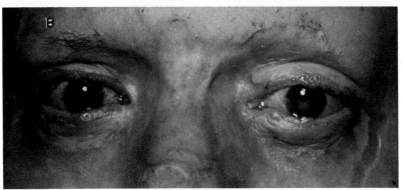

FIG. 40.   Use of the tarsorrhaphy in lid repair.
A.   Position of Tarsorrhaphy.
B.   Appearance of the lids shortly after separation.

2. To immobilize the lids and keep them splinted during plastic repair and to permit better healing afterward.

3. To protect the cornea in cases of corneal pathology or proptosis and thus provide an anatomic patch so to speak.

One paracentral tarsorrhaphy may suffice for minor procedures. However, when a considerable amount of surgery is to be done, and especially in grafting, two tarsorrhapies should be created: one at the junction of the inner and middle thirds of the lids and the other at the junction of the middle and outer thirds. After healing and some stretching, the lids may separate enough to allow the patient to use the openings between the tarsorrhapies for seeing. The inner opening may be used for near vision and the central opening for distant vision.

WEEKS Tarsorrhaphy

The method of the late W. W. Weeks for creating these temporary tarsorrhaphies is a nice procedure. It requires a bit of care because it leaves a thin rim of epithelium on both sides of the lid margin and thus

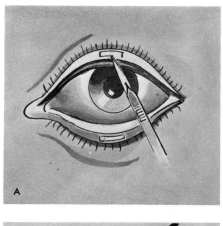
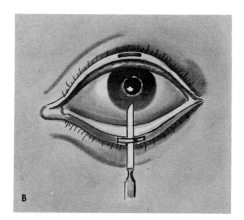
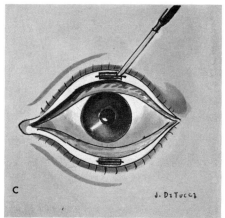
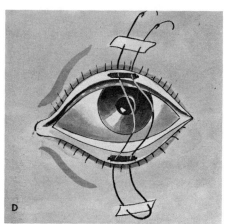

J. DiTucci

FIG. 41. Temporary Tarsorrhaphy (Weeks).
A. The marginal epithelium to be removed is marked off.
B. The epithelium is resected.
C. The raw edges are split.
D. A double-armed suture is inserted over pegs and tied.

helps preserve the normal lid contour and gives minimal marginal scarring.

Procedure (fig. 41): The two lids are pinched together so that the margins are brought close to each other and 6 to 8 mm. areas are marked off with the point of a knife at opposed sites of the upper and lower margins. Misplacement is easy if this is not carefully done and distortion will result unless the lids are exactly opposite each other.

Horizontal parallel incisions are made to outline the amount of mucocutaneous intermarginal tissue to be resected. A thin blade is then inserted on the flat and carried from one end to the other with a fine sawing motion. In this way a clean rectangular raw area is created on both lid margins (figs. 41A and B). The raw areas are split into skin-muscle and tarsoconjunctiva to a depth of 2 mm; this allows the wound to spread and makes for more healing surface (fig. 41C).

Both needles of a double-armed 4–0 braided silk suture threaded on a peg are passed 3 mm. apart through the skin and muscle just below the ciliary margin of the lower lid to come out in the center of the split margin. They are continued through the opposite upper lid split margin to emerge just above the cilia of the upper lid. The sutures are threaded through another peg and tied securely to bring the raw surfaces of the two lids in close apposition (fig. 41D). The sutures should not be tied so tightly as to cut through or cause sloughing. The same procedure is followed with the second tarsorrhaphy if two are needed. One then proceeds with the rest of the contemplated surgery or a patch is applied.

Dressings are done in 48 hours and then daily. The tarsorrhaphy sutures should be left in 10 days to assure complete healing, otherwise the lid adhesions may separate. To remove, one simply cuts the suture over the lower lid peg and pulls it out by the knot over the upper lid peg. (See Comment after Procedure 42.)

This type of tarsorrhaphy takes a little care and time but is bound to leave practically smooth, scarless lid margins.

Simple Tarsorrhaphy

The simplest method of creating a tarsorrhaphy is to mark off the opposing areas of the lids to be fused by means of a scratch mark. The epithelium between the marks is shaved off and the raw surfaces are sutured together. The technic follows:

Procedure (fig. 42): The two lids are pinched together as in the previous procedure and 6 to 8 mm. areas are marked off with the point of a knife. All the epithelium between the marks is shaved off carefully. Thus a rectangular raw area is created in both lid margins. The raw areas are split into skin-muscle and tarsoconjunctiva to allow the wound to spread and make for more healing surface (fig. 42A). Closure is made as in the previous case (fig. 42B).

Frequency of dressings will depend on the surgery done. The tarsorrhaphy sutures should be left in 10 days to assure complete healing, otherwise the lid adhesions may separate.

Comment: In both the above procedures since the adhesion produced is usually somewhat shorter than the area marked off, the raw surface of the lid margin should measure no less than 8 mm. for single tarsorrhaphies and no less than 6 mm. for double tarsorrhaphies. After some time the lids become separated somewhat as the adherent areas epithelialize and stretch. As noted above, tarsorrhaphies often become stretched enough for the patient to be able to see between them. This does no harm and is, in fact, an asset as the limited movement of the lids helps to stretch a newly laid graft, or, at least, prevents its contraction. And if the tarsorrhaphy has been created for corneal protection, it is still quite adequate. This applies to all types of temporary tarsorrhaphies.

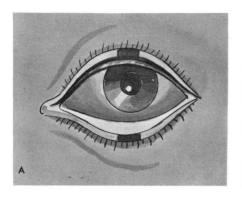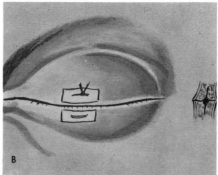

Fɪɢ. 42.   Simple Temporary Tarsorrhaphy.
A.   Area of tarsorrhaphy is marked off and the whole epithelium is shaved off.
B.   The tarsorrhaphy is closed.

Tarsorrhaphies used as adjuncts to grafting procedure should be left in place 6 to 10 weeks. If used to protect the cornea, they should not be opened until the corneal condition warrants it.

Through and Through Tarsorrhaphy (Author's)

Some intermarginal sutures have a disconcerting way of loosening or pulling out long before their function is fully accomplished; and a loose suture is as worthless as an absent one. This may occur in lids whose vitality has been lowered by severe trauma or frequent surgical procedure. It may happen in lids narrowed congenitally or by loss of tissue due to trauma; or in severe exophthalmos with strong lid retraction. Undoubtedly other examples will occur to the reader. In all cases where the tendency to lid separation is so great that it threatens the integrity of the intermarginal suture the following technic has been found rewarding by the author in providing a lid union which is least likely to tear loose.

Procedure (fig. 43): The oposing lid margins are denuded of epithelium for the desired length and split in the gray line shallowly in order to give more healing surface as in the previous procedures.

Both needles of a 4–0 double-armed silk suture are passed through a peg 4 mm. apart and then through the *full thickness* of the lower lid just below the ciliary margin to emerge on the conjunctival surface. The needles are then passed through the *full thickness* of the opposing upper lid 4 mm. apart from conjunctiva to skin surface to emerge above the ciliary margin where they are again passed through a peg (fig. 43*A*).

The lower suture loop is cut and the two ends are firmly knotted and left long. The needles are cut off and the upper sutures tied so that the freshened opposing lid margins come together snugly (fig. 43*B*).

Each of the upper sutures is now firmly tied to one of the lower sutures (fig. 43*C*). The purpose of this is to equalize the anterior and

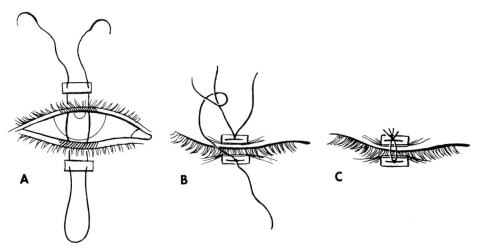

FIG. 43. Author's Tarsorrhaphy.
A. A double-armed suture is passed through a peg and through *full thickness* lower lid just below the ciliary margin from skin to conjunctiva. It is then passed similarly through the upper lid from within outward to emerge on the skin surface above the ciliary border and then through a peg. The needles are 4 mm. apart.
B. The lower loop is cut and the sutures tied. The needles are cut off and the upper sutures are tied so that the freshened areas of the lid margins come together. One of the upper sutures is being tied to one of the lower.
C. Final appearance.
(Fox, S. A.: Courtesy Archives of Ophthalmology.)

posterior tension of the sutures on the lid margins and thus prevent a buckling forward of the lid edges.

Comment. Since most tarsorrhaphy sutures are passed only through the skin-muscle lamina of the lid it is not surprising that they pull through when tissue vitality is low or when the tendency to lid separation is great. Pegs help but are no panacea since such sutures can pull through pegs and all. The above technic uses the full lid thickness which includes the tough tarsal plate and thus withstands tension much better. Also, mattress sutures spaced wide apart—4 mm. in this case—have a wider base and hence hold more firmly than when placed closer together.

The indications for this type of suture with or without tarsorrhaphy have already been mentioned. It is especially useful in lids which have been operated several times and as an accessory in advanced exophthalmos requiring lateral canthoplasty. In such cases not only does the forward position of the globe make closure difficult but upper lid retraction, often present, tends to push the bulb out so much that in rare instances the lid gets stuck *behind* the globe and is replaced only with difficulty. Here the wound edges of the lateral canthoplasty are in constant danger of pulling apart and a reinforcing accessory intermarginal suture, placed medial to the canthoplasty, may mean the difference between surgical success or failure.

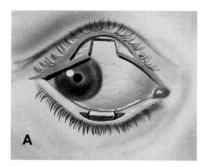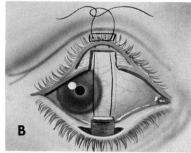

FIG. 44.   Tarsal Sliding Graft Tarsorrhaphy.
A.   The upper and lower lids are split opposite each other in the gray line. A
      tarsoconjunctival groove is fashioned in the upper lid to receive a tongue of
      tarsoconjunctiva from the lower lid.
B.   The tongue of tarsoconjunctiva is being drawn up to fill the groove in the
      upper lid. (The split in the upper lid is exaggerated here to show the
      groove.)

There remains one caveat: This procedure leaves sutures on the
conjunctival surface and these could be a source of corneal irritation.
However, since all the knots are on the skin side this is probably not
a serious danger. It can be completely obviated by placing the sutures
just medial or lateral to the cornea. When two sutures are used there is
no problem since their usual position is to each side of the cornea.

Tarsal Sliding Flap Tarsorrhaphy

Another tarsorrhaphy which provides firm union of the lids is one
in which a little sliding graft of tarsus is used in a tongue and groove
manner.

Procedure (fig. 44): The lids are pinched together and the margins
are marked off as in figure 41. Both lids are then split within the limits
marked off and vertical tarsoconjunctival incisions are made so as to
create tongues of tarsoconjunctiva opposite each other in both lids. A
5 to 6 mm. section is resected from the tarsoconjunctival tongue of the
upper lid to create a groove. The opposite slip of tarsoconjunctiva is
dissected up and freely mobilized by further conjunctival incision and
dissection so that there is no pull on the lower lid (fig. 44A). A 4–0 silk
double-armed suture is passed through the edge of the tarsal slip from
without inward. The sutures are then passed through the upper edge of
the upper lid groove from within outward to come out on the skin surface
(fig. 44B). The tarsal slip from the lower lid is pulled into the upper lid
groove and the suture tied over a peg. A firm dressing is applied to hold
the tarsal tongue in position during healing.

Comment: This procedure works equally well when the tongue and
groove are transposed, i.e., when the tongue is fashioned in the upper

lid and pulled into a lower lid groove. Like the procedure shown in figure 43 it is especially useful in cases where the simpler tarsorrhaphies have failed. After being released it also heals just as well as the simpler tarsorrhaphies. However, it requires more surgery and tissue from an opposing lid—hence its indications will probably not be as frequent as the author's through and through tarsorrhaphy. Also it is of a more permanent character and may be left in place for a much longer time than the preceding tarsorrhaphies.

Opening of Temporary Tarsorrhaphy

When ready to be released, 0.5 per cent tetracaime is instilled into the conjunctival sac and several drops of 1 per cent lidocaine are injected into each area of union which is then snipped across cleanly with a small straight scissors. Irregularities and excess tissue are trimmed off. The conjunctival sac is fitted with a bland sterile ointment and the eye lightly patched. Dressings are changed daily and copious ointment instilled. Any tendency to readhesion should be discouraged by separating the lids with a spatula. The raw surfaces are re-epithelialized rather quickly and are usually completely healed on the second or third day. Little scarring results with any of the above methods.

TEMPORARY INTERMARGINAL SUTURES

All the tarsorrhaphies above are termed temporary because they are all destined to be undone after they have served their purpose. Usually this is in 6, 8, or 10 weeks. In the case of corneal pathology it may be several months or a good deal longer. However, there are cases when closure of the lids is required for a few days only as after the removal of an orbital tumor, when pressure bandages are used to protect the cornea for a few days and for many other reasons. In such cases surgical union of the lids is not needed and only the sutures described above, i.e., without denudation of marginal epithelium, are used. Such sutures can stay in anywhere from 10 to 20 days before reaction or infection sets in. Then they must be removed. However, by then they will have served their purpose.

When corneal protection is needed for a few days only, the simplest of all is the modified Frost suture. This is a double-armed suture passed through a rubber peg, then centrally through the skin-muscle layer of the lower lid just below the ciliary margin to emerge in the gray line (fig. 45A). The lower lid is pulled up over the cornea by means of the suture which is then taped to the forehead (fig. 45B). In the rare cases where the upper lid has to be pulled down (as in ptosis overcorrection) the suture is reversed and taped to the cheek.

The above is a simple modification of the Frost suture. As originally

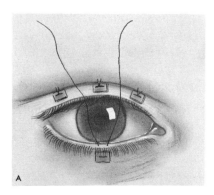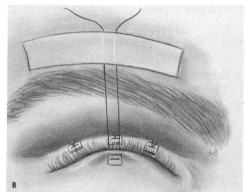

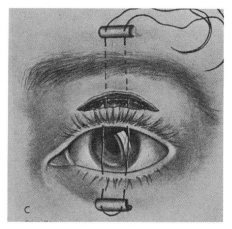

FIG. 45. Temporary Intermarginal Sutures.
A. Modified Frost suture in lower lid after ptosis surgery.
B. The lid is pulled up and over the cornea.
C. Original Frost suture.
    (Frost, A. S.: Courtesy American Journal of Ophthalmology.)

described it was passed through the margins of both lids then subcutaneously to emerge above the brow where it was tied over a peg
(fig. 45C).

Recently a plastic glue (Eastman 90 Monomer) has been suggested
for use as a temporary tarsorrhaphy. It is used by pulling the upper lid
down and gluing the lashes to the lower lid. In entropion the glue may be
used to evert the lid and glue the lower lid lashes to the cheek. Collodion
serves a similar purpose. Nice long lashes help.

LID SPLITTING

Lid splitting used to be not only the most common but also the most
peculiarly ophthalmologic of all the basic technics of lid surgery. There
was hardly a procedure involving the lid margin from the least minor

triangular excision to the most involved total lid reconstruction, in which it was not used. Lid structure being what it is, how could it be otherwise? Few places in the body provide such a tempting cleavage plane between two sets of tissues capable of such complete separation and subsequent union with so little resulting disfigurement or damage.

Lid splitting is centuries old. It was probably first used on the upper lid in an attempt to avoid the ravages of trachomatous cicatricial entropion and has been variously attributed to Antyllus in the second century A.D., Aetius of Amida in the sixth century A.D. and Paulus of Aegina in the seventh century A.D. Undoubtedly it had been used for hundreds of years previously. The modern literature credits Kuhnt with being the first to split the lower lid in his procedure for the correction of senile ectropion but as the elder Fuchs points out ". . . This is nothing but a modification of the old method of Antyllus."

The incision is made in the gray line (fig. 46A) with a knife (fig. 46B) and then carried to any desired depth by careful dissection with a scissors. Extreme care must be used not to injure the roots of the cilia. However, even with the utmost care, cilia may be lost. Usually this is of no great importance, especially in major repairs and in older individuals. But in dealing with the lids of young people, especially female, loss of a few lashes may be magnified into a tragedy despite an otherwise excellent result. Hence lid splitting has its serious drawbacks. For such cases alternative methods of lid splitting are given.

Figure 46C shows a method in which the incision starts not in the gray line but at the posterior edge of the lid margin. The point of the knife is angulated forward away from the posterior edge toward the skin-muscle layer so that it emerges between skin-muscle and tarsoconjunctiva at least 3 mm. beyond the margin and thus avoids the roots of the cilia. From here the dissection with blunt-pointed scissors proceeds between the two laminae. A thin rim of tarsus is thus left attached to the skin-muscle layer.

A third method of lid splitting is illustrated in figure 46D. The lid is everted and an incision of the required length is made directly through tarsoconjunctiva at least 3 mm. away from and parallel with the lid edge. Two vertical incisions are then made at each end of the horizontal incision and the tarsal tongue thus created is dissected up and separated from the skin-muscle layer. This may be done along the whole length of the lid or along any part of it. The disadvantage of this method is that when the lids are separated the excess tarsus has to be dissected up again and allowed to retract and sutured back to its position unless one wants to sacrifice all this tarsus. (It is a bit more work but is worth doing to conserve valuable tarsal tissue.) The method shown in figure 46D is cleaner and even less hazardous to cilia but will furnish 3 mm. or so less tarsus than the method illustrated in figure 46C.

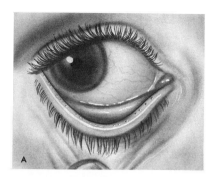
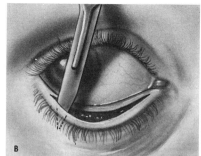
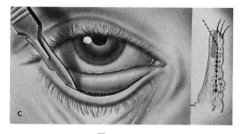
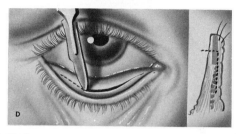

FIG. 46. Method of Lid Splitting.
A. The gray line.
B. Splitting in gray line.
C. Angulated split through the posterior lid edge.
D. Separation of laminae beyond the margin and hair follicles.

LID HALVING

The "halving" principle, based directly on the easy separability of the lids into laminae, has also been an important fundamental in surgery of the lids. Lid halving is a term coined by Wheeler in 1919 when he published his first report on the lid surgery he had done in the First World War. "An important point," he stated, "is that tarsal incisions and skin incisions should never be in the same position, but should be made in such a way that there is overlapping. Thus, what is known in carpentry as halving is accomplished and union is assured. . . . Furthermore, recurrence of the notch formation is prevented."

Reduced to simplest terms, halving means that the lid is split so as to halve the suture line. Hence when the split lid is united in the process of repair, the place of union of the skin-muscle layer does not correspond with that of the tarsoconjunctival layer. This has advantages: (1) The resultant wound is stronger because two thinner layers are under tension rather than one thick layer. (2) Healing is not only by edge to edge contact but also between two laminal surfaces. (3) Most important, scarring and hence notching is less likely, due to the division of the wound edges into two unions of lesser area.

Despite all these manifest advantages halving has fallen on evil days and is being used less and less in lid repairs. There are a number of

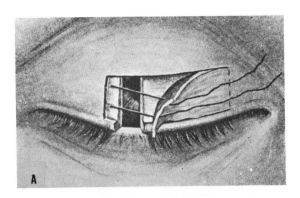

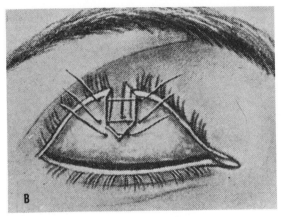

FIG. 47. Direct Half-Halving Technic (Wheeler).
A. Rectangular debridement of notch, resection of skin rectangle only on one
side and preparation for closure by drawing skin flap over from the other
side. Note that lid margin is not split.
B. Separate closure of tarsoconjunctiva on conjunctival surface.
(Wheeler, J. M.: Courtesy Columbia University Press. Original illustration.)

reasons for this. The most important, perhaps, is that we have learned
that full thickness closure of a lid laceration can be made without notching if properly done (fig. 51). (This was the major reason for the halving
closure originally.) Another reason is that to attain halving, healthy
tissue must be wasted whether direct or indirect halving is used (figs.
47, 48, 49 and 50). This is not always available. A third reason is that
halving, which is simply a method of closure, began to be used in the
larger repair technics requiring much lid splitting and thus encouraged
cilia loss. For all these reasons halving has been all but replaced by direct
suture of lid wounds.

However, it still has its occasional uses and is of great value in
special areas such as around the punctum. Halving is of various kinds:

    a. Direct half halving (fig. 47)
    b. Direct full halving (fig. 48)
    c. Modified halving (fig. 49)
    d. Indirect halving (fig. 50)

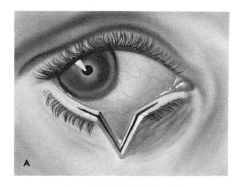 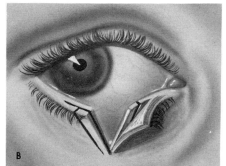
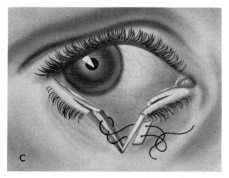 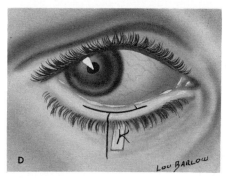

FIG. 48. Direct Full Halving Technic (Wheeler).
A. Tumor is resected or notch debrided. The lid on either side is split.
B. Amount of skin-muscle to be resected from one side and tarsoconjunctiva from the other is indicated.
C. Vertical double-armed suture is placed after resection.
D. Appearance on completion of the repair. Note amount of lid splitting necessary sometimes to draw wound lips together.

Direct Half Halving

This is described in Wheeler's own illustration of his technic (fig. 47). Here it is clearly shown that after the coloboma is debrided it is prepared for closure by resecting only skin-muscle from one side of the wound without further tarsal resection. The tarsal coloboma is then closed and the skin-muscle is drawn over to be sutured beyond the tarsal suture line thus making a halving closure.

Direct Full Halving

This type of halving, also described by Wheeler, has been commonly used for many years and is now also gradually being abandoned for reasons stated above although still used by some.

Procedure (fig. 48): After resecting a marginal lid lesion or debriding a lid notch the lid on either side of the wound is split (fig. 48A). A small triangular segment of skin-muscle is resected on one side and a similar segment of tarsoconjunctiva is resected on the other side (fig. 48B). A double-armed suture is passed vertically from within outward first through the bared tarsoconjunctiva then through the skin-muscle to emerge on the skin surface (fig. 48C). The suture is drawn up snugly and tied over a peg (fig. 48D). Skin and conjunctival sutures are added if necessary to assure good closure. A marginal suture may also be added to assure good approximation. The same technic may be used for rectangular wounds of the lid.

Modified or Indirect Halving

This is an uncommon type of halving usually used in vertical double advancement flaps in which either the skin-muscle or tarsoconjunctival lamina are cut narrower so as to separate suture lines (fig. 49A). Another type of modified halving is also seen in the partial halving type of closure shown in figure 81.

Modified or indirect halving is also used when the portion of lamina resected does not involve the primary wound. This technic is of inestimable value in certain areas, especially around the punctum. Such a repair is seen in figure 50 A. Here resection of healthy tarsus, although not involved in the wound, brings the edges of the primary skin-muscle wound at the punctum closer together when the tarsus is closed. It makes for easier closure and less punctal jeopardy. This is also valuable in the case of double ciliary margin wounds (fig. 50B) where uninvolved tarsus is resected to bring the two resection wounds closer together.

REPARATIVE INTERMARGINAL (FIGURE-8) SUTURES

In 1942 Minsky reported his intermarginal or—as it is now called—figure-8 suture for the repair of lid lacerations. This has been rediscovered and has recently become so popular that it is now being used

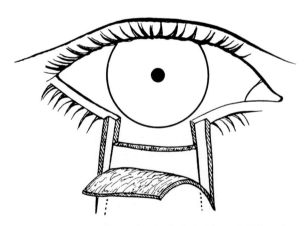

FIG. 49. Modified Halving. Two vertical flaps are fashioned, one wider than the other, to make a halving closure.

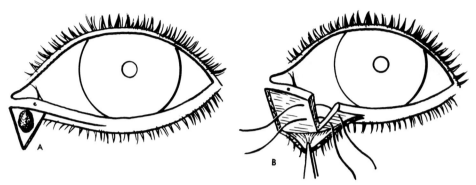

FIG. 50. Indirect Halving.
A. Ciliary lesion in punctal area.
B. After resection the lid is split and healthy tarsoconjunctiva is resected to facilitate closure.

for all types of lid notches and even for lesions not involving the whole lid margin (fig. 84). This type of closure is excellent in cases of lid lacerations or lid notches in which the wound margins can be brought together without tension. The following are modifications of Minsky's intermarginal splinting or figure-8 suture.

Figure-8 Splinting Suture (Modified) for One Lid Notch

The Minsky suture is best used for lesions which are perpendicular to the lid margin or reasonably so. It has been modified here by the author from Minsky's original reported technic.

Procedure (fig. 51A): After suitable infiltration anesthesia one needle of a double-armed 4–0 silk suture is entered in the gray line 3 mm. from one side of the lid break to emerge in the wound 4 or 5 mm. below the lid margin. The needle is entered in the opposite lip of the wound, again 4 or 5 mm. below the margin, to emerge in the gray line 3 mm. from the edge of the laceration. The arms of the two sutures are crossed without tying to check on the alignment of the wound lips to make sure that there is no vertical or horizontal displacement. The suture is then tied with a double knot but the needles are not cut off. The lid is pulled forward by means of this suture and the conjunctiva sutured with 5–0 or 6–0 chromic catgut interrupted sutures as necessary. In similar manner the skin wound is sutured with 5–0 interrupted silk sutures. The two needles of the marginal suture are now passed through the gray line of the *opposing* lid to emerge in the skin above the ciliary margin where they are tied over a peg. Healing is usually uneventful and the skin sutures are removed on the sixth or seventh day. The marginal sutures in the tarsus are left in for 9 or 10 days.

This suture works equally well for upper or lower lid lacerations.

Comment: The procedure may be varied by inserting tarsocon-

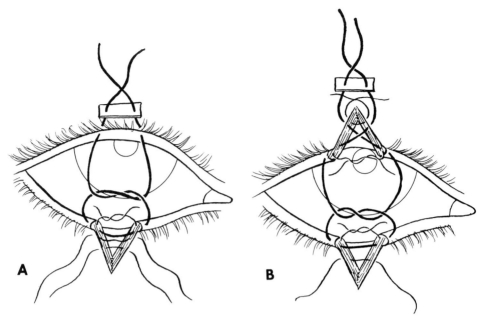

FIG. 51. Minsky's Figure-8 Sutures. Intermarginal (Figure-8) Splinting Suture (modified).
A. A double-armed suture at the border closes the notch and is tied. Accessory sutures close the skin-muscle and tarsoconjunctival layers. The suture is passed through the opposing lid for support.
B. Similar technic is used to close opposing notches of the upper and lower lids with one suture.

junctival sutures from in front before the intermarginal suture is tied. This places the knots on the tarsus and may avoid corneal abrasion if the lid break is near the cornea. Also the lid is sometimes shortened and edematous and not easy to evert to permit insertion of the conjunctival sutures; placing them from in front in such cases is easier. After the tarsoconjunctiva is sutured one then proceeds to complete the intermarginal suture and to insert the skin sutures.

This versatile suture is not only useful in the lesser lesions involving the ciliary (fig. 84) and full lid margin (figs. 87 and 88) but also in the larger lid dehiscences where it may be employed in conjunction with a canthotomy and cantholysis (figs. 97) and an advancement flap (fig. 98).

Figure-8 Splinting Suture (Modified) for Opposing Lid Notches

This is the suture that Minsky originally called his figure-8 suture and not the one just described above. However, both are now loosely called figure-8 sutures.

This suture is used when there are lacerations in both upper and lower lids which are opposite each other and which can therefore be repaired with one suture (fig. 91). This is not common.

Procedure (fig. 51B): The lower lid is repaired exactly as described above (fig. 51A) thus forming the lower loop of the figure-8.

With this repair completed the suture is continued upward and the identical procedure is repeated in the upper lid laceration. Here again the conjunctival sutures may be inserted from in front and tied on the tarsal surface. After forming the upper loop of the figure-8 in the upper lid each needle is continued into the opposite edge of the wound about 2 mm. higher to emerge on the skin surface where the sutures are tied over a peg. The tarsoconjunctiva is then closed with 6–0 chromic sutures and the skin with 5–0 silk sutures as necessary. A patch is applied and changed daily. All skin sutures are removed on the fifth or sixth day. The intermarginal suture is removed on the ninth or tenth day unless it loosens sooner.

Comment: The main virtue of the figure-8 suture is that it allows for full thickness lid closure without notching. This is enhanced by splinting the involved lid to the opposite lid. This does not mean that notching will always occur if splinting is not done. But the additional effort and time expended is small and if notching is prevented in only five or ten per cent of the cases, it is well worthwhile.

There are many ingenious modifications of the original figure-8 suture (see figs. 90*A* and *B*). However, since its primary function is to prevent notching, it must be free to pucker up the wound lips at the lid margin. Secondary loops of the same suture placed lower in the wound or mattressed at the sides prevents this puckering. Hence, I can see no special virtue in trying to do most of the repair with one suture and feel that the result on the average is better with a single loop suture at the margin and a layer to layer closure as shown above.

CANTHOTOMY

Canthotomy is a simple horizontal section at the lateral canthus through the raphé including the palpebral ligament. Its use goes back to ancient times and it is frequently employed in ophthalmic surgery as a temporary measure and almost always at the lateral canthus.

The indications for lateral canthotomy are:

1. As a preliminary step to permanent canthoplasty or permanent lateral tarsorrhaphy.

2. To facilitate exposure of the socket and orbit in plastic repairs and reconstructions.

3. Widening of the palpebral fissure to facilitate enucleation, exenteration, cataract extraction, etc.

4. To relieve pressure on the globe in lid edema, blepharospasm, chemosis, etc.

Procedure (fig. 52):   The lids are pulled well apart and somewhat nasally at the lateral canthus in order to put the canthal ligament on stretch. One blade of a stout blunt-pointed scissors is inserted under the canthus into the conjunctival sac and advanced until it strikes the lateral

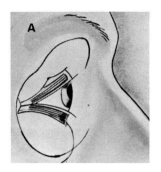 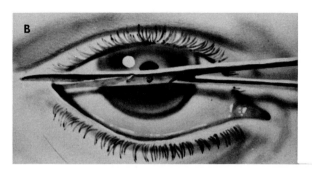

Fig. 52. Canthotomy of the Lateral Canthal Ligament.
A. Diagrammatic representation of the ligament.
B. The canthal incision.

orbital rim. The scissors should be pointed horizontally in line with the
closed palpebral fissure and slightly backward, as the ligament is inserted
about 3 mm. posterior to the lateral orbital rim (fig. 52A). If this is not
done, the ligament will be pushed temporally by the point of the scissors
and not sectioned completely. One firm snip of the scissors should be
sufficient to divide the ligament into upper and lower arms (fig. 52B).
The structures cut are skin, raphé of the orbicularis, orbital septum,
levator attachment, canthal ligament, orbital fat and conjunctiva.

Comment: If the incision is wholly in the fibrous raphé, bleeding
may be minimal. If some of the orbicularis fibers are caught in the
wound, the bleeding is severe but soon stops spontaneously and sutures
are usually not necessary. Some like to crush the tissues with a clamp
before incision in order to minimize bleeding but I prefer not to insult
healthy tissues by using this unphysiologic and barbarous maneuver. The
fissure is lengthened and widened in this way, but this is a temporary
enlargement and if left alone, healing is complete in a few days with the
original canthal angle restored.

CANTHOLYSIS

Cantholysis at the lateral canthal angle is an important fundamental
in ophthalmic plastic repairs and reconstructions. Its object is to relax
the lid and mobilize it so that it may be drawn medially more easily. As
will be seen in the following chapters it is a useful technic and frequently
used.

Cantholysis was first used by Von Ammon for entropion in 1839,
rediscovered by Agnew in 1875, again by Pochisov in 1935 and by many
others since. It is of no permanent value in entropion but it is important
in mobilizing either the upper or the lower lid or both in plastic repairs.

Procedure (fig. 53):   After doing a canthotomy as described above,
the lips of the wound are separated again and the arms of the incised

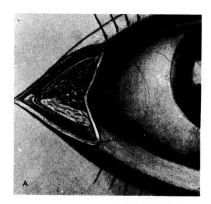
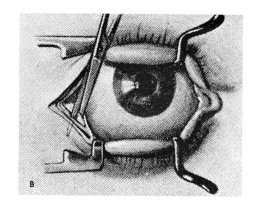

Fig. 53. Cantholysis.
A. Upper and lower arms of canthal ligament after canthotomy.
B. Section of lower arm.

ligament put on stretch nasally (fig. 53A). One blade of a slender
scissors is inserted behind the skin and muscle and in front of the
conjunctiva and the upper or lower arm of the severed ligament is cut
across (fig. 53B). The lid can be felt to slacken thus showing that the
arm of the ligament has been severed. If there is no slackening the
maneuver must be repeated.

Comment: This is a most valuable technic in all sliding graft
repairs of the lids. With it lids can be mobilized and long incisions extending toward the ear may be avoided. About 5 or 6 mm. of mobilization is
gained in this way.

Use of Lid Skin for Lid Repairs

This subject has been fully discussed in Chapter 3. Suffice it to say
here that this is as important a fundamental as any. In lid repairs the
ophthalmic surgeon should give no thought to the use of skin from anywhere else until he has assured himself that no skin from other lids is
available.

Plasties

No discussion of the fundamentals of lid surgery is complete without
mention of the minor plasties commonly used. Of these the Z plasty is the
most common and the most useful. Its origin is lost in obscurity but its
inventor or inventors showed high ingenuity.

The Z Plasty

The specific advantage of the Z plasty (fig. 54) is its ability to
reduce pull in one direction at the expense of a line perpendicular to it.

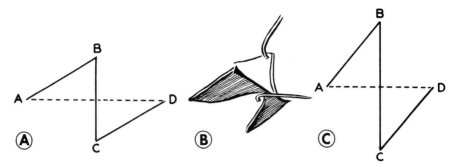

FIG. 54.   The Z Plasty.

A. Construction of the flaps.   C. Result of the transposition.
B. Transposition of the flaps.

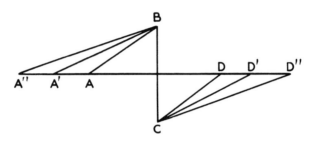

FIG.   55.   Diagrammatic relation of the size of the angle to the relaxation obtained.

Thus if there is tension due to tissue contraction along the vertical line BC and it is desired to reduce it, the Z figure is constructed as seen in figure 54A. This consists of two triangles ABC and BCD based on line BC. It will be noted that the distance AD is longer than BC. After the flaps ABC and BCD have been dissected up and transposed, the figure assumes the form seen in figure 54C. Triangle ABC becomes ADC and BCD becomes BAD.

Thus BC is now longer than AD and the amount of relaxation along line BC is the difference in length between BC and AD in the original figure. The angles ABC and BCD should not be greater than 50 degrees or it will be difficult to transpose the flaps unless the skin is unusually thin and extensible. The angles need not be equal to each other. Sometimes the situation is one requiring one angle smaller than the other. The disparity in size may be as much as 20 degrees but not much more.

It is obvious from figure 55 that the larger the angles ABC and BCD the greater the difference between BC and AD and the more relaxation there will be along line BC. The size of the transposed angles will depend on the amount of relaxation needed and the character of the tissues the surgeon has to deal with.

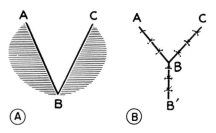

FIG. 56. Wharton Jones V-Y Plasty.
A. Incision.   B. Closure.

The V-Y Plasty (of Wharton Jones)

The V-Y plasty of Thomas Wharton Jones, a physiologist turned ophthalmologist, is another valuable minor plasty in lid surgery (fig. 56). First reported in 1847 for cicatricial ectropion of the upper lid it has found its greatest field of usefulness in minor cicatricial ectropion of the lower lid (fig. 183). It will not work in the extreme cases of ectropion.

The V-Y plasty can also be used to relieve tension but its usefulness has less application here and is restricted to the lesser conditions in which scar tissue pull is relatively minor. It is also of value in conjunctival scarring to relieve adhesions. After the incision ABC is made (fig. 56A) the flap and surrounding skin are thoroughly undermined. The flap is allowed to retract to its new position and the wound is closed as shown in figure 56B, converting the V to a Y.

Inspection will show that the more acute (and longer) the V figure is the more effective the relaxation within the limits of the incision and the better the result. Contrarily, the more obtuse the V the less effective the relaxation. Hence this type of repair is best limited to long narrow scars.

Dieffenbach's Winged-V

In 1845 Dieffenbach, "the father of plastic surgery" and the innovator of extraocular muscle surgery, though not an ophthalmologist, suggested the resection of a skin triangle with upper horizontal incision for the repair of cicatricial ectropion (fig. 57). This "winged-V" incision is useless in such cases because it reduces the skin layer still more vis-a-vis the tarsoconjunctival layer; indeed, the loss of more skin aggravates the condition. Dieffenbach also suggested, more usefully, that his winged-V technic be used in repairs where small areas of tissue, as in the case of small tumors, have to be resected. Figure 57A illustrates the incision and figure 57B the closure in such cases.

One of the curious paradoxes found in the literature is that practically the identical procedure was suggested by von Graefe in 1864 for

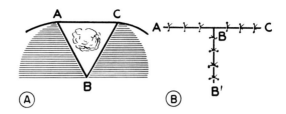

FIG. 57.   Dieffenbach's Winged-V Plasty.
A.   Incision and resection.   B.   Closure.

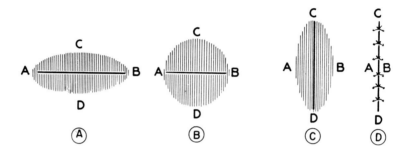

FIG. 58.   Diagrammatic illustration of change of direction of skin pull.
A.   Horizontal excision.
B. and C.   Undermining and conversion of horizontal to vertical wound.
D.   Vertical closure.

cicatricial *entropion* and this is one of its best and most logical indications, i.e., to increase skin-muscle pull to equal that of the cicatrized tarsoconjunctiva (see fig. 201, Chapter 16).

Simple Relief of Tension Lines

The simplest of all technics for relief of skin tensions, where the area involved is small, is the conversion of an incision into a suture line closure which is perpendicular to the original incision (fig. 58). Thus, if there is some tension in the direction of CD, the incision AB is made and the whole area undermined. Closure is made in the direction of CD. This works only in minor injuries where loss of tissue and scarring has been minimal and where the skin is sufficiently lax to permit such a maneuver.

Temporal Advancement Flap—Burow's Triangle

One of the most common of the basic technics is the temporal advancement flap (fig. 59A). It is extremely useful in the handling of repairs involving the temporal half of the lid. Here advantage is taken of the favorable position of the lesion which permits drawing of tissue from the wide open spaces of the temporal region to fill in a lid dehis-

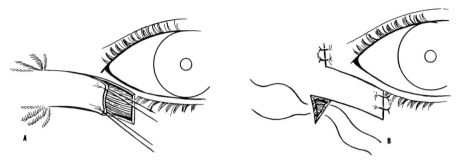

FIG. 59. Temporal Advancement Flap—Burow's Triangle.
A. Advancement flap with wrinkles forming above and below as result of skin pull.
B. Technic of closure with resection of Burow's triangles to counteract skin wrinkles.

cence. This type of repair is seen at its simplest in figure 79, then in increasing complexity in figures 95, 100 and 103.

Burow's triangle (fig. 59B) is a frequent concomitant of the advancement flap.

In 1838 Burow reported his technic for smoothing out skin wrinkles by resection of a little skin triangle. Ophthalmologists have found this constantly useful since. It is of special value in advancement and rotated pedicles where wrinkles are likely to form in the adjacent tissues due to the pull of the pedicle. Thus when a skin pedicle is formed and advanced to cover a bared area, the fixed skin on each side of the pedicle is frequently thrown into wrinkles (fig. 59A). If left alone, these wrinkles may gradually smooth themselves out. However, they are easily resected at the time of operation and thus nothing is left to chance. Resection is always done triangularly with the apex of the triangle pointing *away* from the pedicle flap and the base of the triangle on the pedicle (fig. 59B). When the bared area is closed it leaves a small vertical line perpendicular to the pedicle which heals easily and leaves little or no scar.

Flat-X Plasty

Lid lesions are best resected in spindle-shaped fashion parallel with the lid margin so that the healing scar follows the course of the normal lid wrinkles and does not run across cut muscle fibers. When the lesion is irregular, rectangular or round in shape, a good deal of normal tissue may have to be sacrificed to attain this shape. To obviate this, the following flat-X plasty has been found very helpful:

After resection of the lesion the upper and lower wound lips are extended upward and downward to form two pedicles (fig. 60A). The pedicles are undermined, the points are clipped off and united (fig. 60B). The edges of the resultant two lesions are undermined, drawn together and sutured (fig. 60C). This results in a horizontal X-like figure, hence the flat-X name.

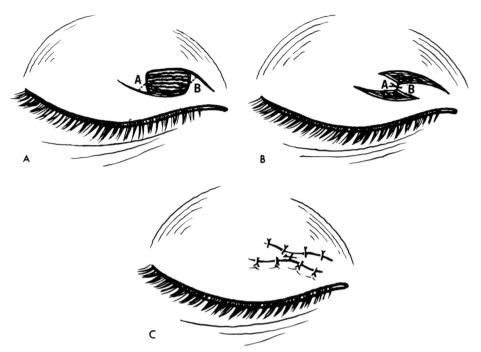

FIG. 60. Flat-X Plasty.
A. After excision of the lesion the upper and lower wound lips are extended downward and upward.
B. The resultant flaps are undermined, the tips are resected and the ends united.
C. The resultant wound lips are undermined and the wounds closed with interrupted sutures. (The closed wound has assumed the shape of an horizontal X, hence the name.)
(Fox, S. A.: Courtesy Archives of Ophthamology.)

Collar-Button Closure

Lid skin neoplasms usually start below the margin then gradually, after considerable time, creep over the margin to the conjunctival surface. Hence, by the nature of things, marginal and conjunctival involvement is usually much less than skin involvement. It has been customary in these cases to do a full thickness lid resection of the whole lesion. This is a waste, since the pathologist's report almost invariably shows no tarsal involvement. One would think that the meibomian gland openings offer ready access to tarsal invasion by marginal neoplasms, but this is not the case as repeated pathologic studies have shown. In the vast majority of cases the surface layers alone are involved and it is only the old, long-neglected cases that show infiltration into the deeper tissues.

Since the amount of tarsoconjunctival involvement is always much less than the skin-muscle (fig. 61A) the resected portion is shaped somewhat like an old fashioned collarbutton (fig. 61B inset) ; hence the name. It need not be emphasized that this technic should not be used in those

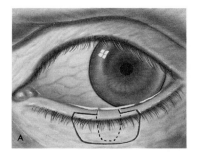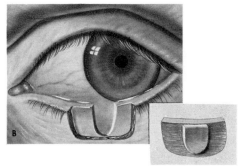

FIG. 61. Diagram of the Collar-Button Resection Technic.

A. Lines of incision around the lesion. Dotted lines enclose tarsoconjunctival portion of lesion.

B. Diagram of dehiscence left when the collar-button shaped section inset is removed.

(Fox, S. A.: Courtesy Archives of Ophthalmology.)

lesions which show an obviously deep infiltration. Also, it is important to make sure that there has been complete excision of the neoplasm. But this is not difficult if sufficient healthy tissue is taken all around as described. Furthermore, this may be ascertainable by frozen section. The application of this technic is shown in figures 99 and 135.

SPONTANEOUS REPAIR

Where large dissections have to be done either for cicatricial contraction or malignancy and where bleeding is difficult to control, it may be wise not to attempt immediate repair. It is not hard to have a long and difficult reconstruction with skin graft completely destroyed by uncontrollable hemorrhage. Discretion, therefore, may dictate secondary repair in such cases.

Areas especially beset by copious bleeding are the nasocanthal angle in which neoplasms have involved the medial ends of the lids and have penetrated deeply into the sac area. I have found that here, if permitted, nature will do a lot of the restorative work with only a minimum of help from the surgeon.

After the lesion is resected the cut ends of the conjunctiva are sutured together to form a new medial cul-de-sac (fig. 62A). One needle of a double-armed 3–0 silk suture is passed through each cut marginal edge of the upper and lower lids. The lids are drawn over medially and the suture fastened to a remaining remnant of nasal periosteum thus putting the lids on stretch (fig. 62B). The suture should be fastened to the periosteum as low down as possible since it is taking the place of the medial canthal ligament. If no periosteum is available

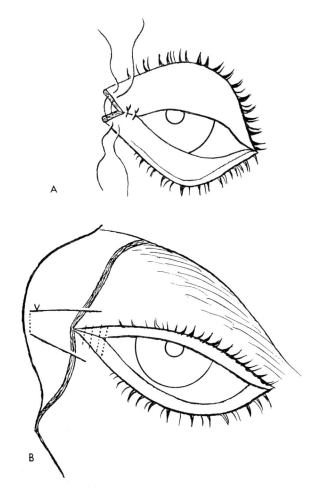

FIG. 62.   Repair by Spontaneous Granulation.
A. After the lesion is resected a new medial fornix is made by suturing the edges of the cut medial conjunctiva.
B. The lids are drawn over medially and sutured to prevent retraction (see also figure 133).

then holes must be drilled in the bone. Due to the loss of tissue the lids cannot be drawn all the way over but they are prevented from retracting. Application of this technic is shown in figures 118 and 133.

REFERENCES

AMDUR, J.: Intermarginal eyelid suture. Arch. Ophth. *69*:556, 1963.
AMERICAN ENCYCLOPEDIA OF OPHTHALMOLOGY: Chicago, Cleveland Press, 1915, vol. 6, p. 4347.
IBID.: Chicago, Cleveland Press, 1916, vol. 9, p. 6703.
AGNEW, C. R.: Canthoplasty as a Remedy in Certain Diseases of the Eye. New York, Putnam Sons, 1875, pp. 1–10.
VON AMMON, F. A.: American Encyclopedia of Ophthalmology. Chicago, Cleveland Press, 1913, vol. 2, p. 1046.

ARLT, C. F. R.: Transplantation des Cilienbodens. Handb. d. Gesam. Augenh. *3*:447, 1874.

————: Inner tarsorrhaphie. Op. cit. *3*:446, 1874.

BEARD, C. H.: Ophthalmic Surgery. Philadelphia, P. Blakiston's Son & Co., ed. 2, 1914.

BOWMAN, W. P.: Collected Papers. London, Harrison & Sons, vol. 2, 1892, pp. 383–386.

BUROW, A.: Zur Blepharoplastik Monatschr. Med. Augenh, & Chir. *1*:57, 1838.

DIEFFENBACH, J. F.: Die Operative Chirurgie. Leipzig, F. A. Brockhaus, 1845. vol. 1, p. 460, 468.

DUVERGER, C., and VELTER, E.: Therapeutique Chirurgicale Ophthalmologique. Paris, Masson et Cie., 1926.

FOX, S. A.: Basic techniques of lid surgery: their origins and their apocrypha. Arch. Ophth. *50*:384, 1960.

————: The flat-X plasty. Arch. Ophth. *72*:204, 1965.

————: Lid halving with variations. Arch. Ophth. *65*:672, 1961.

————: A new tarsorrhaphy suture. Arch. Ophth. *66*:833, 1961.

————: Collar-button resection. Jap. J. Ophth. *42*:410, 1964.

FOX, S. A., and BEARD, C.: Spontaneous lid repair. Am. J. Ophth. *58*:947, 1964.

FROST, A. D.: Supportive suture in ptosis operation. Am. J. Ophth. *17*:1633, 1934.

FUCHS, E.: Text-Book of Ophthalmology. New York, Appleton & Co. 1905, ed. 2, p. 798.

HELMBOLD: Zur Operation gegen Ektropium des unteren Lides. Klin. Monatsb. Augenh. *35*:283, 1897.

JONES, T. W.: A Manual of the Principles and Practice of Ophthalmic Medicine and Surgery. London, J. J. Churchill, 1847, pp. 418–421.

KUHNT, H.: Beitrage zur Operationen Augenheilkunde. Jena, G. Fischer, 1883, pp. 45–55.

LISFRANC, J.: American Encyclopedia of Ophthalmology. Chicago, Cleveland Press, 1913, vol. 2, p. 1052.

MINSKY, H.: Surgical repair of recent lid lacerations. Intermarginal splinting suture. Surg. Gyn. & Obstr. *75*:449, 1942.

MIRAULT, G.: Nouvelle méthode pour la cure de l'ectropion consecutif a la brulére. Ann. d'ocul. *25*:121, 1851.

PANAS, L.: Maladie des Yeux. Paris, G. Masson, 1894. vol. 2, p. 137.

POCHISOV, H.: Operation for spastic entropion. Sovet. Vestnik. *6*:131, 1935.

ROBERTSON, D. M.C.L.A.: The operation of central blepharorrhaphy. Trans-Ophth. Soc. U. K., *4*:423, 1886.

SCHIMEK, R. A. and BALLOU, S: Eastman 90 for plastic lid procedures. Am. J. Ophth. *62*:953, 1966.

SMITH, B.: Plastic surgery in ophthalmology. W. Virginia Med. J. *46*:1, 1950.

WALDAUER, J.: Zur Operation der Trichiasis des oberen Lides. Klin. Monatsbl. Augenh. *36*:47, 1897.

WALTHER, P.: Ectropium anguli oculi externi, eine neue Augenkrankheit, und die Tarsoraphie, eine Augenoperation J. d. Clin. u. Augenh. *9*:86, 1826.

WEEKS, W. W.: Surgery of the Eye. New York, privately published, 1937, p. 9.

WHEELER, J. M.: War injuries of the eyelids. Plastic operations for a few types: Case reports with photographs and drawings. Trans. Am. Ophth. Soc. *17*:263, 1919.

————: Halving wounds in facial plastic surgery. Proc. 2nd Cong. Pan-Pac. Surg. Assoc., 1936.

————: Collected Papers. New York, Columbia Presbyterian Med. Cen., 1919, p. 338.

CHAPTER 5

Extramarginal Lesions

CHALAZION

A CHALAZION is a chronic inflammatory granuloma of a meibomian gland caused by the retention of secretion. It usually occurs singly but may be multiple. It tends to increase in size slowly, but after attaining a certain size it may remain completely stationary. This affection is usually painless unless secondary infection intervenes in which case incision and drainage is required much as in other purulent conditions. Thus the most common chalazion encountered is the chronic painless type. Though painless, it constitutes a cosmetic blemish which usually requires removal.

Lid incision for chalazion is the most common surgical procedure in ophthalmology. Despite its frequency, however, there is lack of agreement as to the choice of technic. Opinions vary all the way from the simple "cut and squeeze" school (without anesthesia) to the more elaborate complete extirpation of the entire lesion. Since not all are identically situated the procedure should be adapted to the particular chalazion in hand. The technics described below are the simplest and, in the author's experience, have given the least recurrences.

Cutaneous Route

Most chalazia can be palpated as hard round nodules beneath the skin surface. These are best approached by the cutaneous route which has the additional advantages of being simplest for the surgeon and least troublesome to the patient since the lid does not have to be everted except for the injection of anesthesia.

104

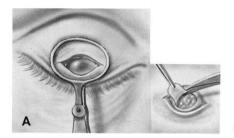
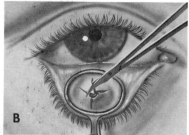
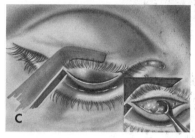

FIG. 63.   Incisions for Chalazion.
A.   Skin route.
B.   Conjunctival route.
C.   Marginal incision and
     curettage.

Procedure (fig. 63A):   After one or two drops of 0.5 per cent proparacaine instillation the lid is everted and a few drops of 1 per cent
lidocaine or procaine are injected along the attached border of the tarsus
opposite the lesion. The needle is then turned and passed toward the lid
margin between orbicularis and tarsus, infiltration of the whole area
to the margin being continued. The lid is turned back and massaged
gently. The chalazion clamp is placed in position and tightened to control
bleeding.

A horizontal incision is made over the chalazion through skin and
muscle. The chalazion is exposed by blunt dissection and the whole
upper half or roof is resected. In the process the contents of the chalazion
are also removed. The remaining half of the cyst wall is curetted and then
cauterized, if desired, with tincture of iodine or phenol. The clamp is
removed and bleeding controlled by pressure. When hemostasis is attained
one or two 5–0 or 6–0 silk skin sutures are used to close the wound. A
firm patch is applied. This may be removed in 24 to 48 hours, the wound
left open or painted with collodion. Sutures are removed on the fifth or
sixth day.

Comment: Incisions heal so well that they become practically
invisible in one or two weeks. There need be no hesitancy to use this
technic or any patient of either sex for fear of leaving scars. Since the
chalazion is simply an enlarged tarsal gland whose walls are part of the
tarsus it is rarely possible to "shell out" the chalazion as described in
some textbooks. Attempts to do so will only result in perforation through

the conjunctiva. The author uses the above method for most of his chalazia with complete satisfaction and no recurrences.

Conjunctival Route

In some cases, especially those of long standing, the chalazion points on the conjunctival surface. There may even have been perforation with a sprouting of granulation tissue. Here one should use the conjunctival route.

Procedure (fig. 63B):   The area is anesthetized as described for the cutaneous route. The chalazion clamp is adjusted and tightened. A vertical incision is made directly into the chalazion cavity and all the adventitious granulations removed, the contents of the chalazion evacuated and the area curetted.

If the chalazion is large a cruciate incision instead of a simple vertical one is made and the points of the four quadrants clipped off. This allows for better drainage before complete healing takes place. The procedure is otherwise as described above. No sutures are used. The clamp is removed and hemostasis attained by pressure. Patching is optional and the patient may be advised to apply cold compresses to reduce swelling and obviate secondary bleeding. Also antiseptic drops such as Sulamyd are used for several days after operation.

*Marginal Route**

For those chalazia which are situated at the margin or just above it the marginal route is simplest.

Procedure (fig. 63C):   After suitable anesthesia the lid margin is everted, an incision is made through the tarsal margin and the chalazion is split. The chalazion lies wholly within the tarsus, hence the incision is made not in the gray line but just behind it, i.e., in the area of the meibomian gland openings. The incision is made sufficiently deep to assure the complete opening of the chalazion. A sharp—or better still—toothed curet is inserted and the walls of the chalazion thoroughly scraped. These may also be cauterized if desired. No sutures are necessary. Bleeding is usually minimal and easily controlled. Dressing of the eye is optional though a patch may be used for a day or two.

HORDEOLUM INTERNUM

Hordeolum internum is an acute infection of a meibomian gland. Like an external hordeolum or stye it is suppurative in character but since it is encased in the fibrous tissue of the tarsus the inflammation

* Discussion of marginal chalazion and stye is included in this chapter for purposes of better organization.

tends to be much more prolonged and severe. The whole lid may become painful and swollen.

It is to be differentiated from the secondary infection of a chalazion by the fact that it *begins* as an acute infection whereas the infected chalazion is usually present in its chronic painless form first. Also the latter type is usually much less acute, less painful and more localized.

Treatment is the same as for any purulent inflammation. Hot fomentations are used until the infection becomes localized, usually on the conjunctival surface. When this occurs the area is incised and drained and hot compresses continued along with chemotherapy or antibiotics until the inflammation subsides.

HORDEOLUM EXTERNUM OR STYE

A stye is a localized purulent infection arising at the lid margin in connection with one or more ciliary follicles and involving the associated Zeis gland. This is an acute inflammation which may be localized or may spread to involve one or both lids. It is much less common than a chalazion or hordeolum internum.

Treatment is by hot fomentations until the area of abscess pointing is localized. The affected cilia are then epilated and, if necessary, drainage is assisted by knife incision of the abscess. Hot fomentations are continued. Chemotherapy or antibiotics are exhibited if the occasion demands.

XANTHOMATOSIS

Xanthomatosis or xanthelasma (*xanthos* = yellow; *elasma* = a plate) is a painless, chronic condition characterized by the deposition of patches of yellowish lipoid material in the skin of the lids. The site of predilection is the inner half of the upper lid although any extramarginal area may be involved. While the cause of the lesion is not definitely known it may be associated with a disturbance of fat metabolism, diabetes and hypercholesteremia. Certainly it occurs most commonly when cholesterol or triglyceride blood levels are elevated. However, it also seems to occur in individuals who are otherwise symptomless and without obvious disturbances of fat metabolism. Lesions associated with hypercholesteremia tend to be yellowish. Those occurring with an elevated serum triglyceride tend to be more orange or reddish.

Xanthomatosis of the lids occurs in two forms:

Xanthoma planum (figs. 64A and 65A) is by far the commoner. It affects females more frequently than males, usually in the later decades of life. The lesion is typically an irregular or oval-shaped small flat plaque, orange-yellow in color, and raised slightly above skin level. It

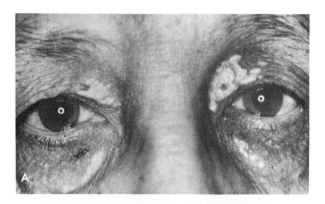

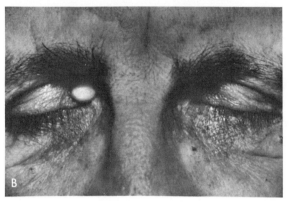

FIG. 64.   Xanthomatosis.
A. Late xanthoma planum.   B. Xanthoma tuberosum

lies within the corium. It is not unusual to have two, three or all four
lids invaded simultaneously by these lesions. Typically the first lesion
is noted in the nasal half of the upper lid (fig. 65A).

Xanthoma tuberosum (fig. 64B) is nodular in type and its site of
predilection is also the nasal half of the upper lid. It is less common than
xanthoma planum and does not usually affect so many lids at once.
Rarely, it is widespread throughout the body. The lesion tends to be
smaller, thicker and more solid than xanthoma planum.

The treatment of choice for both types of xanthoma is resection.
Usually they are small enough to require nothing but simple excision and
closure. However, if the lesions are large (fig. 64A) or if numerous small
ones are present which, in toto, cover a large area, they may be excised
altogether and skin grafted. Another simpler but more prolonged method
is to excise the lesions a section at a time, seriatim, so that the total
loss of surface tissue is not too great at any one time. It is best to let five
to six weeks elapse between operations to allow for skin stretching. This
method may obviate the necessity for grafting if carefully and patiently
followed.

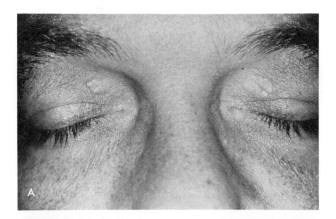

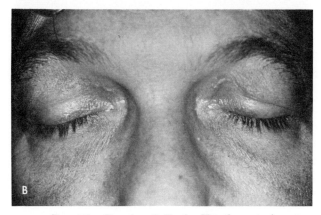

FIG. 65.   Repair of Early Xanthomatosis.
A.   Early typical bilateral xanthoma planum.
B.   After simple resection and repair.

Procedure (fig. 65):   After suitable cleansing of the area it is infiltrated with anesthetic solution containing epinephrine 1:50,000. The skin is put on stretch and the lesion marked out by incisions through clear skin 1 mm. beyond the borders. The marked out area is then dissected up and resected. The edges are undermined slightly and carefully sutured together with 5–0 silk interrupted sutures. The eye is patched and dressed every two days thereafter. Sutures are removed on the fifth or sixth day (fig. 65*B*).

Comment: As stated above, in the case of large or numerous xanthelasmas the surgeon must decide whether to graft skin immediately or dally with several resections. Both methods have their advantages. Electrocoagulation may be employed in all cases instead of surgery. However, this is more time consuming since multiple sittings are required. Also, in dark-complected individuals light patches of depigmentation may be left which take a long time to disappear. Sometimes they are worse cosmetic blemishes than the original xanthomas.

Tumors and Cysts

Benign Lid Lesions

Among the commoner benign lid lesions, usually extramarginal but occasionally marginal, are fibroma (fig. 66*B*), nevus (fig. 66*C*), xanthoma (figs. 64 and 65), verruca, sebaceous cyst, papilloma (fig. 75), keratoacanthoma (figs. 66*F* and 67), molluscum contagiosum, chalazion and other lesions discussed above. To these may be added the rarer cornucutaneum (figs. 66*A* and 68*A*), hidrocystoma (fig. 66*D*), hemangioma (fig. 66*E*) and others.

The nevus (mole) merits a special word. It has been estimated that every adult has 15 to 20 nevi on his body. Of these about 75 per cent are the intradermal nevi or common moles which are not uncommon on the lids. The much less common but more potentially dangerous types are the junctional and compound nevi which are believed to give rise to the malignant melanoma. In general, any previously quiescent nevus which undergoes such changes as enlargement, ulceration, bleeding, loss of hair and increased pigmentation should be treated as malignant. The treatment here is neither x-ray nor radium—but *wide* excision.

In most cases these lesions are small enough so that the surgical problem is simply one of resection and closure. (Although such a lesion as the pigmented nevus seen in figure 66*C* is extensive enough to require grafting.) Thus lesions 66*B*, *D* and *E* are excised spindle fashion with the long axis of the resection paralleling the palpebral fissure (see fig. 38). The skin edges are undermined if necessary and sutured with interrupted 5–0 silk.

Keratoacanthoma is a curious lesion. This is a benign epithelial tumor of unknown etiology which occurs most commonly on the skin of the face and lids. More rarely it may occur on the conjunctiva. It starts as a nodule which proliferates rapidly and may grow to 2 cm. in size. Typically it has a central crater (fig. 66*F*) filled with keratin. Left alone it usually regresses in about four months. It is easily mistaken for a malignant lesion and the certain diagnosis can only be made by biopsy.

Not all these lesions regress so rapidly or completely and they may even recur if incomplete surgery is done. Figure 67*A* shows a complete acanthoma in full flower and in the process of resolution (fig. 67*B*). Some reporters have advised resection if resolution is not complete.

Malignant Lid Lesions

The common malignant tumors which invade the lid are:
1. Basal cell epithelioma.
2. Squamous cell epithelioma.

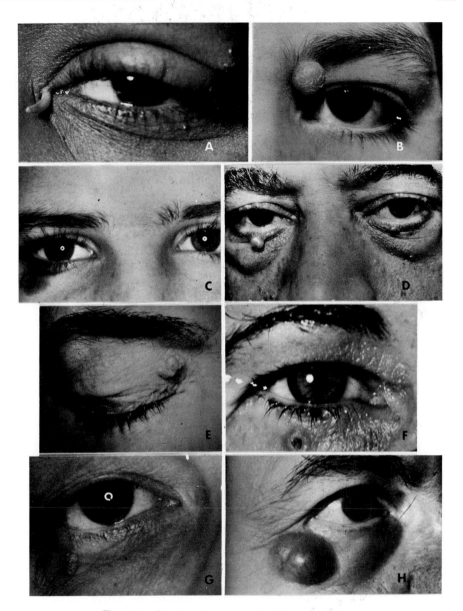

FIG. 66.   Benign Extramarginal Tumors.
A. Cornucutaneum.   E. Hemangioma.
B. Fibroma.   F. Keratoacanthoma.
C. Pigmented nevus.   G. Intradermal nevus.
D. Hidrocystoma.   H. Lipoma.

3. Adenoid epithelioma, i.e., epithelioma arising from the hair follicles, Zeis glands and sweat glands of the lids.

The tumors above are listed in the order of their frequency, not malignancy. (There are others of less frequency.) Thus, according to reports, the basal cell epithelioma occurs at least forty times as often as the squamous but fortunately the former is much less malign. It is only

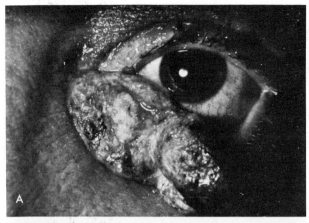

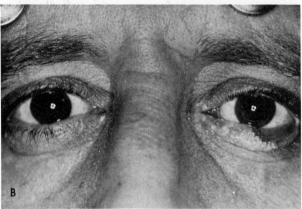

FIG.   67. Keratoacanthoma.
A.   Large keratocanthoma of left lower lid.
B.   Two months after spontaneous involution; note residual lesion and some
    ectropion.

locally invasive and does not metastasize. However, having no capsule,
it invades the surrounding tissue with pseudopodia-like projections well
beyond its apparent border. The reason for wide excision is therefore
obvious. If neglected, it can infiltrate the deeper tissues of the orbit,
bone and even the brain. Squamous cell tumors do metastasize and are
frequently traceable to neighboring young nodes. They can be fatal if
neglected. The adenoid tumors are least malignant and, like the basal cell
epithelioma, are only locally invasive without metastasizing. They constitute only about five per cent of all malignant lid tumors. Malignant
melanoma of the lid is still more rare.

Lid epitheliomas are most common in the older age groups, occurring usually in the sixth decade of life or later. Clinically, basal and
squamous cell epitheliomas are not always easy to differentiate and many
benign lesions such as inverted follicular keratosis, keratoacanthoma,
pseudoepitheliomatous hyperplasia and senile keratosis have been mistaken for squamous cell tumors. The latter because of their keratin con-

tent may show whitish areas and, rarely, may appear pearly white especially on the conjunctiva (fig. 156E). Both usually appear as grayish-white nodules with indurated edges and central depression, without attachment to the subcutaneous tissues. As the tumor grows its surface may become irregular with ulceration and bleeding. All are slow growing although the squamous type grows the most rapidly. A two or three year history of "no growth" is not uncommon.

The site of predilection is for transitional areas, hence they are most commonly found near the lid margin where the skin merges into the mucocutaneous marginal epithelium. At first the usual lesion does not involve the lid margin. At it progresses, however, it spreads to the margin and may continue on to the conjunctival surface. Another common site is the nasocanthal angle. All are much more common in the lower lid than in the upper, the ratio being anywhere from 20 or 40 to 1, or more, judging by reports of incidence. This is fortunate because lower lid repairs are easier to make.

Resection is the ideal method of handling these lesions and it should be done with a generous hand. Pathology sections frequently show nests of tumor cells under intact epithelial edges. Hence excision should be made widely well beyond the apparent edges of the tumor and its visible limits. The factor of subsequent cosmetic repair must always be secondary. It has been reported that only about a third of the cases showing incomplete excision will recur subsequently. However, this is cold comfort when facing a recurrence.

SURGERY OF EXTRAMARGINAL NEOPLASMS

The remainder of this chapter is devoted to the repair of neoplasms not involving the lid margin. Following chapters will discuss the more complicated technics of marginal lid repair.

The problem when the lid margin is not involved is simply one of resection and repair with as little residual scarring as possible. The tumor must be carefully palpated between two fingers and an incision made several millimeters beyond its apparent margins. If small enough, the tumor is excised, the edges undermined if necessary and neatly drawn together. The final wound should be as nearly as possible horizontally spindle-shaped to make closure easy. Furthermore, a wound of this shape heals with less visible scar. If possible, also, the longest diameter of the wound should follow the pattern of orbicularis fibers (cf. fig. 38) for smooth healing as previously indicated.

Resection and Closure

The lesion seen in figure 68A is a cornucutaneum which springs from a papilloma. It is an example of the less common lesions which dot the lid occasionally. These are striking looking tumors of the lid skin with

a predilection for the sites near the margin or lateral canthus. They are
epidermal growths, resembling the horns of animals and are usually
conical in shape. They are seen almost exclusively in older people.
Usually they are short but lesions of 4 to 5 cms. in length have been
reported. (Another example is seen in figure 66A.) They usually arise
from scars, warts, sebaceous cysts and even malignant growths but their
etiology is not definitely known. Their presence is usually without
incident but even trifling trauma may induce inflammation and infection.
If shed spontaneously, recurrence is common and carcinomatous changes
may occur. The best treatment is with resection as for malignancy.

Procedure (fig. 68):   The whole lesion is resected with an incision
circling the base and including a 3–4 mm. rim of healthy tissue all
around. The resection is horizontally spindle-shaped. Skin and muscle
are included in the resection. Since there is ample tissue here, undermining is minimal and closure simple (figs. 68B and C). The final result
is seen in figure 68D).

On the other hand, when an extramarginal lesion which is probably
malignant is in the lower lid, the problem is not so simple. The position
in the lower lid precludes resection of too much tissue especially when the
lesion is larger. Such a problem was posed by the neoplasm seen in
figure 69A. Despite this, since the patient was elderly with an adequate
amount of loose skin, simple resection was done.

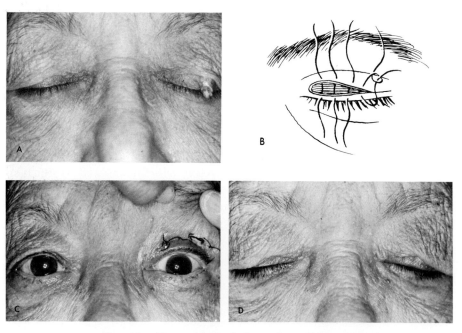

FIG. 68.   Extramarginal Resection—Upper Lid.

A.   Cornucutaneum of left upper lid.   C.   Before suture removal.
B.   Resection.   D.   Final result.

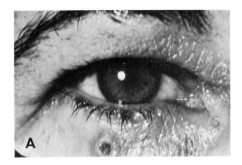
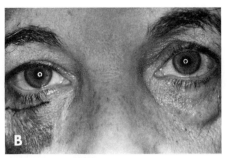
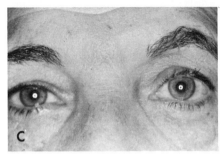

FIG. 69. Extramarginal Repair of Lower Lid.
A. Neoplasm of right lower lid.
B. Horizontal resection and closure.
C. Result.

Procedure (fig. 69): The lesion was resected in the shape of a horizontal spindle with an areola of healthy tissue all around. On closure there was a slight tendency for the lid to pull away from the globe (fig. 69B). Healing, however, was without incident and within 2 weeks the lower lid resumed its normal position against the globe (fig. 69C).

Thus there are cases that require finesse in handling. The fact that the lid margin is not involved does not always mean a quick and easy repair. Sometimes so much tissue has to be resected that skin grafting is required (figs. 73 and 74). Also the size and position of the lesion makes a difference in the technic of repair. Dehiscences at the lateral canthus may be covered by sliding pedicles from the temporal region. Nasally a lesion of equal size will require a skin graft because sliding grafts are not so easily attained in this locality and, if used, may leave so much scarring that it is better to use a graft.

Changing Direction of Skin Closure

The following case illustrates the possibility of converting a vertical or near vertical skin closure to a partially horizontal closure and thus minifying downward pull on the lower lid. The possibility of converting a vertical to a horizontal pull was discussed in Chapter 4, figure 58.

These maneuvers are possible in older people when the lesions are relatively small and the skin is lax.

Procedure (fig. 70): The lesion (fig. 70A) is resected with a rim of healthy tissue leaving an almost vertical wound (fig. 70B). The margins of the wound are treated as follows: The medial half of the upper lip and the lateral half of the lower lip are well undermined (fig. 70B). On closure, the medial lip of the wound is pulled down and the lateral pulled up. The closed wound thus assumes a more horizontal direction (fig. 70 C) and exerts relatively little downward pull on the lid. Healing in this case was uneventful and the final result is seen in figure 70 D.

Flat-X Plasty Repair

Whenever possible lid lesions are best resected in spindle-shaped fashion parallel with the orbicularis fibers and the lid margin. Thus the healing scar follows the course of the normal lid wrinkles and does not run across cut muscle fibers.

The trouble is that lid lesions are nonconformists. Perversely they present round, square, rectangular or irregular shapes which, if resected as a spindle, would sometimes entail the sacrifice of too much healthy skin. This is especially undesirable in cases where the lesion is obviously benign. In all such cases I have found the following little plasty very useful.

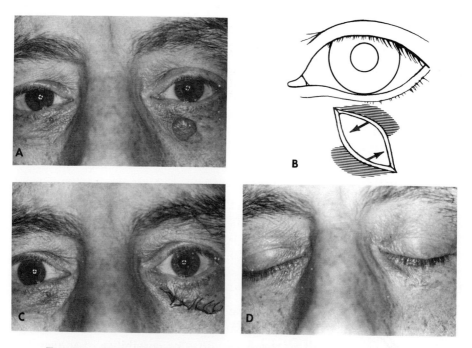

FIG. 70.   Change of Direction of Skin Closure.
A.   Neoplasm below left lower lid.
B.   Schema of wound margin undermining.
C.   Wound closure.
D.   Result.

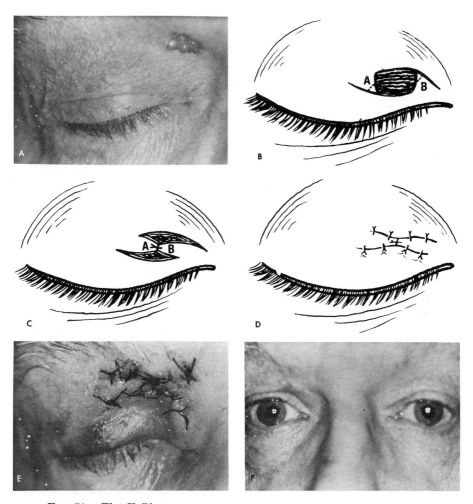

FIG. 71. Flat-X Plasty.
A. Neoplasm of right upper lid.
B. The lesion is resected and the upper and lower wound lips are extended downward and upward respectively.
C. The resultant flaps are mobilized, the tips are resected and the ends united.
D. The wound lips are undermined and the wounds closed with interrupted sutures.
E. Appearance after closure.
F. Final result.
   (Fox, S. A.: Courtesy Archives of Ophthalmology.)

Repair of the lesion in figure 71A is a good example of the value of the flat-X plasty described in figure 60. This was a recurrent basal cell carcinoma roughly rectangular in outline which did not lend itself readily to a spindle-shaped resection without sacrifice of much healthy tissue.

Procedure (fig. 71): After resection of the lesion an incision is made continuing the lower lip of the wound in an upward curve to form the flap A. Flap B is formed in similar fashion by continuing the upper lip of the wound downward (fig. 71*B*). The pointed tips of the flaps are resected for better closure. The flaps A and B are undermined so that they can be advanced centrally and the tips sutured. This converts the original wide wound into two narrow wounds (figs. 71*C*). The edges are undermined sufficiently to permit easy closure (fig. 71*D*).

I have called this the flat-X plasty because of its appearance at the close of the repair (fig. 71*E*). It is effective in preventing excision of normal tissue. Also, since closure finally results in suture lines approximately parallel with the lid margin, healing is good and the resultant scarring minimal (fig. 71*F*).

Canthal Repairs

The point has been made, and will be made again, that lesions at the medial canthus are more difficult of repair than similar lesions at the lateral canthus because of their less favorable position; yet the medial canthus is a far more common site of predilection for tumors than the lateral canthus (figs. 72*A* and 74*A*). If small enough, even medial canthus lesions are amenable to successful repair by simple excision and closure. But somewhat larger lesions, which at the lateral canthus could be closed by small sliding flaps (fig. 79), require free skin grafting (fig. 74).

Repair by Excision and Closure

Procedure (fig. 72): Figure 72*A* presents a small rodent ulcus of the left nasocanthal angle, a common lesion at this site. It was removed by thorough resection with a 4 mm. margin of normal tissue all around. The wound lips could just be approximated after extensive undermining. Healing was without incident and the final result is seen in figure 72*B*.

Repair by Free Whole Skin Graft—Lateral Canthus

When the extramarginal tumor is as large as that shown in the

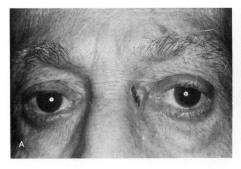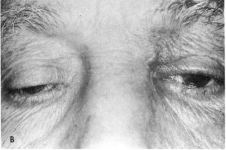

FIG. 72. Nasocanthal Angle Tumor.
A. Rodent ulcer of left nasocanthal angle.
B. Appearance after resection and repair.

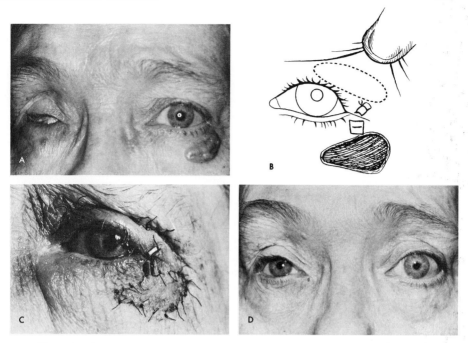

FIG. 73.   Repair at Lateral Canthus by Free Whole Skin Graft.
A.   Basal cell carcinoma of left lower lid near lateral canthus.
B.   The lids are sutured and a free whole skin graft is outlined in the ipsilateral
        upper lid.
C.   The graft in place.
D.   Final result two months later.

left lower lid (fig. 73A) then one must graft skin no matter where it is. As previously stated, the best skin is lid skin, if available. Here it was taken from the ipsilateral upper lid as described in Chapter 3.

Procedure (fig. 73):   The tumor is measured and 3 mm. are added on each side to allow for the resection of a border of healthy tissue. In other words the graft to be taken is 6 mm. wider and 6 mm. longer than the tumor measurements.

After suitable anesthesia the upper and lower lids are united by a simple tarsorrhaphy suture without surgical fusion of the lids as described in Chapter 4. (Since the patient was monocular surgical tarsorrhaphies were deemed inexpedient.) The whole tumor (fig. 73A) with its areola of healthy tissue all around is resected and all bleeding is stopped. A graft of full thickness skin is taken from the upper lid of the same side (fig. 73B) and sewed into position in the lower lid with 6–0 silk interrupted sutures which are placed close to the edge and tied tightly. The donor area in the upper lid is similarly closed (fig. 73C). A pressure dressing is applied for six days. The donor area sutures are removed, loose sutures from the graft picked off, the area carefully cleansed and the dressing reapplied for three more days. At this time the rest of the sutures including the tarsorrhaphy sutures are removed. A simple patch is used until healing is complete. The result, two months later, is shown in figure 73D with the graft blending in completely with the surrounding area.

Comment: Although a large amount of skin was required, it was easily spared by the ipsilateral upper lid without residual lagophthalmos. In fact more could have been taken if necessary. Despite the extensiveness of the lesion, repair is simply made by skin excision and grafting. Basal cell tumors rarely invade deeply and complete resection usually constitutes a cure.

The size of the graft was measured *before* injection and before excision of the lesion. This is done because injection balloons out the tissues and tends to make the measurements inaccurate. Also, after resection of the tumor the wound margins spread; hence, it is better and more accurate to do the measuring before the lesion is resected. However, if this were a resection done on a cicatrix then the measurement would be made after the lesion has been opened and the fibrous tissue resected.

Repair by Free Whole Skin Graft—Medial Canthus

Next to the lower lid lesions, medial canthus lesions are the most

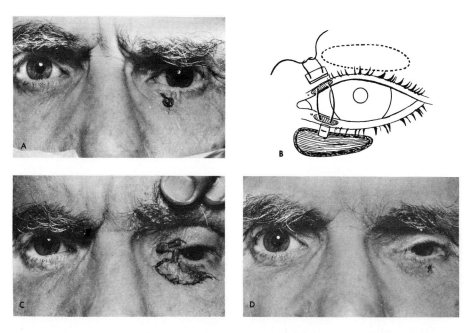

Fig. 74.   Repair at Medial Canthus by Free Whole Skin Graft.
A.   Appearance before tumor resection.
B.   Lesion is resected, a tarsorraphy is made medially and a full thickness skin
      graft from the ipsilateral upper lid is taken.
C.   The skin graft in place.
D.   Two months later—before opening of tarsorrhaphy.

common. They may be so small as to be amenable to resection and closure (fig. 72) or they may spread so much (fig. 74A) that they require skin grafting. The procedure of skin grafting here is the same as above but modified for the medial canthus. If possible, the skin is again taken from the ipsilateral upper lid so that only one eye requires patching.

Procedure (fig. 74):   Complete removal of the lesion (fig. 74A) with an areola of healthy tissue all around left a large dehiscence which required a substantial-sized graft from the ipsilateral upper lid. A surgical tarsorrhaphy was made lateral to the puncta (fig. 74B). A graft was taken from the ipsilateral upper lid and grafted into the lower lid bed (fig. 74C). Healing was good and all but the tarsorrhaphy sutures were removed on the tenth day. The tarsorrhaphy was left for 2 months (fig. 74D) before it was opened.

Comment: Grafts at the medial end of the lid require more careful handling than at the lateral end because of the presence of the puncta and canaliculi. The lower lid, especially, must be carefully watched for a possible tendency to eversion. Hence the surgical tarsorrhaphy was left in here for two months. It will be noted that in contrast, at the lateral end of the lid, a simple suture (fig. 73) without surgical fusion sufficed.

REFERENCES

BEARD, C. H.: Ophthalmic Surgery, ed. 2. Philadelphia, P. Blakiston's Son & Co., 1914, p. 213.

BONIUK, M. and ZIMMERMAN, L. E.: Tumors of the eyelids. Arch. Ophth. *69*:698, 1963.

DUVERGER, C., and VELTER, E.: Therapeutique Chirurgicale Ophthalmologique. Paris, Masson & Cie. 1926.

EINAUGLER, R. B., and HENKIND, P.: Basal cell epithelioma of the eyelid. Apparent incomplete removal. Am. J. Ophth. *76*:413, 1969.

FAYOS, J. V., and WILDERMUTH, O.: Carcinoma of the skin of the eyelids. Arch. Ophth. *67*:52, 1962.

FOX, S. A.: The flat-X plasty. Arch Ophth. *73*:204, 1965.

GIVNER, I., KALLOS, A. MEDINE, M., and ORFUSS, A. J.: Keratoacanthoma. Report of two cases. Am. J. Ophth. *49*:822, 1960.

GOODING, C. A., WHITE G., and YATSUHASHI, M.: Significance of marginal extension in excised basal-cell carcinoma. N.E.J. Med. *273*:923, 1965.

MARTIN, H. E.: Cancer of the eyelids. Arch. Ophth. *22*:1, 1939.

PAYNE, J. W., DUKE, J. R., BUTNER, R., and EIFRIG, D. E.: Basal cell carcinoma of the eyelids. Arch. Ophth. *81*:569, 1969.

REESE, A. B.: Tumors of the Eye. New York, Paul B. Hoeber, Inc., 1953, pp. 1–38.

WHEELER, J. M.: Treatment of tumors of the eyelids. N. Y. J. Med. *39*:870, 1939.

CHAPTER 6

Ciliary (Anterior) Margin Lesions

GENERAL CONSIDERATIONS

SURGERY OF CILIARY MARGIN
LESIONS
DIRECT VERTICAL CLOSURE
HORIZONTAL EXCISION AND CLOSURE

ADVANCEMENT FLAP REPAIRS—
LOWER LID
ROTATED FLAP REPAIRS
HALVING REPAIRS
FIGURE-8 SUTURE REPAIRS

GENERAL CONSIDERATIONS

IN THE PREVIOUS CHAPTER it was shown that the repair of lesions not involving the lid margin is relatively simple. In most cases it is a matter of resection and closure though grafting has to be done to replace lost tissue in the larger repairs. However, once the margin of the lid becomes affected, even if it is only the anterior or ciliary portion, the technic of repair becomes somewhat more involved.

The margins of the lids, fringed by the lashes anteriorly, are important elements in the cosmetic equipment of the eye. The upper lid especially, with its longer, more abundant lashes, can stand little deformity without becoming an obvious cosmetic blemish. It is well to keep this in mind in all surgery of the lid borders for, even when the greatest care is exercised, cilia will sometimes be lost or will grow out irregularly. The surgeon should warn the patient of this possibility in order to avoid later disappointment.

Small epitheliomata, fibromata, papillomata, cysts, melanomas, keratoses and other tumors limited to the marginal surface of the lid are not rare. They usually originate on the skin surface and invade the lid margin secondarily and their handling will vary depending on whether the whole margin or only the ciliary area is involved.

If the lesion is malignant, complete extirpation is necessary. Electrocoagulation should never be used for malignant tumors nor for those having the least possibility of malignancy. Nor is irradiation the method of choice in the author's opinion. As previously noted, since benignity of a lesion is rarely assured, the safest procedure is to treat it as if it were malignant.

122

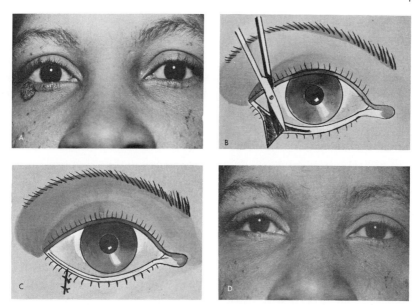

FIG. 75.   Triangular (Vertical) Repair of Lower Lid.
A.   Lesion of the right lower lid.
B.   The lid is split, the lesion resected triangularly and the edges are undermined.
C.   The wound is closed.
D.   Final result.

SURGERY OF THE CILIARY (ANTERIOR) LID MARGIN

Direct Vertical Closure

If the lesion clearly involves only the anterior half of the lid margin without impinging on the posterior half of the lid and *it is small enough*, the tarsoconjunctival layer of the lid need not be disturbed at all or very little. Since the skin-muscle layer is relatively elastic, it may sometimes be drawn across the inelastic tarsoconjunctival layer without too much lid splitting. Such a lesion is seen in figure 75A. It was resected and the wound closed without further dissection and without injury to the cilia.

Procedure (fig. 75):   The lid behind the lesion is split into its two layers and the tumor is resected triangularly (fig. 75B). After resection the wound lips are undermined and vertical closure is made (fig. 75C). The final result is seen in figure 75D.

Comment: If the neoplasm is near the nasal end of the lid, care must be taken to protect the punctum. Only if the punctum itself is involved need it be injured (see fig. 116). When the tumor, as here, is quite small, triangular excision with some undermining suffices and the lid splitting is limited to a minimum. Figures 46C and D show the methods of lid splitting which are least hazardous to the cilia.

Horizontal Excision and Closure—Lower Lid

If the lesion on the anterior lid margin is narrow, a horizontal re-section parallel with the lid margin may be done. Then the skin-muscle layer can be undermined, drawn up and sutured to the lid margin.

Procedure (fig. 76): The lid behind the lesion (fig. 76A) is split in the gray line. The dissection between the two lid laminae is carried downward well below the lesion. The tumor is now resected with several millimeters of normal skin all around (fig. 76B). If necessary the skin-muscle and tarsoconjunctival layers are separated still more until the cut edge of the skin-muscle layer can be drawn up easily and without tension to the lid margin and sutured to the tarsoconjunctiva (fig. 76B, inset). Closure is made with 5–0 silk interrupted sutures (fig. 76C). A simple patch suffices. Sutures are removed on the sixth day (fig. 76D).

Comment: This technic can be used only if the tissue resected is not too wide. Otherwise the downward pull on the lid margin will be too great and ectropion may result. Wide dissection to mobilize the skin-muscle layer so that it can be drawn up without tension is important.

Slight overcorrection is sometimes encountered. This may be due to early edema which subsides in a few days. Sometimes it persists some-what longer as seen in figure 76C. Usually, however, if too much tissue has not been resected, the working of the orbicularis and the stretching

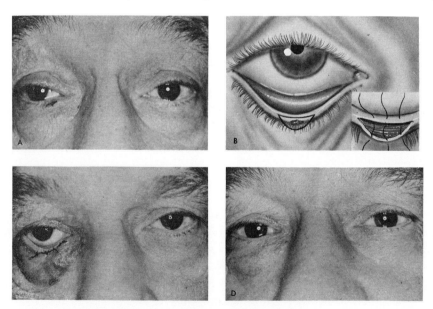

FIG. 76. Horizontal Repair of Lower Lid.
A. Basal cell carcinoma of right lower lid, ciliary margin.
B. The lid is split, the tumor resected, the skin is undermined, pulled up and sutured.
C. Note some ectropion immediately after repair.
D. Final appearance after six weeks.

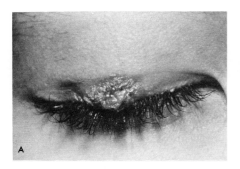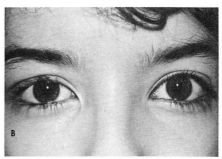

Fig. 77. Horizontal Repair of Upper Lid Lesion.
A. Neoplasm of right upper lid.
B. Final result after resection and repair as in figure 76.

of the aging lid skin will restore the lid to its normal position in a week or two as in this case (fig. 76D). The firm lid skin of younger individuals does not stretch so easily, hence this procedure should be used with caution in the lower lids of the young. Cilia must be lost because they are involved but not beyond the area of the lid split.

Horizontal Excision and Closure—Upper Lid

An identical type of repair is seen in figure 77. Here it was simpler because the upper lid is much wider and offers more area for repair and more tissue with less danger of eversion. The lesion (fig. 77A) was resected in toto, the upper lip of the wound undermined, pulled down and sutured to the margin. The final result is seen in figure 77B.

Vertical Advancement Flap Repair—Lower Lid

Ordinarily lower lids do not lend themselves to vertical advancement flap repairs. However, in rare instances, there is enough redundant skin even in the lower lid to warrant an attempt at a short vertical flap if well undermined.

Procedure (fig. 78): The patient had an ugly intradermal nevus involving the ciliary margin of the right lower lid (fig. 78A). After resection two skin incisions slanting outward slightly were made downward to outline an advancement flap from each side of the wound. The flap was mobilized, pulled up and sutured at the side and to the lid margin (figs. 78 B and C). Healing was uneventful and the final result was good (fig. 78D).

Comment: The danger of these lower lid flaps is the creation of ectropion if they are made too long. Hence the lesion in which this type of technic is contemplated should be carefully studied before it is used.

Temporal Advancement Flap

When a ciliary margin lesion is situated near a lateral canthus, repair is facilitated because an advancement flap can easily be fashioned

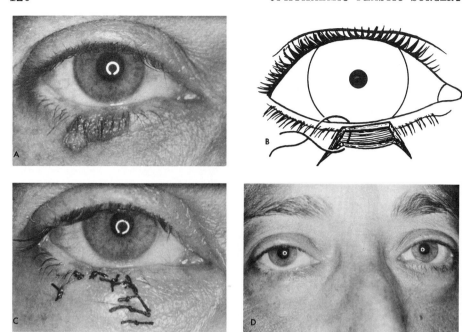

FIG. 78. Vertical Advancement Flap Repair of Lower Lid.
A. Intradermal nevus of right lower lid.
B. The border behind the lesion is split, the nevus resected and a vertical advancement flap is fashioned.
C. The flap is pulled up to the lid margin and sutured.
D. Final appearance after eight weeks.

at the canthus and slid over to cover the dehiscence made by the resection.

Procedure (fig. 79):   This patient had a pigmented lesion situated at the extreme lateral canthus barely involving the lash line (fig. 79*A*). The lesion was resected, the lid was split and a small advancement flap was fashioned by two divergent skin incisions directed laterally from the upper and lower edges of the wound. The flap thus created was undermined, drawn over and sutured medially (fig. 79*B*). The wound was dressed daily and the sutures removed on the fifth day. The final result (fig. 79*C*) was quite adequate.

Rotated Flap Repair

In the lower lid where excess skin is not always as readily available as in the upper, it is sometimes judicious to use a rotated flap in ciliary margin resections to avoid downward pull. This was done in the following case.

Procedure (fig. 80):   After resection of the lesion (fig. 80*A*) the basal incision is extended laterally to create a flap (fig. 80*B*). This is dissected up, rotated to the lid margin and sewed into position (fig. 80*C*). The final result is seen in figure 80*D*.

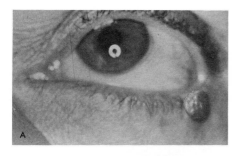
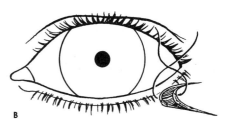
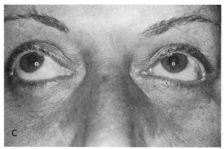

FIG. 79. Temporal Horizontal Advancement Flap Repair.
A. Neoplasm of left ciliary margin of left lower lid.
B. Resection and repair by small advancement flap.
C. Result of repair.

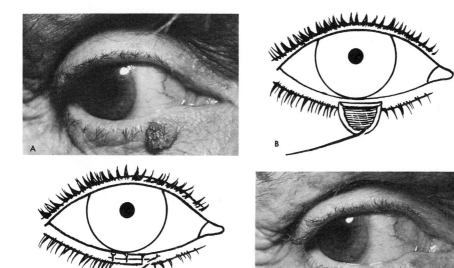

FIG. 80. Rotated Flap Repair.
A. Neoplasm of right lower lid.
B. Neoplasm is resected and flap is fashioned.
C. Flap is dissected up, rotated to margin and sutured.
D. Final result.

Comment: The rotated flap is not a commonly used technic. But it has the advantage of drawing on horizontal, not vertical, skin; hence, there is less tendency to downward pull and ectropion.

Repair by Partial Modified Halving

When the ciliary margin lesion is larger (fig. 81*A*) than that depicted in figure 80*A* and it is desired to avoid much lid splitting, partial modified halving can be done. This reduces the amount of necessary lid splitting and possible lash loss to a minimum.

Procedure (fig. 81): The margin behind the lesion in the left lower lid is split into two layers and the lesion is resected in toto with a border of healthy tissue all around (fig. 81*B* inset). The wound is then prepared for halving by resecting a sector of tarsoconjunctiva at one end and splitting the lid on that side (fig. 81*B*).

The tarsoconjunctival wound is closed with 6–0 chromic catgut tied on the tarsal surface. The skin-muscle lamina is drawn over nasally and closed with 5–0 silk (fig. 81*C*). The eye is patched and dressed daily. The skin sutures are removed on the sixth day. The final result is seen in figure 81*D*.

Comment: As in the previous procedure both skin-muscle and tarsoconjunctiva were resected although the full lid margin was not

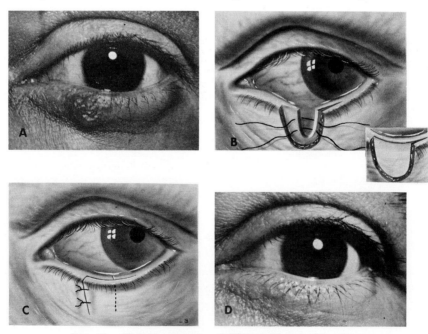

FIG. 81. Halving Repair of Ciliary Margin Neoplasm.
A. Anterior margin lesion of left lower lid.
B. Resection (inset) and preparation for halving closure.
C. Halving closure is made.
D. Final result.

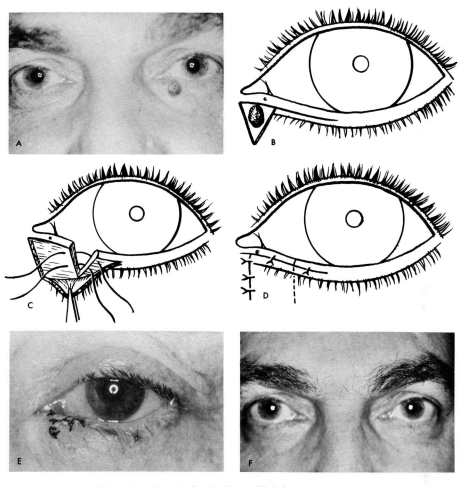

FIG. 82.   Repair by Indirect Halving.
A.   Lesion anterior to punctal area of left lower lid.
B.   Incision lines.
C.   Resection of lesion and of tarsoconjunctiva laterally.
D.   Closure of wound.
E.   Appearance of wound before removal of sutures.
F.   Final result.

involved. When the tumor was resected it was found that the skin-muscle wound edges could not be brought together unless a good part of the lid margin were split and/or cantholysis done. Neither could the skin-muscle be pulled up to the tarsoconjunctival border as in figure 76 because the wound was too wide and ectropion would have resulted. Hence, the simplest procedure was to resect enough normal tarsocon-junctiva to permit closure by the halving technic. In other words, a *modified halving* procedure was justified although the tarsoconjunctiva was not involved, because it made closure easier, prevented lid splitting and avoided lash jeopardy.

The reverse is also true, i.e., when tarsoconjunctiva alone has to be removed it is sometimes found that there is considerable excess of skin-muscle lamina on closure. Here also it may be convenient to halve the wound by resecting enough skin-muscle to facilitate good approximation of the edges and attain a good cosmetic closure without wrinkling.

Repair by Indirect Halving

The most important area of usefulness of indirect halving is around the punctal area where anterior margin lesions are rather frequent. Here closure without tension is important so as not to interfere with tear conduction. Figure 82A presents such a case.

Procedure (fig. 82): The lid in the region of the left punctum is carefully split into its two laminae and the split is extended laterally for several millimeters (fig. 82B). The lesion in front of the punctum is carefully dissected away in triangular fashion. At the lateral end of the lid split a wedge of tarsoconjunctiva is resected (fig. 82C).

The tarsoconjunctiva is closed with 5–0 chromic catgut tied on the anterior tarsal surface. The skin-muscle is closed with 5–0 silk on the anterior surface and a couple of 6–0 sutures on the margin (fig. 82D). Appearance of the repair before removal of sutures is seen in figure 82E and the final result in figure 82F.

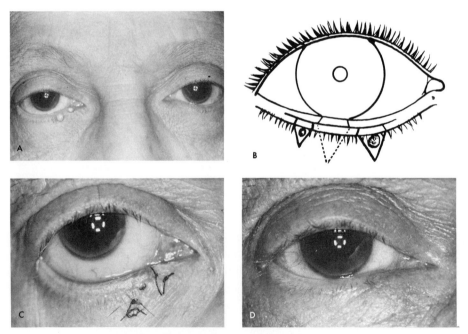

FIG. 83.   Halving Repair of Double Lesion.
A.   Double lesion of right lower lid.
B.   Scheme of resection.
C.   Appearance before suture removal.
D.   Final result.

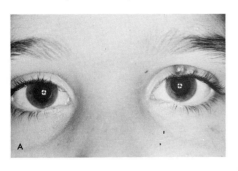
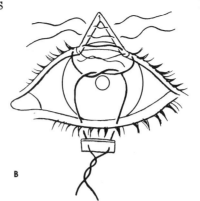
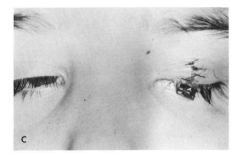
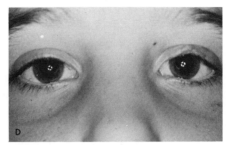

FIG. 84. Repair by Full Thickness Resection and Figure-8 Suture.
A. Hemangioma of left upper lid.
B. Resection and closure by figure-8 suture.
C. Appearance before removal of sutures.
D. Final result.

Comment: Resection and suture of healthy tarsus helps shorten the lid and brings the edges of the skin-muscle wound closer together. This makes for easier closure and avoids more lid splitting and possible cilia loss as in the previous case.

Indirect Halving in Double Lesions

Another indication for indirect halving is in the repair of double lesions which are not close together as seen in figure 83A.

Procedure (fig. 83): The lid is split into its two laminae for the whole distance between and including the lesions. Both neoplasms are resected triangularly. A wedge of tarsoconjunctiva is then resected between the two anterior wounds (fig. 83B). When sewn together this brings the lips of the skin-muscle wound closer together (fig. 83C) enabling easy closure and minifying the danger of cilia loss. The final result is seen in figure 83D.

Repair by Figure-8 Suture

Full thickness resection of a lesion which only involves the ciliary margin would seem heroic treatment. Yet it is being done more and more with good results.

Procedure (fig. 84):   This young lady presented a hemangioma of the left upper lid (fig. 84*A*). After suitable anesthesia a full thickness triangle apex up including the lesion is resected. The wound is then closed according to the modified Minsky technic (fig. 84*B*). The appearance before removal of the sutures is seen in figure 84*C* and the final result in figure 84*D*.

Comment: At first glance resection of uninvolved tarsus seems a waste of healthy tissue. But is it? If tarsoconjunctiva were not resected the margin to each side of the wound would have to be split and the larger the wound the longer the split would have to be to attain mobility and enable closure of the skin-muscle. This means greater and greater possibility of cilia loss. This way no lid splitting at all is required. At the most a canthotomy and cantholysis may have to be done to assist closure (as in figs. 97 and 98), and those heal without scarring. Few other procedures could have given as good a result as that seen in figure 84*D*. The end justifies the means here.

CHAPTER 7

Lesser Marginal Lesions

AFFECTIONS OF THE ENTIRE LID MARGIN make the problem of repair more complex because both laminae of the lid are now involved. But even here the lesser lesions offer no great technical difficulties; the larger lesions may be difficult indeed.

MARGINAL CYSTS

These lesions are almost always benign and can be removed entirely with little dissection. Care must be taken to include the cyst walls which are always quite thin.

After injection around the area (fig. 85A) the cyst covering is gently incised and the inner cyst lining uncovered. As it is grasped the cyst usually collapses, spilling its contents. However, this is of no consequence since the lining can now be entirely removed thus insuring against recurrence. The excessive skin covering the cyst now contracted, is resected and the wound easily closed. Healing is usually rapid and the final result good (fig. 85B).

ANKYLOBLEPHARON

Ankyloblepharon is an adhesion between the margins of the upper and lower lids. It may be congenital or traumatic or surgical. It differs from acquired phimosis in that all lid structure is lost in phimosis (figs. 248 and 249) which by definition is a diminution in both width and length of the palpebral fissure. Congenital ankyloblepharon (see Chapter 18) is most common at the lateral canthus (the filiform type as seen in fig. 228 is less common) and is usually accompanied by other anomalies such as

133

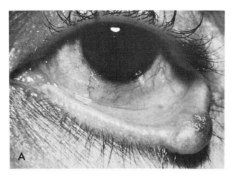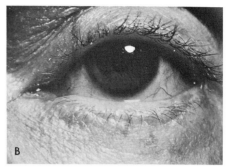

Fig. 85. Resection of Marginal Cyst.
A. Cyst of left lower lid.   B. Appearance after resection.

microphthalmos, anophthalmos, etc. It is rare. Traumatic ankyloblepharon may be due to physical trauma, burns, chemical injuries, etc. and
is frequently accompanied by symblepharon. Surgical ankyloblepharon is
even more rare except when needed tarsorrhaphies are made. To these
causes should be added destructive diseases of the lid margins. When
situated at either canthus it causes an apparent shortening of the
palpebral fissure.

Treatment of ankyloblepharon is surgical. If uncomplicated, repair
is simple.

Repair of Ankyloblepharon

Procedure (fig. 86): The lesion is investigated with a muscle hook
behind the fused lids to see whether there is symblepharon. If absent and
if the lid margin adhesion to be separated is a small one, the blades of
a blunt-pointed scissors are carefully inserted to straddle the adhesion
which is cut across with one snip. If more extensive (fig. 86A), the
separation is first made superficially with a knife, cutting through the
skin and subcutaneous layers and the section completed with scissors.

One blade is inserted into the conjunctival sac at one end of the
bridge of tissue which is straddled and sectioned with small bites of the
scissors. After separation the raw edges of the lids are thinned out, if
necessary, by debridement (fig. 86B) and each sutured, skin to conjunctiva, to prevent readhesion of the margins to each other (fig. 86C).
Ample ointment is instilled and the eye patched. The wound is inspected
daily and adhesions, if any, freed. Epithelialization is usually complete
by the third or fourth day. Figure 86D shows the eye after healing is
complete.

Comment: If symblepharon is present, dissection must be carefully
made to avoid injury to the globe. If the symblepharon is minor, the
conjunctiva can usually be repaired by undermining and drawing the
wound lips together. If the symblepharon is more extensive, repair
should be made immediately as outlined in Chapter 12 or it will recur.

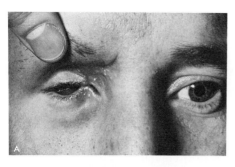
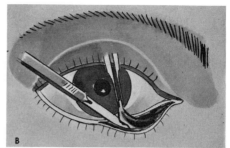
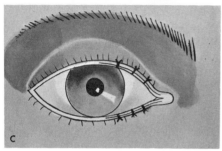
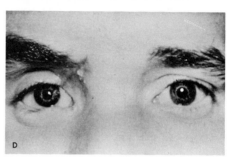

Fig. 86. Repair of Ankyloblepharon.
A. Appearance before repair.
B. and C. Steps in debridement and closure.
D. Final appearance.

It is important to suture the skin and conjunctiva of each lid carefully to each other with multiple sutures and to inspect the wound daily. There is a great tendency in these cases for the lids to readhere. This must be discouraged by constant separation and instillation of ointment until there is complete epithelialization of the margins.

NOTCHES AND COLOBOMATA

Lid notches and colobomata may be due to trauma or produced in the course of tumor excision preliminary to plastic repair. Less frequently they are of congenital origin.

The lid notches and colobomata caused by bullets, shell fragments, land mines, automobile accidents, explosions and similar products of man's civil and military inventive genius for destruction are infinite in size, shape and variety. However, the triangular notch is the most common because the lips of a marginal laceration tend to separate as a result of the horizontal pull of the broken orbicularis fibers on the lacerated tarsus. In the upper lid there may also be some tendency toward upward pull because levator action is now unopposed at this point (provided the levator is intact). This also helps the tendency toward notch formation.

However, where there has been loss of tissue in addition to laceration the coloboma may be lunate, rectangular or otherwise irregular in shape depending on the injury, the amount of tissue lost and the consequent cicatrization. The type of repair used in such defects will depend to a large extent on some of the following factors:

1. The size, shape and position of the defect.
2. The presence or absence of the eyeball.
3. Whether the upper or lower lid is involved.
4. The condition of the surrounding tissue.

But whatever the cause, whether due to trauma, congenital deformity or excision of tumor, the underlying principles and the technics of repair remain the same.

Marginal dehiscences due to trauma or tumor resection with little loss of tissue and little tendency to pull apart will yield to almost any type of repair if done early enough and carefully enough. Simple approximation of the two edges with a marginal suture and closure on both skin and conjunctival surfaces might suffice. However, use of an intermarginal suture is safer and more certain to prevent notching.

The Figure-8 (Intermarginal) Suture
Lower Lid—Modified

The technic used in this and subsequent figure-8 closures is modified and simplified somewhat from Minsky's original technic.

Procedure (fig. 87): After suitable infiltration anesthesia, a full thickness lid triangle, apex downward, containing the lesion is resected from the left lower lid with a rim of 3 mm. healthy tissue all around. Bleeding is controlled and the resulting triangular coloboma is closed as follows: A double-armed 4–0 silk suture is entered in the gray line 3 mm. from one side of the lid break to emerge in the wound 3 mm. below the lid margin. The needle is entered in the opposite lip of the wound, again 3 mm. below the margin, to emerge in the gray line 3 mm. from the edge of the laceration. The arms of the two sutures are crossed without tying to check on the alignment of the wound lips to make sure that there is no vertical or horizontal displacement. The suture is then tied with a double knot but the needles are not cut off. The lid is pulled forward by means of this suture and the conjunctiva closed with 5–0 or 6–0 chromic catgut interrupted sutures as necessary.

Alternatively the tarsoconjunctival sutures may be inserted from in front so that the knots lie on the tarsal surface. In similar manner the skin wound is closed as necessary with 5–0 interrupted silk sutures. The

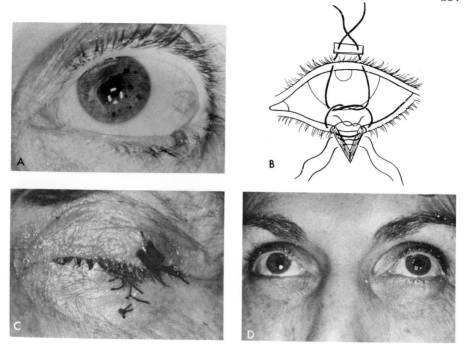

FIG. 87.   Repair of Lower Lid by Figure-8 Technic.
A.   Neoplasm of left lower lid.
B.   Figure-8 suture repair after resection.
C.   Appearance before removal of sutures.
D.   Final result.

two needles of the marginal suture are now passed through the gray line of the opposing lid to emerge in the skin above the ciliary margin (fig. 87B) where they are tied over a peg (fig. 87C). Healing is usually uneventful and the sutures are removed on the sixth or seventh day (fig. 87D).

This suture works equally well in the upper lid as seen in the next case (fig. 88). The lesion in the left upper lid (fig. 88A) is resected triangularly apex upward. Closure is made exactly as described in figure 87 but in reverse (fig. 88B). Sutures are removed in six days (fig. 88C). The final result is seen in figure 88D.

Poorly Applied Intermarginal Suture

The importance of the intermarginal splinting suture in the figure-8 technic is shown in figure 89 where the splinting was improperly done.

In the repair of the laceration in the right upper lid (fig. 89A) the break was sutured properly in layers and the lids were splinted together by means of an intermarginal suture. But the splinting was not done at the *point of lid rupture* (fig. 89B). The result was a lid notch after healing (fig. 89C). This had to be repaired again (fig. 89D).

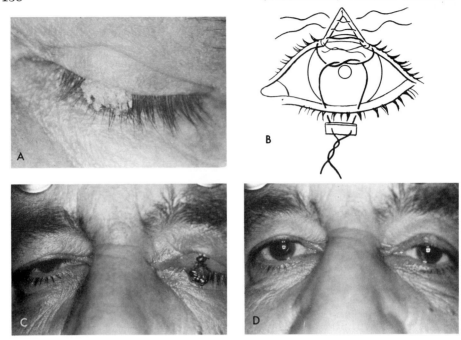

FIG. 88.   Repair of Upper Lid by Figure-8 Technic.
A.   Upper lid lesion.
B. and C.   Repair by figure-8 suture after resection.
D.   Final Result.

It was said above that most notches would probably heal well without opposing lid splinting—and they will. But a small percentage, as in this case, do not heal well. A notch would have been avoided had proper lid splinting been done. It takes so little time and effort to splint the lids properly that it is well worth doing in every case to avoid notches in a few.

Modified Figure-8 Sutures

Since its publication by Minsky in 1942 a number of modifications of the intermarginal (figure-8) suture have been reported by Smith, Amdur, Mustardé and others.

Smith uses a single suture with a preliminary deep buried loop before the ends of the sutures are brought out through the gray line and passed to the opposing lid (fig. 90A). Amdur uses a single "shoelace" suture in which the preliminary loop passes through the full thickness of the lid (fig. 90B). Mustardé uses a running suture to close the tarsus and does not splint the repaired lid to the opposing lid. In view of what occurred in the case pictured in figure 89, it would seem better not to omit the intermarginal splinting portion of the suture.

The technic described in figures 87 and 88 is a simple modification

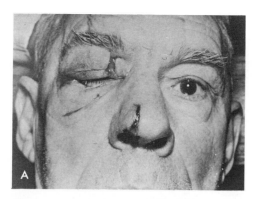

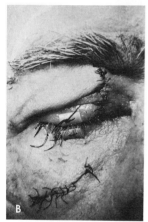
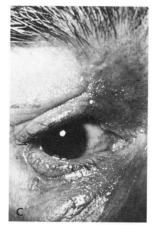
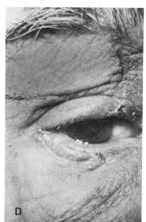

Fig. 89.   Poorly Applied Figure-8 Suture.
A.   Traumatic notch of right upper lid.
B.   Failure to apply splinting suture at point of break.
C.   Resultant notch.
D.   Result after proper figure-8 repair.

of Minsky's more complicated operation. It has served me well and I have no hesitancy in recommending it.

Repair of Opposed Upper and Lower Lid Notches

When there are simultaneous upper and lower lid lacerations which are directly opposite each other (fig. 91A) these are best corrected by the figure-8 splinting suture as described in figure 51B.

Procedure (fig. 91):   The lower lid is repaired exactly as described in figure 87 thus forming the lower loop of the figure-8.

With this repair completed the suture is continued upward into the upper lid laceration. After forming the upper loop of the figure-8 in the upper lid each needle is entered into the opposite edge of the wound about 2 mm. higher to emerge on the skin surface where the sutures are

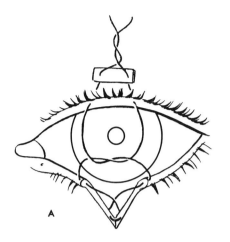
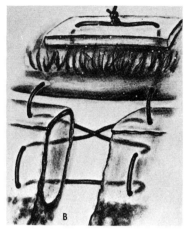

FIG. 90.   Modified Figure-8 Sutures.

A.   (Smith) A deep loop is placed in the plane of the gray line. The sutures are then crossed, passed into opposite sides of the notch, brought out in the gray line and passed up into the opposing lid.

B.   (Amdur) Method of through and through insertion of shoelace suture.

tied over a peg. Here again the conjunctival sutures may be inserted from in front and tied on the tarsal surface. The skin is then closed with interrupted 5–0 or 6–0 silk sutures where necessary (fig. 91*B*). A patch is applied and changed daily. Sutures are removed on the sixth or seventh day. The final result is seen in figure 91*C*.

Repair of Unopposed Upper and Lower Lid Notches

When the upper and lower lid lacerations are not opposite each other (fig. 92*A*) then each notch must be repaired individually.

Procedure (fig. 92):   After suitable anesthesia by instillation and infiltration the notches in the upper and lower lids are each repaired by the intermarginal suture technic described in figures 87 and 88. Each laceration is handled separately as if it alone were present. The tarso-conjunctiva is closed with catgut and the skin with 5–0 silk interrupted sutures (fig. 92*B*).

A simple patch is applied and since the lower lid coloboma is close to the cornea, the eye is inspected daily. Healing is good (fig. 92*C*) and sutures are removed on the sixth day. Figure 92*D* shows the final result ten days after repair.

Comment: This type of injury is rather common. For some reason simultaneous lacerations of the upper and lower lids occur most often at different sites rather than directly opposite each other. Whether the lesion involves one lid or both, whether it is traumatic or due to surgical resection, the same technic may be adopted and will prove successful.

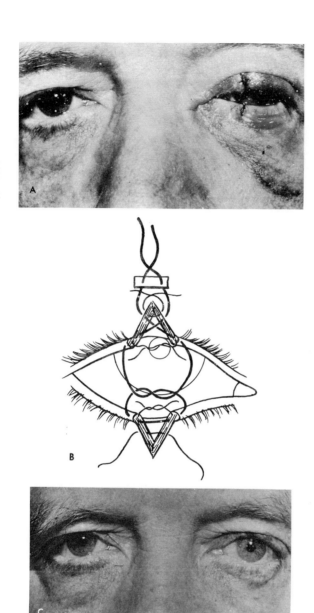

FIG. 91. Repair of Opposed Marginal Notches by Figure-8 Technic.
A. Opposing notches of left upper and lower lids.
B. Repair by single figure-8 suture.
C. Final result.

HALVING REPAIRS

Various modifications of the halving technic also give good results with triangular notches which are not too large. Two types of repair are illustrated below.

Repair by Half Halving

When the notch is small enough it is sometimes possible to attain a

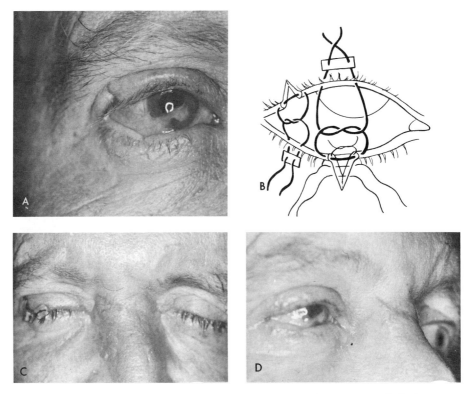

FIG. 92.   Repair of Unopposed Marginal Notches by Figure-8 Technic.
A.   Unopposed notches of right upper and lower lids.
B.   Repair of notches by individual intermarginal splinting sutures.
C.   Appearance before removal of sutures.
D.   Final result.

halving effect by resecting only skin-muscle and leaving the tarsoconjunctiva intact as shown in figure 47.

Procedure (fig. 93):   The notch in the right upper lid (fig. 93*A*)
is debrided and a small triangular segment of skin-muscle is resected
from the lateral lip of the wound. The medial lip of the wound is split
into two layers sufficiently to allow closure of the skin-muscle lamina
without tension. No tarsoconjunctiva is resected (fig. 93*B*).

The tarsoconjunctiva is closed with chromic catgut sutures tied on
the tarsal surface (fig. 93*B*). A vertical double-armed suture of 5–0 silk
is inserted through the lateral lip of the bared tarsoconjunctiva from
behind forward and the needles are then passed through the medial lip of
the skin-muscle layer wound and tied over a peg (fig. 93*C*). Additional
interrupted skin-muscle sutures are added to attain good wound closure
of the skin-muscle layer.

The eye is patched and dressed daily. Sutures are removed on the
sixth day. The final result is shown in figure 93*D*.

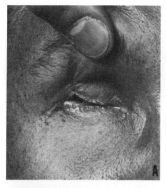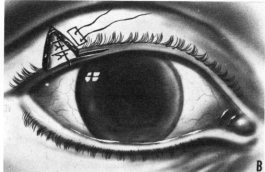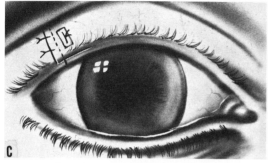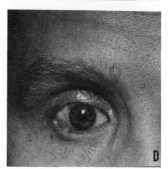

Fig. 93.   Half Halving Repair.
A.   Traumatic notch of right upper lid.
B.   The notch is debrided and the lid is split medially.
     The tarsus is closed without further tarsal resection.
C.   The skin-muscle layer is pulled over the tarsal wound and closed.
D.   Final result (cf. fig. 47).

Comment: As noted, closure is attained here without resection of tarsus. Since the posterior lamina is inelastic, the smaller the notch the easier it is to close. Thus it is the elasticity of the skin-muscle layer which permits a half-halving closure with a minimum of lid splitting.

Repair by Triangular Full Halving (Old Style Closure)

Figure 94 shows a notch repair created by the full-thickness lid resection of a marginal melanoma of the right lower lid (fig. 94A). Although the lesion itself seems small, segments of clear tissue were resected to each side because of its pigmented character, thus making for a larger notch to be repaired than would at first appear.

Procedure (fig. 94):   The lesion is resected in the form of a triangle apex downward. The lid to each side of the notch is split into skin-muscle and tarsoconjunctiva laminae. On one side of the wound a small triangle of skin-muscle measuring 3 mm. at its base in the lid margin is resected. On the other side a similar triangle of tarsoconjunctiva is removed (fig. 94B). A vertical double-armed suture of 4–0 braided silk is passed through the bared tarsoconjunctiva from within outward and

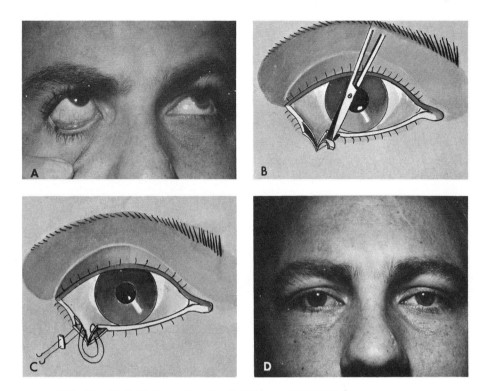

FIG. 94. Full Halving Repair of V-Shaped Lid Notch.
A. Pigmented lesion of lid margin.
B. A full thickness triangular section is resected. Tarsoconjunctiva is resected on one side and skin-muscle on the other to attain a halving closure.
C. A vertical mattress suture is inserted.
D. Final result five weeks later.

then through the skin-muscle of the other side, also from within outward, to be tied on the skin surface over a peg (fig. 94*C*). Additional sutures are inserted to assure good apposition of the skin and marginal lips of the wound. A light dressing is applied. Sutures are removed on the fifth day. The final result is seen in figure 94*D*.

Comment: This type of repair, especially in trauma, is rapidly reaching extinction because it calls for resection of too much normal tissue and lid splitting as seen in figure 48, thus jeopardizing cilia. An even better reason for its abandonment is that the figure-8 technic is simpler and gives better results. Halving is now valuable in modified and indirect form only (figs. 81, 82 and 93).

TEMPORAL ADVANCEMENT PEDICLE

When the lesion is nearer the lateral canthus (fig. 95*A*) much lid splitting may be avoided by taking advantage of the position of the

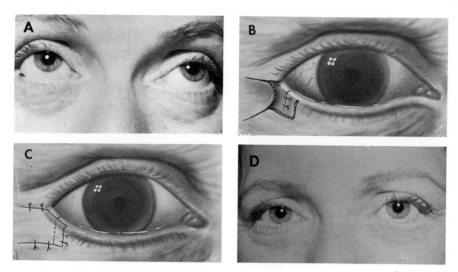

FIG. 95. Temporal Advancement Flap Repair.
A. Melanotic marginal lesion of right lower lid near lateral canthus.
B. Rectangular full thickness resection and closure of tarsus after canthotomy
    and cantholysis of lower arm of lateral canthal ligament. A sliding pedicle
    is fashioned from the temporal region.
C. Appearance after closure.
D. Final result.

lesion and drawing a temporal pedicle over to complete the repair
Thus a lesion, almost identical to the preceding one, can be repaired with
much less lid splitting and cilia loss.

Procedure (fig. 95): The lesion is resected rectangularly with at
least 3 mm. of healthy appearing tissue all around. Canthotomy and
cantholysis (figs. 52 and 53) of the lower arm of the lateral canthal
ligament are done. The tarsoconjunctiva, now freely mobilized, is closed
with 6–0 chromic catgut. A small sliding flap is fashioned at the canthus
(fig. 95B), drawn over and closed with 5–0 silk sutures (fig. 95C). The
wound is dressed after 48 hours and then daily. Sutures are removed on
the sixth day. The final result is seen in figure 95D.

Comment: Although lesions 94A and 95A are quite similar the
position of the latter near the lateral canthus allowed for this advancement
pedicle type of repair. Note that resection here was rectangular to
facilitate closure by sliding pedicle. Here too the segment excised had to
be unusually large because of the pigmented character of the lesion.

Although the basic technic of the advancement flap is the same as in
figure 79, the repairs become more complicated as the lesion grows
larger. Thus the simple skin advancement flap now requires additional
repair of the tarsoconjunctiva. In procedure 103, a still larger repair,
canthotomy, cantholysis and relaxation sutures must be added for
adequate closure.

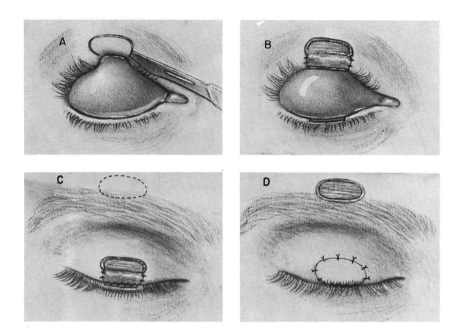

FIG. 96. Hinged Flap Repair of Coloboma (Elschnig).
A. The skin flap is mobilized.
B. The flap is turned down and sutured into the coloboma.
    The opposing lower lid margin is freshened.
C. The flap is sutured to the lower lid and a hair-bearing graft from the brow
    is fashioned.
D. The hair-bearing graft is sutured into place.

REPAIR BY HINGED FLAP (ELSCHNIG)

A modification of the original technic described by Elschnig can be
of value but only when the socket is anophthalmic. The operation calls
for the use of a hinged flap and free graft to restore tissue.

Procedure (fig. 96): A piece of plastic tissue of rubber dam is
cut to pattern to fit the lid coloboma. This pattern is reversed, placed just
above the coloboma and the area marked out on the lid surface about one-
third larger. The edges of the coloboma are freshened and split into two
layers for a few millimeters at the sides only. The skin of the previously
marked out area is incised (fig. 96A), except at the upper edge of the
coloboma to preserve the attachment, dissected up and rotated down
toward the lid margin to fill the original defect in the lid (fig. 96B).
Since the attachment at the upper edge of the coloboma serves as a hinge,
the dissection should be done carefully in order not to endanger the
blood supply to the hinged flap. The flap is sutured laterally to the
freshened edges of the *posterior* layer of the coloboma with interrupted
4–0 plain catgut sutures tied on the conjunctival side. Thus the skin

side of the flap is on the conjunctival surface and the raw side on the skin surface.

A conformer of the proper size and shape is inserted into the socket to supply support for the flap. The margin of the fellow lid opposite the graft is freshened and the marginal edges of the turned down flap are sutured to the tarsal edge of the lower lid margin. A free skin graft cut to pattern is fashioned either from the contralateral upper lid (fig. 96C) or from behind the ear and sutured into place with 5–0 silk sutures to cover the raw area (fig. 96D). This is also sutured to the anterior margin of the opposite lid with a 5–0 running silk suture. If possible, it is well to take the graft from a partial hair-bearing surface such as the brow or temporal region in order to supply lashes for the lid margin at the same time.

A layer of Cilkloid or Telfa is placed over the graft and a firm pressure dressing applied for five or six days. This is then removed, the area cleansed and the pressure dressing reapplied for three or four more days. Sutures are removed at the first dressing if this can be done without disturbing the graft; otherwise they are removed at the second dressing. The eye is patched subsequently until complete healing has taken place.

Comment: When other technics have failed or are not indicated, this is a useful secondary procedure for small colobomata of either lid. It may only be used where the globe has been lost; with an intact globe present the skin lining would irritate the cornea. This method is also contraindicated where there is much scarring of the injured lid, as cicatricial contractions of the surrounding area will make it difficult to obtain a good hinged flap and will jeopardize its vitality. A delayed flap may enhance the chances of success. The small amount of skin used here as socket lining causes little disturbance or discharge.

Like the procedure shown in figure 101 this technic is especially valuble when the deformity is lunate or crescent-shaped, i.e., when the loss of tissue along the lid margin is appreciable but not too wide. When the eye is in place the technic to use is the one illustrated in figure 101.

REFERENCES

AMDUR, J.: A modified intermarginal suture for eyelid lacerations. Arch. Ophth. *69*:556, 1963.

ELSCHNIG, A.: Cited by Spaeth, E. B., Principles and Practice of Ophthalmic Surgery. Philadelphia, Lea & Febiger, 1944, p. 345.

FALCHI, F.: Methode der Blepharoplastik bei zentralem Coloboma des Augenlides. Arch. Augenh. *59*:226, 1918.

FOX, S. A.: Some methods of lid repair and reconstruction. Am. J. Ophth. *29*:452, 1946.

————: Crescentic deformities of the lid margin. Arch. Ophth. *39*:542, 1948.

MINSKY, H.: Surgical repair of recent lid lacerations. Intermarginal splinting suture. Surg. Gynec. & Obst. *75*:449, 1942.

MUSTARDÉ, J. C.: Repair and Reconstruction in the Orbital Region. Baltimore, The Williams & Wilkins Co., 1966, p. 102.

REEH, M. J., and HYMAN, S.: Treatment of lid tumors. Tr. Am. Acad. Ophth. and Oto. *59*:507, 1955.

REESE, A. B.: Partial resection of lid and plastic repair for epithelioma and other lesions. Arch. Ophth. *32*:173, 1944.

SHERMAN, A. E.: Choice of procedure in ophthalmic plastic surgery. N. Y. J. Med. *48*:861, 1948.

SMITH, B.: Plastic surgery in ophthalmology. W. Virg. Med. J. *46*:1, 1950.

WHEELER, J. M.: Lower lid repair. Tr. Am. Acad. Ophth. and Oto. *58*:580, 1954.

CHAPTER 8

Larger Marginal Lesions

COMBINED FIGURE-8
  TECHNIC REPAIRS
  FIGURE-8 AND CANTHOLYSIS
  FIGURE-8 AND TEMPORAL
    ADVANCEMENT FLAP

COLLAR-BUTTON TECHNIC
  REPAIRS

VERTICAL ADVANCEMENT
  DOUBLE FLAP REPAIR

TEMPORAL ADVANCEMENT
  FLAP REPAIR

OPPOSING LID TARSAL
  GRAFT REPAIR

MODIFIED HUGHES TECHNIC
  REPAIR

COLOBOMATA which involve one-third of the lid margin and neoplasms which require resection of at least one-third of full thickness lid usually require more surgery than those described in previous chapters.

However, such lesions may vary considerably in the difficulty or ease of their repair. The difference will depend to a large extent on the age of the patient and the position of the lesion. Older atonic lids have more "give" and can stand the loss of a larger amount of tissue than the firm, tonic lids of the young. Also, a lesion at the lateral canthus from which a pedicle flap may be drawn will give much less trouble in repair than a central or medial lesion involving the punctal area.

COMBINED FIGURE-8 REPAIRS

The figure-8 suture can be useful even in the repair of larger lesions by combining it with other technics to give additional mobility. This is illustrated in the following two procedures (figs. 97 and 98).

Repair by Figure-8 and Cantholysis

Given enough elasticity in the lid, a congenital coloboma of the upper lid can be repaired by a figure-8 suture combined with cantholysis of the upper arm of the canthal ligament.

Procedure (fig. 97): A congenital coloboma (fig. 97*A*) of the right upper lid was resected and repair made by figure-8 suture technic after canthotomy and cantholysis (fig. 97*B*). The resected portion including the lesion measured 12 mm. Healing was good (fig. 97*C*) and the final result is seen in figure 97*D*.

Comment: Probably no other type of repair would give as good a result with such little loss of cilia and with so little surgery. Unfortunately not all colobomata can be handled so easily.

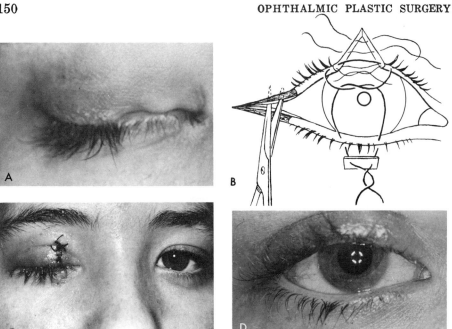

FIG. 97.   Repair by Combined Figure-8 Suture and Cantholysis.
A.   Congenital coloboma of right upper lid.
B.   Repair by cantholysis and figure-8 suture.
C.   Appearance before suture removal.
D.   Final result.

Repair by Figure-8 Suture and Temporal Advancement Flap

Procedure (fig. 98):   The lesion in the left lower lid (fig. 98A) is resected with an areola of healthy tissue all around. A canthotomy is made, the lower arm of the lateral canthal ligament is severed (fig. 98B) and an incision from the lower outer angle of the coloboma creates a lateral sliding flap which is undermined. This gives enough mobility so that the wound edges can be approximated and a figure-8 closure made (figs. 98C and D). Healing here was without incident and the final result is seen in figure 98E.

Comment: Thus the versatile figure-8 suture can also be employed in larger repairs and reconstructions by combining it with other technics.

Repair by Collar-Button Technic

It was pointed out in an earlier chapter that the collar-button technic reduces tarsal excision and hence frequently permits closure directly without the help of cantholysis. This makes complete repair a good deal easier since unyielding tarsus is harder to replace than the more elastic skin-muscle lamina.

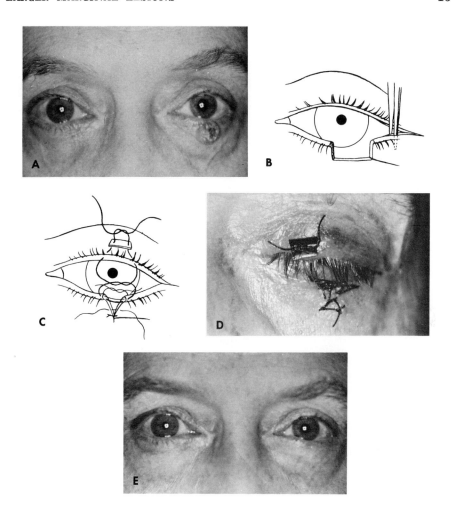

FIG. 98. Repair by Combined Figure-8 Suture and Advancement Flap.
A. Neoplasm of left lower lid.
B. Resection of neoplasm, canthotomy, cantholysis and preparation of advancement flap.
C. Closure of wound by advancement pedicle and figure-8 suture.
D. Appearance before suture removal.
E. Final result.

Central Lesion of Lower Lid

The patient pictured in figure 99A had a malignancy of the left lower lid with only slight conjunctival involvement (fig. 99B). A biopsy done before she was seen had reported basal cell carcinoma.

Procedure (fig. 99): At operation the lesion is resected in toto by the collar-button technic (fig. 61) with a rim of healthy tissue all around.

With the help of canthotomy and cantholysis the tarsoconjunctival edges are drawn together and sutured. Since the resected portion is

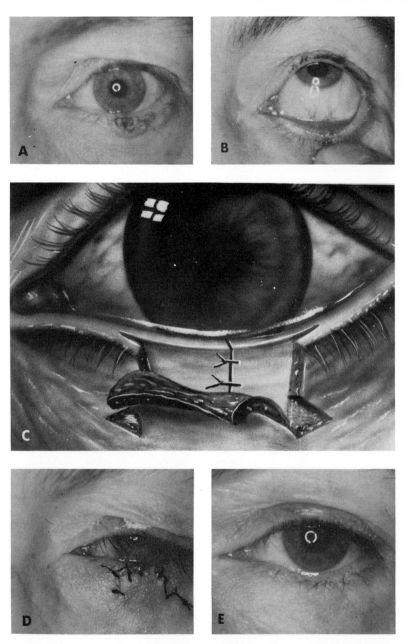

FIG. 99.   Collar-Button Repair by Horizontal Tarsal Closure with Vertical
Skin-Muscle Flap.

A. and B.   Basal cell carcinoma of left lower lid. .Note large skin lesion and
small area of conjunctival invasion.

C.   The lesion is resected and after canthotomy and cantholysis at the lateral
canthus, the tarsoconjunctiva is closed.   A vertical skin-muscle flap is
mobilized.

D.   Appearance before removal of sutures.

E.   Final result.

(Fox, S. A.:   Courtesy Archives of Ophthalmology.)

narrow a vertical skin-muscle sliding flap is fashioned by means of two short vertical incisions (fig. 99C). This is undermined easily, drawn up and sutured to the tarsal edge at the margin (fig. 99D). Thus halving is attained. A patch with monocular bandage is applied for three days. The eye is dressed daily and sutures removed on the sixth day. Pathology report showed complete excision of the tumor. The final result is shown in figure 99E.

Comment: Since the portion of tarsoconjunctiva resected was small the upper lid was not used as a source of tissue although it might have been. At any rate the result was adequate.

Sometimes curious and unforeseen happenings occur with a closure such as the above. Despite the fact that more skin-muscle is resected than tarsoconjunctiva, when the tarsoconjunctival lamina is closed the skin-muscle dehiscence is shortened by that much and is sometimes actually thrown into folds and becomes so loose that little additional surgery is needed for good closure. This is especially true in older individuals whose skin is unusually lax.

One type of closure has already been discussed above, i.e., the creation of a sliding flap by two short vertical incisions (fig. 78). At other times the anterior lamina is so loose that it does not have to be incised at all; it is simply pulled up and sutured to the margin. On occasions the skin laxity is even greater and skin has to be resected at one end to avoid wrinkling.

Temporal Lower Lid Lesion

The lesion shown in figure 100A is quite similar to the one above except that it is much closer to the lateral canthus and hence another technic is available for closure, i.e., the advancing pedicle from the lateral canthus. The lesion on the right lower lid had been present for over three years.

Procedure (fig. 100): The tumor of the right lower lid is resected by the collar-button technic (fig. 100B). Canthotomy and cantholysis of the lower arm of the ligament are done. This permits the two lips of the tarsoconjunctival wound to be drawn together easily (fig. 100C—dotted line) and united with interrupted 5–0 chromic sutures tied on the tarsal surface. A sliding flap is fashioned at the temporal canthus, mobilized and drawn over to cover the bared tarsus (fig. 100C). Wrinkles forming at the temporal end of the flap are resected and the wounds repaired according to Burow's (fig. 59) technic. Postoperative care is as for the previous case. The final result is seen in figure 100D. Pathology report showed complete excision of the tumor which was a basal cell epithelioma.

Comment: As with all other procedures the collar-button technic is simpler when the lesion lies at the lateral canthus. Here also if the

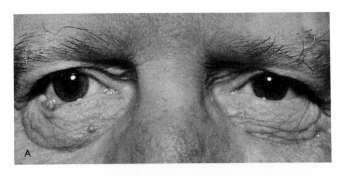

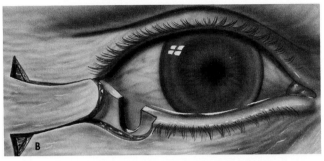

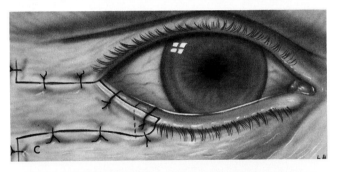

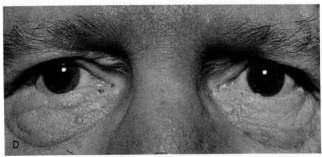

FIG. 100. Collar-Button Repair by Horizontal Tarsal Closure with Temporal
Skin-Muscle Advancement Flap.

A. Neoplasm of right lower lid with tarsoconjunctival involvement.
B. Collar-button resection of lesion and formation of temporal sliding flap.
C. The tarsoconjunctiva is closed after canthotomy and cantholysis. The skin-
muscle flap is drawn over and closure is completed.
D. Final result.

(Fox, S. A.: Courtesy Archives of Ophthalmology.)

usual full thickness lid resection had been made, a sliding graft of tarsoconjunctiva from the upper lid would have been necessary. The use of the collar-button left the upper lid intact.

REPAIR BY DOUBLE VERTICAL PEDICLES

Central Lunate Coloboma—Upper Lid

A rather unusual type of lid deformity following injury is the lunate or crescent-shaped dehiscence of the lid margin. The loss of tissue is not extensive since the dehiscence is usually shallow, amounting to no more than 4 or 5 mm. at its deepest point. But much of the margin may be involved and with it, of course, the lash line. A good example of this type of lesion is the left upper lid shown in figure 101*A*. This injury, although not striking, requires as much planning and as painstaking a technic as do some of the more serious deformities. The following method has given satisfactory results:

Procedure (fig. 101): The affected portion of the lid margin is split into two layers, debrided and the dissection carried sufficiently beyond the tarsus to obtain adequate mobilization. At the ends of the split, two vertical incisions are made in the tarsoconjunctival layer. Similar incisions are made in the skin-muscle layer but these are placed 2 mm. to the outside of the tarsoconjunctival incisions in order to obtain a halving effect (fig. 101*B*). The two flaps, one of tarsoconjunctiva and the other of skin-muscle, are mobilized by further dissection and pulled down beyond the lid edge so that the point of deepest indentation of the deformity is slightly below the level of the normal lid margin. The excess is resected. The flaps are pulled down somewhat beyond the lid margin to allow for retraction if there is any tension on them.

Three double-armed 4–0 silk sutures are threaded through pegs and passed through both flaps near the lid margin from without inward. One is centrally placed; the two lateral ones are inserted so as to straddle the vertical incisions (fig. 101*C*). The edge of the opposing lid is freshened and the sutures are carried through this edge to come out beyond the lash line where they are tied over pegs. One or two additional sutures are used to close the skin-muscle incisions. Where no eye exists a conformer is inserted into the socket. A monocular dressing with pressure bandage is applied. The eye is redressed on the fifth, eighth and tenth days at which time the sutures are removed. The tarsorrhaphy may be opened in four to six weeks; or lash grafting may be done at this time.

Comment: This may seem like formidable surgery for a lid deformity which is not too striking. But attempts at simplifying the procedure have resulted in failure. Trials at pulling down a solid flap (without splitting) have not been uniformly successful. Also, omission

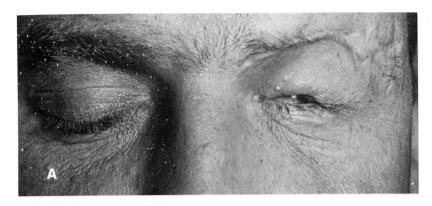

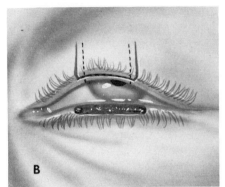
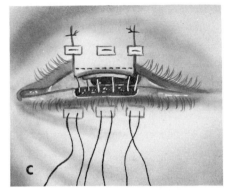

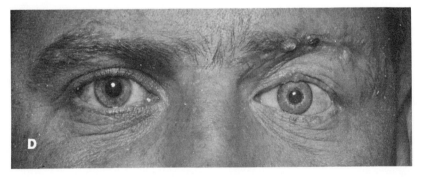

Fig. 101.   Upper Lid Repair by Two Vertical Advancement Flaps (Modified
Halving).

A.   Appearance of lesion of left upper lid with eye closed.
B.   The lid is split and two sliding flaps are created.
     The opposing lid margin is freshened.
C.   The flaps are pulled down to fill the lid coloboma and three double-armed
     sutures are placed. *Broken line,* line of resection of excess tissue.
D.   Result of repair.

of a surgical tarsorrhaphy has resulted in only partial correction with
this technic. As can be seen the result is not beautiful but it is cosmetically useful and functionally acceptable (fig. 101D). Lash grafting
was not done.

Repair of Lower Lid Coloboma

A tumor of the lower lid (fig. 102*A*) was handled by a similar technic because here again the resection was not wide and enough mobility could be attained.

Procedure (fig. 102):   After resection of the lesion the lid is split into its two laminae and two vertical sliding flaps are formed and sutured as in the previous case (fig. 102*B*). The patient is seen before the removal of the sutures (fig. 102*C*). The final result is seen in figure 102*D*.

Comment: Had the lesion been deeper in the lid this technic could not have been used and grafting might have had to be done. Vertical sliding grafts in the lower lid are always hazardous. Unless done in older individuals and unless the resection is narrow, there is always danger of downward lower lid pull. Even here it will be noted that the right lower lid margin is about 1 mm. lower than the left lower margin. On the other hand, *if shallow enough,* even larger lesions may be repaired with this technic. Thus in procedure 134 the whole lower margin was resected and repaired in this way.

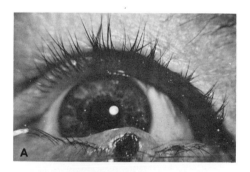
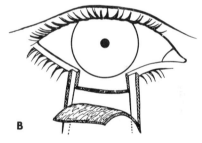
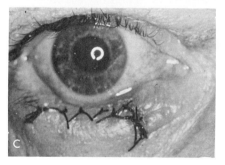
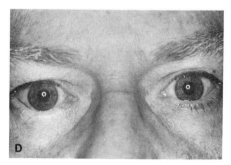

Fig. 102.   Lower Lid Repair by Two Vertical Advancement Flaps (Modified Halving).

A.   Neoplasm of right lower lid.
B.   Resection and preparation of two vertical flaps for halving closure.
C.   Appearance before suture removal.
D.   Final result.

Repair by Temporal Advancement Flap

Figure 103 shows the technic of repair where considerable lid tissue both in length and width has been lost in the temporal half of the lid.

Procedure (fig. 103): The lesion at the lateral canthus of the right lower lid (fig. 103*A*) is resected in toto. A right lateral canthotomy is made and the lower arm of the lateral canthal ligament is severed (fig. 103*B*). The canthotomy incision is extended through skin and muscle outward and slightly upward. At the lower end of the coloboma another horizontal incision is made outward and somewhat downward. The length of these incisions will depend on the length of pedicle necessary to close the defect without tension. It is also important to free the pedicle flap from its attachments to the periosteum and fascia at the orbital margin.

When the pedicle has been dissected up several 4–0 plain catgut relaxation sutures are passed through the base of the raw surface of the pedicle, then more medially through the subjacent bed so that, when tied, the pedicle flap will be pulled medially (fig. 103*C*). One of these sutures should catch up some of the periosteal fibers of the external orbital rim which will serve as a good anchor against backward slippage. The lower incision is closed by diagonal interrupted 5–0 silk sutures placed more medially in the fixed lip of the wound so that, when tied, the pedicle is again advanced medially. Similar sutures are placed in the upper incision as far as the canthus (fig. 103*D*).

When the pedicle flap is approximated and sutured the cut conjunctiva is undermined, brought up and sutured to the upper margin of the skin-muscle pedicle to recreate the lower lateral fornix. The lower wound may be closed by a figure-8 suture to insure against notching. This is not necessary if closure is easy without tension (fig. 103*E*).

The eye is dressed after 48 hours and then daily until the wound is healed. The sutures are removed on the sixth day. The final result is seen in figure 103*F*.

Comment: This method of coloboma repair is applicable to both upper and lower lids and may be used whether the eyeball is present or not. In the latter case, a conformer is inserted into the empty socket to preserve its proper shape while healing.

Opposing Lid Sliding Grafts

Sliding grafts from opposing lids are being used less these days than formerly. However, there are situations where they are still of value and make for a good repair.

Repair of Central Upper Lid Coloboma

Traumatic colobomata sometimes offer bizarre patterns of destruction. Occasionally a case comes along where the skin loss is minimal

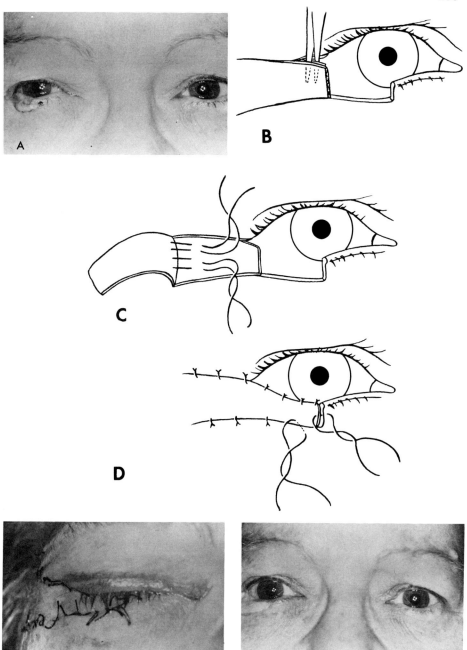

FIG. 103. Repair by Cantholysis and Long Temporal Advancement Flap.

A. Neoplasm of right lower lid.
B. Resection of tumor with canthotomy and cantholysis.
C. Creation of advancement flap and insertion of relaxation sutures.
D. Closure with angulation of skin sutures.
E. Appearance before removal of sutures.
F. Final result.

but where tarsus and conjunctiva are so fibrosed and cicatrized that a good deal of the posterior layer of the lid has to be sacrificed. Figure 104*A* is typical of such a case. Although tissue loss was apparently slight, a large portion of tarsoconjunctiva had to be replaced. If a halving repair had been used, appreciable shortening of the lid would have resulted. The following procedure gives an adequate result in such cases:

Procedure (fig. 104):   The edges of the coloboma are freshened and scar tissue resected; care is taken to remove a minimum of healthy tissue. The lid in the region of the coloboma is split into skin-muscle and tarsoconjunctival layers and the anterior layer is mobilized by dissection. The notch in the tarsoconjunctival layer is converted into a rectangle.

The opposing lower lid is everted and a tongue of tarsoconjunctiva is fashioned to the dimensions of the upper lid coloboma (fig. 104*B*). The flap is mobilized by adequate dissection so that when it is sewed into place there will be no pull on either lid. A double-armed 4–0 braided silk suture is passed through the edge of the flap from without inward (toward the conjunctiva), then through the upper edge of the rectangular dehiscence from the conjunctival to the skin surface and threaded through a peg. If the dehiscence is large, sutures of 4–0 plain catgut may be used on each side to help hold the flap in place (fig. 104*C*). The mattress suture is tied and the flap thus firmly anchored into position.

Another double-armed 4–0 silk suture is threaded through a peg and the needles passed through the marginal edges of the upper skin-muscle lamina from without inward. They are then carried through the skin-muscle layer of the opposite lid from within outward and brought out beyond the lash line and tied over a peg. One or two additional interrupted 5–0 silk sutures are used to complete closure of the skin-muscle wound (fig. 104*C*). A firm dressing is applied with bandage. This is changed on the third day for a patch and the eye dressed daily until complete healing. The sutures are removed on the sixth day.

At the end of six weeks the area of lid fusion is infiltrated with a few drops of procaine and the lids separated with scissors. Ointment is instilled and the eye redressed daily with liberal instillations of ointment until complete epithelialization has taken place. The final result is seen in figure 104*D*.

Comment: If the socket is anophthalmic, as it was here, a conformer should be inserted before closure to assure proper position of the flap and good counterpressure for the dressing. When the notch is near either canthus, the incision splitting the lid is prolonged beyond the canthus to give sufficient mobility to the skin-muscle layer. Whether central or lateral, a canthotomy is not needed.

This was a fortunate repair since the skin only had to be dissected

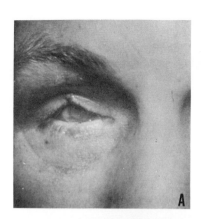
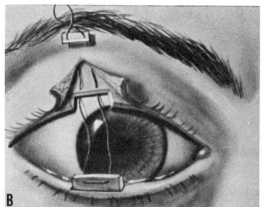
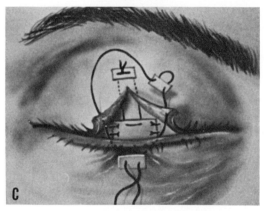
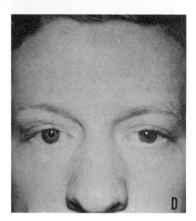

FIG. 104.   Upper Lid Notch Repair by Tarsal Graft from Lower Lid.
A.   Traumatic central notch of right upper lid.
B.   The notch is debrided and converted to a rectangle. A tarsoconjunctival graft is fashioned from the opposing lower lid and drawn up into the upper lid dehiscence. The edges of the skin-muscle wound are mobilized for easy closure.
C.   Closure of the tarsoconjunctival and skin-muscle wounds.
D.   The final result.

up and sutured. It did not have to be drawn up nor brought from elsewhere. Other cases are not so fortunate.

Repair of Central Lower Lid Notch

The technic used in the above case is even better adapted to lower lid repairs. Figure 105A shows a central notch of the lower lid, loss of the eye and shelving of the lower cul-de-sac.

Procedure (fig. 105):   The lower lid is split, debrided and the two lips of the wound mobilized. At this point it becomes evident that there is not enough tarsoconjunctiva. Hence the technic shown in figure 104 is applied here but in reverse. That is, the upper lid opposite the lesion is split and a tarsoconjunctival sliding graft fashioned for the repair

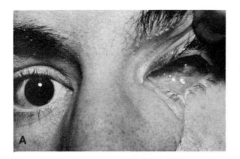
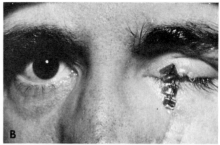
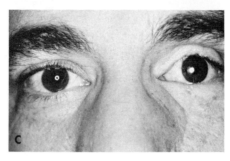

FIG. 105.   Lower Lid Notch Repair by Tarsal Graft from Upper Lid.
A.   Traumatic notch of left lower lid.
B.   Closure with upper lid tarsoconjunctival advancement graft (cf. fig. 104).
Appearance before removal of sutures.
C.   Final result.

of the dehiscence in the lower lid. Figure 105*B* shows the lid at completion of the repair. Figure 105*C* illustrates the final result.

HUGHES PROCEDURE FOR LOWER LID REPAIR

The original Hughes procedure for the repair of lower lid lesions was first reported in 1937. It was popular for many years and is still a useful operation in the armamentarium of lid surgery. As originally done, before modifications began to creep in, repair was made by a tarsoconjunctival graft from the upper lid and a vertical advancement skin flap from below. There was a second stage in the repair in which a lash graft was done as described in Chapter 13. Later this latter step was practically abandoned since the result was rarely worth the effort.

One of the main drawbacks to this procedure is that the repaired lid usually rides lower than the opposite lower lid. This happens no matter how well the skin flap from below is mobilized. Another original drawback was the splitting of the upper lid in the gray line endangering the cilia. As a result, modifications were subsequently made. The upper lid was split as shown in figures 46*C* and *D* and instead of advancing grafts from the lower lid, free grafting was used. These modifications enhanced the value of the technic considerably.

Procedure (fig. 106):   After resection of the lower lid tumor (fig. 106A) the upper and lower lids are united by two tarsorrhaphies (fig. 42). A free whole skin graft is then taken from the ipsilateral upper lid (fig. 106B) and planted into place in the lower lid dehiscence (fig. 106C).

The upper lid lesion is closed and a pressure dressing is applied for 5 or 6 days and then the eye is dressed every other day. Sutures are removed on the first or second dressing (fig. 106D). After 6 weeks the fused lids (fig. 106E) are separated. The final result is seen in figure 106F.

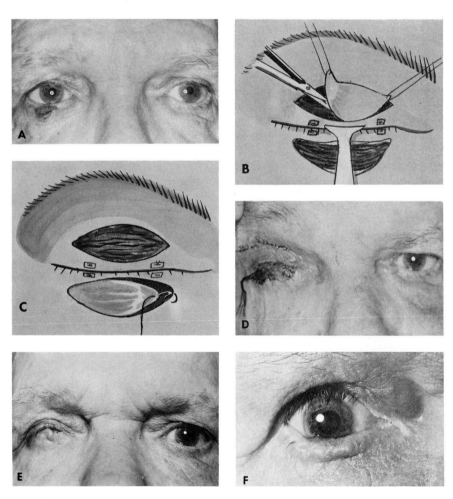

FIG. 106. Modified Hughes Procedure.
A.   Tumor of right lower lid.
B.   Resection of lesion and preparation of skin graft in ipsilateral upper lid.
C.   Suturing of graft.
D.   Appearance before removal of sutures.
E.   Eight weeks later.
F.   Final result.

Comment: Note that the right lower lid margin following this type of correction rides in a normal position as compared with the fellow eye. After six weeks the lid is inspected. If there is a tendency for the upper lid to be pulled down, then it is obvious that there is a shortage of lower lid skin. In such a case the lower lid skin is dissected up and allowed to retract. The dehiscence is then filled with another free-skin graft. If there is no tendency for the upper lid to be pulled down then there is obviously enough lower lid skin present and the lids may be separated and upper lid skin spared.

REFERENCES

Fox, S. A.: Lid halving with variations. Arch. Ophth. *65*:672, 1961.

McLean, H.: Plastic reconstruction of the upper lid. Am. J. Ophth. *24*:46, 1941.

Minsky, H.: Surgical repair of recent lid lacerations. Intermarginal splinting suture. Surg. Gyn. & Obstr. *75*:449, 1942.

Reese, A. B.: Tumors of the Eye. New York, Paul B. Hoeber, Inc., 1951, p. 4.

Wheeler, J. M.: War injuries of the eyelids. Plastic operations for a few types: Case reports with photographs and drawings. Tr. Am. Ophth. Soc. *17*:263, 1919.

————: Restoration of the margin and neighboring portion of the eyelid. J.A.M.A. *75*:1055, 1920.

————: Halving wounds in facial plastic surgery. Proc. 2d Surg. Cong. Pan-Pac. Surg. Assoc., 1936, p. 228.

CHAPTER 9

Surgery at the Medial Canthus

IN GENERAL, medial canthus defects are more difficult to repair than the lateral. This is due to the presence of the puncta and canaliculi which must be preserved if at all possible. A second reason is that the nose is in the way. This leaves little room to maneuver in the nasocanthal angle as compared with the wide open spaces at the temporal end of the lid. If skin is lost at the medial canthus a rotated flap from the forehead may be brought down or a flap from the cheek up. But forehead and cheek skin is much thicker than lid skin and is not a good match; also forehead and cheek scars are quite prominent and take a long time to clear. Free skin grafts are much more acceptable here.

There is one advantage: The medial portions of the lids are rounded and free—or relatively free—of cilia. Hence surgery can be done here without fear of cilia loss.

PERMANENT MEDIAL CLOSURE

Medial Tarsorrhaphy (Arlt)

Temporary tarsorrhaphies are usually medial or paracentral, i.e., somewhere inside the canthi. Permanent lid fusions on the other hand almost always have their greatest locus of usefulness at the canthi.

The medial tarsorrhaphy was used by Arlt in early ectropion to repair eversion of the medial portion of the lower lid along with the punctum. It was also used in old enucleations in which there is shelving of the lower lid with inability to retain a prosthesis. The procedure consists in the resection of a strip of skin all around the margin of the medial canthus nasal to the upper and lower puncta. The raw skin surfaces of the upper and lower lids are then united with 6–0 chromic sutures (fig. 107A). In order to make certain of a permanent result two rows of sutures may be laid down; the inner lips of the upper and lower wounds are closed with 6–0 interrupted chromic catgut sutures. Then the outer lips are closed with 5–0 or 6–0 interrupted silk sutures. The latter are removed on the fifth or sixth day after operation.

Simple Medial Canthoplasty

In unusual conditions where the lower lid is extremely lax it may be necessary to do a small canthoplasty to help bolster an ectropion repair. In such cases the procedure shown in figure 107B is extremely useful.

Procedure (fig. 107B): The lid margins medial to the puncta are freshened as in the previous case and the posterior lips of the wound are sewn together with 6–0 chromic catgut. A rectangle of skin 4 to 5 mm. in width is then resected from the upper lid and a sliding flap of skin is fashioned in the lower lid. The flap is pulled up to cover the bared area in the upper lid and sutured into position with 5–0 or 6–0 interrupted silk sutures.

Since, like the lateral tarsorrhaphy, this procedure narrows as well as shortens the palpebral fissure, another possible indication for it would be advanced exophthalmos in which lateral canthoplasty is not enough to protect the cornea. It has also been suggested for cases of epiphora where the punctal eversion has not responded to other procedures.

It is sometimes used in unusual types of ectropion as a method of desperation. Thus pictured in figure 108 is a case of leontiasis ossea with lower lids so lax that even in closure they hang down exposing the caruncle and plica (figs. 108A and B). Here the regulation Kuhnt-Szymanowski procedure for ectropion did not suffice and bilateral medial tarsorrhaphies had to be done to attain closure of the palpebral fissure (figs. 108C and D). This is one of the rare instances in which this type of tarsorrhaphy is justified.

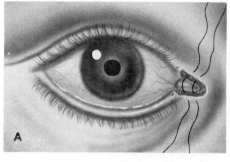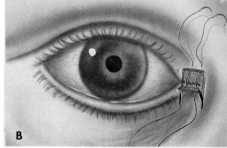

FIG. 107.   Permanent Medial Tarsorrhaphy.
A.   The skin close to and surrounding the medial canthus is resected and upper and lower denuded areas are united. Puncta and canaliculi are preserved.
B.   For a firmer closure the posterior lips of the upper and lower lid wounds are united with a running suture of 6–0 chromic catgut. A rectangle of skin is resected from the upper lid and a sliding skin flap is fashioned in the lower lid, pulled up and sutured to cover the bared area in the upper lid.

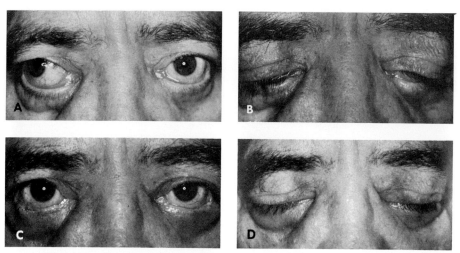

FIG. 108.   Repair of Atonic Ectropion.
A.   Bilateral atonic ectropion.
B.   Exposure of bulb on closure of eye.
C.   Appearance after Kuhnt-Szymanowski ectropion repair and bilateral perma-
nent medial tarsorrhaphy.
D.   Note complete closure now.

To sum up then, indications for a medial tarsorrhaphy are rare.
They include: (1) cases of advanced exophthalmos in which lateral tarsorrhaphy furnishes insufficient corneal protection, (2) cases of unusually lax lower lids which are not responsive to ordinary ectropion reparative technics, and (3) cases of lower medial punctum eversion which
cannot be repaired by other methods of reinversion.

Since the permanent medial tarsorrhaphy covers the caruncle and
plica and hence constitutes a cosmetic blemish, it is used only when all
other methods are contraindicated or have failed.

Medical Canthoplasty (Strampelli and Valvo)

Strampelli and Valvo have developed an ingenious procedure for the
correction of excessive width at the medial canthus as seen in paralytic
lagophthalmos (fig. 109A).

Procedure (fig. 109):   Two conjunctival flaps are resected on the
nasal side of the inner lid surface including the mucosa of the caruncle
itself. However, the central portion of the caruncle which is directly
opposite the palpebral fissure is spared (fig. 109B). A stout double-armed
silk suture is then passed from the skin surface of the upper lid, through
the cut upper conjunctival lip, through the caruncle, through the lip of
the lower conjunctival wound, then out to the skin surface of the lower
lid (fig. 109C).

When the suture is tied, each of the previously excised areas "fold

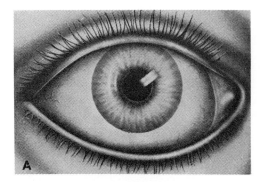
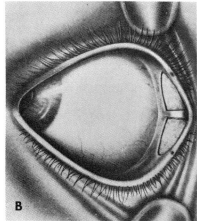
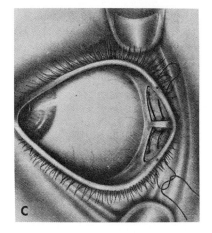
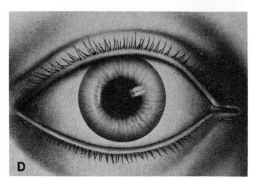

Fig. 109.   Medial Canthoplasty (Strampelli and Valvo).

A. Paralytic exophthalmos with excessively wide medial canthus.

B. Resection of medial conjunctival flaps including mucosa of caruncle except central portion opposite the fissure.

C. A stout double-armed silk suture is passed from the skin surface of the upper lid through the upper conjunctival lip, caruncle, lower conjunctival lip and out to the skin of the lower lid.

D. Final result.

(Strampelli, B., and Valvo, A.: Courtesy American Journal of Ophthalmology.)

like the pages of a book." Correction is obtained by symblepharon between the end of each excised area to its respective part of the caruncle and thus the medial canthus is narrowed (fig. 109D).

This procedure has been used successfully for three years by the authors.

Shortening of the Medial Canthal Ligament

Shortening of the ligament at the medial canthus is sometimes done for blepharophimosis in conjunction with epicanthus. The object of this is to draw the medial canthus nasally since in blepharophimosis there is usually too wide a medial intercanthal space. Shortening is most simply effected by tucking.

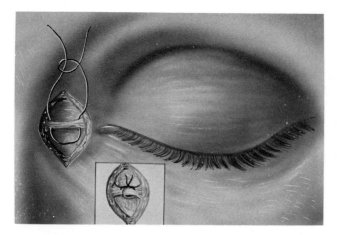

FIG. 110. Tucking of the Medial Canthal Ligament.
An incision is made as for lacrimal sac exposure and the medial canthal ligament is exposed. A stout white silk or linen suture is passed through the ligament and tied, thus creating a tuck with shortening.

Procedure (fig. 110): Exposure of the medial canthal ligament is made as for a sac operation. Once in view, a stout white silk or linen suture is passed close to the bony attachment of the ligament. The needle is then passed through the ligament again about 5 or 6 mm. more laterally. The suture is tied and the ligament thus tucked. If too much of a bite is taken it will not be possible to effect a complete tuck as the ligament only has so much give, especially in the young. However, a shortening of 4 to 5 mm. is usually possible. When done bilaterally a wide medial intercanthal space may be appreciably narrowed.

If, after dissection, there is not enough mobility of the ligament, the orbital fascia is incised above and below the ligament as shown in figure 117. This permits better mobilization and hence more freedom of movement of the ligament. The insertion of a lacrimal probe into the lower canaliculus helps identification and avoids injury to the delicate canaliculi.

Comment: This procedure is usually done in conjunction with a lateral canthoplasty and cantholysis which allows the lids to be pulled medially still more easily and hence facilitates the procedure. (See Congenital Blepharophimosis Chapter 18.)

EPICANTHUS

The most important type of epicanthus is congenital. This is discussed in Chapter 18. Two additional types deserve a word here.

Cicatricial Epicanthus

As its name implies, cicatricial epicanthus is usually traumatic and is frequently accompanied by ankyloblepharon, downward displacement of the canthus, ectropion and injury to the canaliculi. Often the eye is lost. Such repairs are not easy because a complication of conditions usually exists.

In the rare cases where cicatricial epicanthus is present in uncomplicated form the repair may be made by Z plasty as described below (fig. 117).

Senile Epicanthus

Under the heading of "external blepharophimosis" Fuchs has described a type of lateral epicanthus seen in older individuals which he ascribed to chronic conjunctival irritation and senile subcutaneous atrophy (fig. 246). Actually this is more properly an epicanthus senilis lateralis because there is no diminution in the size of the palperbal fissure as in a true blepharophimosis.

A similar type of epicanthus senilis medialis seen occasionally is due entirely to senile skin atrophy (fig. 111). The treatment for both medial and lateral senile epicanthus is simple excision of the excess skin.

Miscellaneous Medial Canthus Repairs

Repair of Upper Lid Coloboma

Figure 112*A* presents an upper lid traumatic coloboma at the medial canthus of the right eye. As stated previously, the choice of procedure here is limited as compared to a lateral or centrally placed lesion. The nose does not offer an ideal site from which to borrow an advancement flap. The forehead offers a rotated pedicle but the thickness of the skin and the resultant conspicuous scar makes this choice a last resort. Also, if a functioning canaliculus is present, careful, finicky dissection is called for and this does not add to the ease of the operation.

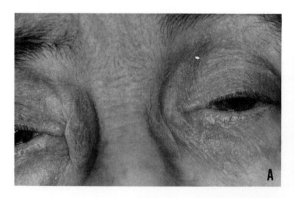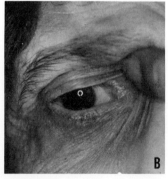

FIG. 111.   Epicanthus Senilis.
A.   Bilateral   epicanthus   senilis   medialis.
B.   Note marked skin relaxation.

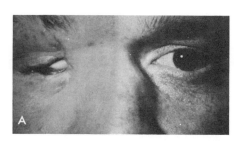
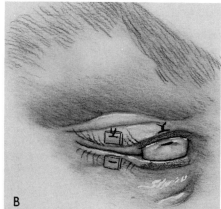
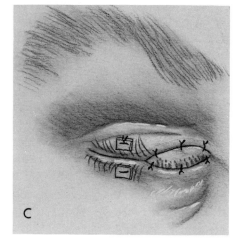
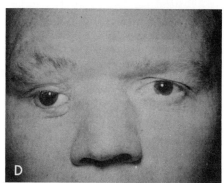

FIG. 112.   Repair of Medial Half of Upper Lid.
A.   Coloboma of medial half of right upper lid.
B.   The medial portion of the upper lid is split as is the opposing lower lid. The tarsoconjunctiva of the lower lid is sutured to the conjunctival remnant of the upper lid. A lateral tarsorrhaphy is fashioned.
C.   A free hair-bearing graft is planted in the upper lid dehiscence.
D.   Final result with prosthesis in place.

Fortunately or unfortunately, both upper and lower canaliculi were destroyed here, hence this aspect of the surgery was simplified. In addition the patient had sustained loss of his right eye. Repair was made as follows:

Procedure (fig. 112):   The remnants of the medial half of the upper lid are split into skin-muscle and tarsoconjunctival layers and all scar tissue is resected. The lower lid is split similarly and a tarsoconjunctival sliding graft fashioned. This is sutured to the remaining tarsoconjunctiva of the upper lid (fig. 112B). The outer halves of the lids are united by a temporary tarsorrhaphy. A hair-bearing skin graft cut to pattern is taken from the left brow and sewed into position over the tarsoconjunctival graft with interrupted 5–0 silk sutures. The lower edge is sewed to the skin-muscle layer of the lower lid (fig. 112C). The wound in the left brow is closed with interrupted sutures, the eye dressed and a firm pressure dressing is applied. On the sixth day the sutures are removed from both wounds and the pressure dressing reapplied for four more days.

Eight weeks later the lids are separated and the edges permitted to epithelialize. The final result is shown in figure 112D.

Comment: In appearance this case is not unlike some of the upper lid notches previously discussed. However, there was much loss of full thickness tissue from the medial half of the upper lid and on dissection so much scar tissue had to be excised from the nasal angle that the best course was to graft both tarsus and skin. The method chosen accomplished the repair with least scarring and least shuffling and distortion of both upper and lower lid tissues. This is also a good example of a hair-bearing graft used for the combined purpose of lash graft and lid margin repair (see Chapter 13).

Avulsion of the Lid from the Medial Canthus

Avulsion of the lower lid from the medial canthus is one of the commoner eye injuries. Unfortunately the continuity of the lower canaliculus is also usually destroyed. The method of repair will vary according to how long a time has elapsed after injury. Needless to say, the sooner the case is seen the easier the repair and the better the result. Early repair of the canaliculus may mean the difference between retention and loss of a functioning tear mechanism. Once cicatrization has set in, welding the ends of a torn canaliculus together to make a functioning tear channel becomes an almost hopeless task; this despite the remarkable cures of old canalicular tears found in the literature. (The repair of canalicular injuries is discussed more fully in Chapter 23.)

Early Repair of Avulsed Lid

Lid avulsion is easier to repair if done early (within 48 hours after injury) before there is cicatrization and retraction. Both the medial and lateral canthi and hence the ends of the lids are inserted at a point posterior to the anterior plane of the eye. The lateral canthal ligament inserts into the lateral orbital tubercle behind the lateral rim of the orbit. The medial palpebral ligament inserts into the region of the anterior lacrimal crest and forms a palpable prominence. In addition, this end of the lid is supported by the lacrimal fascia and Horner's muscle which insert into the *posterior* lacrimal crest and prevent ectropion when the canthal ligament is cut. Hence, in any repair, the medial (as well as the lateral) end of the lid must be fastened sufficiently posteriorly to regain its normal position. In the early cases (fig. 113A) the technic of repair is as follows:

Procedure (fig. 113): Repair of the canaliculus is described in

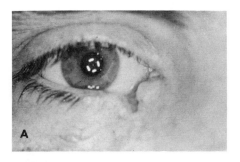

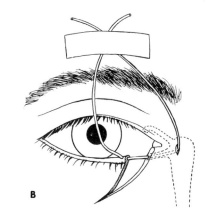

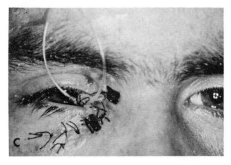

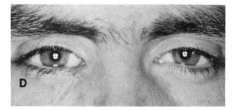

FIG. 113.   Early Repair of Lower Lid Medial Avulsion.
A.   Tear of left lower lid through canaliculus.
B.   Repair of canaliculus as described in Procedure 286.
C.   A double-armed suture, through pegs, fastens the lower lid to the medial
     canthal ligament (see fig. 114C). The skin and conjunctiva are sutured
     separately.
D.   Final result.

Chapter 23 (fig. 286). The conjunctiva is then sutured with 6–0 chromic
catgut while there is good exposure, before the skin is repaired. This may
be done from before backward, i.e., the sutures are passed through the
tarsoconjunctival side, repassed forward and knotted on the tarsus.
This is not only easier than everting the lid and suturing the conjunctival
surface but has the additional virtue of avoiding knots which press on
the globe.

A double-armed 4–0 silk suture is threaded on cutting needles which
are of sufficient size and thickness to be passed through the periosteum.
They are threaded on a peg and are passed through the full lid thickness
of the upper edge of the lateral lip of the wound below the margin so as
to avoid injury to the canaliculus. The needles are continued behind and
above the normal position of the nasal attachment of the medial canthal
ligament and brought out on the skin surface above the normal site
of the ligament where the sutures are tied over a peg. The medial end of
the avulsed lid should now be in a position of overcorrection, i.e., slightly
higher than the opposite fellow lid (fig. 113C). The process of healing
usually causes it to sink a little so that cosmetically the final result is
good.

The skin wound is sutured and the marginal approximation is carefully made to avoid notching. The skin sutures may be angled upward so that the lateral wound lip is drawn higher as well as inward. Subsequent treatment follows as for canaliculoplasty described elsewhere. The final result is seen in figure 113D.

Comment: Destruction may be so severe and bony loss so great that the medial canthus is disorganized and periosteal suturing cannot be done. In those cases the lid must be fastened to the bone by means of steel wire through holes drilled into the bone.

Some surgeons wire the lid end routinely into the lacrimal crest in this type of repair. The author has had satisfactory results with stout silk sutures. The important point is that the wound edges should come together without tension and with no tendency to pull apart. Under such conditions nature will heal the wound whether it is held together by steel or silk sutures.

Late Repair of Avulsed Lid

Procedure (fig. 114): In old cases the first step is to excise all scar tissue no matter how extensive the dissection as subsequent contraction of remaining fibrous tissue can mar the repair. (It is assumed that no canalicular repair will be done here as this is always unsuccessful in old cases. However, there is nothing to stop the surgeon from trying his luck should he so desire.)

An incision from the canthus is made down and outward and the skin well undermined. This incision should not be straight but curved or beveled. The object of this is to minify drag on the lower lid and provide a larger healing area for the flap. If the injury is severe and an appreciable amount of tissue has been lost it will be necessary to do a canthotomy and an inferior cantholysis, i.e., cut the lower arm of the lateral canthal ligament in order to attain better mobility (fig. 114B).

Thus the lower lid is converted into a large sliding flap which should come into position easily without tension. It is important now to see whether any conjunctival defect exists. If present, this is closed with interrupted 6–0 chromic catgut sutures.

At the medial end of the lid margin a double-armed 4–0 silk suture is passed through the apex of the flap. The two needles are then passed deep to the attachment of the medial canthal ligament and slightly above to achieve some overcorrection as in the previous procedure. In this way the lid angle is brought up high enough and posterior enough to lie snugly against the eyeball.

Closure of the skin wound is made with 5–0 silk sutures placed diagonally and starting at the outer end of the wound. The sutures are angled so that they are more medial in the fixed lip of the wound than in the flap, hence when tied, the lid is drawn nasally (fig. 114C).

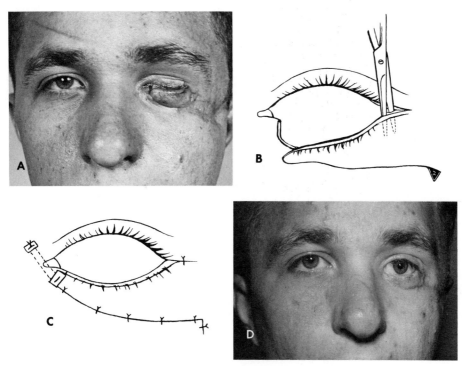

FIG. 114.   Late Repair of Medial Lower Lid Avulsion.
A.   Avulsion and cicatrization of left lower lid.
B.   Canthotomy and cantholysis of lower arm of lateral canthal ligament.   The
     lid is mobilized by wide incision and converted into a sliding flap.   The
     conjunctival cul-de-sac is repaired.
C.   The lid is drawn up under the medial canthal ligament by means of a
     mattress suture.   A Burow's triangle resection counteracts lateral wrinkling.
D.   Result six weeks later with prosthesis in place.

When the nasal area is reached and the wound becomes more perpendicular, the sutures are angled up and medially so as to help pull the lid up and in. Sometimes, if difficulty is encountered in drawing the lid medially, more traction is obtained by subcutaneous relaxation sutures.

At the temporal end of the skin incisions a pucker may form because of the pull of the flap medially. This is corrected by the excision of a small Burow triangle of skin and suture. A pressure dressing is applied for 48 hours and the wound then dressed daily until healed. Skin sutures are removed on the sixth day. The double-armed suture is removed on the ninth or tenth day. The final result is seen in figure 114D.

Comment: If the canaliculus has been repaired, caution must be used not to undo this. Fortunately, the common canaliculus and punctum lie deep to the ligament and can usually be avoided. Obviously, in older cases in which the canaliculus is beyond repair, the operation is simpler—unfortunately.

Repair of Medial Avulsion of Both Lids

The same trauma which so often wreaks havoc at the medial canthus with the lower lid can cause avulsion of both lids. This is not an uncommon injury and, although repair is somewhat more difficult, a good cosmetic result can be attained if the above technic is expanded to include both lids.

Procedure (fig. 115):   Tears in the canaliculi are repaired as described in Chapter 23. The conjunctiva is then sutured since it will be more difficult to get at this layer once the lids have been fastened into position. The repair is made with 6–0 chromic catgut to avoid symblephara and to assure as normal a cul-de-sac as possible postoperatively.

One needle of a double-armed 4–0 silk suture threaded on large curved cutting needles is passed through the upper lateral edge of the lower lid wound taking a good bite. The other needle is passed in similar fashion through the lip of the opposing torn upper lid. Both needles are now passed deep to the attachment of the medical canthal ligament, the lower needle being passed upward and inward, the upper downward and inward. The needles are brought out on the skin surface within a few millimeters of each other and tied over a peg. As the sutures are tied the lids are drawn medially and slightly backward into their normal position (fig. 115*B*). The external skin wounds are closed and again care is taken to line up the margins to avoid notching (fig. 115*C*).

Postoperative care is the same as outlined above for single lid avulsion. The double-armed suture is kept in place at least 10 days to assure good healing. The skin sutures may be removed on the fifth or sixth day. The final result is seen in figure 115*D*.

Comment: As described above, the same double-armed suture used to repair avulsion at the lower lid is used to repair simultaneous upper and lower lid avulsion. And it works just as well, as may be seen in figure 115*D*. Obviously the figure-8 suture cannot be used here because the suture has to be anchored in the medial canthal ligament.

Lower Lid Tumor Repair

Neoplasms at the medial canthus are a double hazard. Not only does adequate tumor resection and repair have to be done but the additional problem of trying to retain a functioning canaliculus is also always present. Frequently, resection of the tumor means cutting into the canaliculus and its probable destruction. This is a problem not easily solved and rarely avoided because neoplasms are common in this area. If the tumor is small and the punctum not closely involved a way out is careful surgery or irradiation. However, even with the greatest care canalicular obstruction by irradiation can and does happen.

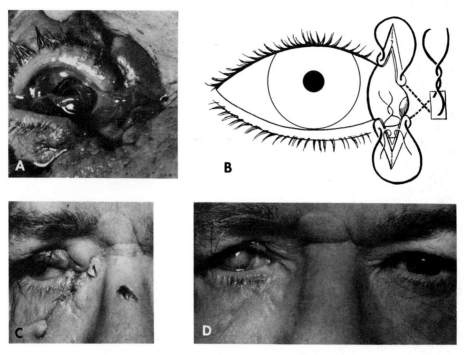

FIG. 115. Repair of Medial Avulsion of Both Lids.
A. Appearance of right upper and lower lids before operation.
B. Schema of repair: Insertion of double-armed suture to repair marginal
   break in both lids. Needles are then passed under insertion of medial
   canthal ligament. Conjunctiva and skin are closed separately.
C. Appearance after completion of operation with all the sutures in place.
D. Final result.

In the case of larger lesions which surround the punctum and
canaliculus both surgery and irradiation will endanger them. The insertion of lacrimal probes and other maneuvers for protecting the
canaliculus against substantial amounts of irradiation are not an
unqualified success. The writer has seen permanent canalicular obstruction after radiation therapy followed by a subsequent recurrence of the
tumor. On the other hand it is possible to resect the whole tumor surgically with some chance of maintaining canalicular drainage as shown
below.

When a tumor involving the lower punctum is resected an attempt
to preserve tear conduction—even though the chances are small—should
be made. Naturally this makes for more elaborate surgery.

The patient (fig. 116A) gave the common history of a growth in the
inner corner of the right eye which had been present for about ten years
and which had begun to increase in size the past year. Inspection disclosed an epithelioma of the medial quarter of the right lower lid margin
involving the punctum.

Procedure (fig. 116): After suitable local anesthesia a lacrimal probe is inserted into the canaliculus and the tumor is resected in toto including 3 mm. of normal tissue all around. Nasally the tissue is dissected around the probe which remains in situ (fig. 116*B*). On completion of the resection the probe is removed and a 4–0 silk suture is immediately threaded through the remaining portion of the canaliculus on a blunt pointed needle which is brought to the skin surface 3 mm. more medially (fig. 116*C*). The technic is described in Chapter 23, figure 283.

The portion of the lid from which the tumor is resected is divided into skin-muscle and tarsoconjunctival laminae. Two vertical sliding flaps are created by vertical incisions, the skin flap being 2 mm. wider on each side than the tarsoconjunctival flap in order to attain halving.

The opposing margin of the upper lid is denuded of epithelium and split for a short distance to create two lips. The tarsoconjunctival flap of the lower lid is pulled up and the vertical conjunctival incisions to each side closed with 6–0 chromic catgut (fig. 116*C*). The flap is then sutured to the posterior lip of the upper lid margin. The skin-muscle flap is pulled up and sutured to the anterior lip of the upper lid margin and the vertical skin incisions are closed with 5–0 silk. Two intermarginal sutures are inserted on each side of the flaps to act as supportive sutures and to assure that the sliding flaps do not retract (fig. 116*D*).

The skin sutures are removed on the sixth day and the intermarginal sutures on the tenth day (fig. 116*E*). The canalicular suture is removed in five weeks. The tarsorrhaphy is opened eight weeks after operation (fig. 116*F*). The final result is shown in figure 116*G*. Note the new large opening into the canaliculus (fig. 116*F*).

Comment: This procedure has its failures and in some cases the new punctum will close no matter what is done, as happened here. On the whole, however, the surgery will be at least as successful as the use of irradiation and will give fewer recurrences.

Downward Displacement of the Canthus

Displacement of the canthus is not seen frequently. This is fortunate because such cases are usually complicated since the trauma causing them must of necessity be extensive and severe. Along with displacement of the canthus, one usually finds cicatricial epicanthus, lagophthalmos and ankyloblepharon, as well as partial lid loss, destruction of the caruncle and canaliculi and, frequently, loss of the globe.

One of the better methods of attaining a repair is by a Z incision which includes the ptosed canthus in the lower angle. It is frequently necessary to do a canthotomy and cantholysis of the lateral canthal ligament to assure adequate mobility of the lids. Figure 117*A* shows a typical case, a war casualty, caused by shell fragments. There is a vertical

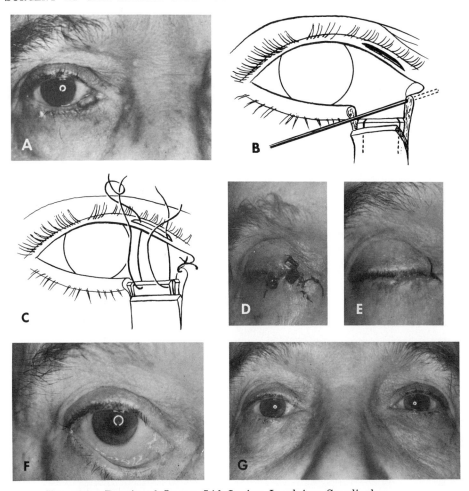

FIG. 116. Repair of Lower Lid Lesion Involving Canaliculus.

A. Tumor involving right lower punctum and canaliculus.

B. A lacrimal probe is inserted into the canaliculus and the tumor is resected with a rim of healthy tissue all around it.

C. A suture is threaded into the remnants of the canaliculus, brought out medially and knotted (cf. fig. 283). The cut edge of the lower lid is split into two laminae as is the opposing lid. The flaps from the lower lid are pulled up and sutured to the homologous laminae of the upper lid.

D. Intermarginal sutures are inserted on each side of the flaps to act as supports. Appearance before removal of sutures.

E. Appearance before separation of the lids with the canalicular suture in place.

F. Showing the new opening into the canaliculus after suture removal.

G. Final result.

scar running across the forehead down through the medial end of the left brow and through the left medial canthus. The canaliculi are severed. The globe had been enucleated. The medial canthus is displaced downward.

Procedure (fig. 117): A Z incision is made with each arm of the incision measuring about 10 mm. The displaced canthus is enclosed by

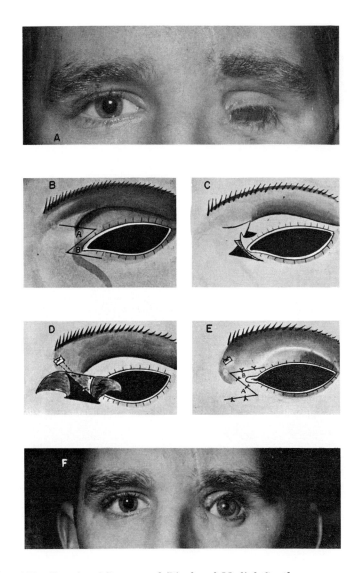

FIG. 117.   Repair of Downward Displaced Medial Canthus.
A. Displacement of left medial canthus downward and outward with blepharo-
phimosis.
B. A Z-incision is made in the skin and muscle.
C. The resultant flaps are dissected up and the remains of the medial canthal
ligament are mobilized from the surrounding tissue.
D. The ligament is sutured into position.
E. The skin flaps are transposed and the wound closed.
F. Result of repair.
   (Fox, S. A.: Courtesy American Journal of Ophthalmology.)

the angle B (fig. 117B). The relative sizes of the angles A and B depend
on how much displacement there is, i.e., the more downward displacement the larger the angle A is as compared with the angle B. However,

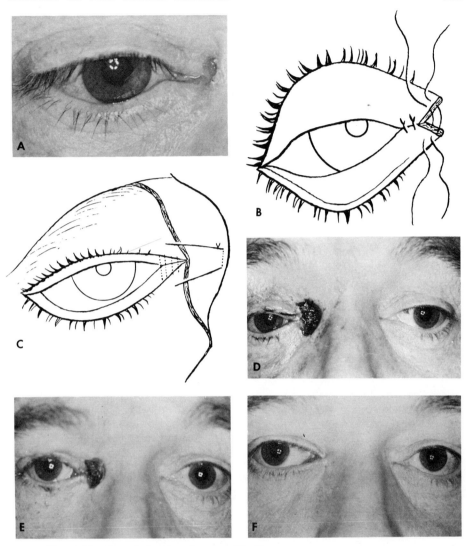

FIG. 118. Repair by Spontaneous Healing.
A. Basal cell epithelioma of right nasocanthal angle.
B. Resection of lesion with medial portion of both lids and repair of medial
fornix.
C. Attachment of lids to nasal periosteum.
D. and E. Appearance four and eleven days respectively after resection.
F. Final result six weeks later.

one must always keep in mind what has been said previously about Z
plasties (Chapter 4), i.e., the triangles should not be larger than about
50° or transposition will be difficult.

The two triangular skin-muscle flaps are undermined and freely
mobilized so that they may be easily transposed (fig. 117C). This is
accomplished by free incision of the orbital fascia and excision of
all fibrous tissue. However, the medial canthal ligament and its surround-

ing tissue is spared and left attached to the lower skin flap. A canthotomy is made and the inferior arm of the lateral ligament cut if necessary for mobility. The skin flaps are transposed and the canthal ligament is drawn medially and sutured to the lacrimal crest with a double-armed 4–0 chromic catgut suture (fig. 117D). Additional subcuticular sutures are used to suture the flaps to the periosteum. The skin incisions are closed with interrupted 5–0 silk sutures (fig. 117E). At the close there should be some overcorrection to allow for subsequent healing back-pull. A firm supportive dressing is applied. The postoperative care is as usual. Sutures are removed on the fifth or sixth postoperative day. The final result is seen in figure 117F.

Comment: See discussion after figures 128 and 129, Chapter 10.

Repair by Natural Granulation

Neoplasms in the nasocanthal angle, when large, offer serious and difficult problems of repair and reconstruction. In the past few years a simplified method for the repair of this type of lesion was reported. This is discussed more fully in Chapter 11, figure 133. The lesion seen in figure 118 is a rather small one and hence is included here.

Procedure (fig. 118): The lesion seen in the right nasocanthal angle is resected in toto and deeply enough to assure complete removal; this may include, as here, the medial portion of the lids with their puncta and canaliculi. The lids are everted and the cut conjunctiva is sutured to recreate a medial fornix (fig. 118B). A double-armed suture is passed through the cut ends of both lids and then through the nasal periosteum and the suture is tied snugly to prevent lid retraction (fig. 118C). The wound is then allowed to granulate in. Figures 118D and E show the condition of the lesion four and eleven days later respectively. The final result seen in figure 118F, attained by allowing nature to do the repair, is probably at least as good as could be gotten by grafting. The reader is referred to figures 62 and 133 for the minutiae of this type of repair.

REFERENCES

ARLT, C. F.: Graefe-Saemisch Handbuch des Ges. Augenh. Berlin, G. Reimer, 1841.
BERGER, E.: Nouveau procédé operatoire pour l'epicanthus. Arch. d'Ophth. *18*:453, 1898.
BLAIR, V .P., BROWN, J. B., and HAMM, W. G.: Surgery of the inner canthus and related structures. Am. J. Ophth. *15*:498, 1932.
CALLAHAN, A.: Reconstruction at the canthi. Tr. Am. Acad. Ophth. & Oto. *51*:485, 1948.
Fox, S. A.: Some methods of lid repair and reconstruction. V. Displacement of the canthi. Am. J. Ophth. *31*:317, 1948.
Fox, S. A., and BEARD, C.: Spontaneous lid repair. Am. J. Ophth. *58*:947, 1964.
FUCHS, E.: Textbook of Ophthalmology, ed. 5. Philadelphia, J. B. Lippincott Co., 1917, p. 953.
HUGHES, W. L.: Surgical treatment of congenital palpebral phimosis. Arch. Ophth. *54*:586, 1955.

JOHNSON, C. C.: Operation for epicanthus and blepharophimosis. Am. J. Ophth. *41*:71, 1956.

SANDERSON, R. S., and RAPPAPORT, I.: Technic of reconstruction of carcinoma of the inner canthus. Am. Surg. *31*:625, 1965.

SPAETH, E. B.: Further considerations of the surgical correction of blepharophimosis (epicanthus). Am. J. Ophth. *41*:61, 1956.

STRAMPELLI, B., and VALVO, A.: Correction of excessive width of the inner canthus. Am. J. Ophth. *63*:330, 1967.

CHAPTER 10

Surgery at the Lateral Canthus

PERMANENT SHORTENING OF
  PALPEBRAL FISSURE
  FUCHS LATERAL CANTHOPLASTY
  ELSCHNIG LATERAL CANTHOPLASTY
  GOLDSTEIN LATERAL CANTHOPLASTY
  WHEELER LATERAL CANTHOPLASTY
  SHORTENING OF LATERAL CANTHAL
    LIGAMENT

LENGTHENING OF PALPEBRAL
  FISSURE
  VON AMMON TECHNIC
  AGNEW TECHNIC
  BLAIR (ET AL.) TECHNIC

REPAIR OF ROUNDED LATERAL
  CANTHUS
  ARROWHEAD (WICHERKIEWICZ)
    TECHNIC
  LATERAL CANTHOPLASTY

REPAIR OF LATERAL CANTHUS
  DISPLACEMENT

NEOPLASMS OF LATERAL
  CANTHUS

T HE LATERAL CANTHUS with its wide open temporal region is an easier area to work in than the medial. There is no lacrimal system to be concerned about and there is plenty of space from which to draw advancement grafts if necessary.

PERMANENT SHORTENING OF THE PALPEBRAL FISSURE

The lateral canthus is not uncommonly the seat of a permanent canthoplasty designed to shorten the palpebral fissure. The most common reasons for this are:

a. To effect closure of the palpebral fissure as in exophthalmos and facial nerve palsy in order to protect the cornea.

b. To shorten too long a palpebral fissure.

c. To repair a rounded lateral canthus for cosmetic purposes.

Several classic procedures for lateral canthoplasty or tarsorrhaphy are available. The variations in technic are minimal and all are useful. Among these are those of Fuchs, Elschnig, Goldstein and Wheeler. The lids are interchangeable in all four procedures, i.e., the skin-muscle flap from lower to upper or upper to lower lid may be reversed to fit the requirements of the case at hand. Thus in the four types of procedures shown the Fuchs and Wheeler show sliding flaps from the lower to the upper lid and the Elschnig and Goldstein technics are examples of sliding grafts from the upper to the lower lid. Any one may be reversed.

Fuchs Lateral Canthoplasty

Procedure (fig. 119): The amount of palpebral fissure to be closed is estimated and measured with a millimeter rule. This may be determined by pinching the two lids together at the outer canthus.

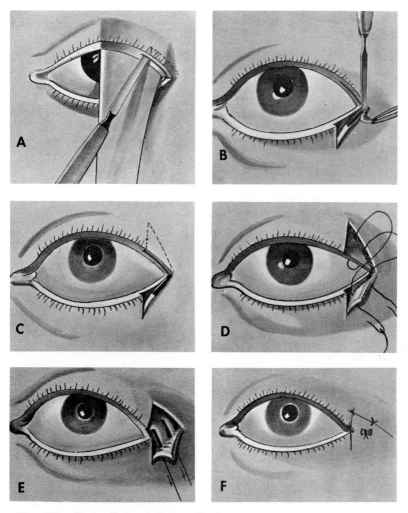

FIG. 119. Fuchs Lateral Tarsorrhaphy.

A. The outer margins of the upper and lower lids are split into two laminae.
B. At the medial end of the lower lid split the anterior layer is incised vertically and the included ciliary margin is resected.
C. The skin-muscle segment to be resected from the upper lid is marked off.
D. After resection a double-armed suture is placed.
E. The suture is tautened and the lower flap drawn up.
F. Additional skin sutures are added to close the wound.

Both lids are split at the lateral canthus into skin-muscle and tarsoconjunctival layers for the previously estimated amount (fig. 119*A*). In the upper lid a split of greater depth is necessary to mobilize a tarsoconjunctival flap. A perpendicular cut of about 8 mm. is made in the anterior layer of the lower lid split at its nasal end and the ciliary margin of this segment is resected (fig. 119*B*). A similar vertical incision is made in the skin-muscle layer of the upper lid and the incision is carried from the upper end of this cut outward and downward to the lateral canthal angle. The skin-muscle flap thus outlined is resected (fig. 119*C*). The involved tarsoconjunctival margins are denuded of epithelium.

The needles of a double-armed 4–0 silk suture are carried through the tarsoconjunctiva of the upper lid from within outward to emerge in the upper part of the denuded area about 3 mm. apart. The needles are then passed through the corresponding skin-muscle flap of the lower lid from within outward and the flap is drawn up to cover the denuded tarsus of the upper lid (figs. 119D and E). The sutures are tied over a peg. Additional interrupted silk sutures are used as needed to close the skin wound (fig. 119F). A simple eye patch is applied. The sutures are removed on the sixth postoperative day.

Comment: There is always a tendency for the lids to separate at the medial end of this union. Hence estimates of amount of closure should be generous. In addition to shortening the palpebral fissure, this procedure tends to raise the lateral canthus and hence is useful in some other types of canthal repair as will be shown later.

Elschnig Lateral Canthoplasty

Procedure (fig. 120):   This is practically the same as the Fuchs procedure except that a tarsoconjunctival flap from the upper lid is pulled down into a triangular defect in the lower lid prepared for it by the resection of a similar tarsoconjunctival flap (figs. 120A and B). Here the involved ciliated edges of the upper and lower lids are denuded of cilia and united by interrupted 5–0 silk sutures. However, the cilia may be left intact if it is expected that the tarsorrhaphy may be undone in the near future.

Goldstein Lateral Canthoplasty

Procedure (fig. 121):   This is probably the most logical and cleanly surgical technic of all. After the lateral ends of the lids are split into their two laminae a triangle of skin-muscle is resected from the lateral

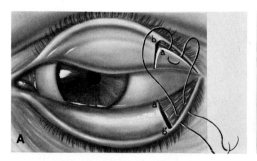 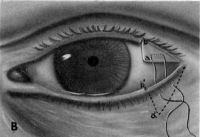

Fig. 120.   Elschnig Lateral Tarsorrhaphy.
A.   The lid margins are split as in the previous procedure and a segment of tarsoconjunctiva is resected from the lower lid. A tarsoconjunctival flap is mobilized in the upper lid.
B.   The flap is drawn down to fill the dehiscence in the lower lid and sutured.

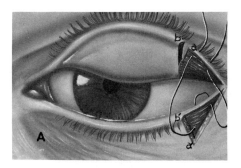 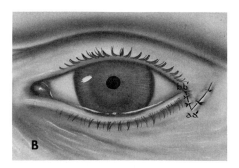

FIG. 121. Goldstein Lateral Tarsorrhaphy.

A. After the margins of both lids are split at the lateral canthus, a triangle of skin-muscle is resected from the lower lid and tarsoconjunctiva from the upper lid. The skin-muscle flap in the upper lid is incised and mobilized.

B. It is pulled down to cover the bared tarsoconjunctiva in the lower lid.

end of one lid and a triangle of tarsoconjunctiva from the other (fig. 121A). The tarsoconjunctival lamina of the one lid may be sutured to the cut end of the conjunctiva of the other lid thus strengthening the union. A vertical incision is then made at the medial end of the bared skin-muscle triangle, creating a flap which is pulled over to cover the bared tarsoconjunctiva of the opposite lid thus mortising the ends of the lids into each other cleanly (fig. 121B). Postoperative care is the same as for the Fuchs tarsorrhaphy.

Wheeler Lateral Canthoplasty

Procedure (fig. 122): This varies somewhat from the above. The upper and lower lids are again split the required amount and the split margins may or may not be freed of epithelium and cilia at the discretion of the surgeon (fig. 122A). A tarsoconjunctival sliding flap is created in the split lower lid by two vertical incisions. A double-armed silk suture is passed from the conjunctival side of the upper lid to emerge in the depths of the lid split. The needles are then brought down through the split and passed through the free margin of the tarsoconjunctival flap of the lower lid from within outward (fig. 122B). They are brought up again through the depth of the upper lid split and through the anterior skin-muscle layer to emerge on the skin surface (fig. 122C). The lower lid tarsoconjunctival flap is thus drawn up into the pocket between skin-muscle and tarsoconjunctiva of the upper lid and the sutures tied over a peg. Additional interrupted sutures are used to close the marginal wound (fig. 122D).

Comment: The four procedures described above accomplish the same thing, i.e., they narrow and shorten the palpebral fissure. However, they have all been included because they differ sufficiently to satisfy varying conditions which may require correction. Furthermore, by leaving the ciliary margins intact, the Elschnig and Wheeler tarsorrhaphies may

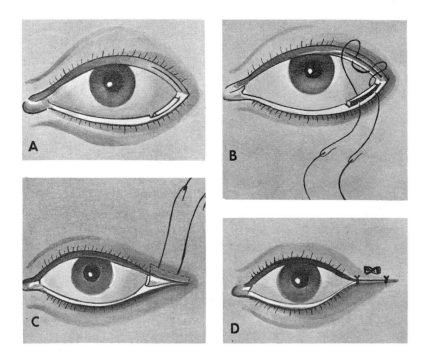

FIG. 122.   Wheeler Lateral Tarsorrhaphy.
A.   The external margins of both lids are split, the laminae of the upper lid are
     separated and a tarsoconjunctival sliding flap is fashioned in the lower lid.
B.   A double-armed suture is passed through the depth of the upper lid split and
     through the edge of the lower tarsal flap.
C.   The flap is drawn up into the upper lid pocket and the sutures passed out
     through the skin.
D.   The wound is closed. The cilia may be left intact.

be undone at any time and the lids restored to their preoperative state if
subsequent improvement occurs. This may not be done if the Fuchs
or Goldstein technics are used.

Summary: The Fuchs procedure shortens the palpebral fissure by
uniting the skin-muscle laminae of the upper and lower lids at the
lateral canthus (fig. 119). The Elschnig technic does the same by means
of the tarsoconjunctival laminae (fig. 120). In the Goldstein procedure a
triangle of skin-muscle is resected from one lid and tarsconjunctiva from
the opposite lid. The resultant bared areas are mortised together (fig.
121). The Wheeler technic creates a pocket between the two laminae of
one lid into which a sliding graft of tarsoconjunctiva from the opposite
lid is drawn (fig. 122). As stated above, in all four technics the lids are
interchangeble, i.e., sliding grafts may be drawn from upper to lower
lid and vice versa.

Shortening of the Lateral Canthal Ligament

Occasionally it is desirable to shorten the lateral palpebral ligament
in addition to shortening the palpebral fissure. This is valuable in some

cases of paralytic lagophthalmos and in exophthalmos, since shortening the ligament causes narrowing of the palpebral fissure as well. (In cases with no lid retraction recession of the levator (fig. 214) is more effective.)

Procedure (fig. 123): The lateral thirds of the upper and lower lids are split into skin-muscle and tarsoconjunctival layers (fig. 123*A*). The

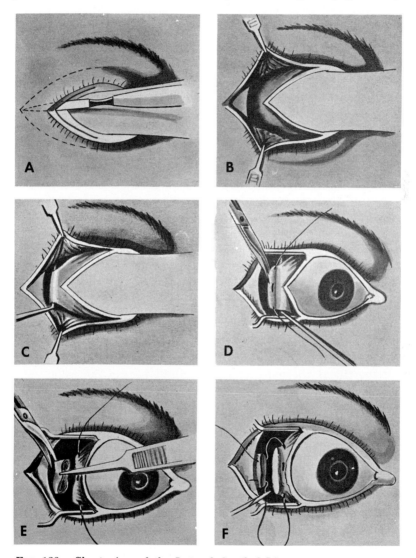

FIG. 123.   Shortening of the Lateral Canthal Ligament.
A.   The lateral thirds of both lids are split.
B.   The skin-muscle layer beyond the external commissure is mobilized and incised and the lateral canthal ligament exposed.
C.   The ligament is brought forward on a muscle hook.
D. and *E.*   A vertical mattress suture is inserted and the central portion of the ligament is resected.
F.   The suture is passed through the lateral stump and tied (After W. W. Weeks.)

skin-muscle layer is undermined laterally well over the external commissure. A horizontal incision through skin and muscle is made over the commissure for better exposure (fig. 123B). The canthal ligament is isolated on a muscle hook and brought forward (fig. 123C). A vertical mattress suture of 3–0 chromic catgut is passed through the ligament from within outward near its tarsal insertion and the middle half of the ligament is resected (fig. 123D). The two needles of the mattress suture are passed into the remaining lateral stub of the ligament and the sutures tied securely (fig. 123E and F). It will be noted that the palpebral fissure is noticeably narrowed as the ligament is drawn laterally and backward. One then proceeds with a lateral canthoplasty as described above if necessary.

Lengthening the Palpebral Fissure

Canthoplasty at the lateral canthal angle may be used as a permanent method of enlarging and lengthening the palpebral fissure. It is so used in blepharophimosis and in plastic repairs and reconstructions. The technic has changed little since von Ammon introduced it over a hundred years ago.

Lateral Canthoplasty (von Ammon)

The easy accessibility of the lateral canthal ligament and the value of canthotomy and cantholysis have already been discussed. Both the latter procedures are preliminary steps in doing lateral canthoplasty.

Procedure (fig. 124):   After doing a canthotomy the temporal conjunctiva is undermined medially (fig. 124A). A 5–0 silk suture is passed through the tip of the conjunctiva, brought out as far as it will come without tension and sutured to the upper lip of the skin wound. Additional sutures are used to unite skin to conjunctiva above and below. Temporally an additional suture unites the two skin edges to each other, since the skin wound is always somewhat longer than the conjunctival wound. Under no condition should the conjunctiva be pulled out forcibly to the lateral apex of the skin wound. This will result in a conjunctival bridle and an unsightly, gaping shallow cul-de-sac.

In order to make certain that the new fornix does not flatten out and gape, a double-armed suture with needles about 4 mm. apart is passed through the conjunctiva of the lateral canthus and brought laterally on the skin surface where the suture is tied over a peg (fig. 124B). This will help deepen the new canthus and keep the edges from everting into a shallow fornix.

It may also be wise at times to interpose a small piece of rubber dam between the two lid margins for two or three days until they epithelialize.

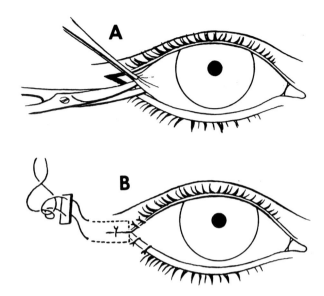

FIG. 124.   Lateral Canthoplasty to Lengthen Palpebral Fissure (von Ammon).
A.   A canthotomy is made and the conjunctiva undermined.
B.   The conjunctiva is pulled out and sutured to the skin edges. The remaining skin incision is closed separately. A double-armed suture is passed through the conjunctiva at the canthus, the needles are brought out lateral to the canthus and tied over a peg.

They sometimes tend to coalesce at the commissure giving a shorter palpebral fissure than planned or expected.

If the amount of fissure lengthening needed is more than the conjunctiva will allow, several methods are available for obtaining more conjunctiva: 1. The conjunctiva may be undermined all the way to the limbus allowing more of it to be pulled over temporally. 2. The bulbar conjunctiva may be extensively undermined and incised as described in figure 144. This will allow still more conjunctiva to be drawn laterally. 3. In cases where the loss of conjunctiva has been still greater a procedure combining free and sliding grafts may be used (fig. 146).

Lateral Canthoplasty (Agnew)

In 1875 Agnew reported his canthoplasty, a modification of the von Ammon procedure. It is interesting to note that this was put forth not as a plastic procedure but as a remedy for treatment in certain forms of corneal and conjunctival diseases especially for phlyctenular or so-called "strumous ophthalmia." Agnew cited 191 cases of eye diseases including panophthalmitis, ectropion and entropion in which the operation was helpful. It was supposed to allow the eye "to have more exposure to air and light."

Procedure (fig. 125):   The first step is a lateral canthotomy as in the von Ammon procedure. Then both arms of the palpebral ligament are sectioned as follows: The arms of the cut ligament are separated and a small blunt-pointed scissors is entered below, between the skin and conjunctiva. The lid is pulled nasally to put the ligament on stretch and the scissors are opened to straddle the ligament which is cut with one snip (fig. 125A). The upper arm of the ligament is cut in similar fashion (fig. 125B). When the arms of the ligament are cut the lid can be felt to give way under the fingers at once. If it fails to yield, another, more careful, attempt is made. Closure of the conjunctiva and skin is exactly as described in the previous procedure.

Comment: This has been a favorite operation for many years. Of course, it is the von Ammon procedure with complete section of the lateral canthal ligament added. But it is a vast improvement on the von Ammon procedure for two important reasons: 1. It increases the length of the palpebral fissure by freeing the attachment of the lids to the palpebral tubercle. 2. It was Agnew who pointed out that the skin incision is always longer than the rest of the canthotomy incision and that no attempt should be made to drag the conjunctiva out to the apex of the skin incision. To do so almost always means obliteration of the lateral fornix and usually results in an unsightly bridle which is especially noticeable in adduction of the eye. This was explained in the previous procedure.

Lateral Canthoplasty (Blair et al.)

Procedure (fig. 126): An incision is made starting at the lateral canthus, running laterally 4 mm., cutting the lateral canthal ligament then curving downward and outward for about 6 mm. The incision then curves upward ending about 7 mm. lateral to and 5 mm. above the

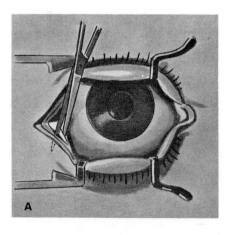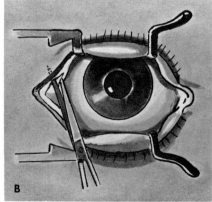

FIG. 125. Canthoplasty (Agnew).
A. Canthotomy and section of the lower arm of the lateral palpebral ligament.
B. Section of the upper arm. Further closure as in figure 124.

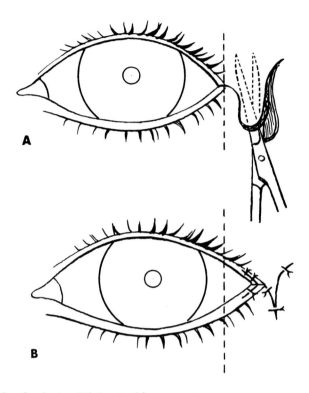

FIG. 126. Canthoplasty (Blair et al.).

A. An incision is made starting at the lateral canthus, curving downward and outward for about 10 mm. and then extended to terminate above the canthus (details are given in text). The resultant flap is undermined and   allowed to retract upward.

B. The conjunctiva is undermined and sutured to its new position at the lid margin and the skin incisions are closed.

canthus. The resultant flap is dissected up, undermined and allowed to retract upward (fig. 126*A*).

The conjunctiva at the canthus is now undermined and sutured to the lower lid without extreme stretching. It is then sutured to the upper lid. Enough sutures are then added to make a good closure of the lid and skin wounds (fig. 126*B*).

It is wise to add here the double-armed suture through the conjunctiva at the lateral canthus as was described in the previous procedure. This will keep the canthus from flattening and help deepen it.

ROUNDED LATERAL CANTHUS

Rounded lateral canthus is occasionally seen as the result of congenital malformation, trauma (fig. 127*C*) or following lid reconstruction. Several methods of repair are available of which two are described below.

Arrowhead Repair (Wicherkiewicz) Modified

Procedure (fig. 127):   About 10 mm. temporal to the outer canthal angle, an arrowhead incision is made pointing outward. The more correction desired, the more obtuse the inner angle is made, for then the pull required to unite the two angles will be greater. Indeed, it may be necessary at times simply to mark out a complete triangle, apex outward, in order to get enough pull laterally to cause acute angulation of the skin at the canthus. The skin and muscle included within the boundaries of the incision are resected (fig. 127A) and the tissue around the canthus is undermined just enough to allow the wound lips to come together without tension. Closure is effected with 4–0 plain catgut subcuticular sutures and 5–0 silk interrupted skin sutures (fig. 127B). Sometimes it may be necessary to use a mattress suture tied over a peg as a stay suture. A firm supportive dressing is applied. The wound is dressed at two-day intervals and the sutures removed on the fifth day. The final result is seen in figure 127D.

Comment: This is a modification of Wicherkiewicz's original technic for the repair of congenital epicanthus. Like most resection technics for epicanthus it is not particularly successful. However, it is quite effective when used to angulate a rounded lateral canthus as in this case.

Repair by Lateral Canthoplasty

Another technic, i.e., use of the lateral canthoplasties, has already been described above. These, of course, also shorten the palpebral fissure but even this is preferable to the unsightliness of a rounded canthus.

Recently Tenzel has reported a method of rounded lateral canthus repair by crossing the tenotomized halves of the lateral canthal ligament. This is not unlike Wheeler's procedure (fig. 227) in which lateral strips of orbicularis are crossed. This gives a good result. However, the technic is more complex and the result no better than with a simple lateral canthoplasty (figs. 119 to 122).

DISPLACEMENT OF THE LATERAL CANTHUS

Displacement of the canthus is not seen frequently. This is fortunate because such cases are usually complicated since the trauma causing them must of necessity be extensive and severe. Along with displacement of the canthus one usually finds lagophthalmos, ankyloblepharon, partial lid loss and, frequently, loss of the globe.

Upward Displacement

Whether a lateral canthus is displaced upward or downward the procedure is essentially the same. It will usually be found that repairs at

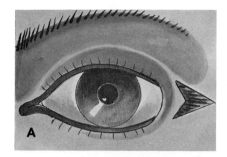
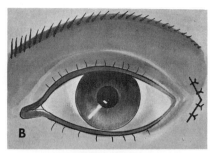
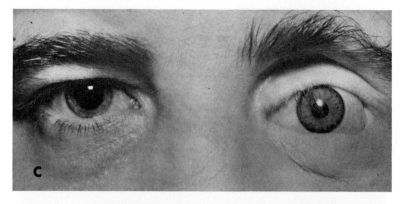
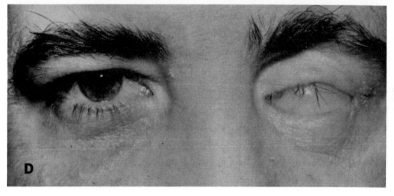

FIG. 127.   Arrow-Head Repair of Rounded Lateral Canthus.
A.   Arrow-head shaped segment of skin-muscle is resected.
B.   The wound is closed.
C. and D.   Rounded lateral canthus of left eye and result of repair.

the lateral canthus are somewhat simpler than the medial unless there
has been much destruction. Figure 128A is an example of upward displacement of the canthus.

   Procedure (fig. 128):   A Z-shaped incision is made as illustrated.
The upper two arms include the displaced lateral canthus between them.
The lower two arms create a flap of skin from the lower lid (fig. 128B).
The incisions are carried down to the orbital fascia and all scar tissue

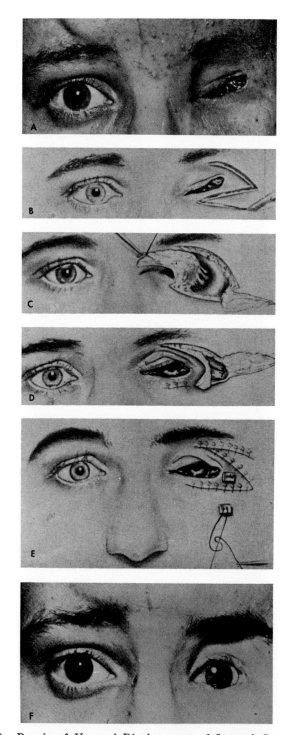

FIG. 128. Repair of Upward Displacement of Lateral Canthus.

A. Upward displacement of left lateral canthus with blepharophimosis.

B. A Z-incision is made to include the displaced canthus.

C. The included flaps are dissected up and the lateral canthal ligament or its equivalent isolated.

is resected. Sometimes, as in this case, the canthal ligament is difficult to identify but plenty of equivalent tough fibrous tissue is usually found to serve. In order to lower the canthus and conjunctival sac to their normal positions, the orbital fascia has to be incised to attain sufficient mobility and the ligament sutured to the zygomatic bone behind the orbital rim at the same height as the lateral canthal ligament of the fellow eye with 4–0 chromic catgut sutures (fig. 128C). The skin flaps are transposed and subcuticular sutures are used to fasten the lower flap to the periosteum of the lower orbital margin. A double-armed stay suture of 4–0 silk is passed through skin, canthal ligament and periosteum of the lower orbital rim, brought out through the skin of the cheek, and tied over a peg (fig. 128D). The skin wound is closed with interrupted 5–0 silk sutures. The sutures are removed on the sixth day (fig. 128E).

Six weeks later a combined marginal lash graft of the outer portion of the upper lid is done. The final result is seen in figure 128F.

Comment: It must be emphasized that unless the ligaments or their equivalent are thoroughly mobilized, the operation will be a failure. This requires sufficient incision of the orbital fascia so that the ligaments can be placed in proper position easily and without tension. Also what has been said earlier about the posterior attachments of both ligaments should be borne in mind. All fibrous tissue must be resected to reduce as much as possible the danger of displacement by scar tissue pull during the healing process. Hence, the ligament also must be firmly anchored in place.

There are two advantages in using the Z incision technic in all such cases: First, it tends to counteract the danger of healing scar tissue pull which may displace the canthus again, by using the skin flaps and skin sutures as well as subcutaneous sutures to counteract this tendency. Second, the transposition of skin flaps supplies skin tissue where most needed from adjacent sites. This is always a good rule in plastic surgery. An additional advantage here is that next to lid skin itself, skin from below the lower lid is nearest in appearance to actual upper lid skin. Furthermore, since it is somewhat heavier and less elastic, it is more likely to counteract upward pull by healing scar tissue.

Downward Displacement

The foregoing case is an extreme example of destruction and displacement. Less severe cases will require only a Z incision with transposi-

---

FIG. 128 *(Continued)*

D. The ligament is sutured into place to the periosteum and the skin flaps are transposed.

E. A stay suture is inserted to fasten the lower flap to the periosteum of the lower orbital rim and the skin wound is closed.

F. Result with prosthesis in place.

(Fox, S. A.: Courtesy American Journal of Ophthalmology.)

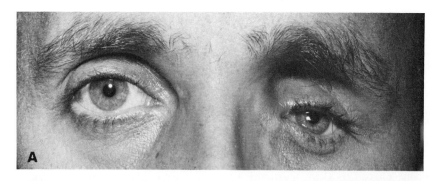

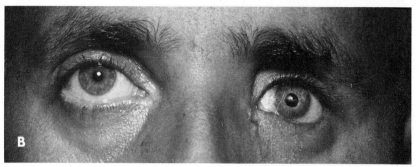

FIG. 129. Repair of Downward Displacement of Left Lateral Canthus.
A. Preoperative appearance of patient.
B. Result of repair by Z plasty as in figure 128 with canthus moved upward,
    instead of downward.

tion of flaps to effect a correction as in figure 129. The technic is essentially the same as in figure 128 except that the transposition is upward and much less dissection and repair is needed.

Another worthwhile method of repair is the useful all-purpose Fuchs canthoplasty or any of its equivalents discussed earlier in this chapter. These may be used in cases of only slight canthal displacement to raise the lateral canthus.

An example of medial displacement of the lateral canthus with traumatic blepharophimosis is shown in figure 248.

NEOPLASMS AT THE LATERAL CANTHUS

The general handling of lateral canthus neoplasms and colobomata, both large and small, is fully discussed in Chapters 6, 7, and 8; notably in procedures 79, 95, and 103, as they increase in complexity. Hence no further comment is needed here except to reiterate the greater facility with which these lesions can be handled as compared with medial canthus lesions. This is amply documented in the descriptions of the above procedures.

REFERENCES

AGNEW, C. R.: Cantho-plasty as a Remedy in Certain Diseases of the Eye. New York, G. P. Putnam's Sons, 1875.

VON AMMON, F. A.: Klinische Darstellingen der angeborenen Krankheiten des Auges und der Augenlider. Berlin. G. Reimer, 1841.

BLAIR, V. P., BROWN, J. B., and HAMM, W. G.: Lateral canthoplasty. Arch. Ophth. June, 1932.

FOX, S. A.: Some methods of lid repair and reconstruction. V. Displacement of the canthi. Am. J. Ophth. *31*:317, 1948.

FUCHS, E.: Textbook of Ophthalmology, ed. 2. New York, Appleton & Co., 1905, p. 798.

HILDRETH, H. R.: The external canthal ligament in surgery of the lower lid. Am. J. Ophth. *18*:437, 1935.

TENZEL, R. R.: Treatment of lagophthalmos of the lower lid. Arch. Ophth. *81*:366, 1969.

WEEKS, W. W.: Surgery of the Eye. Privately printed, 1937, pp. 12, 13.

WHEELER, J. M.: Collected Papers. New York, Columbia Presbyterian Medical Center, 1939, p. 425.

CHAPTER 11

Major Repairs and Reconstructions

FREE FULL THICKNESS
  LID GRAFT
    LEFT TO RIGHT LOWER LID
    RIGHT LOWER TO RIGHT UPPER LID
    LEFT UPPER TO LEFT LOWER LID

SPONTANEOUS GRANULATION

DOUBLE ADVANCEMENT
  VERTICAL PEDICLE

COLLAR-BUTTON TECHNIC

MODIFIED HUGHES TECHNIC

TOTAL UPPER LID
  RECONSTRUCTION

THE CUTLER-BEARD TECHNIC

ROTATED GRAFT FOR LOWER
  LID REPAIR (MUSTARDÉ)

ROTATED GRAFT FOR UPPER
  LID REPAIR (MUSTARDÉ)

THE FOLLOWING CASES of lid reconstruction were chosen because each represents a somewhat different type of injury, or because varying procedures or combinations of procedures were used in each case. This discussion will give the reader an idea of some of the methods available for these larger repairs and how the planning and solution of these problems is carried out.

The line between a repair and a reconstruction can be an exceedingly tenuous one and not always easy to define. Certainly when practically a whole lid has to be restored—as in some cases below—it must be classed as a reconstruction. On the other hand, lesser counterparts, quite similar in technic, will be found in previous chapters. Most often the difference is simply a matter of size and tonicity or atonicity of the lid. Another difference is the difficulty of technic or the combination of technics required in a reconstruction. Finally, there is the arbitrary individual and personal definition of what makes or does not make a case complicated enough to be called a reconstruction; in other words, what's one man's repair is another man's reconstruction.

I have avoided stressing the size of the lesion as a basis for systemizing the types of repair because lids vary in elasticity and tonicity. Some lids cannot be closed easily if only 20 per cent has been lost; others, as in the elderly and infirm (cf. senile ectropion), can lose almost half a lid and permit closure of the wound.

RECONSTRUCTION BY FREE FULL THICKNESS LID GRAFT

This type of repair is one of the few important recent breakthroughs in ophthalmic plastic surgery. It bids fair to replace some of the more complicated multiple-step procedures now in use.

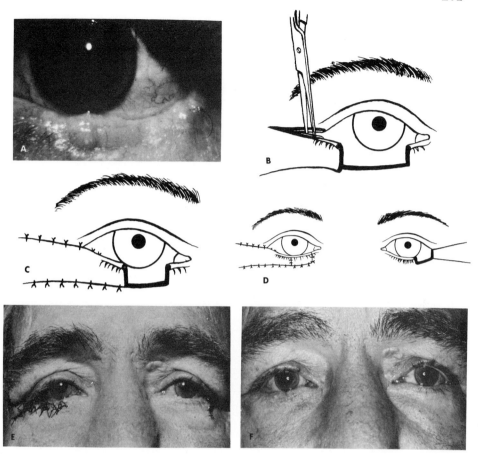

FIG. 130. Repair by Autogenous Full Thickness Lid Graft from Left Lower to Right Lower Lid.

A. Neoplasm of right lower lid.
B. Neoplasm is resected. Canthotomy and cantholysis of lower arm of right canthal ligament are done with formation of advancing pedicle.
C. The pedicle is pulled over and sutured.
D. A full thickness graft is taken from the left lower lid and planted into right lower lid dehiscence.
E. The pedicle is pulled over in the left lower lid and sutured.
F. Final result.
   (Fox, S. A.: Courtesy American Journal of Ophthalmology.)

Graft from Left to Right Lower Lid

Procedure (fig. 130): This patient had a neoplasm involving well over half of the right lower lid (fig. 130A). He had had no previous surgery or x-ray therapy.

Under local infiltration anesthesia, the central 20 mm. of the right lower lid is resected to a depth of 6 mm. A right lateral canthotomy is done and the lower arm of the canthal ligament is lysed (fig. 130B). An advancement flap is fashioned in the right temporal region by means of two diverging incisions. The flap is undermined and mobilized by means of several 4–0 plain subcuticular relaxation sutures. When pulled nasally a coloboma of 10 mm. remains (fig. 130C). A full thickness graft measuring 7 by 12 mm. is taken from the left lower lid at the lateral canthus and sutured medially into the right lower lid wound (fig. 130D). Closure is completed with 6–0 chromic conjunctival and 5–0 silk interrupted skin sutures.

A canthotomy and cantholysis are made at the left lateral canthus and with the aid of an advancement flap the conjunctiva is closed with 6–0 interrupted chromic sutures and the skin with 5–0 interrupted silk sutures (fig. 130E). A supportive dressing is applied. Three days later the graft in the right eye was found pink and healthy. Healing in both eyes was complete on the sixth day and the sutures were removed. The final result is shown in figure 130F.

The pathology report was basal cell carcinoma. (See Comment after Procedure 132.)

Graft from Right Lower to Right Upper Lid

This patient gave a history of a growth on the right upper lid which had been present for 5 or 6 years. It was removed about 3 years previously but recurred and was removed again in August, 1967. The pathology report was epidermoid carcinoma. The lesion recurred again rather rapidly. External examination showed a neoplasm involving about three-quarters of the right upper lid. The medial portion of the lesion had invaded the lid margin; laterally only the skin surface was involved (fig. 131A).

Procedure (fig. 131):   The tumor of the right upper lid is resected. This involves full thickness resection of the medial half; laterally only skin is resected. An advancement flap is fashioned at the temporal region of the upper lid and pulled medially. This leaves a central coloboma measuring 12 mm. which is filled with a free full thickness graft from the right lower lid.

The graft is fastened into position with closely placed interrupted sutures: 6–0 chromic on the conjunctival surface and 5–0 silk on the skin surface (fig. 131B). The donor lid is closed as described in the previous case by means of an advancement flap after cantholysis.

Healing was uneventful with a good take noted on the third day (fig. 131C). The final result is seen in figure 131D. The pathology report was epidermoid carcinoma. The patient was last seen 18 months later; both lids were normal. (See Comment after Procedure 132.)

Graft from Left Upper to Left Lower Lid

This patient gave a history of having had a Ziegler puncture for entropion of the left lower lid with consequent dissolution of most of the lid. External examination disclosed almost complete loss of the left lower

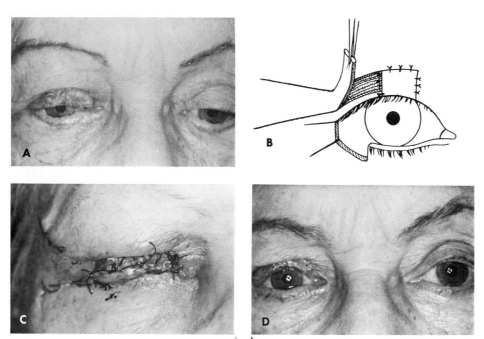

FIG. 131. Repair by Autogenous Free Full Thickness Graft from Right
Lower to Right Upper Lid.

A. Neoplasm of right upper lid.
B. Full thickness resection of medial portion and skin resection laterally are
done. An advancement flap is moved over to cover bared lateral area and
graft is taken from right lower lid to fill coloboma in the right upper lid.
C. Coloboma in lower (donor) lid is closed as in the previous case.
D. Final result.

(Fox, S. A.: Courtesy American Journal of Ophthalmology.)

lid except for some residual remnants at the canthi. The surrounding
area was inflamed and swollen (fig. 132A).

Procedure (fig. 132): After subsidence of all inflammation, a canthotomy is done at the left lateral canthus and the lower arm of the
ligament is sectioned. An advancement graft is fashioned as previously
described by means of undermining and subcutaneous relaxation sutures.
The lid remnants are drawn together and the central coloboma in the
left lower lid is reduced to 12 mm. (fig. 132B). A rectangular graft
measuring 7 by 13 mm. is taken at the lateral canthus of the left upper
lid and sewed into the dehiscence in the left lower lid with closely placed
interrupted 6–0 chromic sutures on the conjunctival side and 5–0 silk
sutures on the skin side. The upper lid coloboma is closed after lysis of
the upper arm of the lateral canthal ligament (fig. 132C).

Healing was uneventful and a good lid margin resulted. However,
so much tissue had been lost that the lid was ectropic (fig. 132D). The
ectropion was repaired by a free full thickness skin graft from the right
upper lid (fig. 132E). The final result is seen in figure 132F.

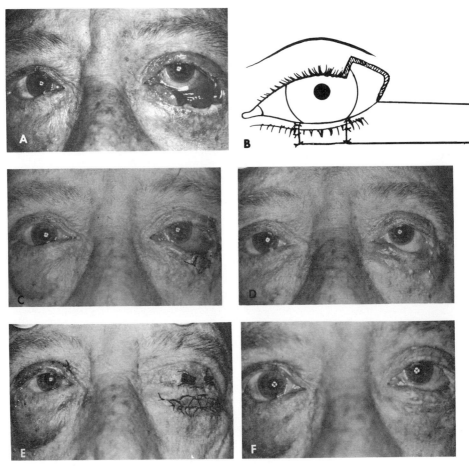

FIG. 132. Repair by Autogenous Free Full Thickness Graft from Left
Upper Lid to Left Lower Lid.

A. Appearance of left lower lid before repair.
B. Canthotomy and cantholysis of left lower lid are done with advancement
flap drawn over. A graft is taken from the left upper lid to close the left
lower lid coloboma.
C. The upper lid coloboma is closed.
D. After healing, ectropion of lid is noted.
E. Skin graft is taken from right upper lid to repair ectropion of left lower lid.
F. Final result.
(Fox, S. A.: Courtesy American Journal of Ophthalmology.)

Comment: The three cases presented above show that grafts from
any lid can be taken to repair a coloboma in any other lid. Since the loss
in all these cases was great, temporal sliding grafts were added to complete the closure. However, in no case would the sliding grafts alone have
sufficed. On the other hand, these grafts were moderate in size and in no
case required rotating a whole cheek (cf. fig. 139).

Full thickness lid grafts are not only feasible but are sometimes
more desirable since they make possible replacement of large lid loss

(more than half a lid) at one sitting thus obviating subsequent surgery. Healing is remarkably rapid with a graft appearing normally pink and healthy on the fifth day. It is my impression that they heal more rapidly than lid skin grafts.

The graft from the donor lid is best taken from the lateral canthal area where canthotomy, cantholysis and an advancement graft are available if necessary. Unlike lid skin these full thickness grafts shrink— hence they should be cut generously and transferred immediately to the recipient lid.

Technically, since this type of repair is relatively easy and requires only one stage, it may ultimately replace even those repairs not requiring sliding grafts for completion. It is of interest to note that Callahan reported one somewhat similar case in 1951.

RECONSTRUCTION BY SPONTANEOUS GRANULATION

The necessity for large repairs may occur at any lid position, canthal as well as central. The tumor pictured in figure 133A is a recurrent basal cell epithelioma of the nasocanthal angle which had first appeared five years previously. Three years after its occurrence the patient received 3400 r of beta radiation in five doses over a period of three weeks. Ten months later the lesion had recurred.

Examination revealed a deep rodent ulcer measuring 14 by 18 mm. occupying the right medial canthus and the right side of the nose. The upper canaliculus communicated with the ulcerous opening. The lower canaliculus was obstructed. X-ray examination showed no involvement of bone. The problem was extirpation of the lesion and reconstruction of the inner third of both lids.

Procedure (fig. 133): Under local anesthesia the lesion was excised down to bone with a 4 mm. margin of normal tissue all around. The resection included the medial thirds of the upper and lower lids, conjunctiva, medial canthal ligament and the lacrimal sac. The lacrimal fossa and the whole surrounding area was curetted down to the opening of the nasolacrimal duct which was probed and irrigated through. (The small lesion in the center of the lower lid was also resected.)

The bleeding was difficult to control. It was therefore decided not to attempt repair at this time. An intermarginal suture was placed to protect the cornea and a pressure dressing applied for hemostasis.

Three days later thin flaps were cut from the adjacent muscle layers to line the bare bone of the lacrimal fossa and medial canthus in order to stimulate granulation (fig. 133B). Also the cut ends of the conjunctiva were sutured together to form a new medial cul-de-sac (figs. 133C and D).

The needles of a double-armed 3–0 chromic catgut suture were passed through each cut marginal edge of the upper and lower lids. The lids were drawn over and the suture fastened to a remaining remnant of nasal periosteum thus putting the lids on stretch. Due to loss of tissue the lids could not be drawn all the way over (fig. 133E) but they were thus prevented from retracting.

Successive photographs taken 4, 6, and 11 weeks later show the repair of the lesion *without* grafting (figs. 133F, G, and H).

Comment: The result of this procedure might be called repair by natural granulation. Minimal surgery was done to help nature along: the conjunctival ends were sewn together, the lids were pulled over medially by a suture fastened to the nasal periosteum to prevent retraction and the bone was lined with a thin layer of muscle to encourage granulation repair. Nature, ever unpredictable, was profligate on the one hand and niggardly on the other. The granulation tissue was heaped up in such profusion that the final result was a canthus somewhat higher on the right side than on the normal left side. On the other hand, epithelium was supplied parsimoniously and there is a tendency to cicatricial ptosis. This can easily be repaired by a small free skin graft from the opposite lid. However, the patient is quite happy with the result and wants no more surgery. He may be right.

This type of repair has now been used in some fifteen cases with little change except that no attempt is now made to line the bare bone with muscle to stimulate granulation; it is not needed. Since the dissection is usually a deep one, if there is any doubt that the whole tumor has been removed, it may be wise to use Moh's paste (see Chapter 26) to follow up the dissection and assure oneself of a clean field. This is one place where this type of chemical diagnosis is of value in ophthalmic plastic surgery.

The lesson to be learned from the above is that in cases where large dissections have to be done either for cicatricial contraction or malignancy and where bleeding is difficult to control, it is wise not to attempt immediate repair. It is not hard to have a long and difficult reconstruction completely negated by hemorrhage; grafting under such conditions is suicidal. In the long run, therefore, discretion may dictate secondary repairs in such cases. This is more time-consuming for the surgeon immediately but may save both patient and surgeon from the need of reoperation subsequently.

Fastening the lids to the medial canthus is a major factor in the procedure. Failure to do so would allow their retraction laterally with a much poorer cosmetic result as a consequence.

Other types of repair are, of course, available. Free grafting may be used or the large forehead flaps which leave deep scars. However, the result here is obtained with a minimum of surgical intervention, a minimum of scarring and at least as good a cosmetic result as with most technics.

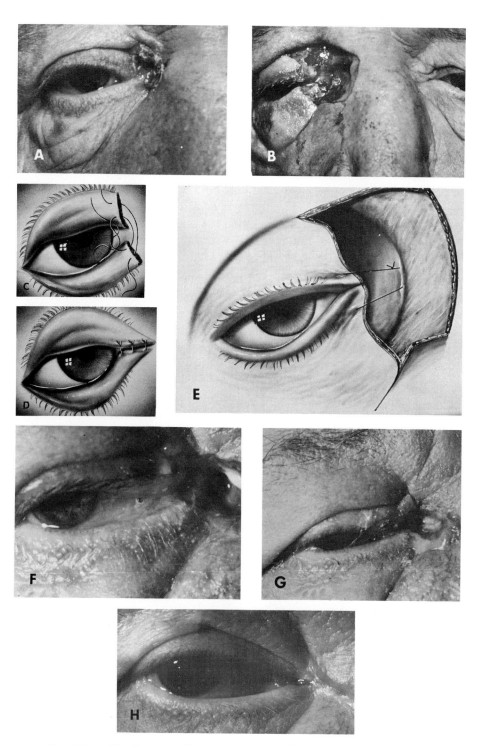

FIG. 133. Simultaneous Reconstruction of Inner Third of Both Lids by
Spontaneous Granulation.

A. Carcinoma involving upper and lower lids.
B. Appearance three days after resection of neoplasm.
C. and D. Repair of medial fornix.
E. Ends of lids are fastened to nasal periosteum.
F., G. and H. Appearance four, six and eleven weeks later.
    (Fox, S. A.: Courtesy Archives of Ophthalmology.)

Repair by Double Advancement Pedicle

A case of malignancy involving almost the whole margin of the left lower lid is seen in figure 134A. The patient gave a history of having had a "pimple" removed from the lid six years previously. In the past two years the eye had been tearing and irritable. Examination disclosed erosion of almost the whole lid margin with obstruction of the lower canaliculus. There was no heaping up of tissue (fig. 134A).

Procedure (fig. 134): After suitable local anesthesia the whole marginal area is excised. The resected portion is 19 mm. long and 5 mm. wide. The remainder of the involved portion of the lid is split into its two laminae and two sliding flaps are created by vertical incisions at each end of the wound. Halving is attained by making the skin-muscle flap 2 mm. wider on each side than the conjunctiva as in the previous procedure (fig. 134B). The opposing upper lid margin is freshened, split shallowly and the flaps of the lower lid sutured to the opposing edges of the upper lid (figs. 134C and D).

A firm supportive dressing is applied. Sutures are removed on the sixth day. The pathology report was basal cell carcinoma with complete tumor excision and the final result is seen in figure 134E.

Comment: It will be noted that the upper lid was only used as an anchor in this case and that no part of opposing lid tissue was used for grafting. Had it been necessary, tarsoconjunctiva from the upper lid could have been easily appropriated. This technic is applicable to lesser lesions as was shown in figures 101 and 102.

Collar-Button Resection of Tarsus with Free Skin Graft

When the skin lesion is very large a free skin graft may be used to complete the repair. This lesion (fig. 135A) had been present for four and a half years and had increased in size during the last six months.

Procedure (fig. 135): After resection of the malignancy in toto by the collar-button technic a canthotomy and cantholysis (fig. 135B) of the lower arm of the lateral canthal ligament are done. The tarsoconjunctival wound is then easily closed with interrupted 5–0 chromic sutures. A free skin graft cut to pattern is taken from the homolateral upper lid and planted into the lower lid dehiscence. The upper border of the graft is sutured to the freshened upper lid margin. The wound in the upper lid is closed with interrupted 5–0 silk sutures (fig. 135C). A firm pressure dressing is applied for six days. This is changed, the area cleansed, the upper lid sutures removed and the pressure dressing reapplied for four more days. At this time all the sutures are removed and a simple patch substituted until healing is complete.

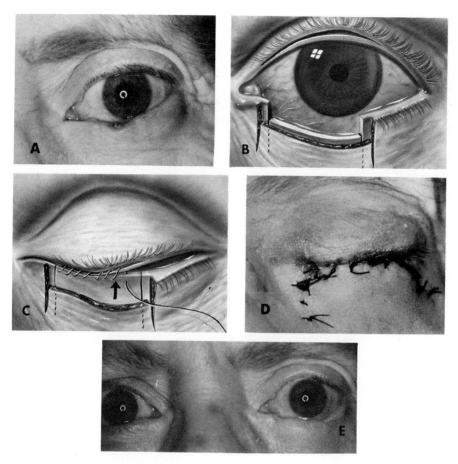

Fig. 134, Modified Halving of Lower Lid by Means of Two Vertical Sliding Flaps.

A. Neoplasm of left lower lid.
B. The lesion is resected and a halving closure prepared by making the skin-muscle flap wider than the tarsoconjunctiva. The upper lid is split.
C. The tarsoconjunctival flap is pulled up and sutured to the upper lid tarsoconjunctiva.
D. The skin-muscle laminae are sutured and closure is completed.
E. Final result.

(Fox, S. A.: Courtesy Archives of Ophthalmology.)

Pathology report was basal cell epithelioma and showed complete removal. The final result is shown in figure 135D.

Comment: A comparison of the lesions shown in figures 136A and 135A shows great similarity. Both are large lesions of the lower lid. The former occupies fully half the lid and invades as much margin as skin. The latter is somewhat smaller and invades only a little of the margin. Hence the collar-button technic could be used here whereas a full thickness resection had to be done in the other. The patient was spared a tarsoconjunctival graft and the surgeon that much more work.

A final word about the collar-button technic: The case presented above could have been repaired just as well by a tarsoconjunctival sliding

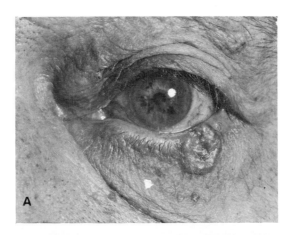

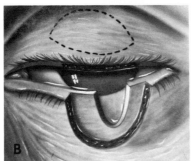
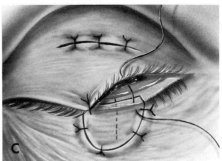

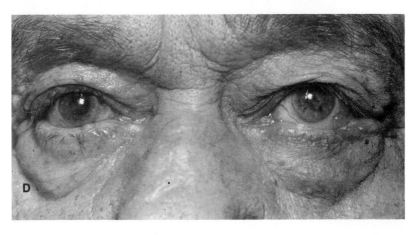

FIG. 135.   Halving by Collar-Button Resection. Repair by Horizontal Closure
and Free Whole Skin Graft.

A.   Large basal cell carcinoma of left lower lid involving margin somewhat.
B.   Collar-button resection of neoplasm with canthotomy and cantholysis. *Dotted
outline* shows skin graft to be taken from upper lid.
C.   The tarsus is closed and the upper lid margin is freshened. The skin graft
is sutured into the lower lid dehiscence and to the upper lid margin.
D.   Final result.
(Fox, S. A.: Courtesy Archives of Ophthalmology.)

flap from the opposing lid. But the collar-button technic made grafting unnecessary, left the integrity of the opposing lid unimpaired and—what is more to the point—gave a good result.

RECONSTRUCTION OF OUTER TWO-THIRDS OF LOWER LID MODIFIED HUGHES TECHNIC

When the temporal lesion is as large as the one pictured in figure 136A a temporal sliding flap, no matter how wide or long, will be insufficient to effect a repair—too much tissue is needed. Hence a modified Hughes technic was used.

Procedure (fig. 136): The tumor is resected with a rim of healthy tissue all around, resulting in the loss of over half the lower lid. The outer half of the left upper lid is split and the margin freshened. At each end of the split two vertical incisions are made in the tarsoconjunctiva and the resulting tarsoconjunctival sliding graft is freely mobilized. This is pulled down and sutured to the remnant of the outer half of the lower lid conjunctiva (fig. 136B).

A large free whole skin graft is taken from the ipsilateral upper lid and sutured into the lower lid dehiscence. A pressure dressing is applied. This is changed on the sixth day, the area cleaned and the dressing reapplied for four more days. At this time the graft has taken well (fig. 136C) and the sutures are removed.

Eight weeks later (fig. 136D) the lids are separated and the final result is seen in figure 136E. Note that the left lower lid margin is not pulled down. Also, despite the large amount of tarsoconjunctiva and skin taken from the upper lid, the ability to close is unimpaired (fig. 136F).

Comment: This case is an example of size affecting the choice of reparative technic. For even if the lesion were situated at the lateral canthus and a temporal canthus type repair were the obvious choice, the large amount of tissue required forced another choice. Two points are worthy of further comment:

1. Total resection of over half the lower lid which left only a remnant of conjunctiva shallowed the outer half of the socket considerably. However, this mattered little since the patient retained his own eye and cosmetically the result was good. Had this been an empty socket, reconstruction of the temporal half of the socket might have been necessary to enable the patient to wear a prosthesis.

2. The whole outer half of the tarsoconjunctiva of the upper lid was converted into a sliding pedicle to replace the resected tarsoconjunctiva of the lower lid. In addition a huge whole skin graft was taken from the same lid to replace lost skin in the lower lid. In all, a large part

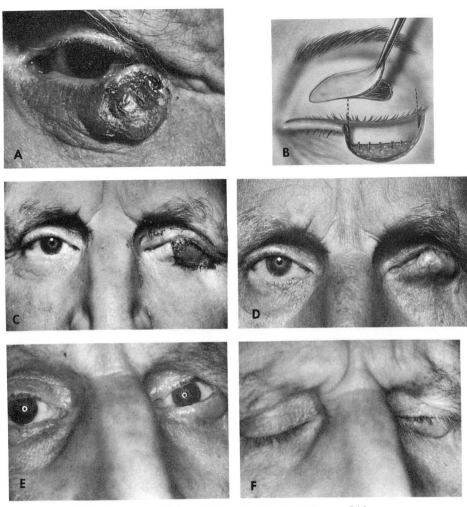

FIG. 136. Reconstruction of Outer Half of Left Lower Lid.
A. Neoplasm of left lower lid.
B. Resection of full thickness lateral half of lid. The outer portion of the upper
    lid is split and a flap of tarsoconjunctiva is fashioned and sutured to the
    conjunctival remnant of the lower lid. A skin graft is taken from the upper
    lid to complete repair of the lower lid.
C. Appearance on first dressing.
D. Appearance before lid separation.
E. Final result.
F. Note that ability to close the eye is unimpaired.

of the upper lid was transferred to the lower lid. Despite this, upper lid
function was unimpaired. The outer half of the lid is pulled up a bit
(fig. 136D) but not enough to make to make it a cosmetic liability and
there is not the slightest trace of lagophthalmos (fig. 136E). One is
constantly amazed at the amount of lid tissue available for transfer to
other areas with the donor lid remaining physiologically functional and

cosmetically acceptable. This is especially true of older people with their relaxed abundant tissues.

This is not a particularly good cosmetic result but it is a satisfactory functional result. If this case came up for repair today a free full thickness graft would have been used from either the ipsilateral upper lid or the contralateral lower lid (cf. fig. 132). This would have enhanced the cosmetic appearance of the left upper lid but not its function since this was not impaired. Although this technic is steadily losing ground, it is still worthwhile and of some use in special instances.

TOTAL UPPER LID RECONSTRUCTION

Reconstruction of the upper lid presents more problems than that of the lower lid. The reasons for this are obvious. The upper lid is the moveable portion of the eye shutter with the lower lid being relatively stationary. Hence in upper lid reconstruction, function as translated into movement becomes a paramount consideration. This means that the levator must be kept constantly in mind and its function preserved wherever possible, even if only a portion of it is present. (Of course, in many cases this is a purely academic consideration. When the eye is lost and destruction is great, only decent cosmetic repair can be the objective.) Lower lid reconstruction for this reason alone is simpler.

The relative widths of the tarsus (11 to 12 mm. in the upper lid and 5 mm. in the lower lid) is another factor complicating upper lid reconstruction. It is easy to borrow tarsus from the upper lid for the lower. It is not so simple to restore lost tarsus to the upper lid. It can be done but not so easily.

Getting skin tissue for the upper lid is more difficult because it is wider than the lower lid and more of it is needed. Because of its position, lower lid skin can be replaced by sliding grafts from the cheek, zygomatic region or upper lid. The upper lid, however, has only the forehead or temple from which to draw a rotated pedicle. This skin is much thicker and less mobile. Hammock flaps from below and free grafts are available, but again, they make for more radical surgery.

Cosmetically, too, the final results of upper lid repair may be poorer because the upper lid is much more conspicuous and shows the scars of injury and repair more easily.

(The following case is probably an object lesson in what not to do; if it were seen today a prosthesis would be suggested which would be much more lifelike and would have spared the patient a good deal of pain and time spent in the hospital.)

Trauma which destroys the entire upper lid and leaves the lower lid intact is a rare phenomenon. The following is one of these unusual cases. This patient sustained a penetrating wound of the right upper lid, right eyeball, fractures of the right orbital bones and a laceration of the right frontal lobe of the brain. The eye had to be enucleated.

When first seen (fig. 137A) the upper lid was completely absent. Except for the palpebral portion of the lower lid, all the conjunctiva had been lost and the socket was lined with granulation tissue. As a result, the lower lid was somewhat entropic. By some trick of fate the caruncle was spared. This was a welcome windfall as the final cosmetic result is always better when this is present. The problem was to reconstruct the whole upper lid and socket.

Procedure (fig. 137): A pedicle flap 12 mm. wide and 30 mm. long was raised from the skin of the right forehead with the lower 4 mm. including the hair of the brow. This was delayed for two weeks to assure a good blood supply (fig. 137B).

Fourteen days later the skin edge around the upper orbital rim was freshened and the granulation tissue covering the upper half of the socket scraped away. The skin of the naso-orbital angle was undermined and mobilized. The pedicle flap from the brow was raised again, rotated down and sutured to the skin below the brow and medially to the naso-orbital angle with interrupted 4–0 silk sutures. The wound above the brow was closed with 4–0 plain catgut subcuticular and 4–0 silk sutures (fig. 137C). The socket was filled with petrolated gauze and the graft pressed against the upper posterior socket wall to insure adequate blood supply. A firm pressure dressing was applied. The graft took well and the skin sutures were removed on the tenth day after operation.

Six weeks later the pedicle graft, now obviously healthy and viable, was dissected away from the socket wall (fig. 137D) and the socket itself lined with a split skin graft taken from the inner aspect of the right arm (figs. 137E and F).

Five weeks later the scar below the brow was excised and subcutaneous tissue resected to thin out the lid (fig. 137G). A free skin graft was taken from the left upper lid and planted in the bed thus prepared for it in the reconstructed right lid (fig. 137H). In this way the lid was widened and its edge brought down to the level of the left upper lid. Both wounds were closed with interrupted 5–0 silk sutures. A conformer was inserted into the right socket and a pressure dressing applied. A simple dressing sufficed for the left eye. The sutures were removed on the fifth day (fig. 137I). The free graft took well and the final result is seen in figure 137J.

Comment: Many methods of repair are open to the surgeon in a case of this sort. These include, among others, the use of a tubed graft from the neck, rotated pedicles from the temple, cheek and lower lid, and multiple free grafts of skin and cartilage. For the following reasons, however, it is believed that the method chosen here was the simplest available for a complicated case.

1. There is comparatively little scarring as a result of the surgery since most of the donor site is buried in the hair of the brow. For cosmetic reasons it is always best to have scars running parallel with the lid margin whenever possible; a tubed graft or temporal pedicle would have been more conspicuous and scar producing.

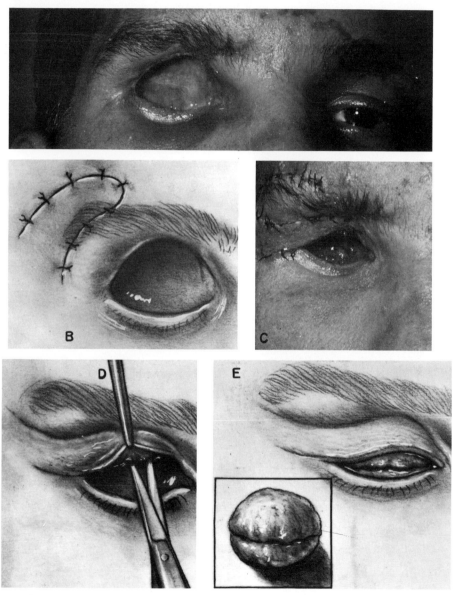

FIG. 137.   Total Reconstruction of the Upper Lid.
A. Loss of entire right upper lid.
B. A delayed flap is raised laterally.
C. The flap is rotated down and sutured into position below the brow.
D. and E. After a "take" the flap is dissected up and the socket relined with split skin.
(Continued)

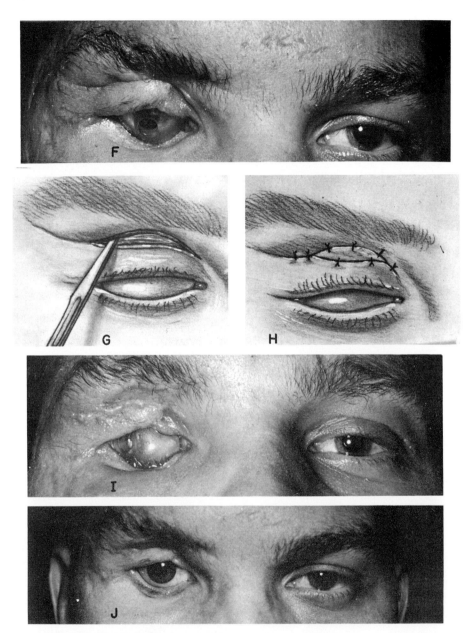

Fig. 137 (*Continued*)

F.   Actual appearance with temporary conformer in place.
G. and H.   A free skin graft is added to widen the lid.
I.   Appearance before completion.
J.   The final result with prosthesis in place.
    (Fox, S. A.: Courtesy American Journal of Ophthalmology.)

    2. The blood supply and therefore the viability of the graft is more certain with a pedicle than with a free graft, especially if it is delayed.

    3. Since brow skin is thicker than the whole lid, the single layer

was enough. Indeed, this single layer had to be thinned out to make the repaired lid conform to the opposite upper lid.

4. In a case of this sort there is no question of restoring lid function. The reconstructed lid is immobile no matter what method is used. The aim of surgery here can only be cosmetic restoration and the result is just as good (or bad) as can be obtained with any other technic.

In cases in which there is so much destruction, the question always arises as to whether the result is worth the effort. Some surgeons of long experience feel that total lid reconstructions are never justified because the patient is so often dissatisfied with the final result. Certainly patients should be warned before operation that one cannot reconstruct a complete lid to match the normal lid in every respect. One must expect and be satisfied with a good deal less than perfection. If one succeeds in reconstructing a lid which is presentable and not too conspicuous, the result is adequate.

In this case lid and socket reconstruction made retention of a prosthesis possible and the patient was not condemned to wearing a patch the rest of his life. The reconstructed lid, although far from perfect, was sufficiently presentable to content the patient.

Cutler-Beard Procedure for Upper Lid Reconstruction

A useful procedure for large upper lid reconstructions is the Cutler-Beard bridge flap technic reported in 1955.

Procedure (fig. 138): The upper lid defect is prepared by tumor excision or freshening of the coloboma's borders. The nearer the shape of the coloboma is to a rectangle the simpler the repair. A full thickness lower lid horizontal incision is made just below the attached tarsal border to match the upper lid dehiscence. Then two full thickness vertical incisions are made to each side down to the lower fornix to create a rectangular advancement flap which is mobilized, pulled up behind the marginal hammock of the lower lid and sutured into position in the upper lid coloboma (fig. 138A). This is best done by a running 6–0 silk conjunctival suture with the ends brought out to the skin and locked. The skin is closed with 5–0 interrupted silk sutures. The raw edge of the lower bridge flap is sutured to the skin of the advancement flap (fig. 138B). The wound is covered with nonadhesive firm supportive dressings without pressure. The eye is dressed in 5 days and loose sutures are removed. All sutures are removed 3 days later.

After 7 or 8 weeks the lower lid bridge adhesions to the skin are separated (fig. 138C). the bridge is pulled down and the new upper lid margin is marked out on the upper lid with an antiseptic dye by a line slightly convex downward to counteract possible retraction. The flap is

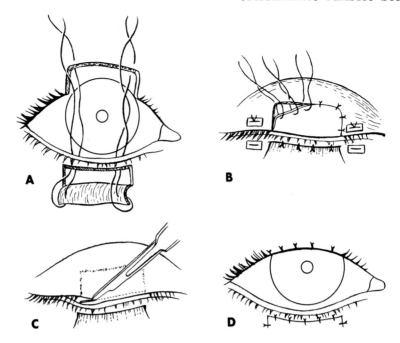

FIG. 138.   Upper Lid Repair (Cutler-Beard).
A.   A rectangular advancement flap is fashioned in the lower lid and pulled up behind the marginal portion of the lower lid to be sutured into the upper lid coloboma.
B.   The raw edge of the lower lid bridge is sutured to the advancement flap.
C.   After healing the lower lid bridge is freed from the flap.
D.   The raw upper lid edge is sutured skin to conjunctiva. The lower lid is repaired by resuturing the lower lid bridge across and at the sides.

divided and the raw upper lid edge is sutured skin to conjunctiva with interrupted silk sutures. The remainder of the flap requires very little freeing and is sutured back to the lower lid bridge and at the sides. Again this is done in two layers as above (fig. 138D). Sutures are removed 5 to 7 days later.

Comment: Little tension is exerted on the flap sutures. In most cases there is adequate lower fornix tissue to provide tissue for an upper lid defect. Notching of the upper lid may occur and is repaired in the usual way. Scar retraction in the lower lid is corrected by resection at a later date. Trichiasis has been noted by Cole which was repaired by a van Millingen mucosal graft.

MUSTARDÉ TECHNIC OF LID RECONSTRUCTION

Mustardé's technics of lid reconstruction are based on the principle that the upper lid must never be used as a source of tissue as this would impair its function. "Sharing," as he calls it, of upper lid tissue for lower lid repair is therefore strictly interdicted. In his own words, "Use the lower lid to reconstruct the upper, but use other tissues to reconstruct the lower."

Hence in the repair of large defects in the lower lid Mustardé is forced back to the huge rotated and sliding flaps of Arlt, Blasius, Dieffenbach, Imré, Elschnig and others, of seventy-five and one hundred years ago. In large colobomata of the lower lid the whole side of the face may have to be moved over to make up the dehiscence (figs. 139A and B) with the mucosal lining provided by nasal mucous membrane.

Large colobomata of the upper lid are repaired by rotated pedicle grafts from the lower lid (figs. 140A-D). Several weeks later the lids are divided and the lower edges revised.

Comment: This belief of Mustardé that use of upper lid tissue for lower lid repair will imperil the function and integrity of the upper lid, and hence should not be done, is contrary to my experience. This is a rule which, among many others, I have broken many times in the past and shall continue to break. The cases reported above in this chapter and elsewhere in this book will show why. Even Procedure 136 in which more than half of the upper lid was used to repair the lower lid, retained excellent functional integrity.

Mustardé's rule does away with a whole armentarium of plastic procedures used successfully for decades by ophthalmic plastic surgeons and would make them the poorer. It is an unjustified interdiction. It is doubtful whether most ophthalmologists would have much use for this outmoded formidable technic of lid repair.

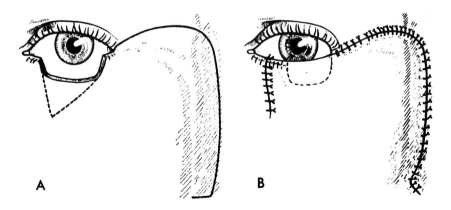

FIG. 139. Rotated Flap Repair of Lower Lid Coloboma (Mustardé).
A. The side of the face is converted into a huge flap.
B. The flap is rotated over and sewed into position.
  (Mustardé, J. C.: Repair and Reconstruction in the Orbital Region. Courtesy Williams and Wilkins Co., Baltimore.)

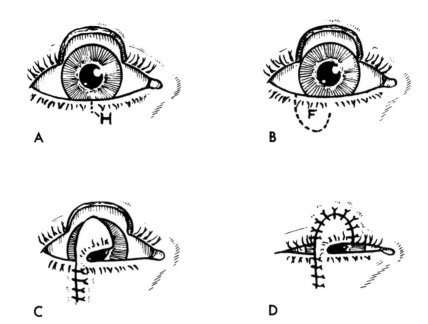

FIG. 140.   Repair of Upper Lid Coloboma by Rotated Flap from Lower Lid
(Mustardé).
A.   Coloboma of upper lid.
B. and *C.*   Flap is fashioned in the lower lid.
D.   Flap is sutured into position in upper lid. After "take" the lids are separated
and irregularities smoothed out.
(Mustardé, J. C.: Repair and Reconstruction in the Orbital Region. Courtesy
Williams and Wilkins Co., Baltimore.)

REFERENCES

BLASIUS: Cited by Zeis, E.: Handbuch der plastichen chirurgie. Berlin, G. Reimer,
    1838, p. 371.
BLASKOVICS, L.: Uber Total plastik des unteren Lides. Bildung einer hinteren
    Lidplatte durch Transplantation eines Tarsus und Bindenhautstreifens aus
    dem Oberlide. Ztschr. Augenh. *40*:222, 1918.
CALLAHAN, A.: Surgery of the Eye—Injuries. Springfield, Ill., Charles C Thomas,
    1950.
CALLAHAN, A.: The free composite lid graft. Arch. Ophth. *45*:539–545, 1951.
COLE, J. G.: Reconstruction of large defects of the upper eyelid. Am. J. Ophth.
    64:376, 1967.
CUTLER, N. L., and BEARD, C.: Reconstruction of upper lid. Am. J. Ophth. *39*:1, 1955.
DUPUY-DUTEMPS, P.: Autoplastie palpebro-palpébrale integrale. Réfection d'une
    paupiere detruite dans toute son epaisseur par greffe cutanée te tarso-conjunc-
    tive prise a l'autre paupiere. Bull. med. *43*:935, 1929.
FOX, S. A.: Some methods of lid repair and reconstruction. IV. Total reconstruction
    of the upper lid. Am. J. Ophth. *30*:1412, 1947.
————: Lower lid repair. Trans. Am. Acad. Ophth. & Oto. *58*:580, 1954.
HILL, J. C., and DAYAL, Y.: Blepharoplasty following tumor surgery. Can. J.
    Ophth. *1*:171, 1966.
HUGHES, W. L.: Reconstructive Surgery of the Eyelids. St. Louis, C. V. Mosby Co.,
    1954.

————————: A new method of rebuilding a lower lid. Arch. Ophth. *17*:1000, 1937.

KALT, J. B. E.: De la restauration de la paupiere inferieure detruite dans son epaisseur aux depens de la paupiere superieure. Bull. soc. d'opht. de Paris, *5*:156, 1892.

LANDOLT, E.: Nouveau procédé de blepharoplastie. Arch. d'opht. *1*:9, 1880.

MANCHESTER, W. M.: A simple method for the repair of full-thickness defects of the lower lid with special reference to the treatment of neoplasms. Brit. J. Plast. Surg. *3*:252, 1965.

MUSTARDE, J. C.: Repair and Reconstruction in the Orbital Region. Baltimore, The Williams and Wilkins Co., 1966, pp. 122, 167.

REESE, A. B.: Tumors of the Eye. New York, Paul B. Hoeber, Inc. 1951, p. 4.

SANDERSON, R. S., and RAPPAPORT, I.: Technic for reconstruction of carcinoma of the inner canthus. Am. Surg. *31*:625, 1965.

SMITH, B., and OBEAR, M.: Bridge flap technique for large upper lid defects. Plast. Reconstr. Surg. *38*:450, 1966.

SPAETH, E. B.: Reconstruction of the upper lid. Surg. Gyn. & Obst. *84*:804, 1947.

SUGAR, S. H.: Technique for eyelid reconstruction. Am. J. Ophth. *27*:109, 1944.

WHEELER, J. M.: Collected Papers. New York, Columbia Presbyterian Medical Center, 1939.

YOUENS, M. T., WESTPHAL, C., BARTFIELD, F. T., JR., and YOUENS, H. T., JR.: Full-thickness lower lid transplant. Arch. Ophth. *77*:226, 1967.

CHAPTER 12

Conjunctival Repairs

THE CONJUNCTIVA is a sheath of mucous membrane which lines the posterior surface of the lids and reflects forward onto the globe where it merges at the limbus with the corneal epithelium. It thus forms a sac of thin transparent tissue which is continuous from the lid margins to the cornea and which is open at the palpebral fissure.

Unlike the mucous membrane of the mouth, conjunctiva does not regenerate. But since it is elastic and there is normally an abundance of it, minor losses due to injury or the excision of tumors, cysts, nevi, pterygia, etc., are easily repaired by simple undermining and suture. Or the raw surface may be covered by small sliding flaps and Z or V-Y plasties.

Tears and cuts in the conjunctiva are cleaned and repaired by undermining and approximation with 6–0 interrupted silk or catgut sutures. Irregular tears should be trimmed before suturing for better healing. The conjunctiva has an excellent blood supply which, together with the antiseptic action of the tears, helps to prevent infection after trauma if ordinary care is taken. For treatment of conjunctival burns see Chapter 24.

CONJUNCTIVAL FLAPS

Rupture of the cornea after trauma, corneal ulcers, iris prolapse, keratoplasty, some technics of cataract extraction, etc., may require a conjunctival flap. The simplest is the limbal flap created by circumcizing

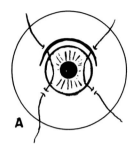 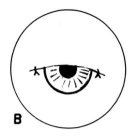

FIG. 141.   Limbal Conjunctival Flap (Kuhnt).
A.   Incision and placement of sutures.   B.   Closure.

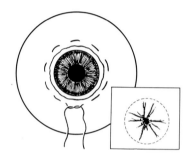

FIG. 142.   Purse-String Conjunctival Closure.
Circumcision of conjunctiva around cornea and placement of suture. Inset shows closure.

half of the adjacent limbus, undermining the conjunctiva, drawing it over the cornea and fastening it to the subconjunctiva on each side (fig. 141).

By undermining the conjunctiva still more and incising it a little medially and laterally it is possible to draw a flap down to protect the whole cornea. It is even possible to draw it down into the lower fornix to correct a symblepharon (fig. 153).

Another method, as in the presence of large corneal ruptures, is to circumcise the conjunctiva entirely around the limbus, undermine it, pass a purse-string suture around the edge and draw it over the entire cornea by tying the suture (fig. 142). A central accessory suture may be used to assure complete closure. Other conjunctival flaps such as bridge or hammock flaps may be used; these leave bared areas which in turn require closure and have no advantage over those described above.

Improvement in corneal needles and sutures have done away to a large extent with the necessity for conjunctival flaps after traumatic corneal rupture. Such rupture can now be sutured directly in most cases and give better final results, both visually and cosmetically, than the conjunctival flaps.

CONJUNCTIVAL GRAFTS

The standard methods of restoring lost conjunctiva are: (1) by free graft, or (2) by sliding or pedicle graft. A third method described below is a combination of these two methods which is useful in canthal repairs.

Free Graft

If possible, conjunctiva should be used to replace conjunctiva. A conjunctival graft from the fornix of the fellow eye or the opposite fornix of the same eye is a simple procedure if it is remembered that conjunctiva is a thin, fragile tissue which, when cut from its bed, will curl up so that it is difficult to unravel and, indeed, to recognize external from raw surface. The following technic will be found useful:

Procedure (fig. 143): The amount of conjunctiva to be taken is estimated and a 6–0 silk suture passed through each end of the proposed

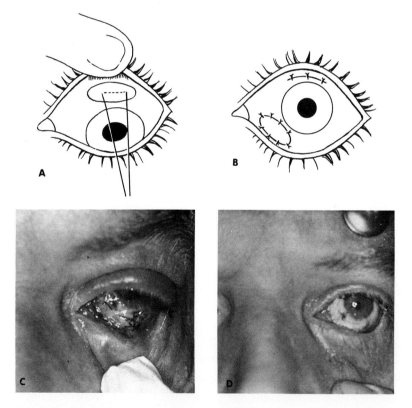

FIG. 143. Technic of Planting a Small Free Conjunctival Graft.
A. The bed to receive the graft is prepared. A central suture is placed in the donor area. The graft to be taken is outlined.
B. The graft is dissected free and sutured into place. The donor area is closed.
C. Appearance before removal of sutures.
D. Final result.

graft (fig. 143*A*). A central suture, preferably white, may also be placed
to assure accurate differentiation of the smooth from the raw surface
after the graft is lifted and has curled up. The graft is excised with
scissors and fastened into its bed by means of the previously placed
sutures which are used to transfer it. Additional 6–0 silk sutures are used
to sew it into place. The lips of the donor site wound are undermined if
necessary and sutured together in the same way (fig. 143*B*). Sterile ointment is instilled and the eye patched. The sutures may be removed on the
fifth day (fig 143*C*). The final result is seen in figure 143*D*.

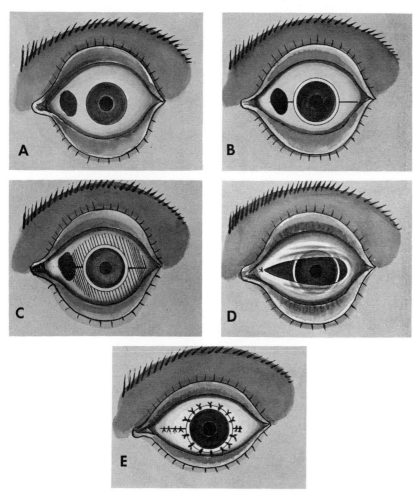

FIG. 144. Technic of Repair by Conjunctival Sliding Graft.
A. The bed to receive the graft is prepared.
B. The conjunctiva is circumcised around the cornea and then incised horizon-
      tally on both sides.
C. The bulbar conjunctiva is undermined.
D. It is drawn over to cover the conjunctival dehiscence.
E. Interrupted sutures are used to close the wound.

Comment: Like buccal mucous membrane, conjunctiva shrinks though not as much. Hence the graft should be cut generously. In case of doubt as to which is the raw surface side a drop of fluorescine is used. The raw surface will stain, the intact surface will not. In the young, catgut sutures used instead of silk simplify postoperative care.

Advancement Graft

Conjunctiva may also be replaced by means of a sliding graft fashioned as follows:

Procedure (fig. 144): The conjunctiva is circumcised around the limbus (fig. 144*A*). It is then incised horizontally at three and nine o'clock from the limbus toward the canthi for a sufficient distance to convert the bulbar conjunctiva into two large advancement flaps (fig. 144*B*). These flaps are undermined, pulled over and sutured together to cover the bare area (figs. 144*C* and *D*). The rest of the conjunctiva is sutured around the limbus to the episclera (fig. 144*E*). Ointment is instilled and the eye patched. Sutures are removed on the sixth day. Figures 145*A* and *B* show the result of such a repair after excision of a large conjunctival tumor involving the plica and caruncle.

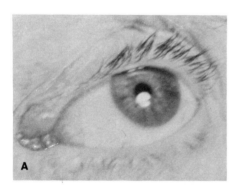 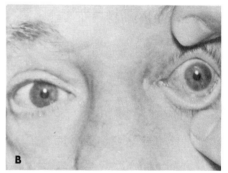

FIG. 145.   Conjunctive Sliding Graft.
A.   Tumor involving caruncle and plica.
B.   Appearance after resection and repair by conjunctival sliding graft.

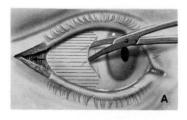 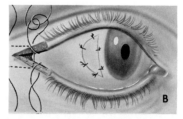

FIG. 146.   Combined Free and Sliding Conjunctival Graft.
A.   After lateral canthotomy, the conjunctiva is undermined medially and a vertical incision is made temporal to the limbus.
B.   The conjunctiva is pulled over temporally and a free conjunctival graft is used to close the dehiscence. The canthus is repaired as shown in figure 124.

Combined Free and Advancement Grafts

When the loss of conjunctiva is appreciable the combined technic of free and sliding grafts will prove useful.

Procedure (fig. 146): After undermining the conjunctiva to the limbus a 15 mm. crescentic vertical incision is made about 5 mm. from and parallel with the temporal limbus. This allows the conjunctiva to be drawn over to complete the repair but leaves a bared area (fig. 146A). This is filled in with a free conjunctival graft from the same or opposite eye (fig. 146B) as previously described in figure 144.

PINGUECULA

The aging process affects the conjunctiva as it does every other tissue of the body. With advancing years the conjunctiva becomes less transparent due to an increased thickening and keratinization of the epithelium. Along with this, hyaline degeneration occurs with atrophy of the subepithelial layers and disappearance of the elastic fibers. These processes are more accentuated in the exposed region of the palpebral fissure on each side of the cornea and ultimately give rise to pinguecula.

A pinguecula (*pinguis* = fat) is a yellowish irregular patch of bulbar conjunctiva appearing on either side of the cornea, but most

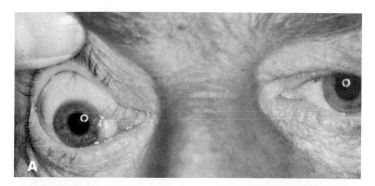

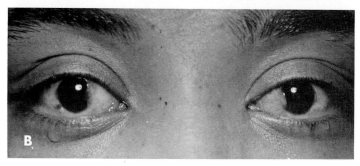

FIG. 147.   Conjunctival Affections.
A.   Large pinguecula of right eye.   B.   Bilateral pterygia.

commonly nasal, brought on by senility and exposure. Pinguecula is misnamed. Because of its yellowish appearance it was considered a fat deposit; actually it is a small mass of subconjunctival dense fibrous tissue imbedded in which are hyaline deposits, hyaline and elastic fibers.

Most often the pinguecula is rather small, flat and practically unnoticeable. Occasionally it gets so large or inflamed that it requires removal (fig. 147A). In such cases it is resected in toto down to the scleral surface and closure made with a couple of fine silk sutures. Scarring is minimal and the cosmetic result is good. The role of pinguecula in the etiology of pterygium is discussed below.

Pterygium

Pterygium (*pteryx* = wing) is a growth of thickened conjunctiva which encroaches on the cornea. The lesion is always situated in the region of the palpebral fissure and almost always on the nasal side of the cornea. It is frequently bilateral and typically described as having a head, neck and body. However, these details are generally hard to make out (fig. 147B). It is usually seen as a triangular-shaped growth with rounded apex encroaching on the cornea and containing a horizontal sheath of blood vessels.

As it grows toward the center of the cornea, it invades the corneal epithelium and Bowman's membrane as well, and is preceded by a grayish halo of superficial corneal opacification. It may be small and nonprogressive for many years and in such cases need only be watched and left alone. Often, however, it progresses rather rapidly and requires removal for visual as well as cosmetic reasons. In recurrent cases scarring may be severe enough to interfere with movement of the eyeball.

Etiology

The elder Fuchs thought that a pinguecula could form the early stages of pterygium. Sugar believes that pterygium is initiated in those cases in which the pinguecula is large enough to involve the edge of Bowman's membrane. Picó believes that there is an unquestionable relation of pinguecula to pterygium; however, it is sunlight which is the chief offender. Pterygium, he points out, is primarily a disease of tropical and subtropical areas and those working in sunlight are most commonly affected. On the other hand, people who start wearing glasses in youth rarely get pterygium. Darrell and Bachrach, working among veterans, also showed that exposure to the ultraviolet light of sunlight increases the incidence of pterygium.

This seems to be confirmed by Cameron who found that the prevalence rate of pterygia varies directly with the latitude. The rate is negligible in the latitudes greater than 40° N or S. Then it increases uniformly to reach its highest value between 30° N or S and the equator. There is some exception to this in equatorial regions where the rate is reduced by cloud cover and the shade of tropical vegetation. This again points to ultraviolent light as being the main factor in the production of pterygia.

Other environmental factors may also be responsible. Detels and Dhur found the incidence of pterygium among sawmill workers to be 25.3 per cent as compared to 7.1 per cent among controls. These were all *indoor* workers who were not exposed to ultraviolet light. They also found that the percentage of incidence increased the longer the employment. Incidentally, 13 per cent of the workers were found to have lateral pterygia—hence they are not as uncommon as was supposed.

Pterygium has been known as far back as man's records go. It was difficult to cure two thousand years ago; it is not easy to cure today. Total excision of the lesion was practiced in ancient times and still constitutes one of the best methods of treatment. Celsus of Rome and Paulus of Greece did a simple ablation and allowed the wound to granulate in. Coccius was apparently the first to undermine, resect and close the conjunctival defect. Until the days of Arlt (1850) this was the favorite method of treating pterygia. In 1855 Desmarres, Sr. opened a new avenue of treatment by transplanting the pterygium into the lower cul-de-sac thus changing the direction of its growth. Desmarres, Jr. (1874) divided the larger pterygia and transplanted half into the upper and lower fornices respectively. McReynolds (1902) was the first to practice burial of the pterygium beneath the conjunctiva. This, with modifications, was one of the most popular methods of treatment until recently.

Surgery of Pterygium (Picó)

A more rewarding procedure for handling pterygia has come to the fore in recent years. Essentially this consists of (1) complete resection of the pterygium, and (2) plastic repair of the resultant conjunctival wound by undermining the lips and closing so as to leave an area of bared sclera next to the limbus. Various modifications of this procedure have been suggested by Newton, Wilszek, Kamel and many others. Leaving bared sclera at the limbus as originally suggested by D'Ombrain, King and others, lessens the possibility of recurrence. The following is the technic of Picó:

Procedure (fig. 148):   A superficial keratectomy is done, dissecting the head of the pterygium away from the cornea (fig. 148*A*). Two horizontal incisions are then made in the normal conjunctiva above and below the pterygium; these incisions converge at the plica (fig. 148*B*). The pterygium is completely resected and the bared sclera scraped clean of any residual tags of tissue (fig. 148*C*). A copper ball cautery is then applied to a 2 mm. wide area adjacent to the limbus and to any residual bleeding vessels.

The conjunctiva above the defect is undermined with scissors and a 10 mm. vertical incision is made in it about 3 mm. from the limbus; this creates a triangular flap (fig. 148D). A 6–0 silk suture is passed through the point of the flap, through the sclera at the lower border of the con-junctival defect, then through the lower conjunctiva about 3 mm. from the limbus (fig. 148E). When the sutures are tied the flap is drawn down (fig. 148F). A second 6–0 suture is passed through the flap, sclera and conjunctiva above (fig. 148F) and tied. Additional sutures are added for conjunctival closure. This leaves a 3 mm. bared area of sclera at the limbus (fig. 148G). Beta radiation is immediately applied to the bared area by means of a strontium 90 applicator (2000 rep) to which a Castroviejo screening mask is attached (fig. 148H). The opening in the mask is shown in the insert of figure 148H.

The eye is dressed and an antibiotic steroid ointment applied routinely. If new blood vessels appear in the area four or five days after operation, they are scraped off and another 2000 rep of beta radiation applied. It is important to prevent formation of granulation tissue in the area until it is covered by corneal and conjunctival epithelium. Picó has only had 3 per cent recurrence in 200 operations.

Comment: There are almost as many technics of pterygium repair as there are ophthalmic surgeons. But most of them now believe in leaving some bared sclera and using beta radiation as described above. Alger adds Newton's groove to the operation, i.e., a groove cut in the affected limbus which is then cauterized. He feels that the conjunctiva should be sutured tightly to the sclera about 6 mm. from the limbus and that sutures should be left in for ten days. Haik applies 900 rad beta radiation to the bared sclera immediately after operation.

FIG. 148. Surgery for Resection of Pterygium (Picó).
A. An incision is made in clear cornea 1 mm. ahead of the pterygium.
B. Superficial keratectomy is done and the pterygium undermined.
C. The pterygium is completely resected, the bared sclera scraped with a knife and the tip of a copper ball cautery is applied to an area 2 mm. wide adjacent to the limbus. The cautery also catches any bleeding vessels on the sclera.
D. The conjunctiva above the defect is undermined with scissors and a 10 mm. vertical incision is made.
E. A needle with a 6–0 silk suture catches up the tip of the lateral triangular conjunctival flap, the sclera at the lower conjunctival border and the lower conjunctival cut edge. The suture is tied and the two conjunctival edges united.
F. A second suture unites the upper vertical cut of conjunctiva. This needle is again passed through the sclera to anchor it.
G. Additional sutures are added for good closure.
H. Beta radiation (2000 rep) to the bared sclera is immediately applied as the last step in the operation.

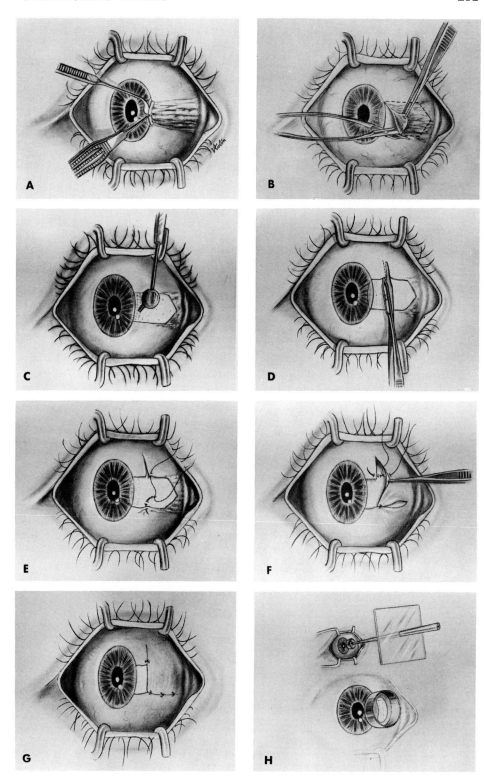

Van den Brenk has reported a series of 1300 pterygia in 1064 patients who received 2 to 3 postoperative beta radiation treatments with a strontium 90 applicator as a prophylactic measure. He reports an over-all recurrence rate of 1.7 per cent.

Recurrence

Recurrent pterygia are a serious problem and may present an almost malignant growth which is difficult to control. Until recently the most optimistic reports have shown something like a 20 per cent recurrence rate with the average higher. Recurrences with the bared sclera technic are less. They are only 3 to 4 per cent with beta radiation. Apparently recurrences are more likely in younger people, in those susceptible to keloid formation and when conjunctiva is left at the limbus.

Most recently the use of triethylene thiophosphoramide (thio-tepa, Lederle) has been found useful in preventing pterygium recurrence. This is a radiomimetic drug which is used instead of beta radiation. It inhibits hematopoiesis locally without affecting general blood composition. Thus it is an inhibitor of capillary and endothelial proliferation.

The drug is used in 1:2000 Ringers solution using 2 drops every three hours during the waking day for six weeks. (It may be and has been used in solutions as strong as 1:100 in oil without ill effects.) The limbus must be watched and the strength of the drug increased if new vessels are noted. The drug is somewhat irritating and a conjunctivitis develops which disappears when use of the drug is discontinued. According to the various reports in the literature postoperative recurrence of pterygium is only 3 to 5 per cent with use of thio-tepa.

PSEUDOPTERYGIUM

Pseudopterygium (cicatricial pterygium; inflammatory pterygium) may occur at any point of the limbus. This is a growth of conjunctiva

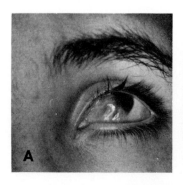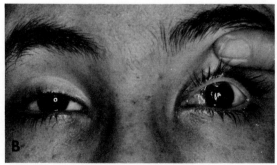

FIG. 149.   Pseudopterygium Repair.
A.   Pseudopterygium due to chemical injury.
B.   Appearance after repair.

over the cornea due to physical trauma, burns, chemical injuries, inflammations, etc. If sufficiently severe, it may impede the movement of the globe and even obstruct vision (fig. 149A).

The procedure of repair is to shave the invading tissue off the cornea as described above. The dissection is carried out beyond the limbus and the excess tissue excised cleanly. If the condition is severe, care must be taken to release all adhesions to assure free movement of the globe and to excise all fibrous tissue which might cause readhesion. The conjunctiva is then drawn over the raw surface and sutured (fig. 149B). Occasionally free grafts of mucous membrane may be needed. The problem differs in no way from that encountered after excision of a cyst, tumor, losses due to cicatrization such as pemphigus, etc.

Recurrence of pseudopterygium is possible as in the case of true pterygium. The best prophylaxis after repair of large pseudopterygia is treatment with beta radiation to destroy newly formed blood vessels. Recurrent pseudoptyergium can run as malignant a course as a true pterygium and the surgeon will be well advised to irradiate postoperatively in the more severe cases. As in the case of true pterygia thio-tepa also works well.

SYMBLEPHARON

Symblepharon is an adhesion between the bulbar and palperal conjunctiva. Partial or incomplete symblepharon, as its name implies, shows effacement of only part of the cul-de-sac. In partial posterior symblepharon (fig. 150A) the attachment between the two conjunctival layers obliterates part of the posterior fornix while in anterior partial symblepharon (fig. 150B) the attachment between bulbar and palpebral conjunctiva does not reach the fornix. In total cul-de-sac symblepharon,

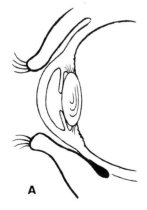

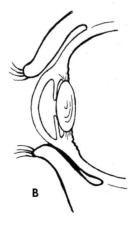

A

B

FIG. 150.   Partial Symblepharon.
A.   Posterior.   B.   Anterior.

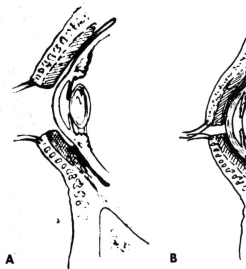
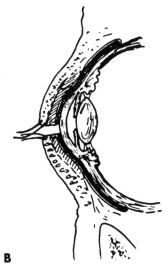

A   **B**

FIG. 151.   Total Symblepharon.
A.   Of fornix.   B.   Of entire conjunctival sac.

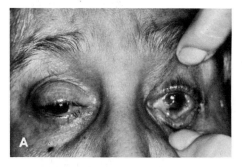
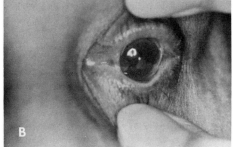

FIG. 152.   Repair of Mild Anterior Symblepharon.
A.   Appearance before correction.
B.   After simple repair by undermining and closure.

as its name implies, a whole fornix is obliterated (fig. 151A) and in complete symblepharon there are no fornices at all left (fig. 151B). In all types the cornea is frequently involved. The causes of symblepharon are most commonly physical trauma or chemical burns. Long-standing acute inflammations such as pemphigus and Stevens-Johnson disease also contribute to its causation.

Mild Symblepharon

When the adhesion is slight, the cornea uninvolved— or only slightly so—and the movement of the eye unimpeded, it is probably best to leave it alone. If a repair is desired in such cases (fig. 152A) the adhesion is cut, the edges of the conjunctiva undermined and drawn together over the raw surfaces and sutured. The wound is dressed daily to assure healing and prevent new adhesions (fig. 152B).

Repair of Symblepharon (Arlt)

When the conjunctival adhesion is larger and the cornea greatly involved, the symblepharon constitutes not only a cosmetic blemish but also a bar to the free movement of the globe (fig. 153*A*). In these cases repair is imperative. The method introduced by Arlt in 1874 is as good now as it was then.

Procedure (fig. 153): The resection is begun in clear cornea just beyond the symblepharon. The conjunctiva attached to the cornea is grasped with forceps and shaved off with a sharp scalpel so that only corneal tissue is left. Often the cornea has been previously ruptured or deeply involved so that scarring is unavoidable. Peripheral to the cornea the dissection is continued with scissors on the under surface of the conjunctiva to the lid margin (fig. 153*B*). One, two, or three double-armed 4–0 silk sutures (depending on the size of the symblepharon) are passed through the conjunctival edge which has been dissected away from the cornea.

All scar tissue in the fornix is resected so that the eye can move freely in all directions. The needles of the sutures are then passed through the fundus of the fornix and out to the skin surface over the lower orbital rim. The single skin suture used here is tightened and tied (fig. 153*C*). These sutures should be threaded on large round cutting needles so that they can be passed easily through the full thickness of the lower lid tissues. The lips of the bulbar conjunctival wound are undermined and united with 6–0 silk or catgut interrupted sutures. If the wound is large, the undermining may have to be extensive. In unusually severe cases, conjunctiva or mucous membrane from elsewhere may have to be grafted. The cornea may also have to be restored by a lamellar graft. The socket is filled with sterile ointment and patched. After 48 hours the eye is redressed daily and the sutures removed on the fifth or sixth day. Patching is continued until the cornea is completely healed (fig. 153*D*). The final result is seen in figure 153*E*.

Comment: Figure 153*C* shows closure of the two sliding conjunctival flaps on the globe according to the Arlt technic. The Teale-Knapp technic shows a different type of closure in which two rotated flaps are used (fig. 154). None of the tissue which has been shaved off the cornea should be wasted. It is all used to reline the anterior wall of the fornix. If the pupillary area of the cornea has been involved and there is residual opacity, an optical iridectomy or corneal transplant may also have to be done later.

In shaving off the conjunctiva from the sclera care must be taken. The condition of the sclera is not always known nor ascertainable preoperatively. The thickened conjunctiva may mask a scleral rupture with exposed ciliary processes and choroid which also require repair. Hence, unless the case has been followed from the very beginning, con-

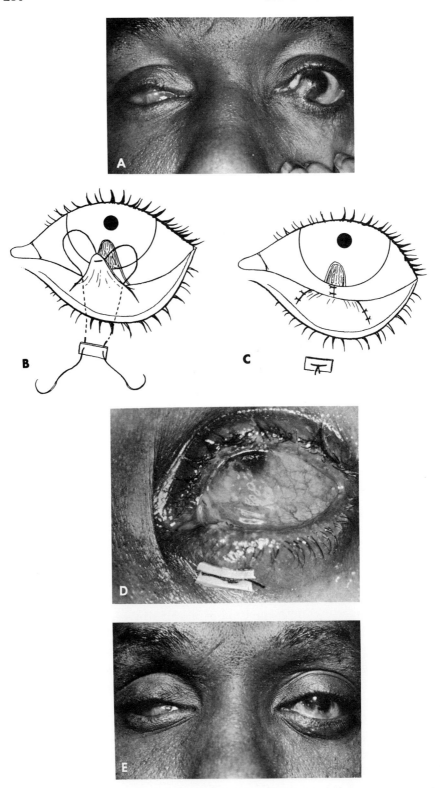

FIG. 153.   Repair of Symblepharon (after Arlt).

A.   Symblepharon of left lower lid with corneal involvement.

B.   The conjunctiva is shaved off the cornea, sutures are passed through the cut edge and then forward to the skin surface of the lower lid at the edge of the lower orbital rim.

C.   The edges of the conjunctiva on the globe are undermined, drawn together and sutured. The edges in the fornix are also sutured. The skin sutures are tightened and tied over a peg.

D.   Appearance before removal of sutures.

E.   Final result.

junctival dissection should be done with circumspection. Also one must be prepared to graft conjunctiva if not enough is available by sliding graft (see figure 145).

Total Symblepharon

In cases of symblepharon involving the whole eyeball the difficulties encountered are sometimes insurmountable. First, such a large amount of conjunctival substitute is necessary that it is not always easily obtainable. Secondly, there is a tendency for grafted oral mucous membrane, if used, to shrink and cicatrize, especially if any host cicatrices are still present. Epidermis is ruled out if the cornea is intact; its use would set up an intractable keratitis which no treatment can control. The use of other tissue such as peritoneum has not proved satisfactory. All in all, unless there is the gravest necessity, such cases had best be left alone if any vision is retained. In the absence of useful vision enucleation of the useless globe and socket reconstruction is to be considered.

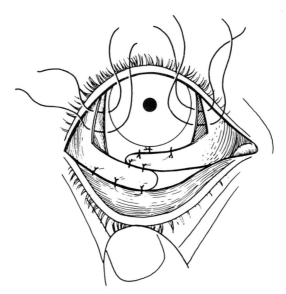

FIG. 154.   Teale-Knapp Technic of Symblepharon Repair.

Conjunctival flaps on each side of the cornea are mobilized and brought down to cover the bared area in the lower fornix.

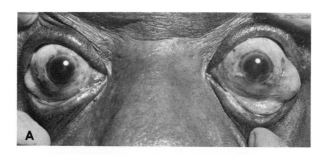

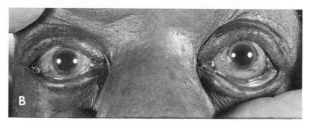

Fig. 155. Fat Hernia.
A. Bilateral lateral subconjunctival fat hernia.
B. Appearance after repair.

SUBCONJUNCTIVAL FAT HERNIA

The appearance of orbital fat beneath the conjunctiva is primarily a congenital condition due to localized weakness of Tenon's capsule which is aggravated with age due to loss of elasticity of the tarsal fascia This is usually bilateral and is characterized by the appearance of a subconjunctival soft, yellow, lobulated mass on the globe most commonly between the superior and lateral recti (fig. 155A). The herniated fat is continuous with the main body of orbital fat and hence its complete removal is impossible.

Usually the condition is nonprogressive and since it is evident only when the lids are raised, nothing need be done surgically. Occasionally the mass becomes large and bulging and sinks so low that it becomes visible and resection of the protruding fat mass has to be done. In such cases an incision is made through the conjunctiva and the thinned out Tenon's capsule and all the presenting fat resected. Tenon's is closed separately with a 6–0 chromic catgut and the conjunctiva over it with 6–0 silk or catgut interrupted sutures. Healing is uneventful (fig. 155B).

CYSTS AND NEOPLASMS OF THE CONJUNCTIVA

Transparent cysts of the conjunctiva are not uncommon (fig. 156A). They contain a slightly viscous clear fluid and appear like migratory

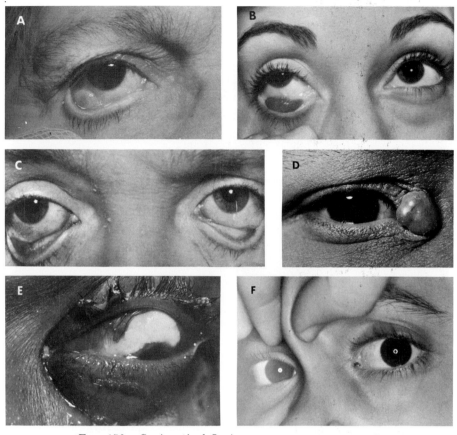

FIG. 156. Conjunctival Lesions.

A. Clear conjunctival cyst.   D. Cyst of caruncle.
B. Hemangioma.   E. Squamous cell carcinoma
C. Melanosis.   F. Nevus of caruncle.

"water blisters" under the bulbar or palpebral conjunctiva. If surgery is desired simple resection and closure is done.

In long-standing chronic inflammation large conjunctival cysts may be found, also glandular retention cysts. Both types are rare. Both are removed surgically. Conjunctival cysts, probably due to epithelial implantation, are also occasionally seen following strabismus surgery. The cyst lining must be removed to be sure of nonrecurrence.

The most common neoplasms of the conjunctiva are nevi, dermoids, papillomas, hemangiomas, lipomas and fibromas. The most common malignant tumors are squamous cell epitheliomata, sarcomas and melanomas (fig. 156). Pigmented tumors and melanosis may be benign, precancerous or frankly malignant. All these require surgical treatment as elsewhere.

A hemangiomatous lesion must be examined carefully (fig. 156B). Often it has deep vascular connections and bleeding after resection may

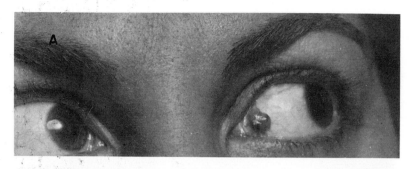

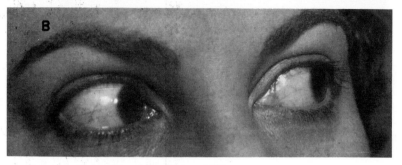

FIG. 157. Affections of Plica.
A. A case of pigmented nevus of the left plica.
B. Appearance after simple resection and closure.

become a serious problem. Some surgeons believe that these are best treated by sclerosing solutions or some other modality rather than surgery.

The incidence of squamous cell epithelioma of the conjunctiva, unlike that of the skin, is much greater than the basal cell. It occurs about ten times as frequently. It is not always easy to distinguish between these two entities although sometimes the squamous tumor may be a clear white due to its keratin content (fig. 156E). Malignant tumors of the conjunctiva require the same careful wide excision as elsewhere, with subsequent repair. Postoperative irradiation must also be considered. In the case pictured in figure 156E, exenteration was done.

AFFECTIONS OF PLICA AND CARUNCLE

The plica and caruncle, covered as they are by conjunctiva, are also heirs to conjunctival pathology. It is not unusual for them to show neoplasms, especially nevi of the pigmented type. The plica is a narrow crescentic fold of tissue lying external to the caruncle and partially covered by it. It is thicker than the bulbar and fornical conjunctiva. A pigmented nevus (fig. 157A) of the left plica is shown which was resected some fifteen years ago (fig. 157B). The caruncle is also covered with conjunctiva, contains hair follicles, sebaceous and sweat glands and

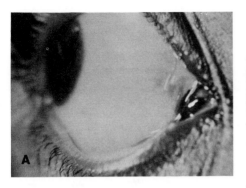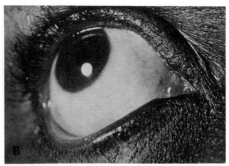

FIG. 158.   Affections of Caruncle.
A.   Melanoma of caruncle.   *B.*   After removal.

hence is also subject to the pathology of all these elements. Figure 158*A*
shows a melanotic nevus of the caruncle removed nine years ago (fig.
158*B*).

In both plica and caruncle, neoplasms are removed by routine wide
excision and closure.

REFERENCES

ALGER, L. J.: Etiology of pterygium recurrence. Am. J. Ophth. *57*:450, 1964.

ARLT, F. R.: American Encyclopedia of Ophthalmology. Chicago, Cleveland Press,
1913, vol. 1, p. 592.

BANGERTER, A.: Pterygium operation and covering of conjunctival defects. Ophthalmologica *106*:316, 1943.

CAMERON, M. E.: Geographic distribution of pterygia. Trans. Ophth. Soc. Austr.
25:67, 1966.

CAMPODONICO, R.: A new procedure in the excision method of pterygium operation.
Int. Cong. Ophth. Washington *1*:20, 1922.

CASSIDY, J. R.: The inhibition of pterygium recurrence by thio-tepa. Am. J. Ophth.
61:886, 1966.

CASTROVIEJO, R.: Plastic and reconstructive surgery of the conjunctiva. Plast.
& Reconstr. Surg. *24*:1, 1959.

CELSUS: Cited by Beard, C. H., Ophthalmic Surgery. Philadelphia, P. Blakiston's
Son & Co., ed. 2, 1914, p. 347.

COGAN, D. G., KUWABARA, T., and HOWARD, J.: The nonelastic nature of pingueculae.
Arch. Ophth. *61*:388, 1959.

DARRELL, R. W., and BACHRACH, C. A.: Pterygium among veterans. Arch. Ophth.
70:958, 1963.

DESMARRES, L. A.: Traité theorique et pratique des maladies. Paris, 1855, ed. 2,
p. 168.

DETELS, B., and DHUR, S. P.: Pterygium. A geographical study. Arch. Ophth.
78:485, 1967.

D'OMBRAIN, A.: The surgical treatment of pterygium. Brit. J. Ophth. *32*:65, 1948.

ESCAPINI, H.: Pterygium excision. Am. J. Ophth. *45*:879, 1958.

GILLIES, H. D., and KILNER, J. J.: Symblepharon: Its treatment by Thiersch and
mucous membrane grafting. Trans. Ophth. Soc. U. K. *49*:470, 1920.

GOLDSTEIN, J. H.: Conjunctival cysts following strabismus surgery. J. Ped. Ophth.
5:204, 1968.

GREER, C. H.: Pigmented tumors of the conjunctiva. Trans. Ophth. Soc. Austr.
15:128, 1955.

242 OPHTHALMIC PLASTIC SURGERY

HAIK, G. M.: The management of pterygia. Am. J. Ophth. *61*:1128 (Pt. 2), 1966.

HILGERS, J. H. C.: Prevention of recurrent pterygium by beta radiation. Ophthalmologica *140*:369, 1960.

JOSELSON, G. A., and MULLER, P.: Incidence of pterygium recurrence in patients treated with thio-tepa. Am. J. Ophth. *61*:891, 1966.

KAMEL, S.: The treatment of pterygium. Bull. Ophth. Soc. Egypt. *51*:493, 1958.

KIFFNEY, G. T.: Large conjunctival cysts. Am. J. Ophth. *54*:458, 1962.

KING, J. H.: The pterygium: Brief review and evaluation of certain methods of treatment. Arch. Ophth. *44*:854, 1950.

KNAPP, H.: Pterygium repair. Arch. Ophth. *14*:1868, 1967.

LANGHORN, M. E.: The inhibition of corneal vascularization by Triethylene thiophosphoramide. Am. J. Ophth. *49*:1111 (Pt. 2), 1960.

LERMAN, S.: Primary lymphosarcoma of the conjunctiva. Am. J. Ophth. *50*:147, 1960.

LIDDY, B. ST. L., and MORGAN, J. F.: Triethylene thiophosphoramide (thio-tepa) and pterygium. Am. J. Ophth. *61*:888, 1966.

LUBKIN, V., and HUGHES, W. L.: The fornix conformer. Arch. Ophth. *61*:248, 1959.

LUBKIN, V.: Lateral and medial fornix conformers. Arch. Ophth. *79*:582, 1968.

MAXWELL, P. W.: An operation for the relief of symblepharon, etc. Ophth. Rev. *12*:189, 1893.

McGAVIC, J. S.: Surgical treatment of ecurrent pterygium. Arch. Ophth. *42*:726, 1949.

McREYNOLDS, J. O.: The nature and treatment of pterygium. J.A.M.A. *39*:296, 1902.

MEACHAM, C. T.: Prevention of recurrence of pterygium. E.E.N.T. Monthly *44*:62, 1965.

NEWTON, F. H.: Operation for recurrent pterygium. Am. J. Ophth. *44*:258, 1957.

PICO, G.: Pterygium: Current concepts of etiology and management. Highlights Ophth. *8*:247, 1965.

ROCK, R. L.: Inhibition of corneal vascularization by triethylene thiophosphoramise (thio-tepa). Arch. Ophth. *69*:330, 1963.

RUIZ BARRANCO, F.: The treatment of pterygium. Arch. Soc. oftal. hisp.-am. *18*:234, 1958.

SPAETH, E. B.: Rotated island graft for pterygium. Am. J. Ophth. *9*:649, 1926.

SUGAR, S. H.: Surgical treatment of pterygium. Am. J. Ophth. *32*:912, 1949.

SUGAR, S., and KOBERNICK, S.: The pinguecula. Am. J. Ophth. *47*:341, 1959.

TAELE, T. P.: On the relief of symblepharon by transplantation of the conjunctiva. Ophth. Hosp. Repts. J. Roy. Lond. Ophth. Hosp. *3*:253, 1857–1859.

VAN DEN BRENK, H. A. S.: Results of postoperative irradiation in 1300 patients with pterygium. Am. J. Roentgen. *103*:723, 1968.

WALTER, W. L.: Pterygium surgery. Am. J. Ophth. *51*:441, 1961.

WHALMAN, H. F.: Mucous membrane grafts in ophthalmic conditions. Trans. Pac. Coast. Oto-Ophth. Soc. *23*:32, 1938.

WILCZEK, M.: Bindenhautplastik. Klin. Monatsbl. Augenh. *135*:822, 1959.

ZAUBERMAN, H.: Pterygium and its recurrence. Am. J. Ophth. *63*:1780, 1967.

CHAPTER 13

Hair-Bearing Grafts

EXAMPLES OF HAIR-BEARING GRAFTS have been mentioned previously and their use touched upon in Chapter 3. It is the purpose of this chapter to present the technics of lash and brow grafting in detail and to discuss them in actual performance.

The grafting of hair-bearing tissue is one of the least satisfying types of grafts. The crop of hair obtained often does not justify the work and trouble of the plowing and seeding operation entailed. For, if the truth be told, less and less lash and brow grafting is being done as time goes on. Lash grafts, especially, are easily and correctly grown only in illustrations and smoothly described in books. But the occasional good result keeps one trying and hoping for a successful harvest when the occasion arises. This is especially true of the upper lid where loss of lashes is most noticeable. Naturally, the examples given here will be those of successful or at least partially successful hair-bearing grafts. This does not mean that the author has not had his full share of failures.

LASH GRAFTING

In general there are two technics commonly used in lash grafting. In one, cilia are grafted as one of the final stages in lid reconstruction. The other type of lash grafting has the double purpose of restoring skin tissue to the lid margin as well as grafting cilia. This is most commonly seen when a hair-bearing brow pedicle is swung down to restore tissue loss at the lid margin.

Simple Lash Graft

Paul Knapp in 1908 was apparently the first to graft hair-bearing skin successfully from the eyebrow when he reported two cases in which he had succeeded in getting "takes" in reconstructed lids. Wheeler reported the same technic in 1920 for the simultaneous repair of an upper and lower lid.

Although no hair-bearing area in the body duplicates lid lashes exactly, the lower medial end of the eyebrow comes closest to actual lashes in length, color and direction and is the first choice as a donor site when cilia are needed. The graft must be wide enough to include four rows of lashes (about 3 to 4 mm.). This usually leaves the two center rows since the border lashes rarely survive surgery. Also the graft must be deep enough to include the root bulbs and this usually means a depth of

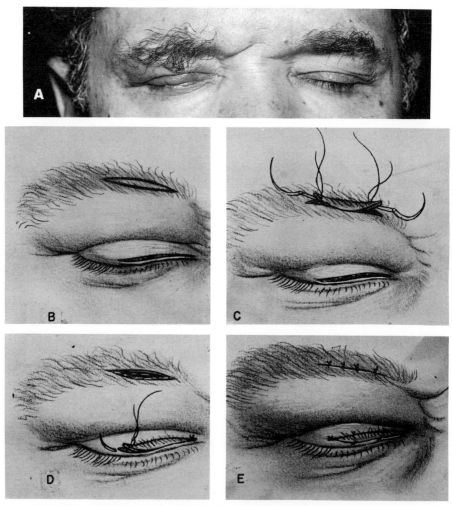

FIG. 159. Technic of the Simple Lash Graft.
A.   Absence of lashes from medial half of right upper lid.
B.   A bed for the graft is made in the lid and the graft area in the brow is outlined.
C.   The hair-bearing graft is raised and a suture is inserted at each end.
D.   The graft is sewed into the bed.
E.   The donor area is closed.

about 3 to 3.5 mm. Care should be taken not to injure these because, at best, their survival is problematic and growth precarious. Even more difficult is getting the hair to grow in the proper alignment and direction.

Since the hair of the brow is directed up and out, cilia transplants for the upper lid are taken from the ipsilateral brow while lower lashes are taken from the contralateral brow and reversed. This is especially important with a normal cornea in place as it helps to direct the hair growth away from the lid margin and eyeball. In the rare cases when brow hair is not available and temporal or occipital scalp hair have to be used, the direction of hair growth must also be watched and the graft properly placed.

Figure 159 is an example of this. The right upper lid was reconstructed following a full thickness resection of the center of the lid. Figure 159A shows the right upper and lower lids fused and healed after the first stage. The next procedure was that of lash grafting of the upper lid.

Procedure (fig. 159): About 2 mm. above the right upper lid edge a horizontal incision is made along the lashless central half of the lid through skin and muscle down to tarsus. The incision is widened by blunt dissection to make room for the graft and all bleeding stopped. A 4 mm. wide hair-bearing graft is taken from the medial end of the ipsilateral eyebrow (fig. 159B). This is 2 mm. longer than the bed prepared for it. A single 6–0 silk suture is placed through each end to facilitate handling (fig. 159C). After excision the graft is picked up by the sutures and fitted into the lid incision. It is sutured at each end by means

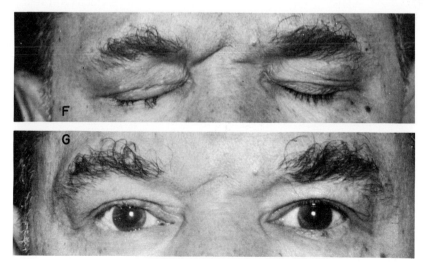

Fig. 159 *(Continued)*
F. Result before the lids are separated.
G. Appearance 10 weeks after separation.

of the carrying sutures (fig. 159*D*). Enough additional 6–0 silk sutures are used to fix the graft in position so that it is on a level with the rest of the lid and does not override the surface. The wound in the brow is closed with 4–0 plain catgut subcuticular and interrupted 5–0 silk sutures (fig. 159*E*).

A firm pressure dressing is applied. At the first dressing six days later the sutures are removed and the pressure dressing reapplied for four more days. A simple patch is used thereafter until healing is completed. The lids are separated twelve weeks later. Figure 159*F* shows the lash growth before the lids are separated and figure 159*G* its appearance 10 weeks after separation (see Comment after next case).

Simultaneous Upper and Lower Lid Lash Graft

Figure 160 illustrates a simultaneous upper and lower lid lash graft. Figure 160*A* shows the right upper and lower lids before lid repair and figure 160*B* incisions for the lash grafting begun after the first stage of the repair.

Procedure (fig. 160): A horizontal incision is made through skin and muscle one mm. above the fused junction of the upper and lower lid margins. A similar but longer incision is made in the lower lid. The lips of both wounds are pushed apart by blunt dissection to make room for the hair-bearing strips of tissue. The graft for the upper lid is taken from the ipsilateral eyebrow. The graft for the lower lid is taken from the right eyebrow and reversed (fig. 160*B*).

The grafts are sewed into position with 6–0 silk sutures and the wounds in the donor eyebrows are closed with subcuticular 4–0 catgut and 5–0 silk sutures (fig. 160*C*). A firm pressure dressing is applied over the grafts. On the sixth day the sutures are removed and pressure reapplied for three more days (fig. 160*D*).

Eight weeks later the lids are separated and the lid edges allowed to epithelialize, being dressed daily with copious ointment instilled in the socket to prevent readhesion (fig. 160*E*).

Comment: It will be noted that in procedure 159 the trough for the graft was made 2 mm. from the lid margin while in procedure 160 the incision was only 1 mm. from the margin. In general, the nearer the grafted cilia are to the lid margin the more natural the appearance and the better the cosmetic result. Hence in procedure 161 where the socket was anophthalmic, the graft was placed as close to the margin as possible. For even if trichiasis developed—as it often does—it would not matter. In figure 159, however, a normal globe was present. To place the cilia graft too close to the margin here would have been to tempt fate. A glance at the result in this case will show that the 2 mm. gap between the lid edge and the graft was none too wide.

The hair originally planted are all lost during the first 2 or 3 weeks and, since it has been estimated that it takes an average of 8 to

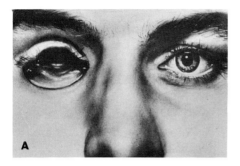 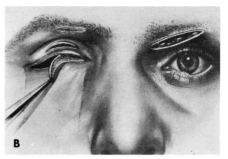

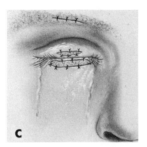

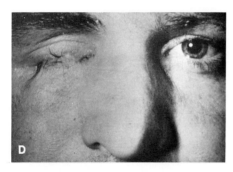 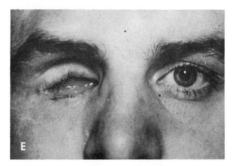

FIG. 160.   Combined Lash Grafts of Right Upper and Lower Lids.
A.   Lids before repair.
B.   Lash graft of repaired right upper lid from right brow; lash graft of right
     lower lid from left brow.
C.   Both grafts sutured into position.
D.   Appearance before lid separation.
E.   After separation.

12 weeks for cilia to regenerate and appear above the skin surface, the
lid margins are bare for what seems a long time. Then, sparsely and
irregularly, the lashes begin to appear. When long enough they should
be pasted down in the proper direction with collodion and kept that way
for some time in an attempt to train them to grow in the proper direction. (It works sometimes.) Pressure dressings for several weeks also
have been advised. However, despite long and careful precautions, it is
difficult to prevent the perverse things from causing trichiasis even in
the most successful cases.

   It is interesting to note that such men as Kuhnt, Sheehan and

Blaskovics all advised tattooing of lashes rather than trying to grow cilia (fig. 166). But hope springs eternal . . . .

Combined Lash Graft and Coloboma Repair—Lunate Coloboma

Crescentic (lunate) dehiscences of the lid margin are colobomata in which there is absence of an appreciable portion of the ciliary border of the lid but the lesion is shallow and rarely extends much beyond the margin (fig. 161A). Although the loss of tissue is not great, the deformity is usually unsightly and, if the upper lid is involved, it leaves an area

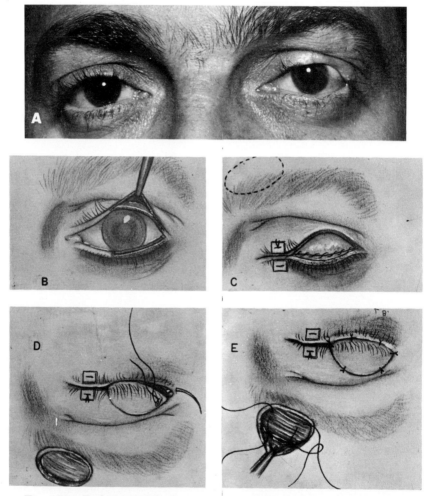

FIG. 161. Technic of Simultaneous Lash Graft and Lid Margin Repair.
A. Partial loss of left upper lid margin.
B. The affected and opposing lids are split.
C. The tarsoconjunctiva of the upper lid is mobilized and sutured to the tarso-conjunctiva of the lower lid. A medial tarsorrhaphy is made.
D. A hair-bearing graft is taken from the ipsilateral brow and sewn into the upper lid dehiscence.
E. The brow wound is closed with subcutaneous and skin sutures.

of cornea exposed when the eye is closed. Repair of this type of defect does not present a major problem and the following method is simple and yields good results.

Procedure (fig. 161):   The involved portion of the lid is split at the gray line into its two layers, the dissection being made sufficiently deep to mobilize both layers adequately. All scar tissue is resected. The opposing lid edge is freshened and also split into its two layers but only to a depth of about 2 mm. (fig. 161*B*). The edges of the tarsoconjunctival layers of the two lids are united by a 6–0 chromic running suture, anchored at both ends. The skin-muscle layer of the injured lid is re-tracted, leaving an area of raw tarsal surface exposed. A mattress suture is passed through the medial portions of the lid margins to complete lid immobilization (fig. 161*C*).

A free graft cut to pattern is taken from the brow of the same lid. This includes about 4 mm. of brow hair to replace the lost cilia of the lid margin and enough clear skin to make up for the rest of the lost skin of the lid. The graft is sewed into place with 6–0 silk interrupted sutures (fig. 161*D*). The donor site is closed with 4–0 plain catgut subcuticular sutures and 5–0 silk sutures (fig. 161*E*). The site of operation is covered with a perforated dressing and firm pressure applied. It is not necessary to patch the fellow eye. The dressing is removed on the sixth day, the area is cleansed, the sutures are removed and the pressure dressing reapplied for three more days. By this time the graft has "taken." The eye is patched daily for a few more days until healing is complete, at

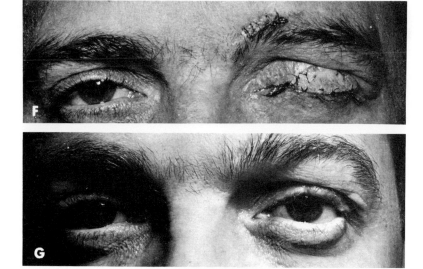

FIG. 161 *(Continued)*
F.   Appearance of the repair before the removal of sutures.
G.   Final result.
     (Fox, S. A.: Courtesy Archives of Ophthalmology.)

which time dressings are discontinued (fig. 161 *F*). The lids are separated six weeks later and the edges allowed to epithelialize with a regimen of daily dressings and copious ointment until completely healed (fig. 161*G*).

Comment: The lid will be somewhat thickened for several weeks but will gradually assume a normal appearance. Cilia should begin to reappear 8 to 12 weeks after operation. In taking a graft, it is preferable to use tissue from the lower medial part of the brow and the skin below it for this is close to the skin of the lid in color and texture. However, because of the direction of the growth of the hair of the average eyebrow this is not always possible and skin above the brow must be taken sometimes as here. This is thicker and somewhat paler than the skin below the brow. But while it is a trifle more difficult to handle, experience shows that the "take" is as certain and, after several weeks, the cosmetic result is about as good. For lower lid repair, tissue from above the brow must be taken and reversed if the globe is present. If the socket is anophthalmic, the direction of cilia is not so important as there is no fear of subjecting the eye to trichiasis and the graft may be taken from below the brow.

EYEBROW GRAFTS

The eyebrow, a good source of hair-bearing tissue for lash grafting, occasionally requires repair on its own account. This may be due to the trauma of battle, accident or burns. The repairs may vary from the correction of displaced eyebrows by means of rotated pedicles to the creation of new eyebrows by free grafting.

Upward Displacement of Eyebrow

Figure 162 shows the technic of correcting the upward displacement of an eyebrow (fig. 162*A*) by a simple Z plasty and transposition of flaps as detailed below.

Procedure (fig. 162): A flat Z incision is made with the upper angle of the Z including the displaced eyebrow. The lower angle includes an area of equal size below the displaced brow (fig. 162*B*). The upper incisions are made through skin and subcutaneous fat sufficiently deep to include the intact hair follicles. (Brow skin is quite thick and one must not hesitate to cut deeply.) All scar tissue is resected. The two flaps are undermined, care being taken not to injure the hair follicles. They

---

FIG. 162. Repair of Upward Displacement of Eyebrow.
A. Cicatricial displacement of right eyebrow.
B. A flat Z incision is made to include the displaced brow.
C. The two pedicles are dissected up, transposed and sutured into position.
D. Appearance before removal of sutures.
E. Final result.

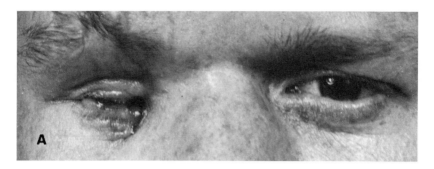

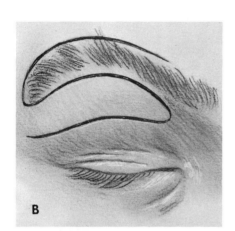

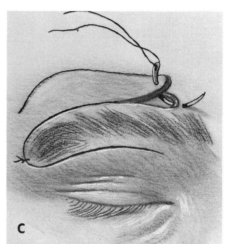

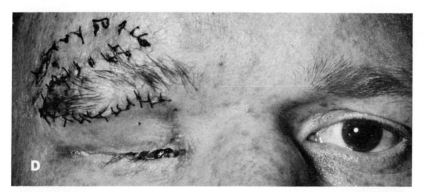

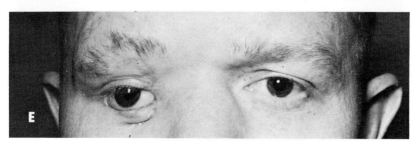

are then transposed and sutured into position (figs. 162C and D). A firm pressure dressing is applied. On the sixth day the sutures are removed and pressure is reapplied for four more days. The final result is seen in figure 162E.

Downward Displacement of Eyebrow

Figure 163 is a similar case. But here the temporal half of the right eyebrow was displaced downward and caught in scar tissue of the lid. The Z plasty was again used but, in this case, the lower angle of the Z included the displaced eyebrow and the upper angle, the skin above the brow (fig. 163A). Repair was completed in a fashion similar to the previous case. Figure 163B shows the completed procedure and figure 163C the final result.

Comment: These procedures are uniformly successful if care is taken not to injure the hair follicles. The blood supply is usually adequate and the graft sure of a "take" if the bed is cleared of scar tissue.

Reconstruction of Eyebrow by Rotated Pedicle

Total absence of an eyebrow is a more difficult and less rewarding procedure for several reasons. The injury which causes complete loss of an eyebrow is usually extensive and severe. Much scar tissue is created and the blood supply of the area is impaired; hence the bed in which the graft is to be seated is not ideal for successful grafting. Furthermore, free hair-bearing grafts are notoriously uncertain under the best conditions. This is not to say that they cannot be done or should not be attempted. But one must not expect too much for they are the least trustworthy of an untrustworthy lot.

Three methods of repair are available. If the contralateral brow is thick and can stand the loss of half its width (fig. 164A) then it may be used as the source of a donor graft from which a pedicle can be rotated over to the opposite bared brow area (fig. 164C). Another method is to use the ipsilateral temporal area as the source for a rotated pedicle to the brow. The third method is repair by means of a free hair-bearing graft from the temporal (fig. 32) or occipital (fig. 33) region. The first method only can be used when scarring of the brow is so great and the area is so avascular that a free graft would have no chance of survival. It is carried out as follows:

Procedure (fig. 164): The hairs of the donor eyebrow need not be shaved but are clipped short. The bed of the recipient brow is prepared by making a somewhat arching horizontal incision in the area of the destroyed brow to match the curve of the fellow brow in height and curvature. This incision is carried down deep enough so that when the graft is in place it will be on a level with the host skin surface. The edges are undermined slightly and separated sufficiently so that the

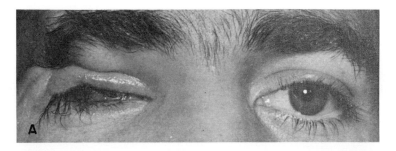

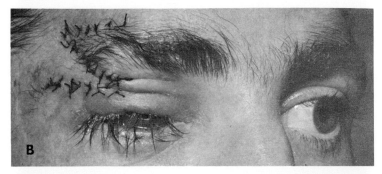

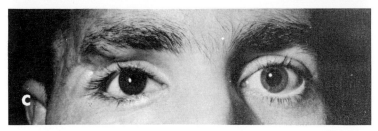

FIG. 163. Repair of Downward Displacement of Eyebrow.
A. The right eyebrow is pulled downward by a cicatrix.
B. Appearance of Z plasty repair before removal of sutures.
C. Final result.

graft may be fitted into its bed snugly. They should not be pushed back so far that they have to be pulled back into position after the graft is planted. Ideally the graft should be held in position by the wound lips. All scar tissue is resected and hemostasis is attained by pressure or ligation if necessary.

The upper half of the opposite eyebrow is split off by two parallel horizontal incisions somewhat inclined toward each other so that a cross section of the graft approximates a triangle apex downward (fig. 164B). These incisions intersect each other at the temporal end of the brow. The two incisions include a strip of hairless skin above the graft so that it will not be too narrow. Thus it contains more vascular supply and has a better chance of survival. The nasal incisions are carried well down toward the glabella to facilitate easy rotation of the graft. The pedicle is dissected up and left attached medially. The fat of the raw surface is cleaned off down to the hair follicles without injuring them. It is rotated into the bed prepared for it and sutured into place with interrupted 5–0 silk sutures (fig. 164C).

The donor site is closed with several 4–0 plain catgut subcuticular and interrupted 5–0 silk sutures (fig. 164D). A pressure dressing is applied to the grafted eyebrow. A simple dressing suffices for the donor brow. The grafted brow is dressed on the sixth day at which time the sutures may be removed. By this time the donor site is well healed and the sutures here may also be removed. The pressure dressing is reapplied to the grafted area for several more days to assure a good take. Figure 164E shows the result of such a procedure to repair the condition seen in figure 164A.

Comment: If a pedicle from the opposite brow is not available then one might be fashioned from the ipsilateral temple region in the same fashion. This is somewhat further away and means a little more scarring but may be worthwhile especially since such an area is usually so disfigured that another incision is of no consequence. Such occasions will not arise often.

Reconstruction of Eyebrow by Free Hair-Bearing Graft

If the blood supply is deemed adequate and the area is not too much scarred a *free* hair-bearing graft from the temporal or occipital region should be considered. Of the two the temporal region is probably the better site.

Procedure: The recipient area is prepared as above and hemostasis attained. A pattern is cut to measure and used as a guide for obtaining the graft. The hairs in the temporal region are clipped short but need not be shaved. After the graft is taken it is turned over and cleaned of all extraneous tissue close to the root bulbs which must not be injured. The graft is then sutured into position with interrupted 4–0 silk sutures. The donor area is closed with interrupted plain catgut subcuticular and 4–0 silk interrupted sutures. Postoperative care is the same as above.

Comment: As in the case of lid grafts the original hairs usually fall out during the first couple of weeks but with a successful take will start growing back subsequently. In the case of pedicle brow grafts the bulbs of the hair follicles may take root immediately and proceed to grow

---

Fig. 164.   Total Eyebrow Reconstruction.
A.   Appearance of right brow before repair.
B.   Brow bed is prepared and opposing brow is split.
C.   The hair-bearing pedicle is dissected up, rotated over and fitted into the recipient bed.
D.   The pedicle is sutured into place and the donor area is closed.
E.   Final result of transplantation from left to right brow.

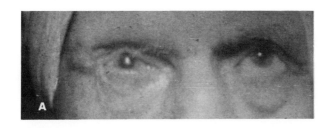

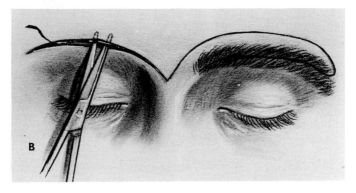

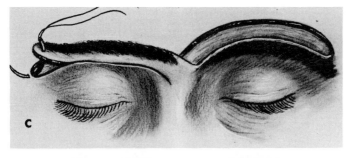

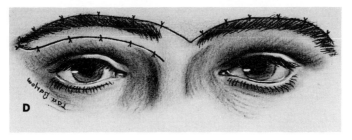

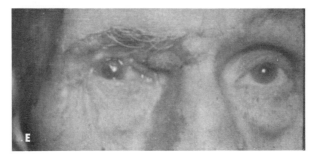

in their new environment without shedding. This is rare. Also rare is such a luxuriant crop of hair as to require occasional trimming. The graft should be cut 25 to 33 per cent larger than the bed to allow for shrinkage and loss of hair at the edges.

Absence of Both Eyebrows

Complete absence of both brows requires free hair-bearing grafts from the temporal and/or occipital regions and is a difficult and unrewarding surgical undertaking. Injuries of such a nature, usually severe burns or explosions, create much scar tissue and impair blood supply to such an extent that the recipient bed is not ideal for "takes." Hence such grafts are not noted for their success and the hopes of the patient must not be raised too high in anticipation. Occasionally, however, success is achieved much to everyone's surprise including the surgeon's.

REFERENCES

Fox, S. A.: Cresentic deformities of the lid margin. Arch. Ophth. 39:542, 1948.
Hughes, W. L.: Reconstructive Surgery of the Eyelid. St. Louis, C. V. Mosby Co., 1954, p. 129.
Knapp, Paul: Zwei fälle von Lidplastik nach Büdinger. Klin. Monatsbl. f. Augenh. 46: Part 2, 317–322, 1908.
Krusius, F. F.: Uber die Einpflanzung lebender Haare zur Wimpernbildung. Deutsch. med. Wchnschr. 40:958, 1914.
Schuessler, W. W., and Filmer, G. A.: A method for restoration of the cilia of the eyelids. Plast. & Recons. Surg. 2:345, 1947.
Toth, Z.: Transplantation of eyelashes. Klin. Monatsbl. Augenh. 116:209, 1950.

CHAPTER 14

Tattooing—Contact Prostheses

TATOOING
  CORNEAL TATTOING
    with Gold Chloride
    with Platinum Chloride
    with Palladium Oxide

           with Corneal Needle
        LID MARGIN TATTOING

        CONTACT PROSTHESES

TATTOOING was known and practiced long before the Christian era. The Maoris of New Zealand, for instance, perfected tattooing to a high art many centuries ago and it has always been prevalent in India, China, Borneo and other parts of the Far East. In primitive cultures tattooing distinguished men of rank and status. More recently tattooing is becoming a dying art especially in Polynesia as part of a general decay of primitive culture due to the onsweep of European civilization.

It was brought to Europe chiefly by sailors and now tattooing emporia thrive in different parts of the world. Essentially it consists of puncturing the skin in desired patterns and rubbing in dyes to fix the pattern indelibly.

It is only in the past few years that permanent color matching of skin grafts and flaps with insoluble pigment has been suggested for medical purposes. It is also used for cosmetic purposes to mask unsightly scars such as a bare hairless patch which is made to blend in with its surroundings. Part of the cosmetic treatment is the *removal* of tattoos in which advances have been made by dissolving them with the laser beam.

On the other hand, tattoo of the cornea for unsightly leukomas is of ancient lineage. Galen in the second century A. D. is known to have rubbed ferric tannate, mixtures of powdered pomegranate bark or salts of copper into the raw corneal surface which had been previously cauterized with a red-hot stylet. And John "Chevalier" Taylor, that notorious quack oculist of the eighteenth century, was apparently the first to make use of a needle and India ink for corneal tattooing.

Around 1870 Abadie and especially De Wecker revived the method and almost immediately thereafter reports of polychrome corneal tattooing began to appear. Thus, in 1872, B. C. Taylor of England and Levis in this country, among others, pointed out the cosmetic and visual advantages of masking corneal leukomas with pigments of various

257

colors. Levis also noted the importance of corneal tattoo in the "palliation or correction of some optical defects of vision such as unnatural opening of the iris" as well as in albinism, permanent mydriasis, conical cornea and irregular astigmatism.

Numerous papers continued to appear from then on noting improvements in method, pigments and instruments for corneal tattooing. By 1906 Chevallereau and Polak had standardized polychrome corneal tattooing sufficiently to recommend the use of a kit of eight basic pigments: yellow, blue, green, red and brown ochre, light and dark gray and black. At present the requisite number of pigments has been reduced to orange, brown, blue, black and white.* Black, of course, is primarily for the pupillary area.

In 1925 P. Knapp of Basel introduced chemical tattooing of the cornea with gold chloride. Again numerous reports immediately followed including those of Gifford and Steinberg in 1927 who were successful in obtaining dark brown or black pupils in four cases by means of 2 to 4 per cent gold chloride solution reduced with tannin. Platinum and silver solutions were found ineffective. In 1929 Pischel reported the use of both gold and platinum chloride and concluded that "tattooing the cornea with gold or platinum is an effective means of coloring the cornea brown or black."

CORNEAL TATTOOING

The common purpose of corneal tattooing is cosmetic: the erasure or masking of unsightly corneal scars appearing in the palpebral fissure. It is most effective in cases of old solid flat scars (fig. 165A). Corneal ectasia, anterior staphyloma, phthisis bulbi, adherent leukoma and glaucoma are contraindications because of the danger of stirring up an iridocyclitis.

From its inception corneal tattooing has also been used to good effect in albinism, aniridia, large iris colobomata, conical cornea and diffuse superficial corneal opacities. In the latter case it is used with or without an optical iridectomy to lessen the amount of irregular dispersion of light into the eye. Nagoya (1905) and A. A. Knapp more recently have reported visual improvement with this method. Two methods of pigmenting the cornea are available: (1) chemical dying of the superficial corneal stroma, and (2) impregnation of the cornea with pigments by needle tattoo. Both methods have their advantages and disadvantages. In chemical tattooage gold or platinum chloride is used to create a black pupil or to obtain a dark brown or black color over a

---

* These pigments are obtainable from Fezandie & Sperrle, Inc., 103 Lafayette St., New York City.

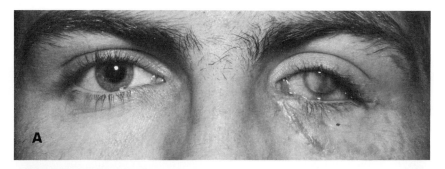

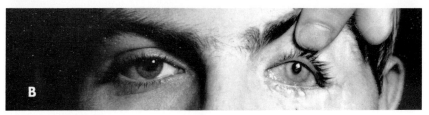

FIG. 165.   Tattoo of Cornea.
A.   Preoperative status of cornea.
B.   Appearance after tattoo of pupillary area with gold chloride.

disfiguring corneal scar. Chemical tattoo is easier and quicker but fading of the color is more rapid; however, the area may be retouched quickly and simply. The chances of setting up a keratitis and iridocyclitis may be somewhat greater but this danger has been overemphasized and the author has had little trouble with the method in this respect.

Corneal tattooage with needles is a longer and more tedious procedure which may require two, three or more sittings for completion. Here also there is some corneal reaction but less than with the chemical method. Fading may also occur, but at a slower rate.

Corneal Tattooing with Gold Chloride

The cornea is anesthetized by the usual instillation of several drops of 0.5 per cent proparacaine or its equivalent. If a central pupil is desired the pupil is outlined with a trephine of the required size and the epithelium is scraped off taking care to keep the boundary of the pupil regular so as not to create a ragged outline. If a scar is to be obliterated the epithelium is scraped off without going too far beyond the scar limits.

A freshly prepared solution of 2 per cent gold chloride (which is normally quite acid) is neutralized to a point of faint acidity with bicarbonate of soda so that litmus paper turns only slightly pink. A tightly wound applicator is dipped in the solution and the excess is wiped off so that it will not spread over other parts of the cornea. The applicator is then firmly applied to the abraded corneal area for a period of from 3 to 7 minutes depending on the color desired. The less the time applied the more brown and less black the ultimate color of the treated area will be. It is wise to prepare fresh applicators every minute or so to assure adequate supply of the chemical. The treated area will be seen to darken.

After the gold chloride solution has been applied the requisite amount of time, a freshly prepared solution of 2 per cent tannic acid is dropped into the eye to reduce the gold chloride and the stained area will be seen to darken to brown or black in about two minutes. If tannic acid is unavailable, then a solution of epinephrine 1:1000 may be used. (Of course, no epinephrine should be used previously for fear of precipitating the gold solution.) Atropine is instilled and the eye patched. Corneal reepithelialization occurs in three to five days (fig. 165B). In most cases ocular reaction is slight except in albinos where Pischel reported slough of the superficial cornea.

Corneal Tattooing with Platinum Chloride

Preparation of the patient is the same as above. A freshly prepared solution of 2 per cent platinum chloride is used which need not be neutralized. The solution is applied as described above but only for two minutes. It is reduced with 2 per cent hydrazine hydrate solution for 25–30 seconds which is then irrigated out promptly. Postoperative care is the same.

In general, platinum chloride gives a darker color than gold chloride and in a shorter time. Both chemicals fade equally but have been known to last for a year or two before requiring repair although earlier fading may be encountered.

Pischel suggests staining the abraded cornea with fluorescine to assure smooth and total abrasion of the area. Others have suggested curettage of the superficial corneal lamellae as well as the epithelium to assure deeper penetration of the chemical and hence more permanence of the stain. In any case restaining is not a difficult matter.

Corneal Tattooing with Palladium Oxide

Vabutta and Toth reported a new operative tattooing method for the cornea. They use palladium oxide which is reduced by vitamin C solution. This is simpler than other methods and is said to give the best cosmetic results. It produces a deep black which "lasts many years."

Corneal Needle Tattooing with Pigments

This is the older method and still favored by some. It requires experience in handling the tattoo needle* and painstaking care of execution but yields somewhat cruder, but more permanent, results than the chemical modality.

---

* Tattoo needles are obtainable from Edward Weck Co., Brooklyn, N.Y.

For a black pupil either lamp black or India ink are used. Both can be autoclaved for sterility. The cornea is anesthetized and the area of pupil trephined as before but not de-epithelialized. A thick paste of black pigment is prepared by adding a few drops at a time of sterile saline to the powder. A little of the black paste is placed on the anesthetized cornea. Then with a multiple tattoo needle held at a slant of about 45 degrees multiple punctures are made into the corneal parenchyma in one small area. The pigment is irrigated off, the effect noted and the process repeated until the whole area has been satisfactorily tattooed. This may be done at one sitting if the corneal area is small.

Atropine is instilled and a patch applied. Corneal and ciliary reaction is usually quite mild.

If scars away from the pupillary area are to be tattooed and it is desired to simulate iris coloration, pigments which are nonirritating, heat and light stable and insoluble are available. In addition to black and white, orange, brown and blue are mixed in various combinations to obtain the desired iris shade. (This requires some experience.) The desired mixture is reduced to a thick paste with saline as with the lamp black and is tattooed into the cornea as described above. Polychrome tattooing is somewhat more laborious and may require several sittings to add the various iris markings and to obtain a good color match.

With this method the whole peripheral cornea may be tattooed in an albino, a large traumatic coloboma may be masked or a large corneal scar covered to reduce glare and improve vision. The effect is usually crude but may become more presentable with experience. From a distance of a few feet it is usually acceptable. There is some tendency to fade here also and this may be repaired by a little additional tattooage.

Tattooing of Lid Margins

As indicated previously lash grafting is at best uncertain and only rarely rewarding enough to warrant the surgery. Tattoo of the lid margin to simulate lashes is more easily done and is, on the whole, at least as acceptable cosmetically as grafting; often more so. However, such tattoo is acceptable cosmetically only in the lower lid. The upper lid is too exposed and noticeable and the result much less satisfactory. Here the artificial lashes mentioned in Chapter 13 are much more to the purpose. The method of tattooing the lower lid is simple.

A thick paste is made of dark brown pigment. (Black tends to turn bluish later hence dark brown is preferred.) The lid is anesthetized and tiny punctures are made close to the margin in the region of normal cilia. Care is taken not to put the punctures too close together. After all the bleeding has stopped the paste is rubbed briskly into the punctured area. The area is wiped clean with a wet sponge and more punctures are made if needed. Another method is to smear the paste on

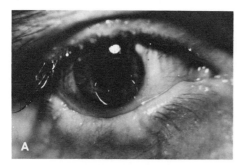 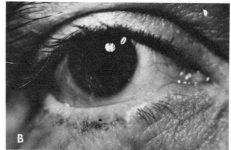

Fig. 166. Lash Tattoo.
A. Preoperative condition.
B. Appearance one year after lash tattoo with dark brown pigment.
(Courtesy Dr. Crowell Beard.)

to the lid and carry the paste into the lid substance with a needle. Bleeding may tend to wash some of the pigment out—hence after bleeding is controlled more may have to be applied. No dressing is required after 24 hours although the patient is instructed not to wash the area for several days until healing is complete.

Whatever method of application is used it is easily carried out as an office procedure. Fading will occur and the lid will have to be retouched from time to time. Figures 166A and B show the right lower lid before tattooing and one year later.

CONTACT PROSTHESES FOR ABNORMAL CORNEAE

With the improvement in prostheses and contact lenses it may well be that the indications for corneal tattooing, rare as they are, may be further reduced. If a disfigured globe has no vision a cosmetic contact shell may be fitted over the eye quite often with excellent results. A corrective cosmetic contact shell with an open pupillary space may be used if some vision is retained in the eye. These have given good results in aniridia, irregular astigmatism and albinism. Tinted contact lenses are also now available in corneal conditions and, for those who can wear them, constitute the best solution of all.

Cosmetic scleral lenses are of two sorts. When fitted for purely cosmetic purposes they require no optical surface and no clearance. Such lenses are used for deformed globes, leukomas, amblyopias and amauroses and such other conditions (fig. 266). Cosmetic optical lenses are used for albinism, aniridia, nystagmus and other conditions in eyes having serviceable vision. Both types should be constantly checked for corneal erosion or vascularization and worn only when necessary.

Therapeutic contact lenses are similarly divided into two groups, those having optical indications including advanced keratoconus, certain aphakias and high astigmatism. The flush fitting therapeutic lenses are fitted to patients with keratopathies, lid deformities, chemical burns and deformed and distorted bulbs.

REFERENCES

AMERICAN ENCYCLOPEDIA OF OPHTHALMOLOGY. Chicago, Cleveland Press. 1914, vol. 5, p. 3475.

_____: Chicago, Cleveland Press, 1920, vol. 16, p. 12521.

CHEVALLEREAU, A., and POLAK, A.: Du Tattooage coloré de la cornée. Ann. d'ocul. 136:26, 1906.

ESPY, J. W.: Cosmetic scleral contact lenses. Am. J. Ophth. 66:95, 1968.

FORBES, S. B.: New pigment for corneal tattooing. Am. J. Ophth. 50:325, 1960.

GIFFORD, S. R., and STEINBERG, A.: Gold and silver impregnation of cornea for cosmetic purposes. Am. J. Ophth. 10:240, 1927.

KNAPP, A. A.: Corneal grafts or tattooing with iridectomy. U. S. Nav. Med. Bull. 42:1366, 1944.

KNAPP, P.: Eine neue Methode de Hornhauttatowierung. Klin. Monatsbl. Augenh. 75:22, 1925.

_____: Die Tatowierung mit Goldchlorid. Klin. Monatsbl. Augenh. 75:693, 1925.

KREIKER, A.: Ein missglückter Versuch bei Albinismus die tarsale Bindenhaut mit Goldchlorid zu farben. Klin. Monatsbl. Augenh. 77:109, 1926.

LEVIS, R. J.: The new operation for coloring corneal opacities. Phil. Med. Times. 3:4, 1872–3.

PISCHEL, D. K.: Tattooing the cornea with gold and platinum chloride. Arch. Ophth. 3:176, 1930.

TAYLOR, C. B.: The art of tinting opacities of the cornea. Brit. Med. J. 2:214, 1872.

VABUTTA, A., and TOTH, I.: New operative method for cornea tattooing. Szemeszet. 97:78, 1960.

DE WECKER, L.: Das Tatowierung der Hornhaut. Arch. Augenh. u. Ohrenh. 2:2 abt. S. 84, 1870.

CHAPTER 15

Ectropion

ECTROPION (*ek* = out; *trepein* = to turn) is a condition in which the margin of the lid is turned outward. This may vary in degree from a slight eversion at the punctum to complete turning out of the lid with exposure of the conjunctival sac.

In ectropion of the lower lid there is epiphora and excoriation of the skin around the lid due to irritation by the tears. If the ectropion lasts for any length of time elongation of the lid with keratinization and hypertrophy of the exposed conjunctiva takes place. Lower corneal exposure may lead to keratitis but this is rare.

Historical Summary

The history of repair of ectropion is old and many methods of correction have come down to us. Some are only of historical interest. Many, as is true of all plastic surgery, are modifications and improvements of previous modifications and improvements. It is not the intention here to attempt to describe or even list the many technics devised since this is not an encyclopedia of historical curios. However, the broad steps taken in the development of the common procedures will be briefly outlined.

In former times, sutures were a favorite form of treating atonic ectropion. Snellen was one of their earliest proponents and his suture is one of the simplest to apply (fig. 167A). A better conceived suture was that of Argyll Robertson which required a small lead plate to be used in conjunction with it. Verhoeff's suture consists of passing and repassing a heavy suture under the skin below the lid margin from one commissure to the other (fig. 167B). At its point of origin it is tied over a peg with a slipknot. This permits later tightening or loosening as required.

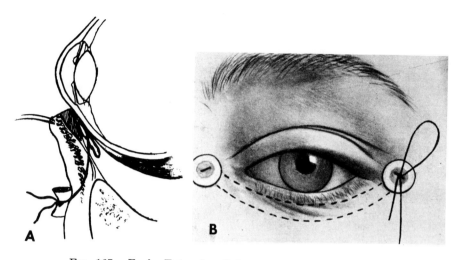

FIG. 167. Early Ectropion Sutures.

A. Snellen suture.   B. Verhoeff suture.

(Beard, C. H.: Courtesy P. Blakiston's Son & Co., Philadelphia.)

The idea behind the repair of lid malposition by suture is to create an irritative inflammation (and suppuration) which in turn will cause fibrous tissue reaction along the suture tracks. These, presumably, contract and bring the lid back into position permanently. Like many cleverly devised procedures, the suture technic is more successful in theory than in practice. If left in long enough, the sutures will undoubtedly cause tissue reaction and sometimes severe suppuration. Unfortunately, however, the lid position usually remains unchanged. This modality has now fallen into deserved obscurity.

The need for strengthening the elongated drooping lid by actual surgical shortening became apparent very early and, as far back as 1812, Adams (fig. 168A) attempted correction by excising a full thickness triangle base up from the center of the lid. This often left a disfiguring scar. Von Ammon improved on the technic somewhat by excising the triangle close to the lateral canthus where it was less noticeable. Kuhnt (fig. 168B) was the first to split the lower lid for the correction of senile ectropion. But since he only resected a triangle of tarsoconjunctiva base upward from the center of the lid leaving the skin-muscle lamina intact, closure resulted in an unsightly bunching which Kuhnt's contemporaries were not slow to point out. Thus Terson termed it a "bourrelet cutané desgracieux," a comment which becomes even more pungent when one realizes that "bourrelet" in the French argot means a swelling on a horse's leg. Müller split the lid laterally and reduced Kuhnt's big pucker to a lot of little ones (fig. 168C). Helmbold overcame this cosmetic blemish by excising additional triangles of skin-muscle (fig. 168D). This did away completely with the skin-muscle pucker resulting from the Kuhnt procedure. (Note the halving type of closure.)

Much earlier Dieffenbach, attacking the problem from another direction, had shortened the elongated lid by excising a triangle of skin-muscle temporal to the lateral canthus. He then pared off the ciliary margin of the outer portion of the lid, undermined the skin and drew it outward to cover the defect. Dimmer combined Dieffenbach's procedure with Kuhnt's into what became known as the Dimmer operation. Szymanowski changed the position of Dieffenbach's triangle and pulled the whole lower lid upward as well as outward by an ingenious realignment of his skin resection lines. This was a distinct improvement on the Dieffenbach technic and was promptly seized upon by Meller who combined it with Kuhnt's triangle into what became known as the Kuhnt-Meller technic until Szymanowski's contribution was acknowledged and the Kuhnt-Szymanowski operation permanently christened. This is one of the few plastic procedures which withstood the test of time for many years without modification.

CLASSIFICATION OF ECTROPION

Clinically six types of ectropion are commonly seen, each of which is a distinct entity.

Congenital
Acquired
    Acute Spastic
    Mechanical
    Senile
    Paralytic
    Cicatricial

A few more rare atonic types such as lateral and marginal ectropion are also discussed below.

CONGENITAL ECTROPION

Congenital ectropion is rare and only a few cases have been reported. It is usually accompanied by other congenital defects (see Chapter 18).

ACQUIRED ECTROPION

Acute Spastic Ectropion

Acute spastic ectropion is seen occasionally in either the upper or lower lid when the lid is forcibly everted. This apparently throws the marginal orbicularis fibers into momentary spasm in the everted state so that force has to be used to reinvert the lid. Most commonly this occurs

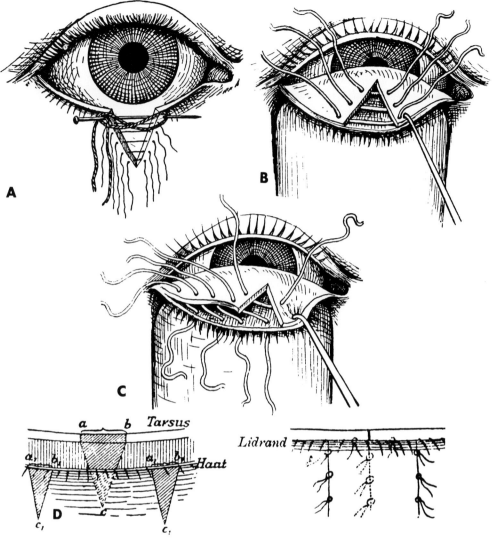

FIG. 168.   Early Ectropion Technics.

A.   Adams' resection of full thickness lid wedge.

B.   Kuhnt's lid splitting and tarsoconjunctival triangle resection.

C.   Müller's modification of Kuhnt's closure.

D.   Helmbold's resection of skin-muscle as well as tarsoconjunctiva. (Note halving type closure.)

(Courtesy American Encyclopedia of Ophthalmology. Cleveland Press, Chicago, 1915.)

in younger individuals or in older patients whose eyes are proptosed. The condition is wholly transient and requires no treatment.

Mechanical Ectropion

Mechanical ectropion, as its name implies, is an actual pulling or pushing away of the lid margin from the globe. It may be pulled away by the weight of edema or tumor; it may be pushed away by exophthalmos, or proptosis of the globe due to an orbital tumor or severe bulbar chemosis. In other words, anything which tends to push or pull the lid away from the globe may cause a mechanical ectropion. Duke-Elder postulates that the normal tonus of the orbicularis fibers acting on the lid below the tarsus at the same time may serve to pull it backward. This type of ectropion is most common in the lower lid with its weaker tarsal plate, though it may also occur in the upper lid if the proptosis or chemosis is severe enough. I have seen a case of mechanical ectropion due to trauma which lasted four months. Six weeks later when the patient was seen again, the ectropion was completely gone and the lid was in normal position.

The treatment of mechanical ectropion is not surgical. As a rule, it merely requires attention to the offending agent and temporary protection of the cornea by patch or bandage until the condition causing the ectropion is corrected. Occasionally, if the conjunctival chemosis or the proptosis is great, canthotomy or even cantholysis may have to be done, thus preventing strangulation of tissue by relieving pressure on the globe. In general, however, treatment is temporary and conservative.

Atonic Ectropion

SENILE ECTROPION. Senile ectropion is by far the most common type of ectropion and occurs more often than all other types of ectropion put together. It is found mostly in the middle-aged and elderly and is frequently bilateral. Its development follows a consistent pattern or syndrome which includes the following stages:

    a. Loss of muscle tonus and relaxation.
    b. Eversion.
    c. Elongation.
    d. Drooping of the whole lid.
    e. Conjunctival hypertrophy and keratinization.

In the first stage the lid is still in good position but it is lax, can be easily pulled away from the eyeball and occasionally a layer of tear film is visible along the margin of the lower lid.

As relaxation develops the medial portion of the lid begins to evert and the punctum gradually becomes visible. This is the first sign of trouble because a visible punctum is a punctum out of position.

The next stage is one of gradual eversion of the whole lid medio-laterally. With this comes elongation and then sagging so that there is not only relaxation but actual lengthening. This explains how it is possible to resect as much as 10 or 12 mm. or even 15 mm. from a lid normally 30 mm. long and still have little decrease in final length.

Conjunctival hypertrophy and keratinization is a final stage seen only in old neglected cases in which the conjunctiva is tremendously thickened due to exposure. Here some of the thickened tissue actually has to be resected before inversion is obtainable.

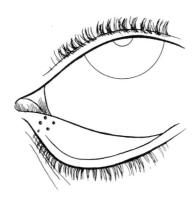

FIG. 169.   Ziegler Puncture for Punctal Eversion.

Many methods are available to the surgeon for the repair of senile ectropion as well as paralytic and mechanical ectropion which are related clinical entities and require a similar type of surgical correction. In the early stages several minor procedures are of value: If the eversion is confined to the punctum then a few cautery punctures may be carefully placed beneath the punctum so as not to injure the ampulla.

Localized Ziegler Puncture for Eversion of Lower Punctum

Eversion of the lower punctum is the most common punctal deficiency and usually seen in early senile ectropion which almost always begins at the medial canthus. If the ectropion has gone on to eversion and elongation, more definitive surgery is indicated. However, in the early cases before eversion has proceeded too far, some benefit may be gained from a localized Ziegler cauterization or a minor conjunctivoplasty.

Procedure (fig. 169):   This is done by everting the medial portion of the lid and injecting a few drops of lidocaine subconjunctivally beneath the lacrimal punctum. With a fine hot muscle hook two rows of two punctures each are laid down behind the punctum sufficiently low so that there is no danger of injury to the canaliculus. After healing and cicatrization this may be enough to cause inversion of a punctum in the very early cases of ectropic eversion.

Conjunctivoplasty for Eversion of Punctum

If the above is unsuccessful and in cases of more advanced punctal eversion, resection of a horizontal spindle of conjunctiva and subconjunctiva below the punctum is indicated.

Procedure (fig. 170):   After suitable anesthesia the medial end of the lid is everted and a horizontal spindle is outlined in the conjunctiva below the punctum which is used as a central point. This spindle should measure about 5 by 8 mm. with the upper incision lying about 5 mm. below the lid margin to avoid injury to the ampulla (which lies 2 mm.

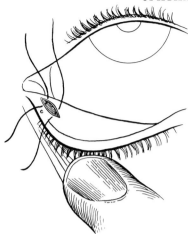

FIG. 170.   Conjunctivoplasty for Punctal Eversion.

below the lid margin). All the included tissue down to the orbicularis
is resected and the wound closed with interrupted 6–0 silk sutures. This
usually suffices to invert the punctum in the milder cases.

Sometimes the medial tarsorrhaphy described in figure 107 may be
successful in cases of punctal eversion where others have failed.

Medial Ectropion Procedure (Blaskovics)—Author's Modification

In 1938 Blaskovics published a procedure for ectropion at the
medial canthus. I have used this—in modified form—with satisfaction
for persistent atonic medial ectropion in all except advanced cases.

Procedure (fig. 171):   A horizontal skin incision is made below the
medial half of the lower lid 3 to 4 mm. from the lid margin. The incision
is carried upward and nasally following the curve of the lower lid. A
narrow triangle of skin is resected in the nasocanthal angle (fig. 171A).
The skin is undermined laterally, and the skin flap is mobilized. The lid
is folded over to estimate the amount of lengthening and the excess of
full thickness lid is resected triangularly, apex downward, about 5 mm.
lateral to the punctum (fig. 171B). The triangular lid wound is sutured
anteriorly and posteriorly. The skin flap is drawn nasally, any further
skin excess is resected and the wound is closed (fig. 171C). Figures 171D
and E show a medial ectropion of the left lower lid and the condition of
the lid after repair.

This procedure usually results in good inversion of the punctum
without covering the plica or the caruncle. There are two important
modifications of the original Blaskovics procedure in this technic: (1)
The skin incision is made close to the lid margin where the scar is
inconspicuous, and (2) a triangle is resected from the lower lid instead
of a rectangle. This makes for a better cosmetic closure and for better
inversion of the ectropic lower lid.

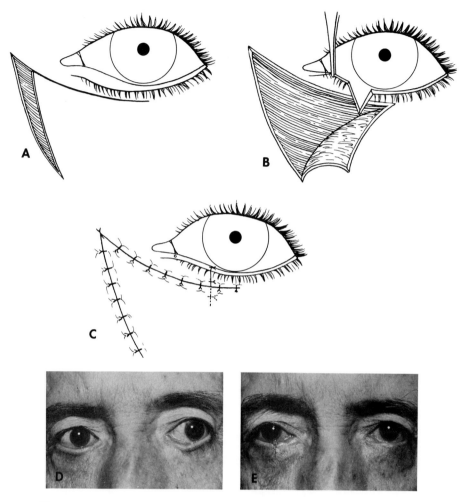

FIG. 171. Repair of Medial Ectropion—Author's Technic.

A. A skin incision below medial half of lid is carried into the nasocanthal angle. A narrow skin triangle is resected.

B. The skin flap is undermined and a full thickness triangle apex downward is resected.

C. The lid wound is closed in layers. The skin flap is drawn up and sutured.

D. Medial ectropion of left lower lid.

E. After correction.

There is one caveat: just enough skin should be resected to cause the lid to lie snugly against the globe and to invert the punctum. Too much resection may produce an epicanthal fold.

Full Ziegler Cautery for Senile Ectropion

In a somewhat more advanced stage of eversion before elongation has taken place, Ziegler cautery puncture along the whole length of the lid may be used. But this will work only before the process of elongation has set in.

Procedure (fig. 172): The lid is anesthetized subconjunctivally at the attached tarsal border along its whole length. By means of the electric cautery or a muscle hook heated to a dull red color in an alcohol flame, six or seven punctures are made just above the attached tarsal border avoiding the canalicular area (figs. 172*A* and *B*). The puncture is made deep into the tarsus. The eye is patched for 24 hours and cold compresses are used several times a day until the reaction subsides. This is rather rapid.

Comment: The correction will occur soon but will probably not be permanent and may need repeating. In general, the Ziegler procedure is more successful in mild ectropion than in entropion. In the former, the lid margin is relaxed and easily affected by cautery. In entropion, the marginal muscle bands may be intact and hence muscle pull must be counteracted; this is not quite so easy.

Wedge Resection and Intermarginal Suture for Ectropion

Some surgeons have gone back to Adams' method of 1812 and excise a full thickness triangle base up from the lower lid and close with a Minsky figure-8 suture exactly as described in figure 51. There is no objection to this providing it is done before there is too much lengthening and drooping; otherwise it is possible to get into trouble.

Comment: To treat a full-blown case of senile ectropion properly one must counteract not only eversion and elongation but also laxity and sagging of tissues. Therefore it is not enough simply to shorten the lid. It must also be hung up higher to counteract the sag and this is why the Szymanowski triangle is so important. To omit this may cause the lid to ride lower and may displace the whole lid margin downward. Figure 173 illustrates this nicely.

Figure 173*A* shows an advanced atonic ectropion with the left lower

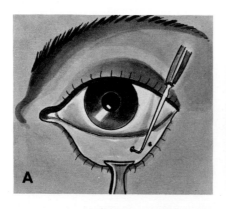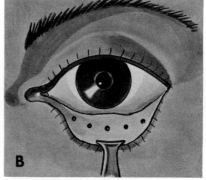

FIG. 172. Ziegler Cautery for Mild Ectropion.
A. Technic of puncture with hot muscle hook.
B. Appearance of the lid on completion.

lid markedly lengthened and everted. Figure 173*B* shows the lid immediately after resection and figure 173*C* shows what happens after a full thickness wedge apex downward is resected from such a lid. The lid is shortened and inverted but, because the Szymanowski part of the procedure has been omitted, the lid is not pulled up to its normal position but

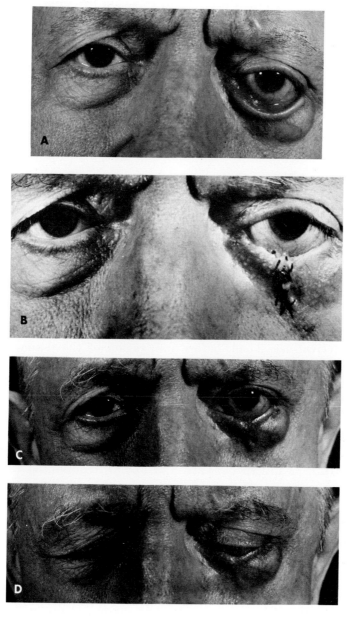

FIG. 173.   Result of Wedge Excision of Advanced Ectropion.
A.   Total ectropion of left lower lid.
B.   Wedge resection and closure.
C. and *D.*   Note notch, pulling down of lower lid and lagophthalmos.

rides well below the lower limbus. Not only that but there is lagophthalmos of the lower lid (fig. 173D) and the eye cannot be closed. The notch is incidental and can be easily repaired but wedge resection alone is obviously not the proper procedure for a full-blown senile ectropion. Where the ectropic process has proceeded to marked elongation the full Kuhnt-Szymanowski procedure or its equivalent has to be done.

Other Methods

Other procedures sometimes used in early atonic ectropion are a medial tarsorrhaphy (fig. 107A) or canthoplasty (fig. 107B) by which the lid fissure is shortened and support for the lower lid attained. These procedures may also be used in combination with the Ziegler puncture, done first to assure inversion of the punctum. Fascia lata has been used to repair paralytic ectropion by passing a strip beneath the marginal skin and fastening it at both canthal ligaments. This keeps the lid margin apposed to the globe much as Verhoeff's suture does (fig. 167B). However, it is highly questionable whether any of these methods have any advantage over the other lid shortening operations described here especially if there has been eversion and lid lengthening.

Kuhnt-Szymanowski Operation for Senile Ectropion

As previously stated the Kuhnt-Szymanowski procedure is the original classic operation for the repair of a full-blown atonic ectropion. With care in carrying it out it will work in most cases where indicated.

Procedure (fig. 174): A few drops of tetracaine are instilled into the conjunctival sac. Then, before infiltration of the tissues the lid is grasped gently with two smooth forceps and folded over in order to get an estimate of how much tissue must be excised in order to bring the lid edge snugly against the eyeball (fig. 174A). The amount of excess lid is measured with a millimeter rule. The triangle of skin to be excised beyond the external commissure is next marked out with an antiseptic dye such as alcoholic gentian violet as follows: Beginning at the lateral canthus, a line is drawn outward and upward continuing the natural curve of the lower lid. This line is as long as the measurement obtained above for lid resection. Starting at the same point at the lateral canthus another straight line is drawn downward perpendicular to the first line. This is approximately one and one half times as long as the first line or slightly longer. The ends of the two lines are united to complete the triangle.

Anesthesia of the area is now obtained by the usual injection of 1 or 2 per cent novocaine or lidocaine with epinephrine and the external half or two-thirds of the lid margin are split in the gray line into skin-muscle and tarsoconjunctival layers to a depth of 10 mm. The greater the eversion, the closer to the punctum the split is carried. The lateral end of the split connects with the short end of the lateral triangle (fig. 174*B*).

The skin included in the triangle beyond the lateral canthus is resected. Some take the subjacent muscle along with it, as this makes for a neater closure; however, this is not necessary. The tarsus is now folded over in the same way as the whole lid was, the excess estimated (fig. 174*C*) and resected triangularly apex downward with the base at the free margin (fig. 174*D*). The more eversion of the punctum there is the closer to the punctum should this tarsoconjunctival triangle be resected. The tarsus is resected conservatively and the edges approximated. If they overlap, a little more tissue is resected until the two wound lips come together snugly without excess pull.

The skin-muscle lamina is next mobilized (fig. 174*D*). The tarsoconjunctiva is sutured on the tarsoconjunctival side with interrupted 4–0 silk sutures with the top suture close to the free margin so as to get good approximation without notching (fig. 174*E*). Alternatively 5–0 chromic catgut may be used and the sutures tied on the tarsal surface. The skin-muscle layer is mobilized, drawn up and out to cover the denuded area beyond the lateral canthus and the excess marginal cilia and hair follicles resected (fig. 174*F*). A 4–0 silk suture unites the new end of the ciliary margin of the lower lid with the canthal angle. Another suture fastens the apex of the skin-muscle flap into the upper angle of the triangular wound beyond the canthus (fig. 174*G*). These are the two most important sutures as the first recreates the canthal angle and the second bears the weight of the skin-muscle flap in its new position. Other interrupted skin sutures are used to close the wound as needed. The lid edge should now lie neatly against the eyeball (fig. 174*H*).

Another suture may be used to close the anatomic dead space between the two laminae of the lid. This is done by insertion of a central mattress suture from the conjunctival side, to emerge on the skin surface where it is tied over a peg. However, a firm pressure dressing usually suffices and makes this suture unnecessary. The dressing is kept on for 48 hours. The wound is then dressed daily and the skin sutures removed on the sixth day. The tarsal sutures are removed on the tenth day. Figures 174*I* and *J* show correction of an advanced senile ectropion by this procedure.

Comment: Silk sutures are preferred to chromic catgut because tarsus is a low-grade tissue which does not heal readily and nonabsorbable sutures are more trustworthy. However, if good approximation of the tarsal ends is obtained, the upper suture which may rub against the lower cornea may be a 4–0 plain catgut which softens and absorbs more readily.

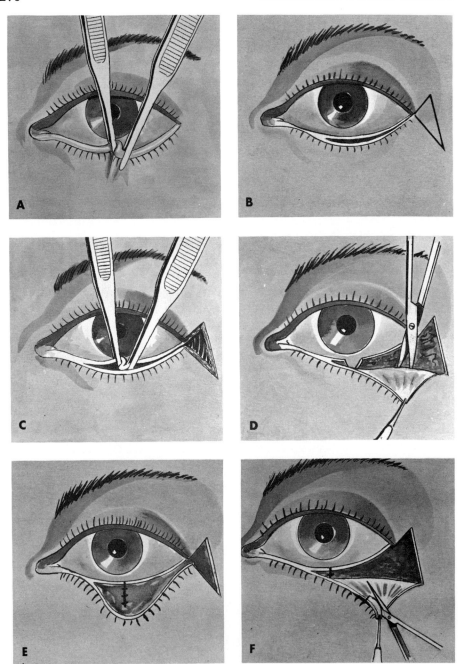

FIG. 174. Kuhnt-Szymanowski Technic.

A. The ectropic lid is folded over and the amount of lengthening is gauged.
B. The lid is split and the lateral skin triangle marked off.
C. The lateral skin triangle is resected and the amount of excess tarsoconjunctiva is gauged.
D. Tarsoconjunctiva is resected and the skin flap is mobilized.
E. The tarsoconjunctiva is closed.
F. The skin flap is pulled laterally and the excess ciliary margin is resected.

Although the results with this procedure are usually good there are occasional complications:

a) The most common complication is undercorrection. This applies especially to the medial canthus in advanced cases. It is difficult to get complete inversion of the punctum here and several postoperative devices such as Ziegler puncture (fig. 169) or resection of conjunctival tissue below the punctum (fig. 170) may be necessary.

In rare cases the conjunctiva is so thickened and keratinized that a horizontal strip of conjunctiva has to be excised along the whole length

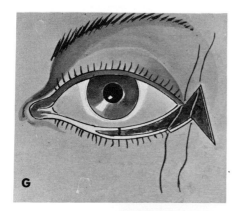 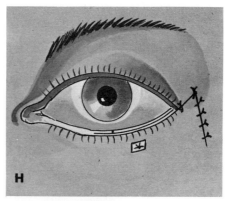

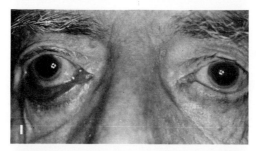

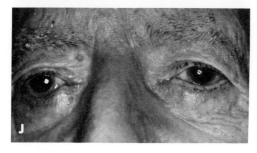

FIG. 174 (Continued)

G. Two important sutures are placed: one marks the new canthus and the other hangs the skin flap up and out beyond the lid.
H. The wound is closed.
I. Senile ectropion of right lower lid.
J. Repair by this technic.

of the lid below the margin in order to permit inversion (Terson's spindle, fig. 180, see below).

b) Overcorrection also occurs. In senile ectropion enough tissue has to be resected to counteract not only lengthening but also loss of tissue tonicity. It is not unusual to resect 12 to 15 mm. of full thickness lid which, considering that the average normal lid length is 26 to 30 mm., is about half the usual length. However, the marked lengthening and loss of tonicity, which many of these lids show, allows for tremendous stretching. And the lid must be stretched in order to attain a normal position against the globe. The lid is sometimes so long and so lax that the temptation is great to resect more tissue than is finally found necessary; as a result, some inversion may occur immediately after operation. This slowly corrects itself and the lid resumes a normal position.

c) As a consequence of the stretching the punctum may be pulled laterally out of position. However, this is rarely of clinical importance and rarely results in epiphora.

d) Shortening of the lower lid may also result in shortening of the whole palpebral fissure. This is of cosmetic not clinical importance. It is not difficult to go back and do an external canthoplasty later in order to lengthen the fissure again.

Kuhnt-Szymanowski Modification (Blaskovics)

In 1938 Blaskovics modified the Kuhnt-Szymanowski technic by making a curving incision in the skin of the lid 4 mm. from the border, starting below the center of the lid and running outward and upward beyond the lateral canthus for about 3 cm. Based on this incision an equilateral triangle of skin is resected (fig. 175A). A full thickness rhomboid is then resected lateral to the center of the lid and the skin between the rhomboid and lateral triangle is completely undermined

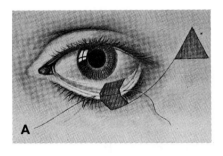 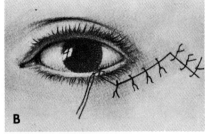

FIG. 175.   Blaskovics Ectropion Procedure.
A.   A rectangle of excess full thickness lid is resected. A skin incision connects the lower end of the rectangle to the medial corner of the skin triangle resected laterally.
B.   The lid wound is closed, the skin is undermined and drawn over laterally to cover the bared lateral triangle.

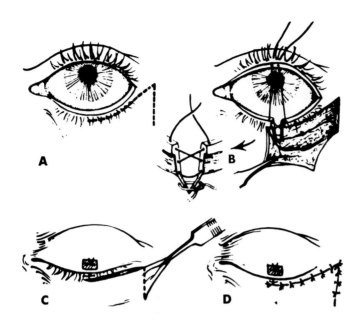

FIG. 176.   Smith Technic of Ectropion Repair.
a.   A skin flap is outlined below the lateral half of the lid.
b.   The flap is mobilized and full thickness wedge of lid is resected.
c.   The lid wound is closed by an intermarginal suture. The skin flap is drawn
     laterally and the excess resected.
d.   The skin wound is closed.
     (Smith, B.: Courtesy Highlghts of Ophthalmology.)

(fig. 175A). The lid is sutured on the anterior and posterior surfaces, then the skin is pulled up to cover the lateral triangle and sutured (fig. 175B). Skin sutures are removed in 4 or 5 days and the lid sutures in 8 days.

Kuhnt-Szymanowski Modification (Smith)

This modification of the Kuhnt-Szymanowski procedure is ingenious and makes it a better operation than the one above. The primary skin incision is not unlike that of Blaskovics but it is closer to the lid margin. Beyond the lateral canthus a vertical incision is carried down (fig. 176a) and the skin dissected down (fig. 176b). A full thickness wedge of lid is then resected and the wound closed with a figure-8 suture (fig. 176c inset). The skin flap is pulled up and the excess resected (fig. 176c) and closed (fig. 176d).

Comment: By and large the complications for the above two procedures are the same as for the classical Kuhnt-Szymanowski operation.

Modified Procedure for Ectropion and Lateral Canthoplasty (Author's Technic)

In an effort to avoid the hazards of lid splitting and yet retain the valuble features of the Kuhnt-Szymanowski technic the following modification has been used with good results.

Procedure (fig. 177):   After instillation of local anesthesia the lid is grasped with two smooth forceps and folded over to gauge how much lid must be resected to bring the margin against the globe. The amount of excess between the forceps is measured and this length of the lateral portion of the lid is split at the lateral canthus. The incision is carried beyond the canthus for an equal distance, continuing the curve of the lower lid. Another incision perpendicular to the end of the first and about one and one-half times its length is made down and out. The split in the lid is extended downward between the two laminae and the tarsoconjunctiva is resected triangularly apex downward (fig. 177*A*).

The skin-muscle lamina is freely mobilized and the tarsoconjunctival wound is closed. The lamina is pulled up and laterally and the excess cilia are resected (fig. 177*B*). At the lateral end of the skin flap the excess skin is also resected by a vertical incision (fig. 177*C*). The skin wound is closed (fig. 177*D*). Figures 177*E* and *F* show a patient whose senile ectropion was repaired by this method.

If the punctum is in good position, and it frequently is in mild or moderate cases, the eye is patched. If the punctum is still everted, a few subpunctal Ziegler punctures are placed or a conjunctivoplasty (fig. 170) is performed.

Comment: Since lid splitting is confined only to that part of the ciliary margin which is resected, this modification has all the advantages of the Kuhnt-Szymanowski procedure without incurring the possible loss of cilia. In addition, there are no incisions on the anterior of the lid. Hence the important Kuhnt-Szymanowski advantages are retained, i.e., lid shortening, lateral and upward orientation of the lid and scars only in the temporal region. This procedure is not as good an inverter of the punctum as the Kuhnt-Szymanowski operation since the tarsoconjunctival triangle is not resected close to the punctum. Therefore, its main indication is in the mild and moderate amounts of senile ectropion, although with the aid of a few Ziegler cautery punctures below the punctum, it is even valuable in more advanced cases. I do not want to denigrate the Kuhnt-Szymanowski procedure. I still prefer it for long-standing cases of senile and paralytic ectropion.

An unexpected bonus, a sort of fringe benefit, has been the efficacy of this procedure as a lateral canthoplasty in cases of stretched, drooping lids which are not ectropic. A not unusual finding is a complaint of tearing due to an atonic lid with the margin well below the lower limbus and the punctum everted but with the lid not ectropic. The advantage of using this procedure here is that, unlike most classic lateral canthoplasties, such as the Fuchs, Wheeler or Elschnig previously shown, this one does

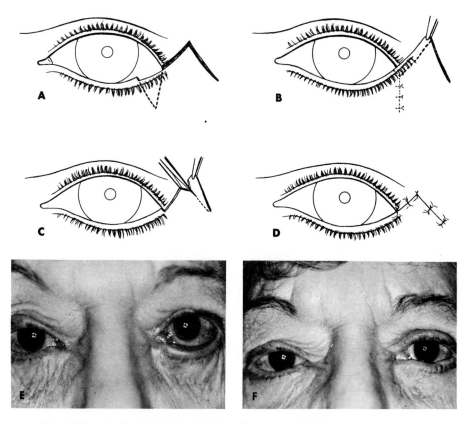

FIG. 177.   Author's Modified Kuhnt-Szymanowski Procedure.

A.   The lid is split at the lateral canthus and the split carried up and out following the lid curve. At the end of this incision a perpendicular skin incision
is made down and out.

B.   The resultant flap at the lateral canthus is mobilized and the excess marginal
tissue, including cilia, resected.

C.   Excess skin tissue is also resected laterally.

D.   The skin flap is pulled up, the lid inverted and the wound sutured.

E.   A senile ectropion of the left lower lid.

F.   Repair by this technic.

not shorten the palpebral fissure. Its effectiveness is shown in Figures
178A and B. I do not know whether this is a better ectropion modification
or lateral canthoplasty. It works well in either case.

Paralytic Ectropion

Paralytic ectropion like the senile type is an atonic ectropion and
here also only the lower lid is usually involved. It is due to paralysis of
the orbicularis which combines with the pull of gravity to give a clinical
picture quite similar to that of senile ectropion. Obviously the loss of
tissue tonus is even greater here so that this may be thought of as
senile ectropion carried to its ultimate degree.

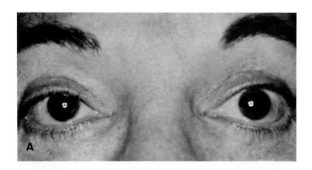

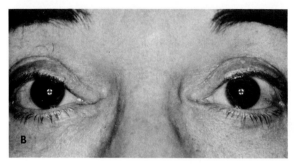

FIG. 178.   Canthoplasty by Technic Described in Figure 177.
A.   Bilateral drooping of both lower lids.
B.   Result of repair.

Paralytic ectropion is not a common condition and in general the surgical problem is the same is in senile ectropion, i.e., to strengthen the lower lid tissues sufficiently so that the lid margin is brought up and stays up against the globe. The procedures used are those described for senile ectropion. Figure 179, a case of paralytic ectropion of the left lower lid. illustrates the repair by the Kuhnt-Szymanowski technic.

RARE AND UNUSUAL TYPES OF ATONIC ECTROPION

Terson's Spindle Resection Technic

This technic is used when the conjunctiva in an ectropic lid is so thick and keratinized due to exposure that inversion of the lower lid is barred no matter how much it is shortened (fig. 180*A*). The remedy is to resect the bulge of the thickened exposed conjunctiva so that inversion of the lid can be accomplished.

Procedure (fig. 180):   After suitable anesthesia a strip of thickened conjunctiva extending the entire length of the lower lid is dissected out (fig. 180*B*). The upper incision outlining the strip is somewhat below the level of the canaliculus and the lower incision at the lower edge of

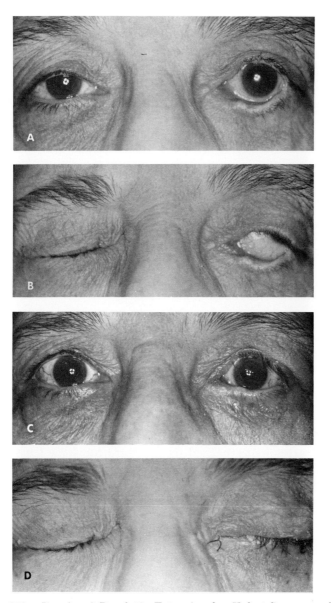

FIG. 179.   Repair of Paralytic Ectropion by Kuhnt-Szymanowski
Procedure.
A. and *B.*   Preoperative appearance with left eye open and closed.
C. and *D.*   Condition after repair.

the exposed conjunctival bulge. The resection is down to tarsus with the
tarsus spared; the conjunctiva may measure as much as a millimeter or
two in thickness. The conjunctival wound is closed with interrupted
chromic catgut or silk sutures. Figure 180*C* shows such a bilateral case
with the Terson spindle resected and (fig. 180*D*) after the repair has

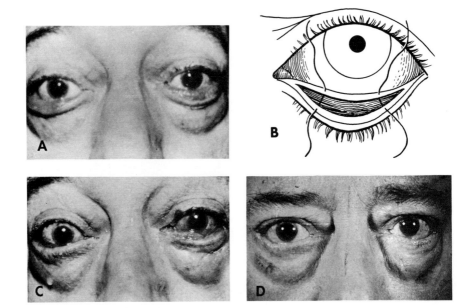

FIG. 180.   Terson Spindle Repair.
A.   Bilateral senile ectropion with hypertrophy and keratinization of both lower lids.
B.   Technic of resection of hypertrophied conjunctiva.
C.   Appearance immediately after resection.
D.   Appearance several weeks later.

been completed. It will be noted that the lids do not reinvert completely at once. But after being bathed by the tears for some time the residual conjunctiva gradually softens and the lids resume their normal position.

Comment: This procedure is usually carried out as a preliminary to the Kuhnt-Szymanowski operation which is then completed in the usual way.

Argyll Robertson "Strap" Operation for Lateral Ectropion (Modified)

A couple of additional rare types of ectropion deserve mention. For atonic ectropion involving only the outer half of the lid (fig. 181) a good operation is the modified Argyll Robertson strap procedure. His full name was Douglas Moray Cooper Lamb Argyll Robertson; he was a great ophthalmologist despite this.

Procedure (fig. 181):   Near the lateral canthus a full thickness lid wedge apex downward is resected after the amount of lid elongation is ascertained. From the apex of the triangular lid wound, a curved skin incision is made which at first is parallel with the lid margin and then extends upward beyond the lateral canthus. A second similar curved incision is made 6 mm. below and parallel with the first (fig. 181*B*). The resultant strap of skin is undermined and mobilized. The lid notch is closed with or without a figure-8 suture. The skin strap is drawn up, the excess is resected and the strap is sutured into place with interrupted 5–0 silk (fig. 181*C*). A firm dressing is applied. Postoperative care is the same as for the Kuhnt-Szymanowski procedure. Correction of lateral ectropion of the right lower lid is seen in figure 181*D*.

Marginal (Tarsal) Ectropion

This is an uncommon, but by no means rare, clinical entity characterized by lower lid eversion which is limited to the tarsal portion only. It differs from ordinary senile ectropion in that (1) eversion does not progress beyond the tarsus and (2) there is no relaxation of the tissues of the lid below the tarsus.

In the early stages there is slight eversion of the punctum with epiphora, giving the appearance of an early common senile ectropion. However, even a cursory examination will show that there is no laxity of the lid tissues; in fact, the skin of the lid is tense and has no "give." In the advanced stages the upper portion is everted on the lower part of the lid like a cuff on a sleeve. Or, to vary the simile, the lower portion of the lid acts as a fulcrum on which the tarsal portion of the lid turns outward, so that even after correction there is a crease just below the tarsus marking the line of eversion. Manual reinversion is always unsuccessful. Hence, this condition is also entirely distinct from the acute spastic ectropion.

Since marginal ectropion is obviously not the common type of senile

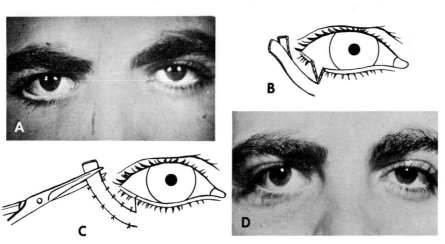

Fig. 181. Repair of Lateral Ectropion (Modified Argyll Robertson Strap Technic).

A. Lateral ectropion of right lower lid.
B. Resection of full thickness lid triangle and preparation of strap.
C. Lid notch is closed and the skin strap is pulled up, the excess resected and incisions sutured.
D. Appearance after repair.

ectropion, it has sometimes been labeled (for want of a better name) chronic spastic ectropion. This has been based on the supposition that it is due to chronic spasm of the orbicularis fibers below the tarsus with or without concomitant relaxation of the pretarsal fibers, the whole process resulting in eversion of the tarsal-containing lid portion. Since in all cases the part of the lid below the attached border of the tarsus is in normal position and shows none of the looseness and lack of tonicity commonly seen in senile ectropion, the clinical picture has strengthened the illusion of spasticity, hence "spastic" ectropion.

The difference in clinical appearance is striking when the two types are juxtaposed. The usual senile ectropion is a loose, flabby lid which is easily pulled up into position. In marginal ectropion, on the other hand, force is required to reinvert the lid and hold it in position. As soon as it is released the ectropion immediately reappears (fig. 182A).

The trouble with the "spasticity" theory is that it is difficult to base on reasonable grounds. It would be difficult enough to explain in unilateral cases (1) what causes the chronic spasm in an otherwise normal appearing eye, (2) how the spasm is limited to the lower orbicularis fibers, and (3) along what arc this spasm travels. In a bilateral case such an explanation would have to border on the supernatural.

A far more tenable and logical explanation is the relaxation of the tarsal sling of the lower lid (i.e., the tarsus with its two canthal connections) while the skin and muscle of the rest of the lid retain their normal tonus. This allows eversion of the tarsal portion only and keeps the rest of the lid in normal position. Hence, whatever lengthening occurs in the lid is limited to the marginal tarsal-contained portion and correction should be and is attainable by limiting the surgery to this area. In the early cases a modified halving procedure is used by Callahan in which part of the orbicularis at the base of the lid is resected and the marginal portion shortened.

In severe cases such as is shown in figure 182A correction may be attained by the following technic:

Procedure (fig. 182):   A Terson spindle is first resected to make inversion possible. Then shortening of the tarsal portion of the lid proceeds. The lower lid is split into its two laminae for about half its central length. The width of the split is about 6 mm. or just beyond the attached border of the tarsus. At the temporal end of the split a vertical incision through the separated skin-muscle layer is made and a similar incision is made through the tarsoconjunctiva at the medial end. A horizontal incision running nasally is then made through the anterior lamina from the lower end of the vertical skin-muscle incision. This runs the whole length of the split. A similar incision is made through the posterior lamina running temporally. In this way two narrow straps are fashioned, one of skin-muscle the other of tarsoconjunctiva (fig. 182B).

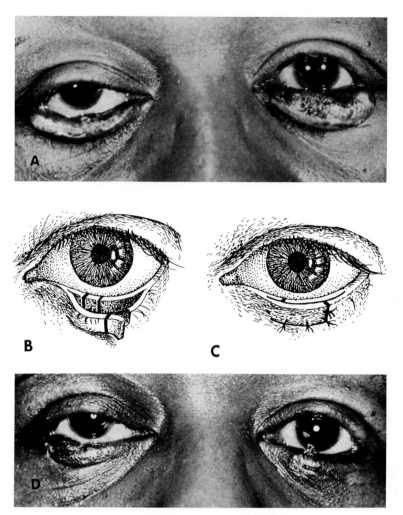

FIG. 182.   Repair of Advanced Marginal Ectropion.
A.   Bilateral marginal ectropion of lower lids.
B.   The lid is split centrally and skin-muscle and tarsoconjunctival straps are
       fashioned. *Heavy vertical lines* show amount to be resected for each strap.
C.   The straps are tautened, the excess resected and sutured into place.
D.   Final result.

The tarsoconjunctival strap is drawn nasally until sufficient inversion of the lid is obtained so that the margin is in normal position. The
excess is resected and the tarsoconjunctiva sutured with 4–0 chromic
catgut. The skin-muscle strap is then drawn temporally, the excess
resected and the wound sutured on the skin surface with 5–0 silk (fig.
182C). The skin-muscle strap should not be tightened too much. It should
be shortened sufficiently to give a good cosmetic closure and no more. It
is the tarsoconjunctival shortening which causes the real inversion.
Tightening the skin-muscle layer too much will tend to counteract this.

It will be found that the skin-muscle layer, despite its greater elasticity, is shortened less than the tarsoconjunctival layer if the directions given above are followed. A firm supportive dressing is applied. Skin sutures are removed on the fifth or sixth day (fig. 182D).

Comment: The three important tissues for the maintenance of the lid in position are skin, muscle and tarsal sling. When all the tissues give way we have the usual senile ectropion. When skin and muscle relax and the tarsal sling remains firm there is senile entropion. When, conversely, the skin and muscle remain firm and the tarsal sling gives way, marginal ectropion results.

Theoretically this is much more reasonable than belief in some apochryphal localized spasm of unknown etiology. Nature in her many faceted manifestations of the aging process has no interest in symmetry. She has a habit of playing these patchy, scurvy tricks on us, and examples of isolated localized islands of senility, pathology and decay throughout the body are myriad. Hence, it should surprise no one that we have *unilateral* entropion, *unilateral* ectropion, etc. By the same token, it is reasonable to suppose that not all the tissues of the lid may give way simultaneously.

Summary of Surgery for Atonic Ectropion

If eversion is limited to the punctal area a localized subpunctal cauterization or conjunctivoplasty may suffice for the time being. Where lid eversion is somewhat greater but there is no elongation of the lid a Ziegler puncture along the whole length of the lid may be enough, although this may have to be repeated. If lid eversion is of still greater degree, with some elongation involving mostly the medial half of the lid, the modified Kuhnt-Szymanowski technic is of value or a wedge resection is done where there is little elongation. If the external half of the lid is involved, the Argyll Robertson strap as modified by the author will work nicely. In cases of total lid involvement the Kuhnt-Szymanowski operation or one of its equivalents given above is the procedure of choice. Here again this may have to be reinforced by a few Ziegler punctures well beneath the canaliculi, or by excision of a strip of conjunctiva if conjunctival thickening is extreme (Terson spindle).

CICATRICIAL ECTROPION

Repair of cicatricial ectropion requires an entirely different set of procedures from that of atonic ectropion. In the latter there is no lack of tissue; indeed, there is too much. In cicatricial ectropion there is scarring and loss of tissue which requires replacement either by mobilization from the surrounding skin or by free grafting. As usual, many procedures exist. In order not to confound confusion, only those which the author has used and found valuable will be discussed fully.

Wharton Jones V-Y Procedure

Where there has been superficial scarring with little loss of tissue, simple excision of the scar with undermining and drawing together of skin edges may suffice. Or, if the loss is minimal, small sliding grafts from the immediate neighborhood obtained by a Z plasty or V-Y incision may be enough. The following case (fig. 183*A*) shows correction of mild cicatricial ectropion by the technic of Wharton Jones, the physiologist who became an outstanding ophthalmologist.

Procedure (fig. 183): A V incision, apex downward, is made to include all the scar tissue of the ectropic lid (fig. 183*B*). The included skin is undermined to the lid margin and subcutaneous scar tissue, if any, excised (fig. 183*C*). The lid border must now be in normal position against the globe if the operation is to succeed. The wound edges are undermined laterally and medially (fig. 183*D*) and sutured together beginning at the lower angle. The undermined skin flap must not be pulled down but must be sutured as it lies in its relaxed position. The closed wound now assumes the form of a Y (fig. 183*E*) with the length of the lower stalk of the Y depending on how much the skin triangle has retracted toward the lid margin. In closing, the skin must be relaxed at the margin. It may even be wise to leave a little loose pucker of skin—i.e., overcorrect—to counteract later contraction. The result is seen in figure 183*F*.

Comment: Long vertical scars are rarely excised with complete relaxation of the lid and replacement to its normal position. The lid margin must be replaced by some such maneuver as the V-Y. Temporary tarsorrhaphies or lid sutures may help during healing. This procedure will work only in mild cases and is worthless in advanced cases of cicatricial ectropion.

Correction of Cicatricial Ectropion by Free Whole Skin Graft

In the average case of full cicatricial ectropion the author's choice is a free whole skin graft rather than a pedicle graft. As stated elsewhere, this is preferred for several reasons: First, it can be of thinner skin usually, hence nearer to lid skin in quality. Second, it makes for less scarring because a rotated pedicle or sliding graft from the area will always leave scars no matter how carefully done. Third, the size of the graft need not be limited for fear of too much scarring as in pedicle grafting. Skin from another lid is almost always available when only one lid is involved. In the following case cicatricial ectropion of the left lower lid (fig. 184*A*) was corrected by a free whole skin graft from the left upper lid.

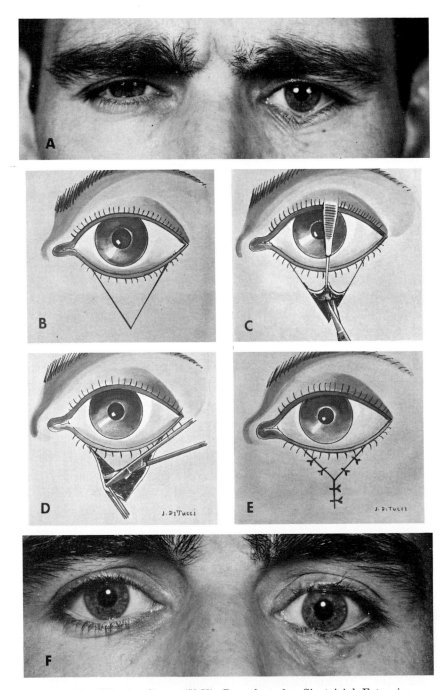

FIG. 183.   Wharton-Jones (V-Y) Procedure for Cicatricial Ectropion.

A.   A case of mild cicatricial ectropion of the left lower lid.
B.   The skin incision.
C.   The skin triangle is dissected up and allowed to retract upward.
D.   The wound edges are undermined.
E.   Closure converts the V incision into a Y.
F.   Final result.

Procedure (fig. 184): A horizontal skin incision is made in the ectropic lid and the lips of the wound undermined. Scar tissue, if any, is excised and the lid allowed to assume its normal position against the globe. Bleeding is controlled and the upper and lower lid margins prepared for two tarsorrhaphies (fig. 184B). These adhesions are important whether the eyeball is present or not, since they not only protect the eye when present but splint the lid and provide an immobile bed for the graft. In the case of an anophthalmic socket, a conformer is inserted before the lids are sutured together in order to fill out the socket and furnish counterpressure for the pressure dressing to be applied later.

The next step is the taking of the graft. If possible, this should be from the ipsilateral upper lid. In that case, the tarsorrhaphies may be left unsutured until after the graft is taken in order not to stretch the upper lid. The amount of skin needed is measured out or, better still, a small piece of gauze or plastic tissue is cut to pattern matching the bed in which the graft is to be laid. The shape taken is usually a spindle. This pattern is laid on the donor lid and outlined with sterile dye solution. The outline should be 1 mm. larger than the pattern and the lid should not be drawn taut or anesthesia injected or else the skin will be stretched and the graft will prove too small. After the pattern is drawn, the area is infiltrated with anesthesia and incised along the drawn outline. The ends are slightly undermined with scissors and 6–0 silk single-armed sutures with needles pointing away from the graft inserted.

A Graefe knife is passed under the central width of the skin spindle from upper to lower incisions and by a gentle sawing motion the skin is cut from its bed. The knife should be visible at all times just beneath the skin; if it cannot be seen it is too deep. When half the graft has been cut from the center to one end the knife is flipped over and the other half is cut similarly. If preferred, a small Stevens scissors with blunt ends may be used to equal advantage. The graft is picked up by the sutures which have been previously placed at each end and anchored into position in the recipient bed (fig. 184C). Additional sutures are added to assure good coaptation of the whole graft. The sutures are placed close to the edges of the wound and firmly tied. The donor site is closed in similar fashion (fig. 184D).

The edges are not undermined unless the graft taken has been so large as to require it. In older people, especially, it will rarely be necessary to undermine since lid skin is ample. A pressure dressing is applied.

If a graft is taken from an upper lid for the lower lid of the same side, the situation is ideal. One dressing only is needed for both. If a contralateral lid has been used as the donor site, a patch for the donor lid will suffice. Care should be taken with the pressure bandage so that the graft is not disturbed; moving it means its destruction. The dressings are untouched for six days. At this time the grafted area is inspected, carefully cleaned with sterile applicators, loose sutures removed and pressure reapplied. The donor lid sutures are removed on the fifth or sixth day and the eye uncovered. On the tenth day all sutures are removed and the site dressed every other day until complete healing has taken place (fig. 184*E*). The final result is seen in figure 184*F*.

Comment: Care while taking the graft will obviate the necessity for further trimming which is a nuisance as all skin, once released from its bed, tends to curl up raw surface inward. And the thinner the graft the surer the take. The sooner the graft is laid in it bed and pressure applied the better. With a good supply of cotton or gauze fluffs under the bandage, pressure may be made as tight as the patient will allow. Machinist waste, which is preferred by some, has no particular advantage over ordinary cotton or gauze fluffs.

The tarsorrhaphy sutures are left in place 10 or 12 days until firm union is assured. Lid adhesions should remain untouched at least eight weeks; longer if the lids are still taut, showing that full contraction has not taken place. The amount of contraction of the graft can also be gauged by the openings between the lids; the more contraction the greater the lid separation. When healing is complete and no further contraction is occurring, the tarsorrhaphies are opened and the lid margins trimmed. The eye is patched for three or four days until marginal re-epithelialization has occurred.

When there is no scar tissue to worry about and there is ample skin to cover the bared area it may not be necessary to create tarsorrhaphies. Intermarginal sutures are enough to keep the lids splinted for two or three weeks. By this time the graft has taken well and the patient will be spared the opening of the tarsorrhaphies.

Involvement of two or more lids usually means the use of skin from a source other than the lids. If the loss is not too great, the lids may be repaired two at a time by free grafts of full thickness skin as described above. The grafts may be taken from the cephaloauricular junction, the supraclavicular area or the inside of the arm in the order named. Or, as discussed in Chapter 3, it might be more advantageous to use epidermis.

Correction of Cicatricial Ectropion with Epidermis

In cases of multiple ectropion, especially following facial burns with much destruction of skin tissue, the use of epidermis is preferred. The advantages are several: First, large amounts are available and can be taken from the thigh or lower abdomen. Second, enough may be taken for all four lids at one time. Third, since burns usually leave the surrounding skin paler than normal, the color match is at least as good as full thickness skin. Fourth, the operation is simpler and shorter since little suturing of the graft is required.

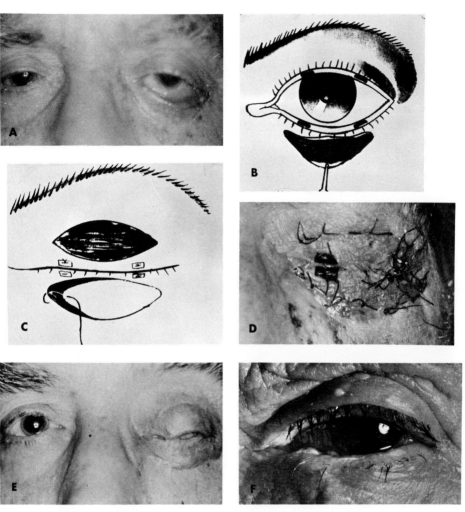

FIG. 184. Repair of Cicatricial Ectropion by Free Full Thickness
Skin Graft.

A. Cicatricial ectropion of the left lower lid.
B. A horizontal incision is made, the lips of the wound are undermined and
   scar tissue resected. Two tarsorrhaphy areas are freshened.
C. The tarsorrhaphies are sutured. A whole skin graft is taken from the
   ipsilateral upper lid and planted in the lower lid dehiscence.
D. Appearance before removal of sutures.
E. Appearance before the lids are separated.
F. Final result.

When the ipsilateral upper and lower lids are involved, they are
corrected together in one procedure.

Figure 185A presents such a case. This man was involved in a gas
explosion resulting in cicatricial ectropion of all but the right upper lid
with scarring and lagophthalmos. Simultaneous repair of the right
lower and left upper and lower lids was done.

Procedure (fig. 185): The lids are united by two temporary tarsorrhaphies. If the contraction is great, this is done after the skin has been undermined and the lids relaxed.

An incision parallel with the lid border and about 3 mm. from it is made in both upper and lower lids (fig. 185*B*). The skin is undermined and all cicatricial tissue is resected (fig. 185*C*). If cicatricial epicanthus or other cicatricial folds exist, they should all be undercut and the skin allowed to retract completely to a normal position. Frequently, burns of the face are only of first degree or mild second degree so that once the skin has been thoroughly undermined and allowed to retract ad maximum, the subcutaneous bed is found to be normal and ready for the reception of the graft. The skin itself need not be excised unless it has been scarred and discolored too badly. This will make that much less grafting necessary. If the burns have been deeper, then the bed should be cleaned of all cicatricial tissue before the graft is laid because subcutaneous scarring will greatly increase the contraction of a graft, whether full thickness or epidermal.

Once the beds are thoroughly exposed and cleaned with the lid margins in normal position, the lids are united by two or even three temporary tarsorrhaphies. The epidermal graft is taken as described in Chapter 3. This should be placed in position immediately (fig. 185*D*). In peeling the graft from the dermatome, it will be found that it tends to curl up. Once this happens it is difficult to separate. To counteract this, it should be grasped by four small hemostats in each corner and transferred to its position in the bed with the clamps still in place and without exerting undue pull on the graft as previously described. (With some dermatomes this technic is simplified by taking the graft directly on a layer of plastic tissue.) This is then placed on the denuded area, raw skin surface downward, and sutured into position with one or two sutures on each side.

A slit is made over the palpebral fissure to allow for drainage from the socket (fig. 185*D*) and the graft is covered with Adaptic or some other type of perforated plastic sheathing. Fluffed cotton or gauze is spread evenly over it (fig. 185*E*) and several adhesive strips are used to hold the dressing firmly in place. The clamps attached to the corners of the graft are removed. More adhesive strips are added if necessary and the whole covered with a firm pressure dressing.

The dressing should not be touched for 5 or 6 days. At this time it is carefully peeled off and the lid cleaned of all extraneous material. The graft should be firmly adherent to the bed at this time. The portions over the margins and beyond the bed will begin to slough but should not be touched unless they are easily removeable. A similar pressure dressing is reapplied for 3 more days. At this time it is removed, the area cleaned and simply dressed with a sheet of petrolated Telfa or

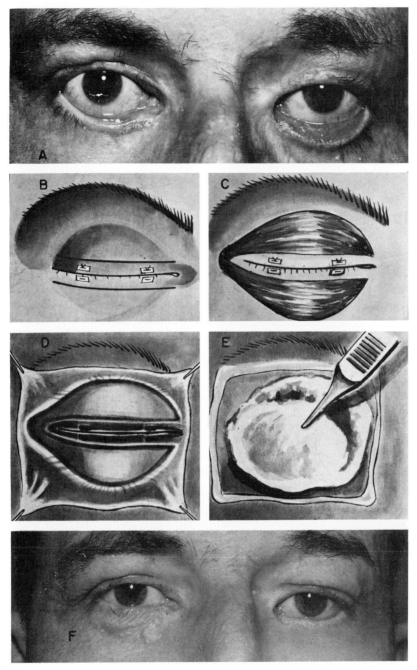

FIG. 185. Repair of Multiple Cicatricial Ectropion by Epidermal Graft.

A. Cicatricial entropion of three lids.
B. The upper and lower lids are immobilized by tarsorrhaphies and the skin incisions made.
C. The skin is undermined and allowed to retract upward and downward.
D. The epidermal graft is placed in position and incised centrally to permit drainage.
E. The graft is covered with a plastic sheet and fluffs before applying a pressure bandage.
F. Final result. Note repair of ectropion and restoration of lid fold in left upper lid.

Adaptic and a patch until healing is fully completed. The lid adhesions are left in place for 6 or 8 weeks. The final result is seen in figure 185*F*.

Comment: Wheeler brought out some excellent points in his discussion of this technic. He stated that the dissection frequently has to be carried well beyond the lateral canthus where it is permissible for the denuded areas of the upper and lower lids to approach each other. He cautioned strongly, however, against establishing a communication at the nasal end where a cicatrical epicanthus may form during the healing process. Experience has shown that these cicatrical epicanthi are difficult to eradicate. Wheeler also warned against the use of catgut sutures or clamps for bleeders and against rough handling of tissues.

Here also if there is ample graft tissue and if little scarring or contraction is expected, intermarginal sutures only may be used instead of tarsorrhaphies. The results are usually good; note the restoration of lid folds in figure 185*F*.

REFERENCES

ADAMS, W.: Cited by Beard, C. H., Ophthalmic Surgery, ed. 2. Philadelphia, P. Blakiston's Son & Co., 1914, p. 286.

VON AMMON, T.: Cited by Beard, C. H., op. cit., p. 286.

BARTLETT, R. E., and McKENZIE, J. W.: Surgery for ectropion. Am. J. Ophth. *62*:298, 1966.

BLASKOVICS, L., and KREIKER, A.: Eingriffe am Auge, 1938. Ferdinand Enke Verlag, Stuttgart, p. 87.

CALLAHAN, A.: Senile ectropion. Am. J. Ophth. *38*:787, 1954.

DIEFFENBACH, J. F.: Die operative Chirurgie. Leipzig, F. A. Brockhaus, 1845–1848, pp. 488–494.

DUKE-ELDER, S.: Textbook of Ophthalmology. St. Louis, C. V. Mosby Co., 1952, vol. 5, p. 4662.

FOX, S. A.: Basic techniques of lid surgery: Their origins and their apocrypha, Am. J. Ophth. *50*:384, 1960.

————: A modified Kuhnt-Szymanowski procedure. Am. J. Ophth. *62*:533, 1966.

————: A medial ectropion procedure. Arch. Ophth. *80*:494, 1968.

VON GRAEFE, A.: Bemerkung zur Operation des Entropium und Ektropium. Arch. Ophth. *10*:221 (Pt. 2), 1864.

HELMBOLD, R.: Zur Operation gegen Ektropium des unteren Lides. Klin. Monatsbl. Augenh. *35*:283, 1897.

IMRE, J.: Operation gegen Ektropium senile. Klin. Monatsbl. Augenh. *95*:303, 1935.

JONES, T. W.: A Manual of the Principles and Practice of Ophthalmic Medicine and Surgery. London, J. Churchill, 1847, pp. 413–429.

KUHNT, H.: Beiträge zur Operationen Augenheilkunder. Jena. G. Fischer, 1883, pp. 45–55.

MELLER, J.: Ophthalmic Surgery (ed. 6). New York, Blakiston, 1953, p. 57.

MULLER, L.: Eine Modification der Kuhnt'sschen Operation zur Behandlung des Ektropium. Klin. Monatsbl. Augenh. *31*:113, 1893.

NEMETH, L.: Surgical treatment of ectropion caused by blepharoadenitis. Opthalmologica *116*:162, 1948.

ROBERTSON, D.M.C.L.A.: A new operation for ectropion Edinb. Clin. & Path. J. *1*:201, 1883.

————: Notes on some points of procedure in the operation of direct transplantation of skin grafts for the cure of ectropion. Practitioner *57*:160, 1896.

————: A note on a method of operating for ectropion of the lower eyelid. Brit.
    Med. J. *1*:1504, 1898.
SNELLEN, H.: Suture for ectropion. Congr. intern. d'opht., Paris, 1862, p. 236.
SZYMANOWSKI, J.: Handbuch der Operationen Chirurgie. Berlin, Braunschweig,
    1870, p. 243.
TERSON, A.: Traitement l'ectropion senile. Arch. d'opht. *16*:760, 1896.
VERHOEFF, F. H.: Cited by Beard, C. H., op. cit., p. 283.
WEEKS, W. W.: Surgery of the Eye. New York, privately printed, 1937, p. 15.
WHEELER, J. M.: Ectropion: A problem for eye surgeons. South Med. J. *29*:377,
    1936.
ZIEGLER, S. L.: Galvanocautery puncture in ectropion and entropion. J.A.M.A.
    53:183, 1909.

CHAPTER 16

Entropion—Trichiasis

ENTROPION

ENTROPION (*en* = in; *trepein* = to turn) is an inversion of the lid margin so that the cilia are in contact with the globe. The danger of entropion lies in the constant irritation to the tissues of the eye which may cause conjunctivitis, keratitis, corneal ulcers, etc.

Entropion differs considerably from both trichiasis and distichiasis. In the former there is either a distortion of the lid border or disarrangement of the lashes toward the globe with the border itself remaining in normal position. Distichiasis is a congenital anomaly with a double row of lashes in which the posterior row is usually turned inward toward the globe (see Chapter 18). In entropion the margin and cilia are both normal but the whole border of the lid is turned inward.

HISTORICAL SUMMARY

The history of entropion is as old as trachoma, and trachoma is one of the oldest diseases known to man. It is not remarkable then that early attempts at surgical repair were aimed at the correction of trachomatous, i.e., cicatricial entropion, usually of the upper lid. For it is this lid with its larger malformed tarsus which is chiefly involved in the disease. Thus Paul of Aegina, some 1300 years ago, split the upper lid into two layers, excised an ellipse of skin above the lash line and pulled the skin-muscle layer with the offending cilia up, leaving the raw tarsoconjunctival layer to hang free over the eyeball.

Over a hundred years ago this horrendous operation was revived in somewhat modified form and became known as the Jäsche-Arlt procedure. An even more monstrous procedure was that of Flarer who simply

298

scalped the lid by amputating away the whole ciliary margin allowing the wound to heal by granulation. Both deserved the early oblivion which overtook them. Anagnostakis and Hotz resected pretarsal orbicularis fibers, pulled up and sutured the lower lip of the skin wound to the tarsus in order to evert the lid border. Spencer Watson, Gayet, Dianoux, Machek and Blaskovics interposed a pedicle of skin between the ciliary and posterior edges of the lid margin thus moving the cilia up out of the way. Van Millingen used a strip of buccal mucous membrane instead of skin for the intermarginal graft (fig. 199).

While all these technics were being developed, Streatfeild had boldly attacked the main seat of the trouble, i.e., the thickened deformed tarsus itself. He modified an older procedure and excised a horizontal wedge of skin, muscle and tarsus and left the wound to heal by granulation. Snellen improved the procedure by suturing the lower skin flap to the tarsus, thus turning the lid edge outward on the tarsal groove as a fulcrum.

Fracture of the tarsus was suggested by Green, Ewing, Williams and Lagleyze among others. Panas in 1882 was probably the first to do horizontal section of the full thickness of the upper lid (fig. 186C) routinely for cicatricial entropion. This has been improved and modified recently by Wies for the lower lid and Ballen for the upper lid again. All the above procedures and many more were devised for the upper lid since the upper tarsus is wider, thicker, in broader contact with the cornea and hence more likely to cause trouble than the lower lid when distorted and misshapen.

Most operations for entropion of the lower lid were directed toward unrolling the lid. It is rather interesting to note that no great distinction was made between senile and cicatricial entropion in these repairs. Graefe in 1864 suggested resection of a triangle of skin for cicatricial entropion of the lower lid (fig. 186A) and added excision of tarsus for the upper lid (fig. 186B). The tarsal triangle has survived to the present day in various forms and has been modified into various shapes in addition to being transposed to the lower lid. Among the more recent is Butler's triangular resection of 1948 and this author's in 1951. More recently it has assumed rectangular and trapezoid shapes. Resection of pretarsal orbicularis fibers and tenotomy of the lateral canthal ligament were also suggested.

Early repairs of senile entropion ran to sutures, and here history seems to go way back to Hippocrates who inserted a vertical suture beneath the free border of the lower lid, tied it and left it in place until it sloughed out. Over a hundred years ago Gaillard, Arlt, Snellen, Stellwag and Graefe, among others, devised methods of passing sutures through the various structures of the lower lid which, on being tied,

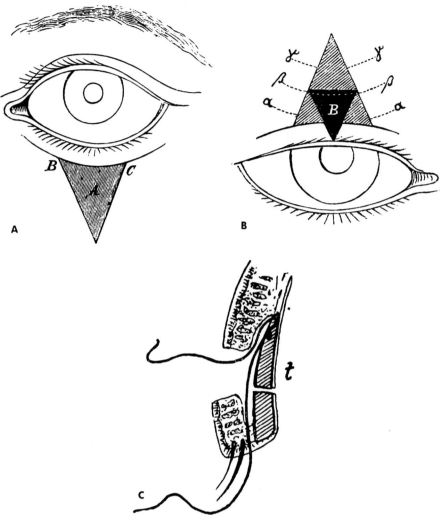

FIG. 186.   Early Entropion Repairs.
A.   Graefe repair of lower lid "entropium spasticum."
B.   Graefe repair of upper lid "entropium spasticum."
     (Graefe, A.: Courtesy Archives für Ophthalmologie.)
C.   Panas repair of upper lid entropion.
     (Panas, P.: Courtesy Encyclopedia of Ophthalmology, Cleveland Press,
     Chicago.)

pulled the lid margin away from the globe. The object was to cause
cicatrization so that the lids would stay in position after the sutures had
been removed or extruded spontaneously. Like the sutures for ectropion,
this modality seems to have lost most of its popularity—probably because
of its general ineffectiveness. Excision of skin and skin-cum-muscle in the
form of ellipses, triangles and rectangles has been used since the time of
Celsus with varying degrees of success, mostly poor.

Back in 1858 Busch did a canthotomy and resected a triangle of skin at the lateral canthus to tauten the skin of the lower lid and thus keep it from rolling in. Goldzieher in 1908 and Blaskovics in 1923 revived the operation in turn and Fuchs described it in the fifth (1917) edition of his textbook.

Cautery for the cure of entropion has an old and honorable if rather unsuccessful history. Thus the Egyptians of ancient times are said to have used red-hot gold plates to destroy the cilia. The Arabians of the eleventh and twelfth century, less affluent, used red-hot irons for entropion. More recently Galezowski, Trousseau and Terrien used the thermo- and galvano-cautery to create a horizontal cicatrix 3–4 millimeters from the lid border. The Ziegler eponym is the most recent one applied to this procedure in 1909. However, it has proved more effective in ectropion than in entropion. Escharotics such as caustic potash, sulphuric acid, etc. have not been overlooked but their use has been abandoned. Injection of alcohol has the same rationale as cantholysis. All of these have been used singly and together with indifferent results.

One of the more successful procedures has been Wheeler's orbicularis strip imbrication from *below* the tarsus which has as its object not the pulling down of the lid so much but holding the lower border of the tarsus against the globe by the tautness of the tarsal strip. This was based on Birch-Hirschfeld's procedure (fig. 187) which was quite similar. In fact Wheeler published two procedures for the correction of entropion in the same paper. In the first he attached a strip of orbicularis to the lateral periosteum. In the second he dissected up a 4 mm. orbicularis

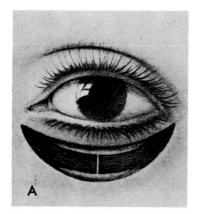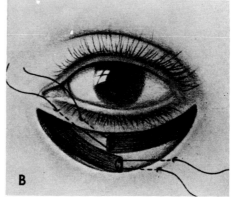

Fig. 187. Birch-Hirschfeld Orbicularis Strip Technic for Senile Entropion.
A. The subtarsal orbicularis strips are mobilized.
B. The tarsal strips are imbricated and the sutures are brought out on the skin surface.
(Cited by Blaskovics, L., and Kreiker, A.: Eingriffe am Auge. Courtesy Ferdinand Enke Verlag, Stuttgart.)

strip, split it vertically, overlapped the ends 4 to 5 mm. and sutured it to the orbital fascia. Hill has combined this procedure with tarsal resection (fig. 194). Meek used two similar strips to pull the lid edge away from the globe but instead of overlapping them he pulled them straight down and attached them to the orbital fascia on each side of the lid. More recently Wessely has used a flap of skin to unwind the lower lid and pull the margin down and away from the globe. In 1960 Jones resected the orbital septum. In 1963 Jones, Reeh and Tsujimura added excision of skin and orbicularis muscle. Thus all the tissues of the lower lid have been shortened in one way or another in order to unwind the lid and correct senile entropion.

Surgical treatment of entropion in general has been less successful than that of ectropion as proved by the many more procedures available for the former. It has always been the case that the more difficult and unsuccessfully treated the condition the more numerous the attempts at its cure. There is no intention here to describe or even list all the procedures extant for the correction of entropion. Many are similar except for details.

CLASSIFICATION OF ENTROPION

Entropion may be classified as follows:
Congenital
Acquired
    Spastic
    Mechanical
    Senile
    Cicatricial

CONGENITAL ENTROPION

Primary congenital entropion is a rare anomaly. It is much rarer than the secondary type which is usually associated with anophthalmos, enophthalmos and microphthalmos. It occurs most commonly in both lower lids and about twice as often in females as in males. The most common cause is an overdevelopment of the marginal orbicularis fibers.

Congenital entropion must be differentiated from epiblepharon though this is not always easy. In the former the whole lid margin is inverted as in all true entropia and it tends to become aggravated with the passage of time. Epiblepharon is characterized by an accessory fold or folds of skin which pushes the cilia against the globe. It may disappear by the end of the first year (see Chapter 18 for complete discussion and treatment of these conditions).

ACQUIRED ENTROPION

Acute Spastic Entropion

Spastic entropion is an acute condition usually due to acute ocular inflammation or prolonged patching of the eye (fig. 188*A*). It may occur at any age and affects only the lower lid because of the smaller, thinner tarsus. The upper lid, because its tarsus is too wide to permit inversion, may show a concomitant blepharospasm.

This condition is usually transient. Temporary measures such as pulling the lid down into place with strips of adhesive or fixing it into place by the liberal application of collodion may be tried. Skin clips have also been suggested but these leave permanent skin marks and are not advised. All efforts should be bent toward eliminating the causative factors, i.e., inflammation, chronic irritation, patching, etc. No surgery is indicated unless the entropion becomes chronic in which case the treatment is as for senile entropion.

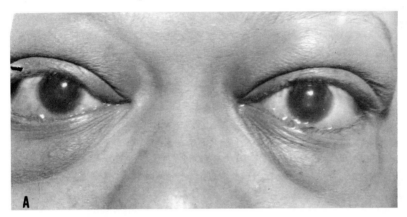

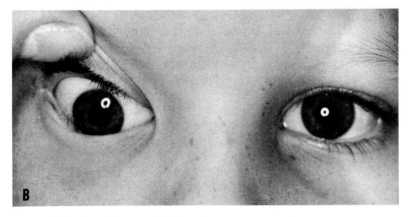

FIG. 188. Rare Types of Entropion.
A. An unusual case of bilateral acute spastic entropion.
B. Mechanical entropion of right lower lid due to lack of support from improper prosthesis.

Mechanical Entropion

Mechanical entropion may occur at any age. It is seen most commonly in the lower lid with anophthalmos (fig. 188*B*), enophthalmos, microphthalmos, etc—i.e., in all those cases in which the lower lid has lost support due to an absent or shrunken globe.

Since the etiology and pathology of this type of entropion is somewhat akin to that of senile entropion, the lines of repair in most cases follow the procedures outlined below for the repair of senile entropion unless it can be helped by a better prosthesis.

Senile (Atonic) Entropion

ETIOLOGY OF SENILE ENTROPION. For years the etiology of senile entropion has been a mystery. It still is to some extent but we are learning more about it. This is important because the more we know about its etiology the more intelligently we can correct it surgically.

Senile entropion (commonly miscalled "spastic") is by far the most common type of entropion. It appears only in the lower lid of older individuals without obvious cause. It has commonly been ascribed to some form of spasm of the muscle of Riolan, in the mistaken belief that this muscle forms part of the pretarsal fibers of the orbicularis. The spasm is presumed to be brought on by ocular inflammation and irritation. However, a history of inflammation is rarely obtainable and careful questioning will usually elicit the fact that the irritation of the globe was caused by and followed the spontaneous turning in of the lid margin and the rubbing of the cilia against the eyeball.

No one has ever explained accurately what initiates the spasm in "spastic" entropion, along what arcs it travels or why and how it is confined to the upper three or four millimeters of the lower lid. But "spastic" it remains. Many explanations have been assigned: (a) Irritation of the cornea or conjunctiva, (b) spasm of the muscle of Riolan, (c) malposition of the insertions of the canthal ligaments, (d) spasm of the marginal fibers of the orbicularis and so forth. It is not hard to dispose of most of these theories:

a. A half dozen drops of local anesthetic dropped into an entropic eye will abolish all surface irritation but the entropion will remain.

b. A look at any anatomy book will show that the muscle of Riolan lies mostly on the lid margin in the neighborhood of the openings of the meibomian glands and is distinct from the fibers of the orbicularis. Thus, not only is it in the wrong position, but it is a weak, scrawny muscle, too feeble to do any bending, spasm or no spasm.

c. If this type of entropion is due to malinsertion of the canthal ligaments, why does it show up only in the loose, atonic lids of elderly people and never anywhere else?

d. Then how about the possibility of spasm of the upper pretarsal orbicularis fibers initiated in some apochryphal way after the efferent fibers leave the conjunctiva? It is difficult to explain a spasm so localized, so selective and so specialized that it affects only the border fibers of the orbicularis while the rest of the lower lid remains uninvolved. Furthermore, there is nothing in the neurologic anatomy of the lower lid to bolster this theory. However, to rule out even the slightest possibility the following experiment may be performed.

After complete instillation anesthesia of the conjunctival sac of an eye with senile entropion an O'Brien akinesia is done, care being taken not to approach the lid area. Despite the fact that both the efferent and afferent fibers are thus blocked out the entropion persists (figs. 189A and B). On the operating table with the patient lying down this is even more striking. So much for spasm.

In 1963 Jones, Reeh and Tsujimura suggested another theory for the etiology of senile entropion: They agree that absorption of orbital fat weakens the support of the globe to the atonic lid and allows the lower border of the tarsus to swing out. But, according to these authors, the most important cause of the entropion is *overaction of the lower preseptal muscle* which, when contracting, "rises up between the pretarsal

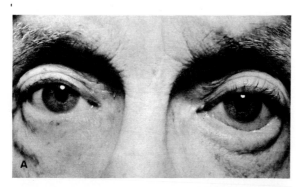

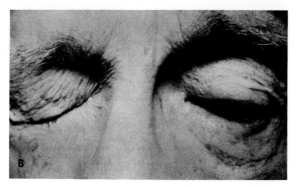

Fig. 189. Effect of Akinesia on Senile Entropion.
A. Senile entropion of the left lower lid.
B. Akinesia leaves lid unaffected.

muscle and pretarsal skin." The tarsus is an "innocent bystander" here. Just how the preseptal muscle becomes detached from the overlying skin and underlying fascia is not explained.

I have never yet seen a case of senile entropion in which the preseptal muscle was free to curl up on the pretarsal muscle; nor, as far as I know, has anyone else. In every case it has to be *cut* away from skin and fascia. I find this theory just as irrational as the "spastic" theory of senile entropion which I rejected twenty years ago.

A recent report by Dalgleish and Smith, who performed an important series of experiments with metal markers, shows that the tarsus, far from being an innocent bystander bends on its horizontal axis with the upper border swinging in and down and the lower border out and up (figs. 190*A* and *B*). As a result, the preseptal muscle arcades do indeed ride up, as they must with the bending of the tarsus, but these authors point out that "there is little tendency for these arcades to invade the tarsal portion of the lid as the close adherence of the dermis to the underlying pretarsal muscle tends to preclude this." To this might be added the adherence of the skin to the preseptal muscle.

Then what causes the entropic lid to turn in? As in senile ectropion, the lid in senile entropion is usually atonic rather than spastic. As Fuchs pointed out in 1890, "Entropion . . . develops mainly in elderly people with flabby lids and its production is favored by deep placing, diminution in size, or absence of the eyeball." It is probable that the same factors which cause senile ectropion also cause senile entropion. These are loss of tonus, relaxation of skin, muscle and fascia and absorption, or what is more probable, the sagging of orbital fat lower into the orbit (hence the "bags") permitting retroplacement and a relative enophthalmos of the globe with consequent loss of support to the lid. All these signs of the aging process appear in both senile ectropion and entropion. The lids in figure 192*E* are certainly not spastic.

But in senile entropion, *the aging process has not involved the tarsal sling*, i.e., the tarsus with its canthal connections (fig. 5). The result is that when the lid closes, as during the normal blinking process, the lower border of the tarsus, because of relaxation of the lower lid tissues, rolls out instead of hugging the globe. The upper border, still taut, rising somewhat with lid closure and having lost support of the globe, tends to roll in as the orbicularis contracts and the lower border rolls out. Add to this the bending of the aged and weak tarsus on its horizontal axis and you have one of the pathogomic signs of senile entropion: the bulge in the lower lid caused by the rolling out and bending of the tarsus. Duke-Elder states, "Indeed, the lower lid is frequently so lax and flabby that it has to sag in one or the other direction: if the orbicularis retains a reasonable amount of tone it will tend to sag inwards, more particularly if the skin is atrophic and redundant and the eye has become deeply placed."

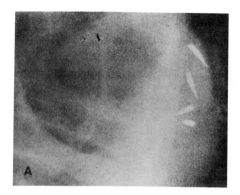 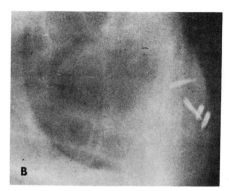

FIG. 190. X-ray Study of Entropic Lid Action.

A. Lower lid in normal (nonentropic) position. The upper two more or less vertical markers are in the tarsal plate. The two lower horizontal markers are in preseptal orbicularis.

B. The same lid is now in the entropic position. The upper edge of the tarsus is now seen to be in a horizontal position and the lower has swung forward. It will be noted that the preseptal markers and the lower tarsal plate marker have approximated each other.

(Dalgleish, R., and Smith, J. L. S.: Courtesy British J. of Ophthalmology.)

It is not the orbicularis which retains its tone in senile entropion but only the tarsal sling.

Since the normal position of the lower lid margin in the average individual is at the lower limbus, the cornea may remain intact for a long time. Conjunctival irritation, however, is common and may be a source of constant discomfort to the patient. The upper lid is never involved.

Surgery of Senile Entropion

Since time immemorial surgical correction of senile entropion has been of two schools: (a) the unwinding or pulling down school and (b) the tautening school. The former treats entropion by the resection or shortening of skin, orbicularis muscle and orbital fascia—one or all—horizontally, i.e., it shortens the lid vertically. In this school is included the various cautery procedures. The tautening school believes in tightening the lid horizontally by vertical resection so that the atonic lid is pressed closer to the eyeball.

Probably the earliest type of treatment was the use of heat cautery to cause lid eversion. Later, correction took the form of sutures of various sorts to unroll the lid and pull it down as previously described. These, along with collodion and adhesive strips, are largely ineffective. Excision of horizontal strips of skin or muscle or both are at best temporary but are used by some in the early mild forms of senile entropion. Also since the pathology of senile entropion is not a "spasm" of the muscle but an actual weakening and atony of all the lid tissues, any procedure aimed at simply unwinding the lid and pulling it down is bound to have only a transitory effect and pulls the lid down out of position as Wheeler showed many years ago.

Another technic used by some is canthotomy with or without cantholysis, i.e., section of the external canthal ligament to weaken orbicularis action. This goes back to von Ammon who first performed it in 1839. It is ineffective. External tarsorrhaphy is another primitive procedure contraindicated here. Alcohol injection at the lateral canthus to weaken orbicularis action is really a milder form of cantholysis which usually has to be repeated and is not permanent.

Cautery for Senile Entropion (Ziegler)

Cautery for lid eversion goes back to the ancient Egyptians. Over the centuries since then, cautery punctures have been used in various modes and patterns. The most popular of these in recent years has been Ziegler's method.

Procedure (fig. 191):   With an electrocautery needle or muscle hook heated in an alcohol flame, five or six equally spaced punctures are made through skin and muscle deep into the tarsus about 4 mm. from the lid margin (fig. 191). The eye is patched for 24 hours, then cold compresses may be applied twice a day. There is usually little reaction.

Comment: The use of this modality has its aficionados and detractors. Thus Dunnington and Regan among others report only six failures in seventy-five cases. Wheeler and many since (including this author) have been something less than enthusiastic. Wheeler pointed out many years ago that Ziegler puncture caused lid contraction and if repeated too often will ultimately pull the lid down so that the margin rides well below its normal position. I have found it ineffective as a permanent cure in advanced cases. However, in early cases it will cause eversion for some time.

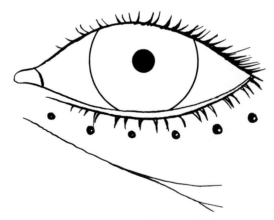

FIG. 191.   Ziegler Cautery for Entropion.   Appearance after completion of full lid cautery.

Double Triangle Procedure for Senile Entropion (Author's)

After a number of modifications the following procedure has been evolved and has now been used successfully for a number of years. It is recommended for all cases of senile entropion.

Procedure (fig. 192):   About 2 mm. beyond the lateral canthus an equilateral triangle apex down, measuring 10 to 12 mm. on each side, is marked off with an antiseptic dye (fig. 192*A*). If the entropion is severe and long-standing, the base line may be made 12 mm. long. The whole lid is anesthetized and the included skin and muscle resected down to the orbital fascia (fig. 192*B*).

The lid is everted on a chalazion clamp and a triangle *with its apex on the free border in the gray line* is marked off on the conjunctival surface of the tarsus. This should be just lateral to the center of the lid with the base at the attached tarsal border measuring 6 to 8 mm. depending again on the severity of the entropion. The tarsoconjunctival triangle is resected (fig. 192*C*). In cases of severe entropion a spindle of orbital fascia is also resected (fig. 192*C* inset).

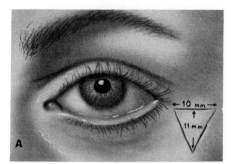
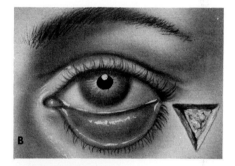
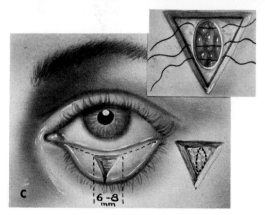

FIG. 192.   Correction of Senile Entropion (Author's Method).
A.   A triangle is marked out at the lateral canthus.
B.   The skin-muscle triangle is resected.
C.   A central tarsoconjunctival triangle with the apex in the gray line is resected. A vertical spindle of orbital fascia is also resected in advanced cases (inset). *(Continued)*

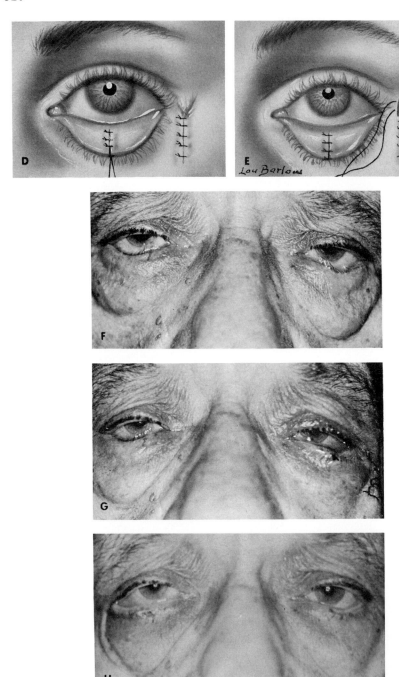

FIG. 192 (*Continued*)

D. The tarsoconjunctival and skin-muscle triangles are closed.
E. A skin pucker which forms above the skin triangle is resected and closed.
F. A case of bilateral senile entropion.
G. Note the transient marginal pucker after left lower lid repair.
H. Final result.

The tarsal wound is closed with three or four interrupted 4–0 silk sutures. The apex on the lid border may be closed with a 4–0 plain catgut suture. This sometimes causes some irritation of the cornea if the ends are left too long. Plain catgut softens rapidly and this suture has never been found to cause severe or prolonged irritation (fig. 192C). The skin-muscle wound at the lateral canthus is closed with 5–0 silk sutures, care being taken to catch up the muscle fibers as well. Alternatively the muscle may be closed separately with 4–0 plain catgut and then the skin with 5–0 silk (fig. 192D). If a wrinkle should form at the top of the wound a small skin triangle (Burow) is excised and the wound closed with silk (fig. 192E).

Following surgery a firm supportive dressing is applied. Further dressings are done in 48 hours and then daily. Skin sutures are removed in six days and tarsal sutures in ten days unless obviously loose before then. Figures 192F, G and H show a bilateral case of senile entropion before, three days, and four weeks after operation.

Comment: This operation has now been performed by the author himself or at his direction in over 400 cases with gratifying results. Its advantages are:

a. The surgery is quite simple.

b. It strengthens the tarsus which is the only firm supportive structure of the lid. Since this does not stretch, recurrence is less frequent. Furthermore, it shortens and strengthens the tarsus where it is needed most, i.e., *at the base*, not at the apex, thus preventing the attached border from rolling out.

c. It also strengthens the other less rigid tissues of the lid, i.e., the skin and muscle (and when necessary the orbital fascia) not vertically to pull the lid down but horizontally in order to stiffen their support of the lid to the globe.

d. The only resultant scar is external to the lateral canthus where it is inconspicuous and gradually fades out.

e. If necessary it can be repeated.

In some of the earlier reports it was suggested that a tarsoconjunctival triangle measuring only 5 mm. at the base and no more be resected. Later experience has proven this precaution unnecessary. Thus when the tarsus is thick and the bulge severe, a 6, 7 or even 8 mm. base triangle may be resected. Furthermore, an immediate overcorrection is not catastrophic. Given a couple of weeks all postoperative overcorrections tend to right themselves and disappear. In only two instances have a few Ziegler cautery punctures been necessary to counteract an overcorrection.

Undercorrection is possible and should be repaired on the operating table if noted immediately. An additional 2 or 3 mm. of tarsus should be resected from one side of the tarsoconjunctival wound.

On closure a small bump will often form at the lid margin where the tarsal triangle has been resected (fig. 192*G*). This always disappears within a week or ten days.

As noted above tunneling between the skin-muscle and tarso-conjunctival laminae between the two triangles has been omitted by the author for a long time. This simplification of the earlier technic has given a better and more permanent correction. There is so much "give" in these lids that there is no trouble in closing the two triangular wounds without undermining.

As a matter of fact, an additional strengthening step of the lid wall has been added to the technic by the resection of the exposed orbital fascia in the lateral triangle (fig. 192*C* inset). This is closed along with the orbicularis muscle. Sometimes some of the orbital fat presents and prolapses. This is simply resected (to the cosmetic benefit of the patient, it might be added). These two steps, i.e., omission of the tunneling between the triangles and the resection of orbital fascia have added to the strengthening of the lid wall and to the lessening of recurrences in severe cases.

Since all operations for senile entropion can only treat the results of the aging process and not the cause there will probably always be some recurrences. Hence the true value of any operation depends on the frequency of recurrences. In the author's experience the above procedure has given the least. The fact that the operation may be easily repeated enhances its value.

In recent years modifications have crept into the literature in which rectangles of tarsus have been resected instead of apex-up triangles (fig. 194). Since the upper border of the entropic lid is up tight against the globe and since it is the lower border of the tarsus which swings out, it seems to me more logical to tighten the *attached border* rather than the whole tarsus by triangular rather than rectangular resection.

Wheeler Orbicularis Strip Procedure (Author's Modification)

Until the procedure immediately preceding was adopted because of its greater simplicity and lesser recurrence rate, the author used Wheeler's orbicularis strip operation. It had been modified for reasons which are explained below. The technic follows:

Procedure (fig. 193): A horizontal incision just below the ciliary margin is made the full length of the lid and the skin is undermined downward. A strip of orbicularis 8 mm. wide is dissected up from the upper part of the exposed muscle (fig. 193*A*). A double-armed 4–0 chromic suture is inserted in the center of the lower tarsal border taking a good bite in the tarsus (fig. 193*B*). The two needles are passed through the strip of orbicularis from behind forward about 2 mm. apart and 3 mm. lateral to the center. Each of the needles is then passed similarly through

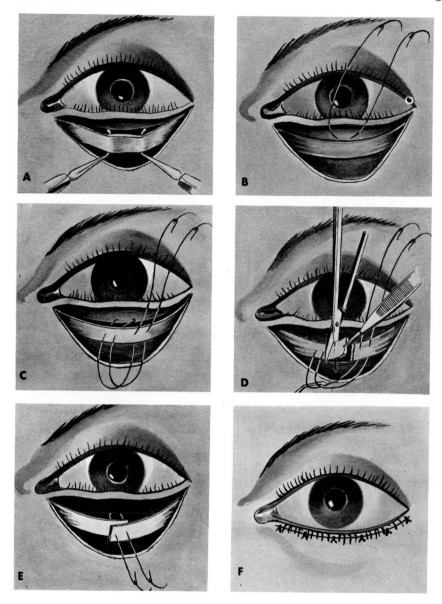

FIG. 193. Orbicularis Crossing Technique for Senile Entropion
(Wheeler, Modified).
A. The orbicularis strip is dissected up and mobilized.
B. A double-armed suture is placed in the central lower border of the tarsus.
C. The suture is passed through the orbicularis strip to either side of the center.
D. The central portion of the orbicularis strip is resected.
E. The suture is tautened and the ends of the strip overlapped.
F. The skin is closed.

the muscle strip from behind forward to the other side of midline so that
about 6 to 8 mm. of muscle strip separates the sutures (fig. 193C). This
central portion of the muscle is resected (fig. 193D) and the suture

pulled up and tied (fig. 193E). If the needles are inserted correctly, the two segments of the muscle strip will overlap each other neatly and fall into line without the slightest difficulty. The skin wound is sutured (fig. 193F) and a firm supportive dressing applied.

The modifications of the original Wheeler procedure are:

a. Incision of skin just below the ciliary margin where the scar is less conspicuous instead of 6 mm. below the margin.

b. The muscle strip is 8 mm. wide instead of the 4 mm. Wheeler suggested because the strip shrinks and frays if too narrow and becomes difficult to handle and valueless as a support for the tarsus.

c. The muscle strip is anchored at the *lower border of the tarsus* rather than to the orbital fascia as Wheeler suggested. This gives a firmer support and is more certain of result because it presses on the lower border of the tarsus and helps keep it against the globe.

d. All the sutures are inserted before the muscle strip is cut because, after division, the muscle strip contracts and it is difficult to estimate the amount to resect.

Comment: This operation is effective not only because it exerts pressure on the lower border of the tarsal plate, thus tipping the upper border outward, but also because the orbicularis fibers are strengthened by shortening and overlapping. Wheeler warns against over- and under-correction, i.e., excision of too much or too little muscle. This is not easy to estimate. In cases of overcorrection, i.e., surgical ectropion, Ziegler puncture usually suffices to reinvert the lid if overcorrection has not been too great. Recurrences occur more frequently than with the author's double triangle procedure. They are due to the weakening and further stretching of the thin muscle strip which is the inherent weakness of this procedure.

Recently Schimek and Newsom have modified Wheeler's type I operation by using collagen tape instead of orbicularis strip to tauten the orbicularis by fastening it to the lateral periosteum. It is to be hoped that the collagen tape has a longer survival life than in ptosis surgery.

Modification of the Wheeler Operation (Hill)

Hill modified and divided Wheeler's orbicularis crossing procedure into two operations.

Procedure (fig. 194): In the first operation for "chronic spastic entropion without horizontal lid laxity" he combines the Wheeler technic with a Hotz skin-muscle resection. He fashions a band of orbicularis about 5 mm. wide just below the tarsal border and curettes away all other adherent muscular tissues from the tarsus. He then imbricates the muscle strip, shortening it by about 5 mm. (fig. 194A) and fastens it securely to the tarsus (fig. 194B) as this author has done since 1951. The upper skin lip is pulled down and sutured to the lower border of the tarsus (fig. 194C) and the skin edges are then sutured to each other.

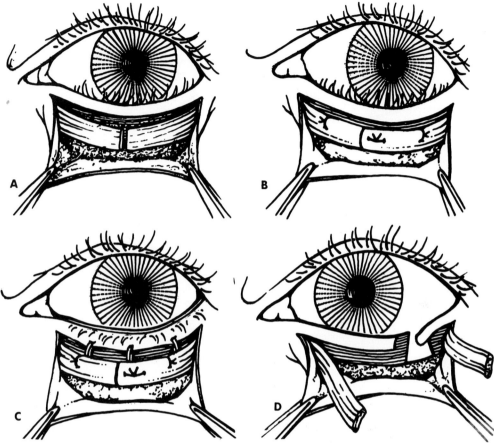

Fig. 194.   Repair of "Chronic Spastic" Entropion (Hill).

A.   A 5 mm. band of orbicularis is dissected up from the tarsus and the tarsus is
      curetted. The orbicularis is cut vertically.
B.   The resultant straps are overlapped 5 mm. and reattached to the lower border
      of the tarsus. Wing sutures are added to each side to prevent "upriding."
C.   The upper edge of the skin incision is sutured to the lower border of the
      tarsus.
D.   Trapezoid excision of tarsoconjunctiva added to the above for "senile"
      entropion.
      (Hill, J. C.: From Manual of Ophthalmic Plastic Surgery. Courtesy Am.
      Acad. Oph. & Oto.)

Hill states that this procedure creates a full tissue barrier "to prevent preseptal orbicularis muscle from moving over the tarsus to the
tarsal plate." It is highly doubtful whether the preseptal muscle does this
as shown above (fig. 190).

For senile "persistent entropion with horizontal lid laxity" Hill adds
a trapezoid excision of tarsoconjunctiva to the above at the lateral third
of the lid (fig. 194D). In both procedures the cilia are glued to the cheek
with collodion and a pressure dressing is applied for from 10 to 21 days
which is changed every 5 days.

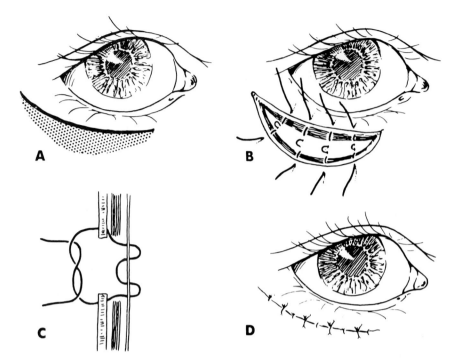

FIG. 195. Repair of Senile Entropion (Jones, Reeh and Tsujimura).
a. The outer two-thirds of the lid is incised.
b. Skin and muscle is resected. Sutures are inserted in orbital fascia.
c. Scheme of suturing.
d. Closure.
    (Jones, L. T., Reeh, M. J., and Tsujimura, J. K. Courtesy American Journal
    of Ophthalmology.)

Lower Lid Shortening for Senile Entropion (Jones, Reeh and Tsujimura)

A good example of a lid shortening or unrolling procedure for senile entropion is that of Jones, Reeh and Tsujimura. In this operation preseptal orbicularis muscle is resected, orbital fascia is tucked and skin resected if necessary.

Procedure (fig. 195): A skin incision is made 6 mm. below and parallel with the outer two-thirds of the lid margin. It is carried upward beyond the lateral canthus (fig. 195a). The skin is undermined upward and downward to expose orbicularis muscle which is split horizontally at the base of the tarsus. A strip of skin and preseptal orbicularis is resected, depending on the severity of the entropion; the width resected usually measures 5 or 6 mm. The orbital fascia is now tucked with 4–0 cotton or silk double-armed sutures to make a pleat in the fascia of about 5 or 6 mm. (fig. 195b). The needles catch up the skin edges going in and as they emerge (fig. 195c). Additional skin sutures are added for good closure (fig. 195d). The usual postoperative care is given. Sutures are removed in 10 days.

Comment: Like all unwinding procedures this, as Wheeler pointed out long ago, usually gives a shortened lid with scleral exposure at the lower limbus. Also, since the skin is sutured to tarsus with no intervening orbicularis muscle, in order "to prevent the preseptal muscle from riding up" the indented scar in the lower lid is slow to disappear, if it ever does. The skin incision is made in the lateral two-thirds of the lid because the authors feel that an incision in the medial third would interfere with the normal function of the lacrimal pump. Fortunately, unless the integrity of the punctum and canaliculus are compromised this does not happen. Otherwise there would be a lot more weepy eyes than there are after any lid surgery.

Fascial Shortening for Senile Entropion (Jones)

Another unrolling type of procedure is the fascial shortening operation of Jones. In a 1968 communication Jones discusses the comparative anatomy of the orbital septum. He sees an analogy between senile ptosis and senile entropion when the body is in the supine position. He feels that both are caused primarily by the marked senile changes in the orbicularis fascia. This, together with fat absorption, reduces pressure on the lids against the globe and results in loss of control of the tarsal base. In the case of senile entropion this is overcome by resecting a strip of fascia and conjunctiva 20 mm. wide and 10 mm. long beneath the tarsus. Jones still insists that a barrier must be created "to prevent the preseptal muscle from overriding the pretarsal" (see page 305). This is done by attaching the cut edge of the orbital fascia with its conjunctiva to the pretarsal skin. This is the third modification of a procedure suggested by Jones in 1960. Skin and muscle are no longer resected here.

Comment: It is interesting to note that the above technic requires the "preseptal muscle dissected free from the septum." If the preseptal muscle is free to override the pretarsal, as Jones claims, why should it be necessary to dissect it away from the septum? Or is the septum also free to ride up?

From the clinical viewpoint the analogy of senile ptosis to senile entropion is a mite too facile. Senile ptosis is a lid drooped out of position due to degenerative changes in the levator muscle. Senile entropion is an inverted lid which is in normal position otherwise. The inversion is due to degenerative changes of the lid layers: skin, muscle and fascia which allow the tarsus to bend on its horizontal axis (see page 306). Senile ptosis is corrected simply by shortening the levator and pulling the lid back into position. By shortening the fascia of the lower lid, Jones straightens the lid in senile entropion but he also shortens it and pulls it down out of position. Shortening of the lid by resecting horizontal strips of any of its tissues will always do this. Such technics go back to the time of Celsus if not earlier.

A more permanent way to correct senile entropion and leave the lid in normal position is not to shorten the lid but to tauten and strengthen it (fig. 192).

CICATRICIAL ENTROPION

Cicatricial entropion is one of the oldest scourges known to man. Some of the earliest surgical procedures which have come down to us have dealt with this stubborn—and sometimes malignant—clinical entity. This is not surprising considering the widespread presence of trachoma.

Until recently trachoma was the most important cause of cicatricial entropion. Strides in the medical control of this disease have reduced its incidence. But enough remains along with the products of physical and chemical trauma to challenge the ophthalmic surgeon. In cicatricial entropion, unlike senile entropion, it is the upper lid which offers the more serious problem as has already been mentioned.

Upper Lid Cicatricial Entropion Surgery

In many cases of upper lid cicatricial entropion the conjunctiva is thickened, rough and shrunken and the tarsal plate is thickened and malformed. Scores of procedures have been devised for the correction of the trichiasis and entropion of trachoma. These procedures aim at restoring the normal relations of (1) tarsus to globe and (2) the skin-muscle to tarsoconjunctiva.

The basis of most of the procedures in the first group is the eversion of the lid margin so that the cilia do not come in contact with the globe. This is attained by resecting, thinning or sectioning of the tarsus horizontally so that the lower horizontal segment is turned up on the incision as a fulcrum thus pulling the ciliary margin upward and away from the globe.

Streatfeild-Snellen "Tarsoplasty" for
Cicatricial Entropion of Upper Lid (Author's Modification)

Horizontal grooving and section of the tarsus for cicatricial entropion is over a hundred years old. Streatfeild reported his procedure for grooving the tarsus in 1857. Snellen added Anagnostakis' sutures to Streatfeild's "tarsoplasty" in 1863 and it became the well-known Streatfeild-Snellen operation. The following is a modification of this procedure which I have found useful in many cases of upper lid cicatricial entropion.

Procedure (fig. 196): A horizontal incision is made through skin and muscle at the upper tarsal border from one end of the tarsus to the other. The skin-muscle lamina is dissected down almost to the ciliary margin to uncover the tarsus (fig. 196A). A horizontal wedge of tarsus 3 mm. wide at the base with the apex toward the conjunctiva is resected

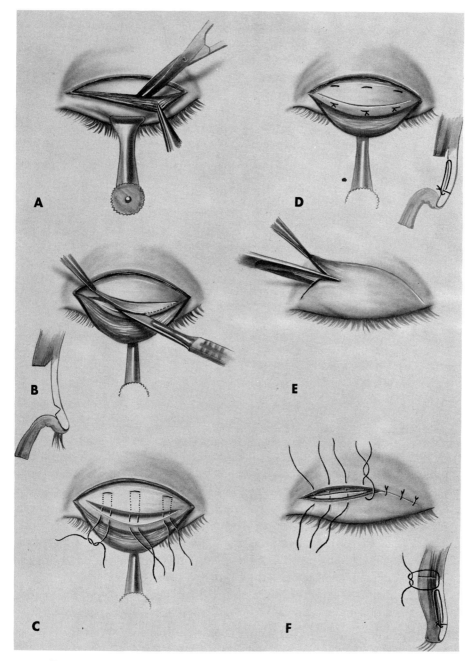

FIG. 196.   Streatfeild-Snellen Technic (Author's Modification).
A. Incision through skin and muscle at upper tarsal border. The skin-muscle lamina is dissected down to uncover tarsus.
B. A horizontal wedge of tarsus is resected.
C. Three chromic sutures are anchored in the upper tarsal border and pass through the edges of the tarsal split.
D. The sutures are tied everting the lid edge.
E. The skin flap is pulled up and the excess is resected.
F. The skin incision is closed with sutures anchored in the upper tarsal border.
    (Continued)

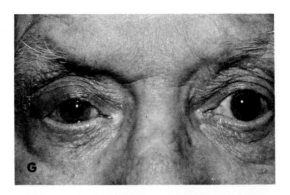

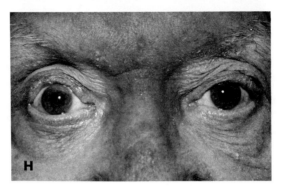

FIG. 196 (*Continued*)
G. and H. shows a cicatricial entropion of the right upper lid with result of
repair.
(Fox, S. A.: Courtesy Archives of Ophthalmology.)

3 mm. above the lid border. The wedge is formed by making two horizontal incisions on the anterior surface of the tarsus. The first is 3 mm.
from the tarsal border and the second 3 mm. above the first. The tarsal
wedge is then created by beveling or inclining these incisions toward each
other so that they meet just before conjunctiva is reached (fig. 196B).
Admittedly this is easier said than done. However, the thickened cicatrized tarsus of trachoma or other inflammation offers a better opportunity for such tarsectomy than a normal tarsus. Should the conjunctiva
be penetrated, immediate closure by plain 6–0 catgut is advised.

Three double-armed 4–0 chromic catgut sutures are anchored
equidistantly in the tarsus just below the upper border. They are then
passed through the cut tarsal edges and firmly tied (figs. 196C and D). As
this is done the lid border becomes everted and the cilia are pulled away
from the globe.

The lower skin-muscle lamina is now grasped, pulled up and enough
tissue is resected horizontally so that the edge just reaches the upper
tarsal border when taut (fig. 196E). The wound is closed with interrupted 4–0 silk sutures by passing the needle through the lower skin-

muscle edge, the upper border of the tarsus and the upper skin-muscle edge (fig. 196*F*). Enough sutures are inserted to make a thorough cosmetic closure.

A firm supportive dressing is applied for 48 hours. The eye is dressed daily and the sutures removed on the sixth day. Figure 196*G* shows a case of right upper lid cicatricial entropion with the postoperative result (fig. 196*H*).

Comment: Most cases of cicatricial entropion of the upper lid, especially those due to trachoma, have two pathologic elements requiring repair: (1) inversion of the lid margin with all that it portends for the integrity of the globe, and (2) loss of conjunctival tissue relative to skin-muscle tissue due to cicatrization. It is this loss of conjunctiva which causes the inversion. Both must be corrected if relief is to be attained. The equilibrium between skin-muscle and tarsoconjunctiva can be restored in two ways, either by grafting mucous membrane to make up for the loss of cicatrized conjunctiva (Procedure 198) or by resection of skin-muscle to restore the balance between the two tissues. It will be noted that the method chosen here was the second and simpler of the two.

Streatfeild's guttering of the tarsus is a clever idea. It divides the thickened tarsus into a hinge with two horizontal leaves so that the lower leaf with its entropic border swings upward and away from the globe using the upper leaf as a fulcrum. But Streatfeild left it there, depending on cicatrization to fix the lid into its new position. This is not enough. His technic cried out for modifications and they came rapidly—by the scores. However, the fundamental principle, that is, the excision of a horizontal wedge-shaped strip of tarsus has been retained in many operations for the relief of upper lid entropion. Hence its retention here.

The important components of this procedure are as follows:

The tarsal gutter—which is at least 3 mm. wide at the base—is placed near the lid border with the sutures anchored in the upper tarsal edge. This gives better marginal eversion than if it were higher up. Closure of the tarsus separately with firm bites also assures adequate tarsal eversion under direct vision. Resection of enough skin and muscle restores the skin-muscle vs. tarsoconjunctival balance which has been upset by conjunctival loss due to inflammation and cicatrization. In addition it helps the upward pull on the lid border and helps keep the everted lid margin in position. This is further assured by suturing the lower skin-muscle lamina to the upper tarsal border to prevent subsequent sag which is the main objection to the classic Streatfeild-Snellen procedure. Incidentally this also assures a good lid fold.

Burow, Panas, Green, Ewing, Lagleyze and many others, brought out modifications of this basic tarsectomy operation with greater or less success. In all of these procedures, resection of strips of tarsus may be omitted if tarsal deformity is not present or is minimal. The effect presumably being obtained by the everting affect of the sutures alone. According to the authors, however, this reduces the surgical effectiveness. Also, these procedures affect the center of the lid more than the ends and additional subsequent excision if skin or muscle or both may have to be done. All these procedures shorten the lid somewhat but not enough to make it cosmetically objectionable.

Horizontal Tarsal Section ("Fracture") for
Upper Lid Cicatricial Entropion

Burow in 1873 was apparently the first to report complete horizontal section of the tarsus although he included orbicularis and sometimes even skin in advanced cases. Many others soon followed with modifications including Green (1880), Panas (1882), Ewing (1902), Lagleyze (1905) and many others. Panas' procedure of full thickness lid section has recently been modified and improved and has become the Wies procedure in the lower lid and the Ballen procedure in the upper lid. Figure 197A is a case repaired by this technic.

Procedure (fig. 197):   After suitable anesthesia an incision through the full thickness of the lid is made 3 to 4 mm. above the lash line running the full length of the tarsus starting at a point lateral to the superior punctum (fig. 197B). Three or four double-armed 4–0 silk sutures evenly spaced are passed through the tarsus from the conjunctival side of the superior tarsal border then between the tarsus and orbicularis, across the cut, and then again between tarsus and orbicularis, to emerge on the skin surface just above the lash line. Here the sutures are tied over pegs.

As the sutures are tied, the upper portion of the tarsus acts as a fulcrum and the lower portion of the lid swings up with the lashes being pulled away from the cornea (fig. 197C). Additional skin sutures are added for good closure (fig. 197D). The eye is dressed daily. The tarsal sutures should be left in 10 to 14 days to allow the tarsoconjunctival split in the lid to granulate in well. The skin sutures are removed in 5 or 6 days. The final result (fig. 197E) is seen two months later.

Comment: This is a good procedure and should be used especially when other operations have failed or in cases of extreme entropion. Due to the unsutured opening in the tarsoconjunctiva, granulation tissue may be overproduced and may appear below the lid margin. This is easily handled by simple resection. Bringing out the sutures above the ciliary margin instead of through the lid border, as Panas did, is an improvement and makes for greater patient comfort. The procedure is uncomplicated and works well with little tendency to recurrence of the entropion.

Tarsal Resection with Mucosal Graft

In trachoma and in such conditions as pemhigus, vernal catarrh and

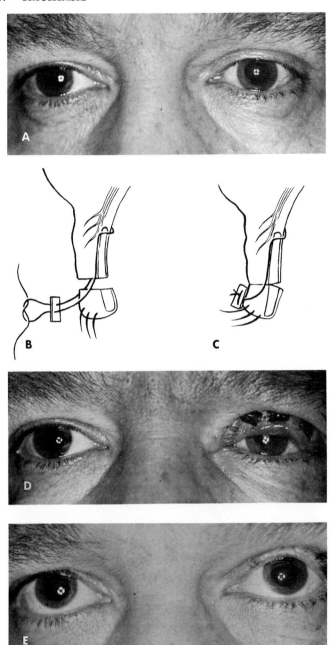

FIG. 197.   Cicatricial Entropion Repair by Tarsal Fracture.
A.   Cicatricial entropion of the left upper lid.
B.   A horizontal incision is made through full thickness lid 3 to 4 mm. above the
     lash line. Three double-armed sutures are passed from the conjunctival
     surface of the attached tarsal border, between tarsus and orbicularis to
     emerge just above the lash line.
C.   The sutures are tied over pegs and the lid margin everted.
D.   Appearance before removal of sutures. Note desired overcorrection.
E.   Final result. Note lid margin eversion.

lye burns, extensive cicatrization of conjunctiva and corneal pathology is
frequently seen. Usually there is excessive thickening, cicatrization and
roughening of the tarsus and one may well have to consider a tarsectomy
(fig. 198) and resection of all the offending tarsoconjunctiva with immediate grafting of buccal mucosa.

Procedure (fig. 198):   The lid is clamped and everted. An incision
is made in the tarsoconjunctiva 3 mm. from and following the curve of
the lid margin (fig. 198*A*). The tarsus is dissected up from the underlying orbicularis and resected leaving a narrow rim of tarsoconjunctiva
at the attached border. Buccal mucosa is obtained (figs. 28 and 29) and
sutured into place (fig. 198*B*). Thus the thickened and distorted tarsus
is replaced by smooth mucous membrane which should be cut generously
to counteract the usual shrinkage.

Comment: Unless mucous membrane is grafted before closure,
entropion is sure to recur due to the loss of so much tissue from the
conjunctival side of the lid. In some of the older procedures conjunctiva
from the upper fornix was mobilized and drawn down to the lid border.
This should not be done as it will bring about recurrence of the entro-

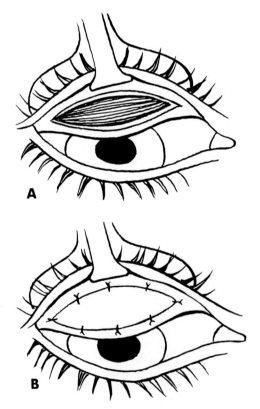

FIG. 198.   Tarsal Resection.
A.   The cicatrized tarsus is resected leaving a 3 mm. rim all around.
B.   Buccal mucous membrane fills the dehiscence.

pion almost inevitably. An ingenious but ineffective technic of Blaskovics was to mobilize the tarsus sufficiently so that it could be inverted front to back with the raw surface now lying against the globe. This procedure not only called for complicated surgery but again required covering the raw tarsal surface by mucous membrane. The surgery described above is simpler and effective.

Van Millingen's Tarsochiloplasty (Modified)

In some early cases of cicatricial entropion it is not always easy to distinguish between mild entropion and trichiasis: There is some lash displacement and the position of the border—strangely enough—may be so equivocal as to give a surgeon pause. This applies to both upper and lower lids—more often, perhaps, to the lower. In such cases it sometimes suffices to separate the offending cilia from the globe by interposing a strip of mucous membrane. This procedure is based on the previous work of Gayet who split the border of the lid and planted a thin strip of skin into the margin. Van Millingen wisely substituted buccal mucous membrane for skin with a great improvement in result and greater comfort to the patient.

Procedure (fig. 199): The lid border is split into skin-muscle and tarsoconjunctival layers. The dissection is carried upward for 3 or 4 mm. to obtain good separation. A 4 mm. strip of buccal mucosa is taken from the lower lip as described in Chapter 3. This should be somewhat longer than the marginal wound because of shrinkage. It is then carefully tucked into the marginal lid split, epithelial surface outward. Sutures at each end and a few on each side are optional (fig. 199*A*). Many surgeons prefer to use no sutures, and indeed, if the graft is tucked in snugly and the eye well bandaged with a good supportive dressing, healing without sutures takes place readily and without incident.

The wound is dressed on the third day and every second day thereafter until healing is complete. Care must be taken to assure the cessation of all bleeding before closure, otherwise the graft will be forced out and the operation nullified.

An excellent modification of this technic is the substitution of a 2 to 3 mm. strip of tarsoconjunctiva from the upper border of the tarsus for the mucous membrane (figs. 199*B* and *C*). This is a stiffer tissue with practically no tendency to shrinkage and is the preferred material for this procedure.

A still more effective modification of the Van Millingen procedure is the resection of a 3 mm. strip of skin 3 mm. above the ciliary margin after the lid has been split. The ciliated strip is moved upward and sutured to the skin edge above. The strip of tarsoconjunctiva is then sutured into the space in the lid border (fig. 199*A*).

This modification also embodies the advantages of the Dianoux pro-

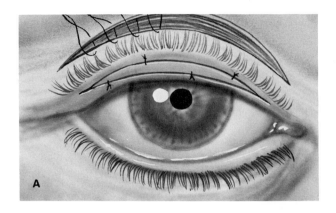

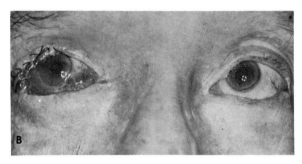

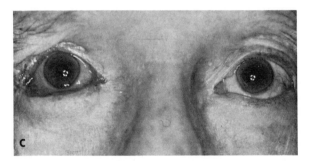

FIG. 199.   Van Millingen Technique for Trichiasis.
A.   The lid margin is split and a narrow strip of mucous membrane or tarsocon-
     junctiva is planted. At the same time a strip of skin is resected above to help
     evert the lid.
B.   Trichiasis of the outer half of the right upper lid and the repair.
C.   Final result.

cedure (fig. 205) since it leaves the cilia high enough on the skin surface
to obviate interference with the cornea. This may well be one of the best
and simplest modified procedures of all for both upper and lower lid
trichiasis and early cicatricial entropion which is not too severe.

   Comment: One minor postoperative complication is that the conjunctival or tarsoconjunctival strip retains its pink color. In most cases
this minor cosmetic blemish is unimportant compared to the relief
attained from the trichiasis.

LOWER LID CICATRICIAL ENTROPION

The problem of cicatricial entropion of the lower lid is somewhat simpler because both lid and tarsus are narrower. Also since the lower lid lies below the lower limbus, corneal involvement is not as frequent a factor. Rarely is the tarsal deformity so great as to require a great amount of tarsal surgery.

The trichiasis of cicatricial entropion here is treated exactly as in the upper lid by electrolysis or marginal plasty, if minor, i.e., if only a few lashes are involved. For greater amounts of entropion, skin and muscle excision is somewhat more effective here than in the upper lid, although tarsectomy is not contraindicated; neither are the marginal interposition procedures of Spencer Watson and Van Millingen and their modifications.

The procedures of Panas and von Graefe have been found most effective here. The Celsus technic which is simpler and perhaps somewhat less effective is of greater value in congenital entropion (fig. 236).

Excision of Skin and Muscle (Panas)

Procedure (fig. 200): Just below both the lateral and medial canthi of the affected lid, 12 to 15 mm. vertical incisions are made in the skin. The lower ends of the incisions are united by a horizontal incision and the included skin flap is dissected up to the ciliary margin. The flap is pulled down until the inverted lid assumes a normal position and the

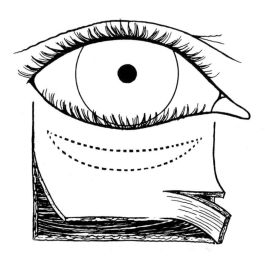

FIG. 200. Panas Procedure for Cicatricial Entropion of the Lower Lid.
The skin below the lid is incised to form a flap and dissected up. A horizontal spindle of orbicularis is resected close to the border (dotted line). The skin flap is pulled down, excess skin is resected and the flap sutured into place.

amount of excess skin necessary to produce permanent eversion of the lid in a normal position is estimated and resected. Also a 5 mm. horizontal strip of orbicularis fibers lying close to the lid margin (fig. 200, dotted line) is resected along the whole lid length. The muscle is closed with 5–0 plain catgut interrupted sutures. The skin is closed with interrupted 5–0 silk sutures.

Comment: This procedure would be inadequate in a senile type of entropion. But in cicatricial entropion of the lower lid it restores the relative quantitative tissue equilibrium between the skin-muscle and tarsoconjunctival layers and is therefore of value.

In earlier days resection of orbicularis fibers was considered "an important feature of some of the best operations for entropion, whether of the spastic or cicatricial variety, for even in the latter variety, owing to the constant irritation of the eye there is usually more or less spasm of the muscle and the removal of a portion of it tends to check the spasm." We now know that the eye in which spasm exists is that of the beholder. Correction of cicatricial entropion of a lower lid is done either by restoring lost tissue, i.e., by grafting tarsoconjunctiva if much has been lost. Or, if only a little has been lost, by counteracting tarsoconjunctival pull by shortening the skin-muscle lamina and thus equalizing the tension on both sides of the lid.

Excision of Skin and Muscle (Graefe)

An operation which is as successful as the Panas procedure and perhaps more so is one suggested by von Graefe more than 100 years ago for cicatricial entropion of the lower lid (fig. 201A).

Procedure (fig. 201):   A skin incision extending nearly the whole length of the lid is made 3 mm. from and parallel to the free border. Two converging skin incisions are now made downward using the first incision as a base and so placed as to outline a central triangle with the apex down in the center of the lid. The size of this triangle will depend on how much correction is desired. Naturally the more tissue excised, the greater the effect will be. The triangle of skin is excised (fig. 201B) and, if necessary, a 5 mm. horizontal strip of orbicularis may also be resected the whole length of the wound to enhance the everting effect (fig. 201C). The skin on each side is undermined and the wound is closed with interrupted 5–0 silk sutures (figs. 201D and E).

A firm pressure dressing should be applied for three days. The wound is dressed daily thereafter and the sutures removed on the sixth day. The final result is seen in figure 201F.

Comment: This is practically identical to the winged-V procedure of Dieffenbach (fig. 57) suggested by him for the resection of small tumors. The result of this operation is to bring additional pressure on the base of the tarsus and cause eversion of its margin. Although one of the oldest, this is perhaps the best of the procedures using skin and muscle excision for the correction of cicatricial entropion of the lower lid.

Tarsal Section for Lower Lid Cicatricial Entropion

Tarsal section may also be used in the lower lid when another procedure has failed. Wies has modified and improved the old Panas technic and uses it for senile entropion. However it is better applicable to cicatricial entropion.

The procedure is approximately the same as described in figure 197. There is a tendency for it to cause some overcorrection in the lower lid due to its narrow tarsus. Hence it should be reserved for the extreme cases of lower lid cicatricial entropion where other procedures have failed.

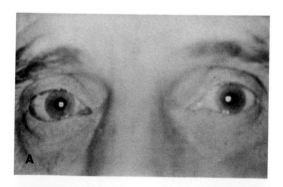

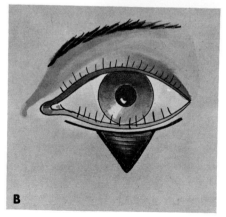
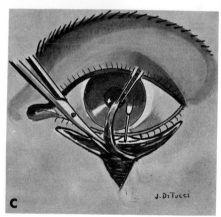

FIG. 201. Graefe Repair of Lower Lid Cicatricial Entropion.
A. Cicatricial entropion of the right lower lid.
B. Incision below lid and resection of skin triangle.
C. Resection of orbicularis strip.
(*Continued*)

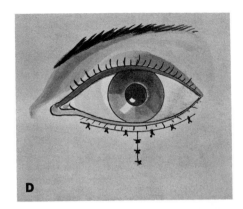

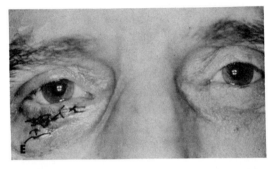

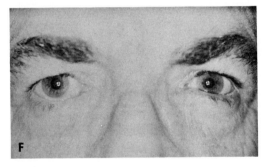

Fig. 201 (*Continued*)
D. and *E.*   Skin closure.
F.   Final result. Note eversion of lid margin and cilia.

TRICHIASIS

Trichiasis is an acquired affection of the lid margin in which the cilia are misdirected, usually backward, causing corneal and conjunctival irritation. It differs from entropion in that the lid margin itself is in normal position but, because of fibrosis and cicatrization, the cilia are misplaced. The most common cause of this condition has been trachoma; it is also a frequent accompaniment of cicatricial entropion. Other rarer causes are severe blepharitis, styes, burns, pemphigus, etc.

The treatment of trichiasis is not simple and has given birth to many ingenious technics for its cure. Although the clinical distinctions between trichiasis and mild cicatricial entropion is not always simple, it is of tremendous importance in the surgical treatment of these two conditions. If the lid border turns in, then none of the procedures described below are acceptable.

Epilation (Friede)

If only a few cilia are at fault, manual epilation or Friede's technic of actual resection may be used. He eliminates the lashes by actual resection of the follicles as seen in figure 202. However, this is only applicable when no more than a few cilia are involved; otherwise entropion is always a dangerous possibility.

Epilation by Electrolysis

Epilation by electrolysis is permanently effective. However, here again, it is applicable where there are only a few misdirected cilia. If too many are removed at once, especially if they are close together, cicatrization and further distortion of the lid margin may ensue. Also in the case of fine hairs it is not always easy to parallel exactly the direction of the hair shaft, hence the root bulb is not always easy to find. Under these conditions surgery is the better choice. Where a few scattered cilia are to be removed by electrolysis the technic is as follows:

Procedure (fig. 203):   The lid border is anesthetized by infiltration. With good light and under ample magnification a very fine needle (fig. 203*A*) attached to the negative pole of a galvanic current is inserted into the hair follicle following the direction of the cilium (fig. 203*B*). The positive pole is held by or attached to the patient. The current is turned on very slowly until bubbles are seen to appear at the point of entrance

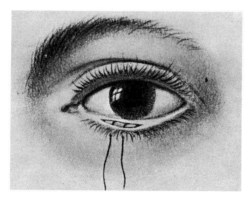

FIG. 202.   Friede's Resection of Marginal Cilia. (From Blaskovics, L., and Kreiker, A.: Eingriffe am Auge.   Courtesy Ferdinand Enke Verlag, Stuttgart.)

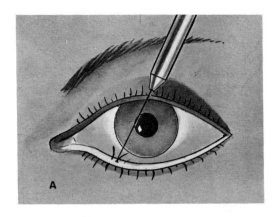

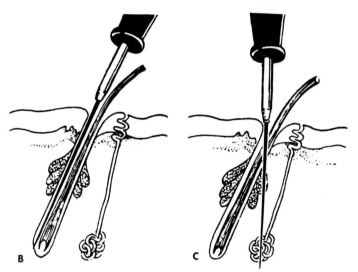

Fig. 203.   Epilation by Electrolysis for Trichiasis.
A.   Application of electrolysis needle.
B.   Proper insertion of needle.
C.   Improper insertion of needle.

of the needle. The lash is then easily withdrawn and will not recur. If it does not come out easily then the needle was not placed properly (fig. 203C) and the process must be repeated.

Comment: The apparatus used may be any source of galvanic current, even a couple of dry cells connected in series. Diathermy current may also be used. This is more rapid and just as effective. If this is used, the needle is inserted and a current of 150 ma. is applied for two seconds. Usually this is enough to loosen the lash. If not, a little more coagulation is needed or the follicle has not been reached and the needle should be reapplied.

Scheie and Albert have found the operating microscope useful for the epilation of the fine cilia of trichiasis. This would seem to be an important improvement especially where very thin, colorless lanugolike lashes are involved.

Tenzel uses a Proelectro epilator under the slit lamp. This instrument employs a galvanic current from a battery source with an output of 2.5 ma. advised. It is effective when used with local anesthesia since the mild galvanic current minimizes scarification even in multiple epilations, according to the author.

Repair of Partial Trichiasis (Spencer Watson)

When the trichiasis is more extensive and involves an appreciable part of the lid margin without tarsal deformity, more definitive surgery becomes necessary. The group of marginal plasties devised by Spencer Watson, Gayet, Dianoux and others, are of value. These plasties aim at displacement of cilia away from the globe by the interposition of tissue at the margin. Modification of Van Millingen's marginal plasty has already been described (fig. 199) and is probably the best of the lot. The Z plasty devised by Spencer Watson in 1873 is excellent for trichiasis of part of the lid, whether upper or lower. It is interesting to note that this was first reported by him for the cure of a case of distichiasis.

Procedure (fig. 204): The affected area of lid margin is split into skin-muscle and tarsoconjunctival layers to a depth of 6 mm. From the temporal end of this marginal incision another horizontal skin incision is made parallel to the first and about 3 mm. above it. From the medial end of the second incision a similar one is made temporally. Thus a flat Z figure of two pedicles about 3 mm. wide is created with the lower pedicle including the misplaced cilia (fig. 204A). Care should be taken that the free ends of these pedicles are somewhat rounded. Otherwise they will be too narrow for suturing or will fray. The pedicles are dissected up (fig. 204B), transposed (fig. 204C) and sutured into place with 5–0 or 6–0 silk (fig. 204D).

A firm dressing is applied. The dressing is changed on the second day and daily thereafter. The sutures are removed on the sixth day.

Repair of Total Trichiasis (Dianoux)

When trichiasis affects the whole lid margin and the pathology is due to ciliary irritation of the cornea and not to lid inversion, the method of Dianoux is of some value.

Procedure (fig. 205): The lid margin is split into skin-muscle and tarsocojunctival layers to a depth of about 8 mm. Two horizontal skin incisions are then made from canthus to canthus 4 and 8 mm. above the lid margin. The flaps are undermined leaving them attached at the ends, thus creating two hammock flaps (fig. 205A—a,b). These are transposed

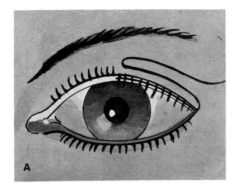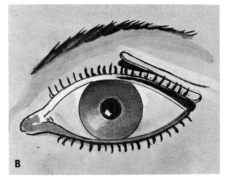

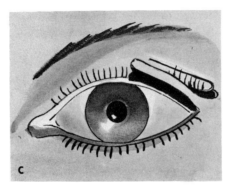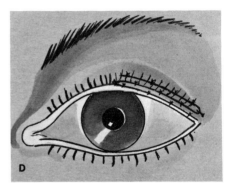

FIG. 204.   Spencer Watson Flat-Z Technique for Partial Trichiasis.
A.   A flat-Z is outlined over the area of entropion.
   The lower leg of the Z splits the lid margin.
B.   The resultant flaps are mobilized.
C. and *D.*   The flaps are transposed and sutured into position.

and sutured (fig. 205*B*). The skin flap (b) is sutured at the margin. The ciliated flap (a), now above, is placed into position above the skin flap and sutured to the upper lip of the wound. The two flaps are then sutured to each other. A firm supportive dressing is applied. Postoperative care is the same as in the preceding procedure.

   Comment: At the time of their introduction, marginal plasties intended to displace the row of irritating cilia were a distinct forward advance. However, there are drawbacks. The first is that such procedures are applicable only to trichiasis or to the milder cases of entropion in which there is no or minimal tarsal distortion and deformity. Another drawback is that it brings skin right down to the lid margin; and skin epithelium alone or along with its fine lanugolike hair may be quite as irritating as the original cilia. Hence, Procedures 204 and 205 are to be avoided where there is any tendency for the lid to turn in. Van Millingen's modification (fig. 199) or Procedures 200 and 201 are then the better choices.

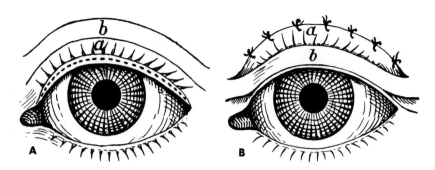

FIG. 205. Dianoux Procedure for Total Trichiasis.
A. The lid is split and two skin hammock flaps (*a* and *b*) are outlined.
B. The flaps are transposed and sutured into position.
   (Courtesy American Encyclopedia of Ophthalmology, Cleveland Press, Chicago.

REFERENCES

AETIUS OF AMIDA: AMERICAN ENCYCLOPEDIA OF OPHTHALMOLOGY. Chicago, Cleveland Press, 1913, vol. 1, p. 111.

ANAGNOSTAKIS, A.: Remarques pratiques sur la traitment du trichiasis. Ann. d'ocul. *38*:5, 1857.

ARLT, C. F.: Die Krankheiten des Auges fur praktische Aertze geschildert. Prague, C. A. Credner, 1854, vol. 3, p. 368.

BALLEN, P. H.: A simple procedure for the relief of trichiasis and entropion of the upper lid. Arch. Ophth. *72*:239, 1964.

BEARD, C. H.: Ophthalmic Surgery, ed. 2. Philadelphia, P. Blakiston's Son & Co. 1914, p. 253.

BESNAINOU, R.: L'entropion-trichiasis trachomateux et sa cure chirurgicale. Int. Rev. Trach. *1*:120, 1956.

BIRCH-HIRSCHFELD: Cited by Blaskovics, L. and Kreiker, A. Eingriffe am Auge. Stuttgart, E. Enke, 1938, p. 59.

BLASKOVICS, L.: Eine operation zur Beseitigung des Entropium habituale. Zeitschr. Augenh. *49*:94, 1923.

————, and KREIKER, A.: Eingriffe am Auge. Stuttgart, E. Enke, 1938, p. 59.

BUROW, A.: Bemerkungen zur Operation des Entropium und der Distichiasis. Berlin Klin. Wchnschr. *10*:295, 1873.

BUTLER, J. B. V.: A simple operation for entropion. Arch. Ophth. *40*:665, 1948.

CELSUS: Cited by Zeis, E., Handbuch der plastischen Chirurgie. Berlin, G. Reimer, 1838, p. 12.

DALGLEISH, R. and SMITH, J. L. S.: Mechanics and History of Senile Entropion. Brit. Med. J. *50*:79–91, 1966.

DIANOUX, E.: De l'autoplastie palpebrale par le procédé de Gayet. Ann d'ocul. *2*:132, 1882.

DIEFFENBACH, J. F.: Die operative Chirurgie. Leipzig, F. A. Brockhaus, 1845, p. 484–487.

DUNNINGTON, J. H., and REGAN, E. T.: Ziegler cautery for noncicatricial entropion. Am. J. Ophth. *61*:1090 (Pt. 2), 1966.

EWING, A. E.: An operation for atrophic entropion, especially of the lower lid. Tr. Am. Ophth. Soc. *9*:15, 1900–1902.

FFOULDS, W.: Surgical cure of senile entropion. Brit. J. Ophth. *45*:678, 1961.

FOX, S. A.: Relief of senile entropion. Arch. Ophth. *46*:424, 1951.

————: Correction of senile entropion. Arch. Ophth. *48*:624, 1952.

————: Repair of senile entropion. Arch. Ophth. *71*:501, 1964.

FUCHS, E.: Textbook of Ophthalmology, ed. 5. Philadelphia, J. B. Lippincott Co., 1917, pp. 678, 951.

GAILLARD, A. L.: Suture pour l' entropion. Ann. d'ocul *18*:241, 1847.

GAYET, A.: Sur un procédé nouveau d'autoplastie des paupieres, applicable aux entropions graves. Cong. Period. Internat. Sc. Med. Compt. Rend. (Amsterdam) *6*:265 (Pt. 2), 1881.

GIFFORD, H.: On the use of Thiersch flaps in the treatment of trichiasis and entropium. Am. J. Ophth. *9*:1, 1892.

GOLDHEIZER, W.: Uber Entropium spasticum senile und seine Heilung. Klin. Monatsbl. Augenh. *46*:426, 1908.

VON GRAEFE, A.: Bemerkungen zur Operation des Entropium und Ektropium. Arch. Ophth. *10*:221 (Pt. 2), 1864.

GREEN, J.: An operation for entropion. Tr. Am. Ophth. Soc. *3*:167, 1880.

HILL, J. C., and FELDMAN, F.: Tissue barrier modification of a Wheeler II operation for entropion. Arch. Ophth. *78*:621, 1967.

HOTZ, C. C.: Operation for entropion. Arch. Ophth. *8*:249, 1879.

HUGHES, W. L.: Reconstructive Surgery of the Eyelids. St. Louis, C. V. Mosby Co., 1954, pp. 201–204.

JASCHE, E.: Jäche's Operation für Entropium und Distichiasis. Klin. Monatsbl. Augenh. *11*:97, 1873.

JONES, L. T.: The anatomy of the lower eyelid and its relation to the cause and cure of entropion. Am. J. Ophth. *49*:29, 1960.

————: A new concept of the orbital fascia and rectus muscle sheaths and its surgical implications. Trans. Am. Acad. Ophth. & Oto. *72*:755, 1968.

JONES, L. T., REEH, M. J., and TSUJIMURA, J. K.: Senile entropion. Am. J. Ophth. *55*:463, 1963.

————: Senile enropion. Am. J. Ophth. *60*:709, 1965.

KIRBY, D. B.: Surgical correction of spastic senile entropion: A new method. Am. J. Ophth. *36*:1372, 1953.

KUHNT, H.: Zur beseitigung des Entropium organicum am unteren Lid. Ztschr. Augenh. *24*:154, 1910.

LAGLEYZE, P.: Operacion del entropion y triquiasis. Arch. de oftal. hispano-am. *5*:1–6, 1905.

MACDONALD, A. E.: New treatment for entropion. Tr. Am. Ophth Soc. *43*:372, 1945.

McKENZIE, J. W., and BARTLETT, R. E.: Surgery for entropion. Am. J. Ophth. *58*:983, 1964.

MEEK, R. E.: An operation for spastic entropion. Arch. Ophth. *24*:547, 1940.

MILLAR, G. T.: Surgical treatment of senile entropion. Trans. Ophth. Soc. U K. *87*:775, 1967.

MÜLLER, L.: Eine neue Operation Methode zur Heilung des Entropium spasticum. Klin. Monatsbl. Augenh. *69*:288, 1922.

PAGENSTECHER, H.: Uber Verlagerung der Levatorsehne Ein neues Operationverfahren fur Entropium und Trichiasis des Oberlides. Arch. Ophth. *36*:265, 1890.

PANAS, P.: D'une modification apportée au procédé dit de transplantation du sol ciliare. Arch. d'ophthal. *2*:208, 1882.

————: Traite de Maladies des yeux. Paris, Masson et Cie, 1894, p. 153.

————: Lecons de clinique ophthalmologique professe a l'Hotel-Dieu. Paris, Masson et Cie, 1899, p. 132.

POCHISOV, N.: Operation for spastic entropion. Sovet. vestnik Opht. *6*:131, 1935.

POULARD, A.: Entropion d'origine angulaire externe. Traitement chirurgicale. Am. d'ocul. *172*:97, 1935.

ROBERTSON, D. M. C. L. A.: The treatment of severe senile entropion. Edin. Med. J. *36*:497, 1890.

SCHEIE, H. G., and ALBERT, D. M.: Distichiasis and trichiasis; origin and management. Am. J. Ophth. *61*:718, 1966.

SCHIMEK, R. A., and NEWSON, S. R.: Horizontal buried collagen tape for senile entropion. Arch. Ophth. *77*:672, 1967.

SCHIMEK, R. A.: A simplified entropion operation. Am. J. Ophth. *43*:245, 1957.

SNELLEN, H.: Suture for entropion. Cong. Internat. d'opht. (Paris) 1863, p. 236.

STELLWAG, VON C.: Ein neues Verfahren gegen einwartsgekehrte Wimpern. Allgem. Wien. Med. Ztg. *28*:527, 1883.

STREATFEILD, W. H. Grooving the fibro-cartilage of the lid in cases of entropion and trichiasis. Ophthl. Hosp. Reports and J. Royl. Lond. Ophth. Hosp. *1*:121, 1857–1859.

VAN MILLINGEN, E.: De la guérison radicale du trichiasis par la tarso-chieloplastie. Arch. d'opht. *8*:60, 1888.

WATSON, T. S.: A new operation for distichiasis with a successful case. Royl. Lond. Ophth. Hosp. Rep. *7*:440, 1873.

WEEKERS, L.: Traitement de l'entropion spasmodique par l'alcoholisation des terminaisons du nerve facial dans la paupiere. Arch. d'opht. *45*:20, 1928.

WESSELY, K.: Beitrag zur Entropium Operation. Graefe's Arch. Ophth. *148*:358, 1948.

WHEELER, J. M.: Spastic entropion correction by orbicularis transplantation. Tr. Am. Ophth. Soc. *36*:157–162, 1938.

WIES, F. A.: Surgical treatment of entropion. J. Int. Coll. Surg. *21*:758, 1954.

ZIEGLER, S. L.: Galvanocautery puncture in ectropion and entropion. J.A.M.A. *53*:183, 1909.

CHAPTER 17

Ptosis

THE UPPER LID MARGIN normally lies somewhere between the upper limbus and upper undilated pupillary border. Its average location therefore is halfway between the limbus and pupil or about 2 mm. below the upper limbus.

When the upper lid droops below its normal position and there is a tendency toward smoothing out of the lid fold, the condition is termed blepharoptosis (*blepharon* = lid; *ptosis* = a drooping). In ophthalmic nomenclature the more abbreviated term ptosis has been given general acceptance and will be used here.

Elevation of the lid is accomplished mostly by the levator palpebrae superioris muscle to which Müller's muscle is a weak accessory. Hence ptosis is most commonly the result of absent or weak levator action and may be complete or partial, depending on whether there is total paralysis of the levator or whether some function is retained.

HISTORICAL SUMMARY

The history of ptosis repair is replete with brilliant, sometimes fantastic, attempts to find some method of raising the ptosed lid permanently. It is a long history and only the highlights will be included here.

Early primitive operations shortened the lid by excising skin, skin-cum-orbicularis, tarsus, tarsus-cum-orbicularis and even whole lid thick-

338

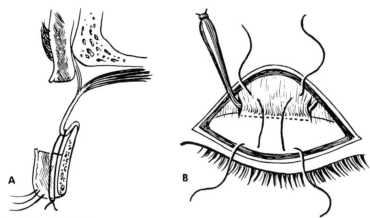

FIG. 206. Early Levator Operations.
A. Everbusch's Levator Tucking Operation. The tarsus and levator are exposed and three double-armed sutures are placed in the levator. The sutures are passed between the tarsus and orbicularis to come out on the lid margin. The levator is thus drawn down on the tarsus and tucked.
B. Lapersonne's Levator Resection and Advancement Technic. The levator is cut (dotted line) and advanced on the tarsus.

ness. Failures encountered with simple excision soon led to the search for other modalities.

In 1857 Bowman published the earliest report of levator resection including skin and conjunctival routes, with and without tarsal resection. Since then this operation with many modifications has been repeatedly rediscovered and has acquired many eponyms. Everbusch in 1883 tucked and advanced the levator (fig. 206A) and since then his name has been attached to the anterior levator approach. Over the years there have been innumerable modifications of Bowman's levator resection technic. It was de Lapersonne, however, who in 1903 first mobilized the levator, resected it and advanced it on to the tarsus (fig. 206B). Everbusch had simply tucked it. Angelucci not only shortened the levator tendon but also attached it to the frontalis, thus assuring a double action. More recently Hildreth, Leahey, Johnson and Berke have also contributed significantly to the transcutaneous approach for ptosis repair.

In 1923 Blaskovics repopularized the conjunctival approach to the levator and his name has been attached to this technic ever since. Recently Berke, Iliff and Fasanella and Servat have also contributed modifications to the posterior approach. But whatever the technic, if it is anyone's operation, anterior or posterior levator resection is Bowman's by right of precedence and original publication.

Another early development was the attempt to establish a surgical connection between the upper lid and the frontalis. Hunt as far back as 1831 resected a spindle of skin beneath the brow thus providing an increased frontalis lifting force to the lid (fig. 207A). Dransart, in 1880, reported the first successful attachment of the ptosed lid to the frontalis by means of sutures (fig. 207B). In short order Pagenstecher, de Wecker, Hess, Koster, Wilder and numerous others "improved" on the Dransart procedure. Mules used gold and silver wire instead of sutures. Bishop employed a fine gold chain.

Lack of complete success with the suture method led Panas to devise his blepharopexy operation in 1894. In this procedure a wide skin flap from the lower half of the lid is buried under the upper half and fastened to the frontalis muscle. Machek modified the technic by using a narrow skin flap from each end of the lid. The Tansley operation uses one central skin strap and was an important improvement over the Panas procedure.

Other modifications followed: Fergus and Roberts brought the mountain down to Mahomet and fashioned long strips of frontalis muscle

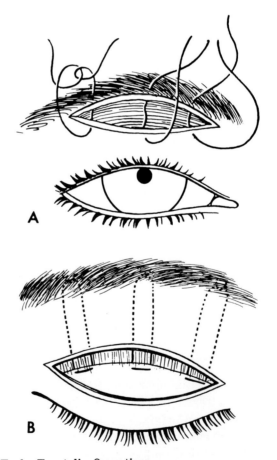

FIG. 207.   Early Frontalis Operations.
A. Hunt's Skin Resection just below the brow for the correction of ptosis.
B. Dransart's subcuticular suture slings from tarsus to frontalis.

which they sutured to the tarsus—a formidable operation in which the result is no better than with the simpler technics. Probably the most logical procedure is that suggested by the elder Reese in 1924 in which diverging strips of pretarsal orbicularis and a central suture are used to attach the lid to the frontalis muscle (fig. 218).

Parinaud and Motais in 1897 each devised a method for using the lifting power of the superior rectus to raise the ptosed lid. Parinaud placed a suture around the superior rectus tendon, tucked it into a tunnel between tarsus and orbicularis and fastened it by sutures to the skin above the lid margin. Motais fashioned a long narrow tongue from the middle third of the superior rectus and pulled it down between tarsus and orbicularis. Thus the greater part of the muscle was left undisturbed. Both these corrections were effected from the conjunctival side of the lid. Since then, there have been numerous modifications and "simplifications" of modifications.

Shoemaker and Kirby exposed the tarsus through the skin for easier access. Young, Greeves, Jameson, Trainor (fig. 219) and others sutured the superior rectus directly to the upper tarsal border or created tarsal flaps to attach to the superior rectus tendon. Dickey used a fascia lata sling and Wheeler attached orbicularis strips to the superior rectus tendon.

The fascia sling in frontalis surgery is a relative latecomer. Payr in 1909 was apparently the first to report such a repair of a case of congenital ptosis. He obtained fascia lata from the upper part of the patient's thigh and attached the lid to the frontalis through a central subcutaneous tunnel (fig. 208A). Wright in 1922 and Derby in 1928 also reported procedures using autogenous fascia (figs. 208B and C).

CLASSIFICATION OF PTOSIS

Cases of ptosis may be divided into a large group of congenital ptoses and a smaller group of acquired ptoses. While there are no exact figures for the incidence of these two categories, a fair estimate is that at least 90 per cent are congenital and 10 per cent acquired.

According to most estimates about 25 per cent of congenital ptosis cases are bilateral and 75 per cent are unilateral. Over 50 per cent have enough levator action to warrant levator resection. This means that if all cases of ptosis—acquired and congenital—are included, well over half of them can be benefited and should be done by levator resection. In other cases correction must be made by transferring elevating function to the frontalis (or superior rectus) muscle.

Acquired ptosis is due to the effects of trauma, disease and the aging process. The trauma may be due to injury to the levator itself or, more commonly, to its nerve supply as in the case of cerebral injuries,

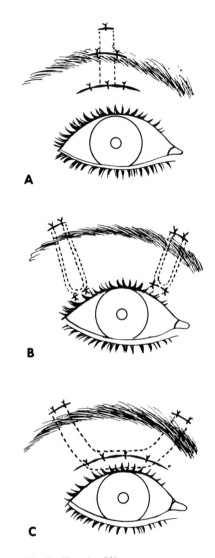

FIG. 208.   Early Fascia Slings.
A.   Payr's single sling.   C.   Derby's single sling.
B.   Wright's double sling.

birth trauma, penetrating wounds, etc. Intraorbital inflammations, hemorrhages, tumors and muscular atrophies are some of the other possible etiologic factors. Finally the aging process with its diminution of muscle tonus may affect the lid muscles and cause a drooping of one or both lids (fig. 221).

Pseudoptosis, or apparent ptosis, is due to weakening of the support furnished to the upper lid by an absent or shrunken globe. Other causes are mechanical conditions such as traumatic scarring (fig. 220) and heaviness of the lid due to neoplasms (fig. 222) or trachoma.

Classifications of ptosis are notoriously variable and no two agree. The following includes the types most commonly seen clinically:

Congenital
    Simple
    Complicated
        With ophthalmoplegias
        With other anomalies
        Synkinetic (paradoxical) ptosis
Acquired
    Senile
    Traumatic
    Neurogenic and myogenic
Pseudoptosis

Congenital Ptosis

SIMPLE. Simple ptosis without other complications comprises 75 to 80 per cent of all congenital ptoses. These cases are due primarily to poor development or lack of peripheral differentiation of the levator muscle, although in some cases central developmental nerve defects may be the cause. They may vary in severity from a barely perceptible drooping of the lid to complete paralysis.

COMPLICATED. Ptosis with ophthalmoplegia comprises another 10 to 15 per cent and is usually due to central nerve defects. The most common muscle anomaly being loss of elevation of the globe due to palsy or paralysis of the homolateral superior rectus. This is not surprising considering the close embryologic and anatomic association between the levator and the superior rectus. Other muscles such as the inferior oblique may also be involved although complete ophthalmoplegia is rare. These cases are usually unilateral.

Ptosis with other lid deformities, such as blepharophimosis, epicanthus, microphthalmos and lid coloboma, is usually hereditary. Here also there may be associated muscle pareses. It is usually bilateral and constitutes only about 3 per cent of all congenital ptosis cases.

A still smaller group of paradoxical ptoses constitutes a heterogeneous collection of cases including the synkinetic, sympathetic, periodic and intermittent ptoses which are relatively uncommon and of which the best known is the Marcus Gunn jaw-winking phenomenon. In this condition there is a unilateral ptosis of the lid when at rest and a retraction above the level of the opposite lid when the mouth is opened. Other forms of paradoxical ptosis include reverse jaw-winking, the raising and lowering of the upper lid on horizontal movement of the eye and raising of the upper lid of one eye on downward movement of the other eye. The etiology of this bizarre group of phenomena is not definitely known but is assumed to be due to aberrant nervous connections between the external eye muscles and the levators.

Acquired Ptosis

SENILE PTOSIS. Senile ptosis is a phenomenon of the aging process manifested by a loss of levator tonus and drooping of one or both lids to a greater or less extent. It may be an inherited characteristic which shows up late in life.

TRAUMATIC PTOSIS. Traumatic ptosis is due to direct or indirect injury to the levator or its nerve connections by cuts, concussion, hemorrhage, etc. Injuries to the superior orbital rim or frontal bones are also causative factors.

NEUROGENIC AND MYOGENIC PTOSIS. Paralytic ptosis may be due not only to peripheral involvement of the third nerve but also to rare basilar, cortical or nuclear lesions. Cerebral hemorrhages, tumors, abscesses, inflammations and degenerations are less usual etiologic factors. Myogenic ptosis may be due to involvement of the levator in a generalized muscular dystrophy, myasthenia gravis, Horner's syndrome and progressive external ocular myopathy. Both neurogenic and myogenic ptosis are rare.

Pseudoptosis

Pseudoptosis is not due to levator pathology. It is seen when the upper lid has lost the support of the globe as in anophthalmos, enophthalmos, microphthalmos, phthisis bulbi, etc. This is not a true ptosis since the fitting of a proper prosthesis where possible or indicated may serve to abolish the ptosis. However, there are cases of long standing in which there has been so much levator atrophy that a levator resection has to be done to correct the deformity. It may also occur in lids with trachoma, other inflammations or weighted down by tumors (fig. 222).

PREOPERATIVE EXAMINATION

A thorough preoperative examination of the patient is imperative before any type of ptosis surgery is undertaken. Pictures will be found extremely helpful and should be taken where possible with the patient looking up and down as well as straight ahead.

In complete ptosis, examination will show the deep brow furrows, arching of the eyebrows and back-tilt of the head. This is the characteristic facies of absent or poor levator action in which the frontalis is used in an effort to uncover the pupil. In certain cases prostigmin may be necessary to rule out a possible myasthenia gravis.

The record of the examination should include a complete catalogue of findings including vision, amblyopia, fusion and congenital anomalies, if present, such as epicanthus, blepharophimosis, microphthalmos, etc. Even more important is a thorough examination of the extraocular musculature especially the superior rectus muscle. Not only is this important in the choice of ptosis procedure but it would be embarrassing after correcting the ptosis to find a squint which had been overlooked.

Corneal sensitivity should also be checked; anesthesia or hypesthesia may mask a later corneal involvement. The presence of a good Bell's phenomenon is important for the same reason. The position of the lid fold and the amount of dermachalasis should be noted. Sometimes excess skin has to be resected to attain symmetry with the fellow eye.

Measurement of Ptosis

Judging the amount of ptosis by the classic method of comparing the width of the palpebral fissure with the normal eye in straight ahead, upward and downward gaze is full of pitfalls as Duke-Elder pointed out long ago. There are many reasons for this; a few will suffice. (1) The *lower* lid also moves up and down with the eye, (2) the position of the brow in the *normal* eye affects upward and downward gaze and hence the position of the lid, (3) it is not always easy to assure the immobility of the brow in such measurements and (4) in cases of severe ptosis the presence or absence of minimal levator action is not always easy to determine. The prudent surgeon should therefore not attempt to use width of palpebral fissure as a yardstick. In cases of bilateral ptosis it is of course hopeless.

Measurement of the amount of corneal overlap is simpler, quicker and, on the whole, more exact. But even here it should be remembered that the *normal* position of the lid margin may be anywhere between the upper limbus and upper pupillary margin. On the whole, the amount of corneal overlap is a better indicator for the degree of monocular ptosis.

Measurement of Levator Action

Far more important than the measurement of the amount of ptosis is the measurement of levator action. The simplest and best procedure is to measure the difference in the position of the upper lid margin in upward and downward gaze.

The patient is told to look down at the floor as far as he can without moving his head. A millimeter rule is held at the lateral side of the eye and the position of the upper lid margin of the ptosed lid is noted (fig. 209*A*). Firm pressure is exerted backward—not downward—on the brow and the patient is instructed to look up to the ceiling (fig. 209*B*). The difference in the levels of the lid margin gives the total excursion of the upper lid and hence the total action of the levator. In the normal eye such an excursion usually measures about 15 mm. (It increases to 18 to 20 mm. with the use of the frontalis.) In ptosis the measurement will

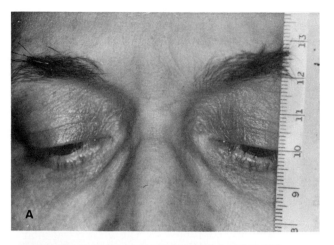

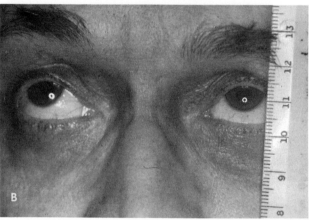

FIG. 209.   Measurement of Levator Action.
A.   Patient looking down with upper lid margin at 10 mm.
B.   Patient looking up with upper lid margin at 11.3 mm.

vary anywhere from zero to almost 15 mm. depending on the severity.

The examiner will have little trouble with an adult or older child. With the young child, 3 years or under, he may have a good deal of trouble. A formal examination is usually impossible. One must then fall back on observation: when the child comes into the room, when it feels that it is not being observed. One must look for a difference in position of the lids and for the appearance or absence of a fold in the suspected lid, no matter how small or evanescent. If the fold at any time seems to increase or decrease in size this is an indication of the presence of levator action and levator resection should be considered.

On the other hand, if the child has to throw its head back and use the frontalis in order to clear the pupillary area, the chances of levator action are not good and some type of frontalis suspension will have to be done. In any case, examinations should be repeated several times and one should not depend on a single observation for diagnosis.

CHOICE OF SURGICAL PROCEDURE

Now what is to be done with these measurements which have been so painstakingly obtained? Unfortunately the answer is neither clear nor unequivocal.

At the present time two classes of procedures for the correction of ptosis are in general use, a third is gradually being abandoned. The choice of modality depends on the presence or absence of levator action to a large extent:

1. Strengthening the levator muscle of the lid. This is applicable if any appreciable levator action is present and is the only procedure giving a result which is akin to a normal lid.

2. Attaching the lid to the frontalis so that arching of the eyebrow will raise the lid. This is the only method available in complete ptosis in which there is also loss of superior rectus action. It is the simplest of all ptosis procedures technically and this may account for its general popularity.

3. Attaching the lid to the superior rectus if it is functioning. The advantages of this technic are that the lid moves with the eye. The disadvantages are loss of the wink reflex, an open eye in sleep and possible diplopia and hypotropia. This modality is moribund and is rarely used now.

There are literally scores of operations for the correction of ptosis. Many of them are excellent; most of them can be substituted for each other without affecting the result materially. The few indications there are apply mostly to the choice of the *main type* of procedure, i.e., shall one strengthen the levator or employ the frontalis? Even these broad indications are not accepted by all. Thus, all surgeons agree that when levator action is present this action should be strengthened. Where no levator action is present, most resort at once to the frontalis to lift the lid. But others will first try levator resection even in complete ptosis because of the complications attending use of the frontalis.

Obviously, given similar cases, choice of procedure will vary with the predilection of the surgeon, his early training, his later experience and his skill attained with a certain technic. After many years of trial and error, my choice is as follows:

If there is 2 mm. or more of levator action, levator resection should be done in both monocular and binocular cases.

With levator action less than 2 mm., frontalis suspension is done with autogenous skin or fascia.

In acquired ptosis the above rules apply but surgery should be conservative. Overcorrection is easy in such cases.

In cases of jaw-winking the levator is resected completely first. This is followed by frontalis suspension. If the jaw-winking is minimal, levator resection alone might be tried first.

If the lid is thick and heavy as in the cases of some reconstructions, elephantiasis and neurofibromatosis, a fascial sling procedure is favored (fig. 215). In cases of complete ptosis with anophthalmos the author's skin sling (fig. 216) is used. The same skin sling is used with the eye present in a lid of normal width.

Where congenital ptosis is accompanied by other deformities such as blepharophimosis, tropia or epicanthus, the latter should all be repaired first. It is best to stabilize all other globe and adnexal anomalies before any ptosis surgery is undertaken.

In all cases of traumatic ptosis, it is well to wait at least 12 to 18 months, and at least 6 months after all improvement has apparently ceased, before repair is undertaken. Function continues to improve for a long time after trauma and sometimes improvement is enough to make surgery unnecessary. It is better to wait too long than not long enough.

In the congenital ptosis of infancy and early childhood, repair may be attempted any time after the age of two or three. By this time tissues are sufficiently strong and mature in their development to withstand the trauma of the extensive surgery required. If one waits too long, amblyopia due to obstruction of the pupil by the lid may become intractable although this is rare as long as the child can clear the pupil. Secondly, the child may develop bad postural habits, such as head tilt, which are difficult to eradicate. The brow wrinkling, eyebrow arching and other facial grimaces necessary for clear vision are cosmetic detriments which should not be allowed to exist any longer than necessary.

The exception to this is a case of bilateral ptosis in which both pupils are covered and the child is unable to see and function. Usually there is very little or no levator action in these cases and lid elevation becomes an emergency. Here repair—even temporary repair—should be done as soon as general anesthesia can be administered. These days this can mean at the age of only a few months. In such cases it is advisable to raise the lids with frontalis slings using such plastic materials as silastic, supramid, methyl methacrylate, etc. In the past few years new materials such as homografts of cobalt irradiated fascia and sclera have been used as frontalis slings. These can be undone at a later date if necessary. Levator resections may even be done if levator action is discovered.

Crutch glasses are a last resort but a valuable one in those rare cases of inoperable ptosis which accompany such conditions as complete external ophthalmoplegia, etc. They are posterior wire spring projections from the spectacle frame which prop up the lid. They can be fashioned by some opticians. Not all patients can tolerate them but they may help make the life of some patients more bearable if they can.

The procedures given in detail below are quite frankly the preference of the author. There are many other operations just as good. But it is believed that it is preferable to outline a few in detail rather than include many and cause confusion. They are the simplest, which will accomplish their object satisfactorily; more complex procedures do not necessarily mean better results. On the other hand, the choice is wide and others may and do prefer different technics.

How Much Levator to Resect?

With levator resection decided upon, how much is to be resected? There is no exact rule. The trouble is that measurements obtained with the patient active in the upright position often have to be applied to an unconscious supine patient whose muscles are completely relaxed. Or, if conscious, his tissues are infiltrated with anesthesia and hence distorted and immobile. This does not take into consideration the difficulties of gauging exact lid position as described above. The wonder is that so many good results are obtained. However, for those who want some sort or concrete measurements the following is offered without guarantee:

If levator action is 2 mm. or less, no levator resection.

If levator action is less than 5 mm., overcorrect 2–3 mm., i.e., at least 20 mm. levator is resected.

If levator action is 6 to 9 mm., correct fully—up to 16 mm. of levator is resected, more if the levator is of poor quality.

If levator action is 10 to 12 mm., the ptosis is undercorrected—no more than 8 to 10 mm. is resected. The horns are not cut.

STRENGTHENING THE LEVATOR

Levator resection is the most satisfactory and physiologically normal of all ptosis procedures and, where applicable, gives the best results. The indication for levator resection is clear. There should be at least 2 mm. of levator function, i.e., an incomplete ptosis whether congenital or acquired.

I have abandoned levator resection where there is no levator action. Sufficient grief has been experienced with these cases and enough have had to be undone to force the conclusion that, at least in my hands, levator surgery in a case of complete levator paralysis is a bad risk. So much levator has to be resected to achieve a decent cosmetic correction that the resultant lagophthalmos or entropion or both which follow— with either undercorrection or overcorrection—is too high a price to pay.

On the other hand, I feel that it is wrong to do anything but strengthen the levator when some levator action exists. Anything else is a Procrustean method in which the patient is made to fit the limitations of the surgeon and is to be deplored. It is a grave injustice to the patient to condemn him to the brow wrinkling and severe lid lag of frontalis surgery with a functioning levator present. It is equally reprehensible to subject a patient with levator action to the loss of the wink reflex and the dangers of corneal exposure in sleep which are frequent concomitants of superior rectus surgery.

Levator resection is also of value in the acquired ptoses of old enucleations, for the atonic ptoses of old age and for the traumatic ptoses where the paretic lid retains some movement. It has also been recommended for the ptosis of trachoma. However, here tarsal resection with mucous membrane grafting is preferable because the tarsus in these cases is thickened, deformed and scarred, and the cornea is the better for its removal (fig. 198).

There is little difference between the skin and conjunctival approaches to levator resection as far as indication is concerned; both work well. The effect of both is enhanced by tarsal resection although in recent years I have done very little of this.

The anterior approach is simpler technically and is preferred because the lid does not have to be everted and the tissues are more easily exposed. On the other hand, the posterior approach leaves no skin scars to show postoperatively and tarsal resection with clean conjunctival closure is effected more easily by this route.

Levator Resection by the Anterior (Skin) Approach (Author's Technic)

This procedure was popularized by Everbusch and has borne his eponym since 1883 although his technic called for a *tucking* of the levator, not a resection. It was Lapersonne who first resected the levator and carried it down to the tarsus.

Procedure (fig. 210): The lid is everted and a traction suture is passed through the superior rectus to help identify it later. The lid is reinverted, the blade of an Ehrhardt clamp is placed under the lid and the clamp tightened just above the ciliary margin. A horizontal incision along the whole length of the lid is made just *below the upper border* of the tarsus through skin and muscle (fig. 210A). These are dissected downward for several millimeters to expose the tarsus and upward for about 15 to 20 mm. to get good exposure of the fibrous membrane which comprises the orbital fascia and the levator aponeurosis (fig. 210B). The orbital fascia is incised horizontally allowing it to retract, thus exposing the levator aponeurosis beneath it (fig. 210C). (The operator can orient himself by locating the orbital fat which lies *behind* the fascia.)

The lid is everted and the conjunctiva is ballooned out with a 1 per cent procaine solution. Two double-armed 4–0 silk traction sutures are passed through the ballooned conjunctiva horizontally with the needles widely spaced. The object of this maneuver is to pull the conjunctiva away from Müller's muscle in order to facilitate separation and minimize the danger of buttonholing it when Müller's and the levator muscles are dissected free (fig. 210D). With the conjunctiva ballooned up and pulled

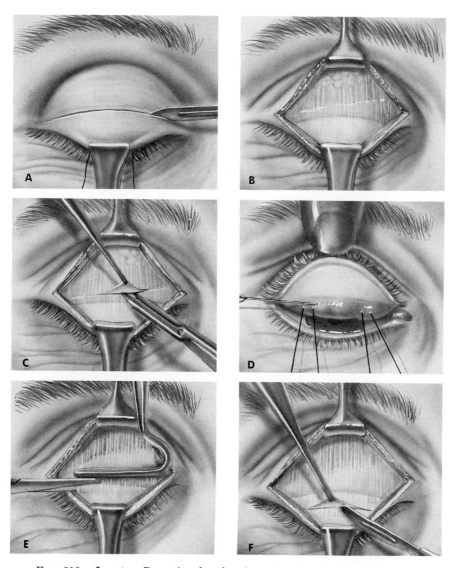

FIG. 210. Levator Resection by the Anterior Approach—Author's Technic.
A. A suture is passed under the superior rectus muscle and an incision is made
through skin and muscle just below the upper tarsal border. (The suture is
omitted in subsequent drawings.)
B. The skin-muscle lamina is dissected upward and downward to expose tarsus
and levator.
C. The orbital fascia is undermined, cut away and allowed to retract. If fat
presents, it is resected.
D. The lid is everted and injected to separate conjunctiva from Müller's muscle.
E. The lid is reinverted and the levator is cut away from the upper tarsal border.
The injection makes separation of the levator easy and makes cutting away
the conjunctiva unnecessary.
F. Alternatively the levator is dissected up from its attachment to the anterior
surface of the tarsus.
(Continued)

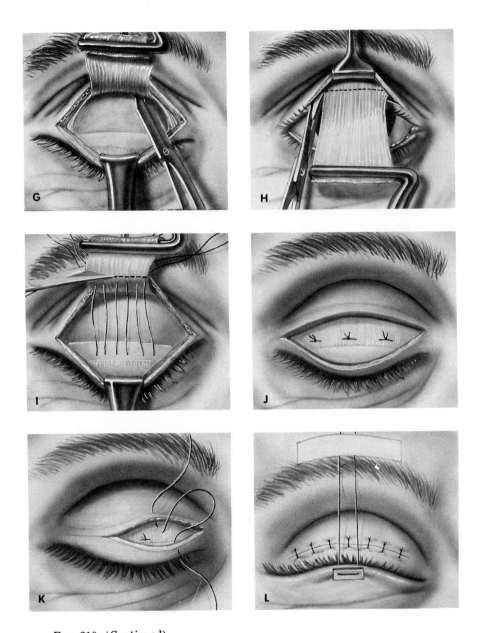

FIG. 210 (*Continued*)

G. The dissection is carried upward freeing the levator.

H. The horns are cut.

I. Three 4–0 chromic sutures are anchored in the tarsus and are passed through the levator from behind forward (see text). The excess levator is resected.

J. The sutures are tied thus drawing the levator down on the tarsus.

K. Four equally spaced 5–0 silk sutures are passed though the lower lip of the skin wound, through the levator and upper tarsal border and then through the upper lip of the skin wound.

L. Additional skin sutures are added and a modified Frost suture is used to draw the lower lip up and protect the cornea.

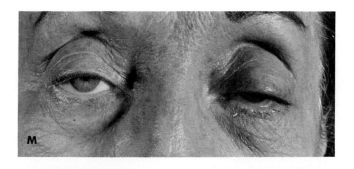

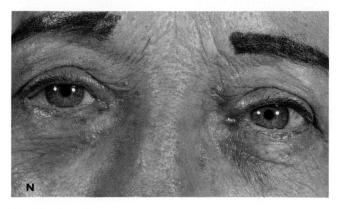

FIG. 210 (*Continued*)
M. and *N.* Bilateral ptosis and its correction by the anterior approach.

away the lid is turned down again and the tissue at the upper border of
the tarsus is buttonholed at one end, undermined, grasped in a ptosis
clamp and cut away from its attachment to the tarsus (fig. 210*E*). The
dissection is carried upward with blunt scissors, separating the levator
muscle from the underlying conjunctiva up to the upper cul-de-sac (fig.
210*G*).

Alternatively about 3 mm. below the upper border of the tarsal
surface a careful shallow incision is made and the fibrous attachment of
the levator dissected up (fig. 210 *F*). Care is taken not to buttonhole the
conjunctiva. If this is done, the opening should be closed at once with
6–0 chromic catgut; the buttonhole is harder to find later. The levator is
raised and its attachments to the medial and lateral horns are severed by
a scissors directed upward toward the orbital roof (fig. 210*H*). In the
mild grades of ptosis it is not necessary to cut the horns of the levator.

The muscle is raised still further and freed from all its fascial
attachments including Tenon's membrane, the superior rectus and the
pulley of the superior oblique, if necessary. The muscle should now come
forward freely. If not, it is inspected and all residual fascial connections,
if any, are carefully dissected away so as to cause no injury to adjacent
or underlying structures. When free the levator is easily movable and

retractable. Three double-armed 4–0 chromic catgut sutures are firmly anchored in the tarsus about 2 mm. from its upper border or lower if more effect is desired. One suture is centrally placed, the other two are spaced about 8 to 10 mm. to each side of the central suture (fig. 210*I*).

The sutures are carried upward and passed through the levator from behind forward to include at least 2 or 3 mm. of tendon between each pair of needles. Again these sutures are spaced so that one is centrally placed in the levator and the other two equidistant to each side. The distance from the cut edge of the levator at which the sutures are inserted will depend on how much correction is desired. The levator is cut across at least 2 mm. beyond the sutures and the sutures loosely tied. The effect is gauged to see that the lid margin lies at the upper limbus or slightly above. If not, the levator may be advanced somewhat lower on the tarsus or more levator resection may be indicated. The sutures are now tied tightly (fig. 210*J*).

The skin is closed with interrupted 5–0 silk sutures or 4–0 plain catgut in youngsters. In order to assure a good lid fold the lower skin-muscle flap lying on the tarsus is pulled up taut and the closing sutures catch up a few fibers at the upper border of the tarsus (fig. 210*K*). If this is done no special sutures to assure a lid fold are necessary.

A double-armed 4–0 silk suture is passed through the center of the lower lid margin (modified Frost suture). The lower lid is drawn up over the cornea, and the suture fastened to the forehead with adhesive tape (fig. 210*L*). Sometimes a lid is so heavy and edematous that it hangs down over the cornea so that a simple patch suffices; with the cornea thus protected no Frost suture is necessary. The eye is dressed daily and the cornea inspected. The Frost suture, if used, is removed in two or three days as it becomes painful due to the constant effort of the eye to open. Skin sutures are removed on the sixth day and a bland unguent ordered until complete healing is assured.

The lid will remain heavy and edematous for three or four weeks sometimes. Figures 210*M* and *N* show the original condition and the result of surgery with a good lid fold.

Comment: Residents sometimes find it difficult to identify the various lid structures especially the fascia and levator since they may be quite thin and friable. Identification is aided when the lid is blown up with local anesthesia. It also helps to think of the upper lid as a laminated structure built up of layers of tissue: skin, orbicularis muscle, fascia, levator, Müller's muscle and conjunctiva. Some are almost diaphanous, it is true, but all are identifiable. Two additional facts will help if recalled here. The orbital fat separates the suprajacent fascia from the infrajacent levator aponeurosis as noted above. Also the fascia and levator fuse in a thickened horizontal band which may lie at the upper tarsal border or several millimeters above (fig. 210*B*). Once this is identified and the fascia reflected upward the levator cannot be mistaken.

The conjunctiva is not cut here, hence it does not have to be resutured, which leaves intact conjunctiva without sutures to molest the cornea.

Levator Resection by Posterior (Conjunctival) Approach

Procedure (fig. 211): The lid is pulled up, the globe down, and a black silk suture is passed behind the superior rectus for identification. An Ehrhardt clamp is applied with the blade on the skin surface at the center of the lid, and tightened securely. The lid is everted and a curved incision made with a knife through conjunctiva, tarsus, Müller's muscle and levator from one canthus to the other. The width of tarsus included will vary with the amount of ptosis and the correction desired. At *least 6 mm. of tarsal width should always be left* in any case so that the relation of the posterior lid margin to the eyeball may not be disturbed. In recent years the author has taken no more than one or 2 mm. of tarsus, i.e., just enough for levator identification (fig. 211A).

With blunt scissors the conjunctiva is then severed from its attachment to the upper border of the cut tarsus and dissected free from Müller's muscle. The levator is also freed from the orbicularis anteriorly (fig. 211B). The orbital fascia is dissected away from the levator (fig. 211C). The horns of the levator are freed medially and laterally from their canthal attachments and all other fascial attachments above and below the tendon should be severed as described in the previous procedure (fig. 211D). The levator muscle should now be freely mobile and should come forward easily.

Three double-armed 4–0 chromic catgut sutures, equally spaced, are passed through the levator aponeurosis from the conjunctival toward the orbicularis side, one through the center of the levator and one about 8 or 10 mm. to each side as in the previous procedure. The distance of the sutures from the tarsal attachment again depends on the amount of correction desired (fig. 211E).

The levator with its attached rim of tarsus is resected at least 2 mm. below the sutures (fig. 211E) and the clamp removed. The needles of the central double-armed suture are passed through the orbicularis and skin to emerge above the ciliary margin on the skin surface. The medial and lateral sutures are similarly brought out to the skin surface (fig. 211F). The sutures are now tautened so that the cut end of the levator is drawn into the slot between tarsus and orbicularis. If the effect obtained is as desired, the sutures are slightly loosened to permit eversion of the lid sufficiently so that the conjunctiva can be sewed to the cut end of the tarsus with a 4–0 *plain* catgut running suture (fig. 211G). However, every time the needle takes a bite, it is passed into orbicularis and skin.

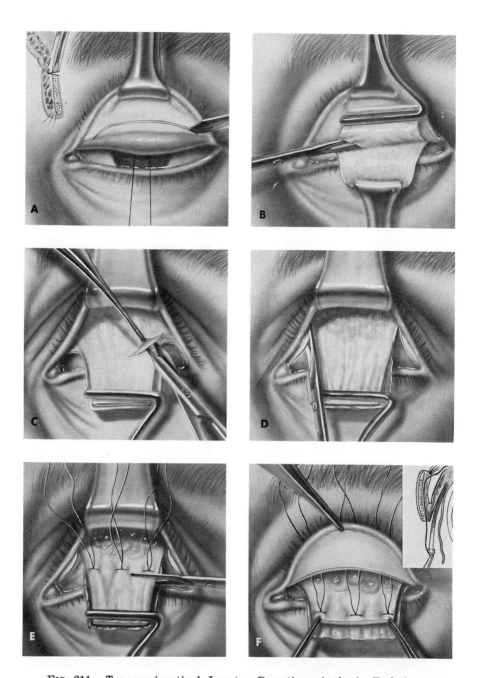

FIG. 211. Transconjunctival Levator Resection—Author's Technic.

A. A suture is passed under the superior rectus muscle. The lid is everted and an incision is made through the tarsoconjunctiva just below the attached tarsal border (the suture is not shown in subsequent drawings.)

B. The levator is freed from the orbicularis anteriorly and the conjunctiva posteriorly.

C. The orbital fascia is dissected away from the levator.

D. The horns and check ligament are cut.

E. The amount of levator to be resected is determined and three double-armed

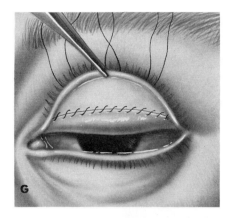

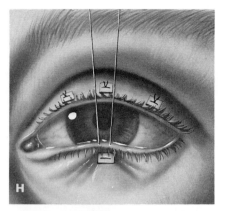

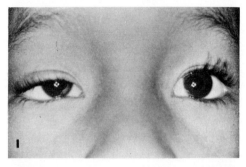

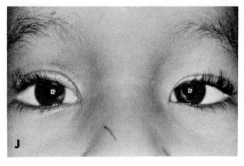

Fig. 211 (*Continued*)

4–0 chromic catgut sutures are passed through the levator from behind forward and *behind* the line of resection. Excess levator is resected.

F. The sutures are passed into the pocket between tarsus and orbicularis and brought out on the skin surface about 3 mm. above the ciliary margin and are tied.

G. The conjunctiva is resutured to the upper tarsal border with plain catgut. At the same time the needle bites into the anterior orbicularis and skin to create a lid fold.

H. The lid is reinverted and the sutures tied. A modified Frost suture is passed through the lower lid which is drawn up over the cornea.

I. and J. Ptosis and its correction by the posterior approach.

This provides the line for the new palpebral furrow and lid fold. No other lid fold sutures are required. The three double-armed skin sutures are now drawn up and tied over pegs. If necessary a Frost suture is passed through the center of the lower lid, drawn up over the cornea and fastened to the forehead with adhesive tape (fig. 211*H*).

Further postoperative routine is the same as for the external approach described above. Figure 211*I* shows a congenital ptosis repaired (fig. 211*J*) by this method.

Comment: The reader is referred to the Comments on the previous procedure most of which are applicable here. The technic just described has, however, several novel features which should be explained. The initial incision is made at once through tarsus and levator rather than peeling the conjunctiva away first. The object of this maneuver is to free the tissues from the tension caused by the eversion of the lid thus facilitating all subsequent surgery. The conjunctiva is not included in the sutures until the levator has been attached. The conjunctiva is then firmly secured by a separate running suture from one end of the tarsus to the other to prevent symblepharon and granulation tissue (see *Complications* below).

Since the skin-muscle lamina lying over the tarsus has not been materially disturbed, there is not as much interference with the normal anatomy of the lid fold as in its case of the anterior approach. However, the fold is adjusted so that it falls into its natural shape and the dressing then applied over it. The shortening of the levator which is a part of the posterior lid lamina may result in a relative excess of the skin-muscle lamina and too much fold. If on closure this is the case some skin-muscle is resected.

Transconjunctival Levator Resection (Iliff)

Another Blaskovics modification is the Iliff operation which has become quite popular in recent years. This technic was first reported in 1954 and received wide acceptance. It was modified by Iliff in 1963. His latest technic follows:

Procedure (fig. 212):   In adults 2 per cent xylocaine with Wydase is used for lid block and for retrobulbar injection. The lid is everted and a solution of 1:100,000 adrenalin is injected along the retrotarsal border to minimize bleeding. A small stab incision is made in the lateral side of the retrotarsal edge through conjunctiva, orbital septum and levator aponeurosis into the potential space between tarsus and orbicularis. Blunt scissors advance across the tarsus to the nasal edge of the retrotarsal margin to create a tunnel. This space is enlarged by blunt dissection and the scissors are brought out nasally through a second stab incision. One jaw of a ptosis clamp is passed into the tunnel and the clamp is tightened at the attached tarsal edge to enclose conjunctiva, tarsus, and the fascia-levator membrane. These tissues are incised distal to the ptosis clamp (fig. 212*A*). Both ends of the arcuate artery are cauterized.

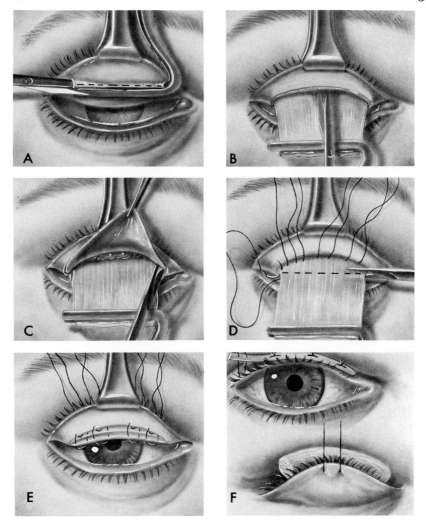

FIG. 212. Iliff's Transconjunctival Levator Resection Technic.

A. The lid is everted and a tunnel is made with a blunt pointed scissors between the orbicularis and fascia-levator membrane at the upper tarsal border. A ptosis clamp is inserted and the edge of the tarsus with its attached tissues is clamped. The tissues in the clamp are cut away from the tarsus.

B. The dissection is carried upward to free the fascia-levator membrane.

C. The orbital fascia and horns are cut to free the levator, Müller's muscle and conjunctiva.

D. A row of four double-armed 4–0 silk sutures is placed through the levator 8–20 mm. from the cut tarsal edge from behind forward through the clamped tissues (conjunctiva, Müller's muscle and levator). The distance of the sutures from the cut edge is determined by the degree of ptosis (see text). The levator is resected.

E. One needle of each of the double-armed sutures is passed through the cut edge of the orbital fascia, the other through the cut tarsal edge, then both needles are passed to the skin surface close to the cilia.

F. The sutures are tied over a 2 mm. wide silicone strip. The redundant skin of the upper lid is invaginated with a cotton roll to create a lid fold. The cotton roll is held in place by a suture from the lower lid to the forehead.

The ptosis clamp is pulled down and the dissection is carried between the levator and orbicularis (fig. 212B). The septum orbitale is cut away from its attachment to the levator exposing the fat which lies between them. The septum is pulled forward with forceps and inspected to assure no further connections. If present, they should be cut. The levator is also pulled to each side and the horns cut (fig. 212C).

The structures in the clamps are pulled down and a row of four 4–0 silk sutures is passed through them and tied anywhere from 18–20 mm. from the cut edge. All the tissues distal to the sutures are resected (fig. 212D). The amount of tissue resected depends on the amount of ptosis. In patients with a large degree of ptosis, 18–24 mm. of levator-cum- Müller's muscle cum conjunctiva is resected. In patients with senile ptosis, only 8–12 mm. resection is needed.

One needle of each double-armed suture is passed through the edge of the cut septum and then between orbicularis and tarsus and brought out on the lid surface just above the ciliary margin. The second needle of each double-armed suture is passed through the cut tarsal edge and then out on the lid margin close to its fellow. The author stresses that the needles be placed close to the cilia "because the skin here is closely bound to the tarsus" (sic!) and will not stretch (fig. 212E).

The sutures are tied over a silicone strip, beads or rubber pegs. In order to form a good lid fold, the redundant skin is invaginated with a tightly wound cotton pollywog. The lower lid is pulled up over the cornea with a loop suture through the skin of the lower lid and fastened to the forehead. This suture helps hold the pollywog in place (fig. 212F). A firm dressing is applied for 24 hours (which, according to the author, is enough to produce a good lid fold) at which time the lower lid suture is removed. The patient is discharged without an eye dressing and instructed to use a bland ointment twice a day. Other lid sutures are removed after ten days. The full effect of the operation is obtained in five or six weeks.

Comment: This is obviously an ingenious and successful procedure which is not difficult technically. However, there are several practical and theoretical exceptions which might be taken: When the orbital fascia is fastened to the lid margin, it is inevitably being shortened. Since it is originally attached to the levator, sometimes well above the upper tarsal border, this may amount to a good deal of shortening. In the higher degrees of ptosis, this might give a lagophthalmos. Since the septum is attached to the orbital rim and not to the frontalis, it cannot "increase the secondary action of the frontalis." The author states that the resection of the conjunctiva enhances "secondary elevating action of the superior rectus and the levator" because it puts a stretch on the fibrous attachments from the sheaths of these muscles to the superior cul-de-sac.

It can be argued just as easily that this "stretch" inhibits the full excursion of the levator and superior rectus. I am afraid that the conjunctiva is just wasted. However, it must be acknowledged that the loss of conjunctiva does not cause any deleterious effects.

Originally the initial stab wounds went through the tarsus just above the attached border. Since the levator is laminated against the tarsus, this is a much better approach than the later incisions which do not seem to go into the tarsus. By stabbing into these softer tissues, it would be rather difficult to estimate just how deep and where the knife is going and would seem to be a "by guess and by God" approach. The original 1954 incisions were a better bet for the casual operator. Also, pressing a cotton peg against the skin for 24 hours is a rather casual way of creating a lid fold. Lid folds are not come by so easily in all cases. Iliff's use of a retrobulbar injection seems superfluous. I have never felt the need for one.

Despite these minor technical cavelings, this is a good operation and, from all reports, generally successful.

Schimek and Cusick (1958) also include the septum in their closure to utilize "the elastic tension of the the septum" (sic!). They use an ingenious method of trying to modify overcorrections: After a few postoperative days, the sutures are loosened and the levator is allowed to retract with the aid of massage. Later under anesthesia the lid is forcibly pulled down. They report excellent or good results in 75 per cent of 93 cases of congenital ptosis, over 60 per cent good results in traumatic ptosis and about 70 per cent good results in acquired hereditary ptosis.

Levator Resection for Minimal Ptosis (Fasanella and Servat)

In 1961 Fasanella and Servat suggested a simple modification of the Blaskovics procedure "for cases of minimal ptosis (3–4 mm.) with some function of the levator showing a fair lid fold and in the absence of the jaw-winking phenomenon of Marcus Gunn."

Procedure (fig. 213):   After suitable anesthesia the upper lid is everted and the upper border of the tarsus is grasped in two curved hemostats so as to include about 3 mm. of the attached tarsal border and 3 mm. of conjunctiva and levator cum Müller's muscle. The curve of the hemostats is parallel to the curve of the lid border (fig. 213A). A 6 mm. strip of tarsus and levator (3 mm. of each) is resected away. As the resection proceeds, the cut edges are sutured either with interrupted or a running 5–0 chromic suture. This serves the double purpose of minimizing bleeding and retaining control of the levator at all times (fig. 213B).

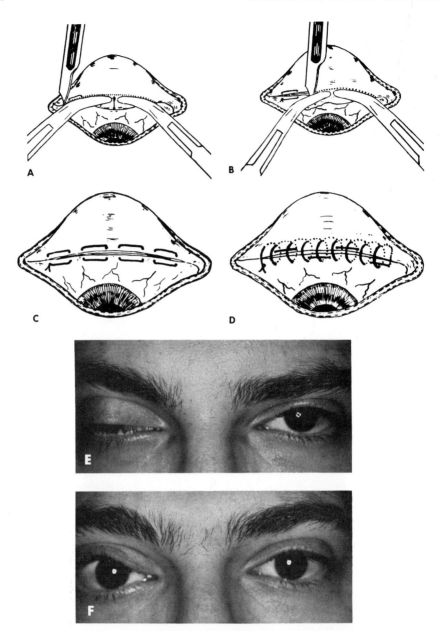

FIG. 213. Transconjunctival Levator Resection Technic of Fasanella and
Servat (original drawings).

A. The upper lid is everted and the upper tarsal border is clamped in two curved
hemostats to include 3 mm. of tarsus and 3 mm. of conjunctiva and levator.

B. The strip of tarsus and levator cum conjunctiva is cut away. The cut edges
are sutured as the resection proceeds.

C. and D. Types of sutures which obviate knots in the region of the cornea.

E. Ptosis of right upper lid with good levator action.

F. Repair by this technic.

(Fasanella, R. M., and Servat, J.: Courtesy Archives of Ophthalmology.)

The authors suggest inserting the suture and knotting it at the temporal end before the resection is begun so that control of tissues is always maintained. A running suture which is tightened at the end of the operation will obviate knots in the corneal region altogether (figs. 213C and D). The eye is closed with two modified Frost sutures and a firm bandage

Figures 213E and F show a ptosis before and after correction by this method.

Comment: The authors stress the fact that this procedure is only for minimal amounts of ptosis. They have had no trouble reinverting the lid postoperatively probably because so little width of tissue (6 mm.) is sacrificed.

This operation is easier and simpler to perform if the following modifications are made: (1) Small clamps should be used. Large clamps obscure the field too much especially in young children with their narrow tarsi. (2) It is more convenient to place the clamps, when possible, *behind* the line of incision. Thus the whole strip of levator-cum-tarsus may be cut away and sutured at once without resorting to the snip and sew technic. (3) A *plain,* running catgut suture should be used since plain gut softens and absorbs faster than chromic. A suture rubbing against the cornea can and frequently does make a patient very unhappy.

In general, I have found this procedure more useful in the acquired than in the congenital ptoses. McCord has reported success with a similar operation for minimal ptosis in which he resects only 4 mm. of levator and Müller's muscle.

Common Postoperative Complications of Levator Surgery

UNDERCORRECTION.   There are several causes for undercorrection in levator surgery. Most frequently it is due to simple failure to resect enough levator. As previously stated, 8 mm. of levator resection is required to obtain any effect; most often 12 or 14 mm. has to be taken. In the more severe cases it is not unusual to resect 16, 18 or 20 mm. for a good result.

Undercorrection should not be diagnosed too hastily. The lid may be heavy and edematous for three or four weeks postoperatively and complete elevation may not be attained until the full effect of the surgery has worn off.

If the undercorrection persists after several months and is slight, the cosmetic result may be sufficient to require no further surgery. If the undercorrection is greater and cosmetically unacceptable, there is no contraindication to a second levator resection. If the external route was employed in the primary procedure, it might be expedient to use the conjunctival route secondarily to avoid too much scarring of one area. The process may be reversed when the conjunctival route is used initially. However, reoperation by the same route is not contraindicated and has been used by the author with satisfaction.

Poor levator tissue due to maldevelopment or fibrosis is another cause of undercorrection. A thin friable or fibrosed levator will require more resection than one which is obviously healthy and well developed.

Pulling out of sutues is rare but may occur. If the levator is sutured to the tarsal surface with chromic catgut, a good deep bite should be taken. The tarsus is not a first grade tissue and sutures may cut through unless firmly anchored. Silk sutures brought to the skin surface and tied over pegs are less likely to slip or cut through.

Undercorrection may occur in cases of minimal or no levator action no matter how large the levator resection. In such cases it is best to resort to another modality if further surgery is done. Paradoxically, despite undercorrection, lagophthalmos, entropion, or both, may occasionally result as noted below.

OVERCORRECTION. This is less common than undercorrection. The most common causes are resection of too much levator, advancement of the levator too far down on the tarsus, resection of too much tarsus, or any combination of these factors.

If the overcorrection is slight, it may disappear spontaneously in time. This has been seen to happen. The process may be aided by having the patient squeeze his lids together 20 or 30 times several times a day. This is effective and works well if started early enough and if the overcorrection is not too great.

Where the overcorrection is of greater degree and persists, there is only one remedy and that is reoperation with some type of levator recession. Berke has described a simple procedure in which he everts the lid and makes a horizontal incision along the whole length of the upper tarsal border through conjunctiva and levator, undermining upward and allowing the levator to retract. No closing sutures are used. I have found this technic inadequate except in the mildest of overcorrections.

Callahan has devised a procedure for overcorrection of ptosis which he has found useful. For overcorrection of 4 to 5 mm. he recesses the levator 7 to 8 mm. using pretarsal orbicularis as a levator extension. In more severe overcorrections he uses a sheet of collagen film suturing one edge to the freed levator and the other to the upper tarsal border. The width of the film depends on the amount of recession desired. These are preferred to the Berke procedure.

This procedure also may be inadequate in the severest cases of overcorrection with lagophthalmos and here I prefer levator recession ad maximum.

LEVATOR RECESSION—AUTHOR'S METHOD. *Procedure (fig. 214):* The levator is exposed by a skin-muscle incision at the upper border of the tarsus (fig. 214*A*). It is freed anteriorly from all attachments to the orbicularis and orbital fascia and posteriorly from the conjunctiva. Usually it also becomes attached medially and laterally and these attachments should be freed so that it retracts completely (fig. 214*B*). If it does not, inspection will show fibrous attachments which are freed.

Three double-armed 4–0 silk sutures, equally spaced, are passed about 2 mm. from the cut edge of the levator from behind forward. The

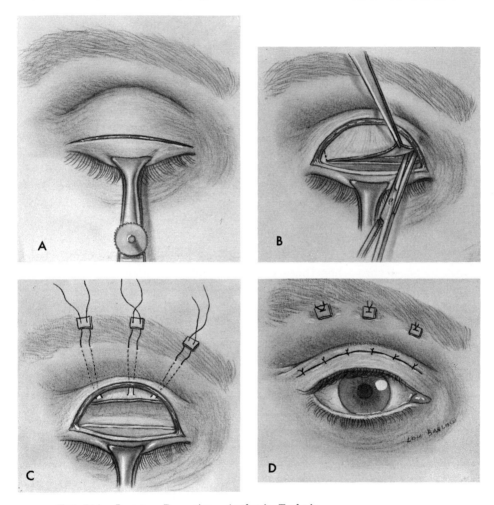

FIG. 214. Levator Recession—Author's Technic.
A. A horizontal incision is made through skin and muscle just below the upper tarsal border.
B. The levator is exposed, freed of all attachments and allowed to retract ad maximum. Three double-armed 4–0 silk equally spaced sutures are passed through the levator edge from behind forward. The sutures are continued through the skin-muscle lamina to emerge on the skin surface.
D. The sutures are tied over pegs and the skin wound is closed.

needles are continued through orbicularis and skin and emerge just below the eyebrow (fig. 214C) where they are tied over rubber pegs. The skin wound is closed with interrupted 5–0 silk sutures (fig. 214D). The eye is patched and dressed daily. Sutures are removed on the sixth day.

Comment: Overcorrection is one of the most difficult conditions to repair in ptosis surgery. One would think that all one had to do would be to locate the attachment of the levator to the tarsus, detach the levator, allow it to retract the amount of overcorrection and then suture it back. It does not work that way.

Overcorrection requires more levator recession than the original resection in many cases. As a matter of fact, some men advocate suturing the upper and lower lids together after the recession to prevent the upper lid from retracting again; this is not a bad idea. Others advocate passing a suture through the upper lid margin, pulling the lid down over the cornea and taping it to the cheek for at least a week to prevent retraction. This has also been useful in some cases.

I have rarely seen a return of the ptosis following complete levator recession. But I have seen a persistent residual lagophthalmos, though of lesser degree; such cases may even require more levator recession. The reason for this difficulty is not clear but it is encountered often enough to make overcorrection with lagophthalmos one of the most dreaded of postoperative complications.

It is possible to have an apparent overcorrection in cases where none exists. This occurs when there is bilateral ptosis which is slight in one eye and more severe in the other and it is only when the worse of the two eyes is corrected that the milder ptosis becomes manifest and the operated eye seems overcorrected by contrast. The procedure here is to correct the second eye also. Such cases are not too rare especially in the acquired senile ptoses.

LAGOPHTHALMOS.   Inability to close the eye completely may accompany overcorrection in cases of ptosis with poor levator function. It may even be present with a cosmetic undercorrection as noted above. It is true that with the passage of time the lagophthalmos tends to diminish. But it rarely disappears completely to the chagrin of both patient and doctor.

A much rarer cause of lagophthalmos is failure to separate the levator from its connection to the suprajacent orbital fascia. The reason this does not happen more often is that levator and fascia are frequently separated from each other automatically during the course of the dissection and resection especially when the anterior approach is used.

In rare instances reoperation of a previous site may cause scarring with sufficient shortening of the upper lid skin to cause lagophthalmos. In such cases skin grafting is required.

ENTROPION. This is the third and least common of the unholy triad of complications including overcorrection and lagophthalmos occurring most commonly in cases with poor levator action. Since the levator forms a part of the posterior lid lamina, the condition here is similar to a cicatricial entropion in which the tarsoconjunctival layer has become too short for the anterior skin-muscle layer with a resultant inversion of the lid margin. Once this is manifest, levator recession is mandatory if corneal injury and possible permanent visual damage is to be avoided.

THE LID FOLD. The upper lid sulcus lies at the upper tarsal border marking the upper line of levator attachment to the skin. Since the skin above this furrow is loose, the normal pull of the levator up and back forms a fold which increases on looking upward and disappears in downward gaze. When the levator is dissected away from the skin and muscle the normal anatomy of the lid fold is destroyed. When healing takes place the lid fold is reformed. Thus there is rarely absence of a lid fold after the levator has been shortened; frequently there is too much and some of it has to be resected. However, the lid fold can come to settle in the wrong place unless properly controlled. If the anterior route is used and the skin muscle over the tarsus is undermined toward the lash line, it should be pulled up taut when the wound is closed and several of the sutures used to close the skin incision should bite into the upper edge of the tarsus. This anchors the lower skin-muscle flap at the upper tarsal border where it belongs and prevents a downward sag.

Another common reason for malposition of the lid fold is misplacement of the skin incision. Hence, the upper lid furrow should be marked out with a colored dye before local injection of anesthesia to match the opposite lid and to assure equal positioning of the folds postoperatively.

If the conjunctival route is used and the pretarsal tissues are left undisturbed, there is usually less difficulty with the lid fold. However, if a wide piece of tarsus is resected (this should never be more than 4 mm.), the lid fold should be adjusted on the anterior surface either by sutures or by positioning it properly before the dressing is applied. Here also skin may have to be resected if too much fold results.

Occasionally pressure on the lid by postoperative dressings will cause the lid fold to heal into position so that it is present even when the patient is looking down or has his eyes clsed. This is almost as unacceptable cosmetically as absence of a lid fold. It may also be caused by pulling the lower lid up over the cornea and leaving it in place too long thus allowing the upper lid skin to heal in its folded raised state so that the furrow becomes permanent.

Unless there has been an excessive amount of levator resection the upper lid after surgery is frequently sufficiently heavy and edematous to come down over the cornea so that a Frost suture is not required. Daily dressings with not too much pressure will allow the lid to move as soon as function is restored and will discourage "freezing" of the lid fold.

LID LAG.   Failure of the lid to follow the eye normally on looking downward is a common, unavoidable, almost inevitable, result of levator resection. This must be distinguished from lagophthalmos (i.e., inability to close the eye completely), which is an entirely different clinical entity. Most cases of levator resection, no matter how little, show some lid lag in the operated eye when the patient looks down. The probable reason for this is simply shortening of one of the important lid layers. Levator shortening enables the lid to rise into normal position but it does not increase or restore the normal elasticity or tonicity of the levator. Hence, after resection, the levator is still long enough and elastic enough to allow normal eye closure when the orbicularis contracts but it is now too short to permit normal lid movement when the eye moves down. In time lid lag tends to diminish; rarely does it disappear completely.

Some operated eyes show a combination of lid lag and lagophthalmos. Thus, though a patient may have no trouble closing his eye, it may remain open during sleep. This may happen in every kind of ptosis repair even with the most successful levator resection technic. In the absence of a Bell's phenomenon (i.e., in poor elevation due to superior rectus palsy) this can become important due to corneal exposure and may exhaust the therapeutic ingenuity of the surgeon.

Lid lag is not preventable, but fortunately it is also of no great consequence either cosmetically or functionally in most cases because it is usually of slight degree and not evident except in extreme downward gaze.

NOTCHING OR TENTING OF THE LID MARGIN.   Two technical errors may be responsible for notching or tenting of the lid after levator surgery. One is too energetic a resection of the tarsus, thus depriving the lid of its skeletal architecture and reducing it to a soft, yielding mass of tissue layers which sags of its own weight on being elevated. Hence, the trend away from tarsal resection in ptosis surgery is a salutary one.

The other cause of notching is an uneven placement of the sutures which refasten the levator to the tarsus after resection. If misplaced so that there is more pull on one (usually the central one) than the other two, the lid will rise too high in the center, the regular lid curve will disappear and notching will result. This is avoided first by tying the sutures loosely with single or slip-knots and noting the position and curvature of the lid margin. If a tendency to notching is noted the knots are readjusted to restore the normal curve of the lid margin. After healing, the correction of notching is a much more formidable problem.

CORNEAL INVOLVEMENT.   Exposure keratitis, although not common, may occur after any type of ptosis repair even where the postoperative result is excellent and there is no overcorrection, lagophthal-

mos or entropion. Apparently some corneas which have always been more
or less covered by the lid react poorly to their suddenly acquired naked
state. Rarer causes are the abrasive action of the sutures used in the
conjunctival approach and too vigorous patching. The keratitis may be
mild and show a quick response to conservative medication such as
frequent instillation of methylcellulose drops and patching at night.
Other cases react much more violently and become therapeutic problems
requiring long and careful coddling before they finally yield to treatment.
If the keratitis develops in the presence of lagophthalmos the sooner the
latter is corrected the better.

Other Postoperative Complications

Other less common postoperative complications of levator surgery
have been noted. Some are of no great clinical consequence; others are
serious but fortunately rare.

Symblepharon may develop unless care is taken to resuture the conjunctiva to the tarsus completely. It may be slight or it may involve the
whole incision. It occurs oftener than suspected. Sometimes granulation
tissue appears in the unsutured parts of the wound and proves troublesome. It is worth the extra time and effort to close the whole length of
the conjunctival wound with a plain catgut running suture to avoid
symblephara. This occurs only in the conjunctival approach.

Postoperative edema occurs rarely—fortunately. When it does, one
must wait several months sometimes before the edema resorbs and the
lid rises up to its proper level. Injection of hyalouronidase solution has
been suggested but that has not always been effective. Careful massage
after all inflammation has subsided may prove more effective.

Conjunctival ectropion or prolapse may occur especially in the
higher grades of ptosis where the dissection has to be carried far up into
the fornix and the conjunctiva has been separated from its loose fibrous
attachments. If left alone the conjunctiva tends to contract and the
ectropion may disappear spontaneously in time. However, it is unsightly
and it is better to prevent this by a careful inspection of the wound at
the conclusion of the operation. If the conjunctiva has prolapsed it should
be pushed up into position gently. If it does not lie in position easily one
or two double-armed sutures should be passed through it, then through
the full thickness of the lid to emerge on the skin surface below the
brow and tied loosely. In the case of an anophthalmic socket, a well-fitting
conformer makes an ideal guarantee against conjunctival prolapse.

Muscle involvement such as hypotropia and diplopia due to accidental cutting of the superior rectus muscle or the superior oblique are
serious complications which are fortunately rare. Unless the eye is am-
blyopic, corrective surgery is required.

Loss of lashes may be caused by carrying the dissection too far down toward the ciliary margin. The remedy is prophylactic not therapeutic.

Infection may occur as anywhere else but is fortunately rare. Unless vigorous action is taken immediately it not only nullifies the operative result but leaves permanent scarring and malformation hard to counter-act. It is a curse of the gods which requires no special discussion—only commiseration.

FRONTALIS SUSPENSION

In the total absence of levator (and superior rectus) action one must resort to the frontalis as an elevator. It is also employed in cases where other procedures have failed. Indeed, most surgeons prefer to use the frontalis now even in the presence of an intact superior rectus.

Of course, the patient is condemned to corrugation of the brow and arching of the eyebrow in order to achieve lid elevation. For the frontalis is an abnormal lifting mechanism which substitutes a lesser physiologic defect for a greater one. It gives unequal width of the palpebral fissure in case of unilateral ptosis unless the patient learns to lift only one brow. There is lid lag on looking down and ptosis on looking up unless the brow is arched. There is also lagophthalmos in sleep as in superior rectus surgery although exposure keratitis is quite rare.

However, in these cases frontalis suspension is so much easier tech-nically than superior rectus suspension and its complications are so much less, that it has displaced superior rectus surgery almost completely. A number of operations exist which are satisfactory; a few of the more commonly used are described.

Autogenous Fascia Sling—Author's Technic

For a number of years I have been using an autogenous fascia sling which has given me satisfaction and good results.

Procedure (fig. 215): Autogenous fascia is obtained from the lower outer aspect of the thigh, as described in Chapter 3 (figs. 36 and 37). A 5–0 silk suture is passed through each end of the strip, tied and the needles are cut off. The fascia is wrapped in a piece of gauze moistened with warm saline until ready for use.

The brow and lid are prepared for the reception of the fascia sling as follows: Two short 3 mm. horizontal incisions are made through the skin and orbicularis of the lid 3 mm. above the margin. One is at the junction of the medial and middle third of the lid and the other at the junction of the lateral and middle third.

Three similar incisions are made just above the brow through skin and muscle. One incision is placed 3 mm. above the center of the brow and one about 12–15 mm. to each side of the central incision. The skin of the central brow incision is undermined upward for about a centimeter to provide a subcutaneous pocket for later use (fig. 215C inset).

After bleeding has been controlled, a Reese ptosis knife or Wright needle is passed horizontally between orbicularis and tarsus from one of the lid incisions to the other. It is poked through until the fenestrated end appears. The instrument is moved back and forth a few times so that the fascial strip may be drawn through easily. The suture at one end of the strip is threaded through the fenestrated end and the fascia is pulled through so that equal lengths protrude from the lid incisions (fig. 215A).

The Reese knife or Wright needle is now inserted into the lateral brow incision and pushed downward carefully behind the orbicularis to emerge in the homolateral lid incision (fig. 215B). When the fenestrated end emerges, it is again moved back and forth to create an adequate tunnel. The suture at the end of the fascial strip is threaded into the fenestration and the strip is pulled upward to emerge in the lateral brow incision. The medial end of the fascial strip is drawn up medially in similar fashion.

The instrument is now passed from the central brow incision to the lateral and medial incisions respectively and the ends of the fascial strip are each brought out through the central brow incision (fig. 215C). The fascial strip is pulled up and tied so that the lid margin lies slightly above the upper limbus with the eye in the primary position (fig. 215D). The fascial strip is knotted twice and the knot is reinforced by a chromic suture passed through the knot and firmly tied (fig. 215D inset). (Fascia is slippery and may become undone if the knot is not reinforced.) In addition, both needles of a double-armed 4–0 silk suture are passed through the fascial knot. The needles are then carried upward beneath the skin in the pocket previously made to emerge on the skin surface about a centimeter above the central brow incision where the suture is tied over a rubber peg (fig. 215D). The brow incisions are closed with 5–0 silk or 4–0 plain catgut in infants. The lid incisions need no suturing.

A modified Frost suture is passed through the lower lid which is pulled up to cover the cornea. The suture is fastened to the brow with adhesive.

Postoperative care: The eye is dressed daily and the Frost suture is removed on the second or third day. By then the lid is somewhat heavy and swollen so that it comes down over the cornea and lower lid protection is not needed. The skin sutures are removed on the fifth day and the brow suture which has been passed through a rubber peg is removed on the tenth day, earlier if it is obviously loose. The patch may be removed on the fifth or sixth day.

A six-year-old boy with total congenital ptosis is shown in figure 215E. Figure 215F shows the boy before suture removal. The final result is seen three months later (fig. 215G).

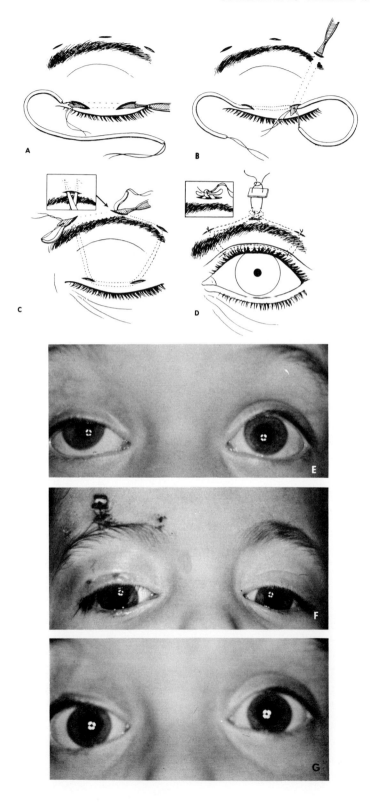

Should there be any sign of keratitis, however mild, the patient is placed on methyl cellulose drops instilled every three or four hours during the waking day. These are gradually curtailed as healing progresses. Ointment should be instilled into the conjunctival sac at night and, if necessary, the eye is patched until exposure is obviously no longer a danger to the cornea.

Comment: For one or two weeks—sometimes longer—the lid may remain disappointingly low due to its edematous condition. However, as the swelling subsides the lid rises gradually and assumes a normal position.

When a bilateral ptosis is corrected simultaneously the fascial strip should be cut 7 or 8 mm. wide and then simply split in half lengthwise. This is ample fascia for two ptosis procedures.

Care should be taken in passing the Reese knife or Wright needle from the brow to the lid incisions. Injury to the globe can be caused, hence the course of the knife or needle should be carefully watched by lifting the lid and watching the conjunctiva.

Under anesthesia the eyes tend to roll up, hence in the case of an infant the globe should be grasped by an assistant and held so that it points straight upward. This will help to position the lid in its proper place.

The advantages of the autogenous fascia frontalis sling are considerable: (a) "Take" is assured, (b) the incisions are minimal and heal rapidly, (c) the tensile strength of the fascia is excellent, hence there is little stretching (cf. muscle slings), (d) the technic is not difficult, (e) best of all, there is no absorption of the fascia hence recurrences are few.

Good fascial slings have also been reported by Crawford (1956) and Johnson (1962). The latter is less complicated. Iliff has suggested the use of reconstituted collagen. However, recurrences with this are frequent. More recently Bodian has suggested using preserved sclera as a sling.

Fig. 215. Autogenous Fascia Sling—Author's Technic.

A. Two short lid and three short brow incisions are made as shown. The fascia is drawn through the two lid incisions.
B. The fascial strip is drawn up laterally.
C. The strip is drawn through from the lateral to the central brow incision and the medial end is being drawn through similarly. Note that a skin pocket is prepared above the middle brow incision (inset).
D. The lid is drawn up. The fascial strip is tied and the knot reinforced with a chromic suture (inset). A double-armed silk suture is passed through the knot and then up behind the skin to emerge high above the central incision where it is tied over a peg. The lower lid is drawn up with a Frost suture to protect the cornea.
E. Complete ptosis of right upper lid.
F. Fascial sling repair before suture removal.
G. Final result.

Double Skin-Strap Sling—Author's Technic

Another procedure which I have found useful where the taking of fascia is contraindicated is a skin sling which I have been using for the past four years.

Procedure (fig. 216): A horizontal line is marked out with an antiseptic dye from canthus to canthus 6 mm. above the lid margin. A second line, parallel to the first, is drawn 4 mm. above.

If the operation is being done under local anesthesia, the lid is now injected and gently massaged to reduce anesthetic swelling. An Ehrhardt clamp is inserted under the lid and the skin is incised along the marked out lines. The skin straps thus formed are dissected up leaving the central 6 mm. attachment intact. The exposed orbicularis fibers are resected (fig. 216*A*).

The skin flaps are smoothed out, epithelial side up, over a protective sheet of plastic or gauze and painted with 30 per cent trichloracetic acid. As the acid is applied the epithelium will turn a grayish white. This is left on for a few minutes, the epithelium is then scraped off with a knife (Bard Parker No. 15 or its equivalent) and the straps are wiped and flushed off with saline. The skin will retain its gray color but this is of no consequence.

A single-armed 5–0 silk suture is passed through the end of each strap and the needles are cut off. Two small incisions are made through skin and muscle above the brow about 12–15 mm. medial and lateral to center respectively. The central part of the skin-muscle lamina between the brow and lid incisions is undermined.

A stout double-armed 3–0 silk suture is passed through the center of the lid engaging the orbicularis and tarsus below the area of attachment of the skin pedicles. The needles are carried up behind the orbicularis and are passed deep into the muscle layer of the brow to come out above the brow (fig. 216*B*).

A Reese ptosis knife or Wright needle is passed deep under the brow through the temporal incision and under the orbicularis to emerge at the point of attachment of the lateral skin pedicle. The instrument is moved from side to side to assure a sufficiently wide tunnel to permit passage of the pedicle. The suture attached to the lateral skin pedicle is threaded through the fenestrated end and the pedicle is drawn up into the lateral brow wound. The medial pedicle is drawn up medially under the orbicularis in similar fashion (fig. 216*C*).

The lid is drawn up by the central suture to a point slightly above the upper limbus and the suture tied securely over a peg. The medial and lateral pedicles are then drawn up, the lid margin is inspected to assure its proper curve and position and the pedicle ends are sutured subcutaneously. The lid and brow wounds are closed with interrupted

5–0 silk sutures or 5–0 plain catgut in the case of the young. A modified Frost suture is inserted in the lower lid which is drawn up over the cornea and taped to the forehead (fig. 216D).

Postoperative care is handled as described for the Tansley procedure (fig. 217). However, the central brow suture is left in for at least two weeks.

Case History

A. B., a 55-year-old woman, had had bilateral congenital ptosis since birth. There were no lid folds and no levator action in either eye. In the past few years the ptosis had gotten worse so that her pupils were covered most of the time. Frontalis action was fair and the lid width normal (fig. 216E). A bilateral skin sling repair was done (fig. 216F). The final result was quite good (fig. 216G) with voluntary closure of the eyes unimpaired (fig. 216H).

Comment: This procedure resembles the Reese technic (fig. 218) except that skin instead of muscle flaps are used. In some ways this is a simpler and even better procedure than the Tansley technic (fig. 217). No skin is wasted here by resection and the skin fold is much more natural whereas the vertical skin strap in the Tansley procedure makes a good lid fold hard to attain.

The two horizontal incisions are placed in such a position that the original furrow of the lid is retained. The incisions must be extended medially and laterally far enough to make adequate pedicles for drawing up the lid.

The skin flaps are cauterized with trichloracetic acid as in the Tansley procedure and de-epithelialized to obviate the possibility of cyst formation. I have never seen such cysts and it may be that cauterization is not necessary but it is easy to do and I have always done it because it seems a wise precaution.

Skin pedicles make a much more substantial sling than orbicularis muscle and are useful in all except the congenitally narrowed lids. They neither dry out as quickly nor do they fray. Hence the danger of subsequent recurrence is considerably lessened. Despite this, I have used a central suture to minimize postoperative droop during the healing period. The exposed orbicularis fibers are resected to prevent bunching as the lid is drawn up. It also helps make a better lid fold. At closure there is slight central bunching at the point of origin of the pedicles. This smooths out in two or three days.

All frontalis slings should be attached to the brow *muscles* and not to the periosteum which is a static structure. Much better movement of the lid will be obtained if the muscle is made the lifting agent.

Despite their undoubted efficacy, skin slings have never proved very

popular for several reasons: a) They are contraindicated in congenitally
narrowed lids which have no skin to spare for slings. (In such cases,
autogenous fascia should be used.) b) The burial of epithelium under

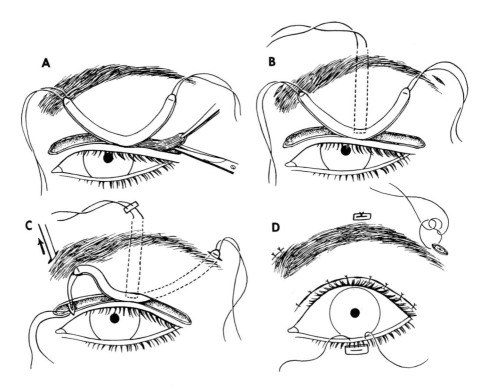

Fig. 216.   Author's Skin Sling Technic.
A.   A horizontal skin incision parallel with the tarsal border is made 5 mm.
     above the lid margin. A parallel incision is made 4 mm. higher. The resultant
     skin straps are dissected up leaving the central 6 mm. intact. The exposed
     orbicularis fibers are resected.
B.   The epithelium of the skin straps is cauterized with 30 per cent trichloracetic
     acid and scraped off (see text). Sutures are passed through the end of each
     skin strap. Two 4 mm. horizontal skin incisions are made above the brow.
     One is placed 12–15 mm. to each side of the brow center. The central part of
     the skin muscle lamina between the skin straps and brow is undermined. A
     stout double-armed 3–0 silk suture is passed into the tarsus under the
     centrally attached skin between the two skin straps. It is then passed upward
     behind the orbicularis and the brow to emerge above the brow.
C.   By means of a Reese ptosis knife or Wright needle the skin straps are drawn
     up medially and laterally.
D.   The central suture is drawn up so that the lid margin lies about 2 mm. above
     the upper limbus. The suture is tied over a peg. The skin straps are fastened
     into position. The brow and lid wounds are closed and the lower lid is drawn
     up over the cornea by means of a modified Frost suture.
E.   Myopathic ptosis.
F.   Repair by author's skin slings.
G.   Final result.
H.   Ability to close eyes unimpaired.

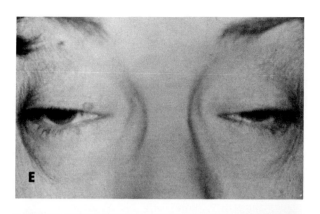

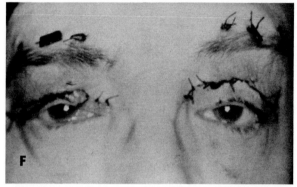

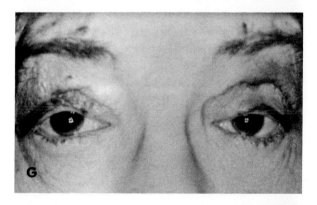

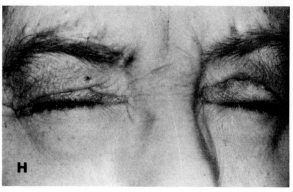

epithelium which was especially objectionable with the cruder early technics has been repugnant to surgeons because of the possibility of epithelial cyst formation. c) It seems to be contrary to normal healing processes. d) Good as the hitherto popular Tansley procedure is, it does not lend itself to adequate lid fold formation: This is an important reason for the unpopularity of any ptosis procedure.

However, autogenous skin slings also have advantages: They work as well as the autogenous fascia slings and do not require extra operative procedures for obtaining fascia. Thus they spare the patients incisions and scars in the thigh. Considering modern fashions in clothes, this is quite a cosmetic advantage, especially for females.

The procedure which I use supplies an adequate lid fold. At first there is a fullness centrally which gradually disappears. Also there are no areas where skin pierces skin creating redundant pockets, since all of the cauterized skin is completely covered. I believe that where indicated, i.e., in lids of normal width with no levator action, this operation is as desirable as a fascial sling—perhaps more so.

The Tansley Technic

Tansley's procedure, published in 1895, incorporates some of the elements of the early Hunt and Graefe procedures with that of Panas. This is a useful technic in congenital ptosis cases without levator action in which the lid is not narrow and ample skin for the flap is available.

Procedure (fig. 217): With an antiseptic dye two vertical lines are drawn 5mm. apart in the center of the lid from just beneath the brow to 5 mm. from the lid margin. The upper ends of the two vertical lines are united by a horizontal line.

Using the lower end of the temporal vertical line as a base, a narrow triangle is drawn with apex pointing toward the lateral canthus. The sides of the triangle are curved somewhat to conform to the curve of the lid margin. A similar triangle is drawn medially. The length of the *base* of the triangles will depend on how much lid lifting is needed. The greater the degree of ptosis the higher the base will obviously be and the wider the triangles.

If the surgery is to be done under local anesthesia, the lid is now injected and gently massaged to reduce the swelling. The marked out lines are incised (fig. 217A). The two triangles to each side of the skin flap are resected (fig. 217B). The vertical skin flap is undermined and mobilized and the pretarsal orbicularis fibers are resected. A suture is passed through the end of the flap (fig. 217C). The strap is draped over a layer of plastic sheeting or a thick gauze pad and the epithelial side is painted with a solution of 30 per cent trichloracetic acid until the whole surface is gray. After a few minutes the epithelium is scraped off and the flap is flushed thoroughly with saline to get rid of all the acid, care

being taken not to contaminate the rest of the field. This is much less of
a a chore than would at first appear.

A stab incision is made deep into the muscle layer under the center
of the eyebrow with a Reese ptosis knife which is passed down behind the

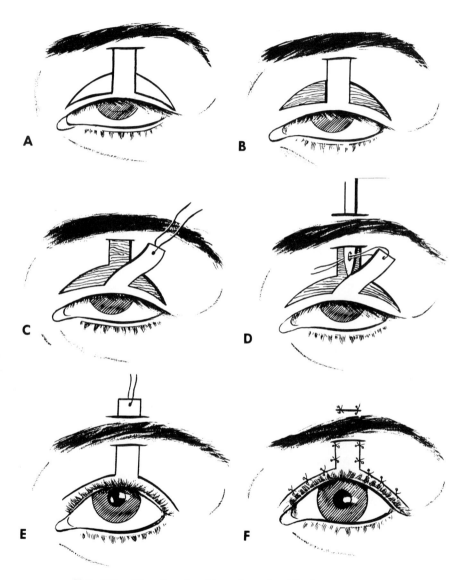

Fig. 217.   The Tansley Procedure for Ptosis.
A.   The skin is incised to outline flap and triangles.
B.   The lateral skin triangles are resected.
C.   The skin flap is raised.
D.   The tunnel for the skin flap is made.
E.   The skin flap is drawn up.
F.   The excess skin is resected and the flap sutured into place.

orbicularis. The knife is moved from side to side to provide ample room for the skin strap to be drawn through (fig. 217D). The suture at the end of the strap is threaded through the fenestration at the end of the knife, and the strap is drawn up under the brow so that the lid margin lies just above the upper limbus (fig. 217E).

At this time the area of the lower triangles is inspected and if there is overlapping of skin a little more skin is resected. However, the lid should not be narrowed too much. The excess skin strap extending above the brow is resected and the end sutured deeply. The lid incisions are closed with interrupted 5–0 silk sutures in the adult or 5–0 plain catgut sutures in the case of a child. The brow wound over the skin strap is closed similarly (fig. 217F).

Sterile ointment is instilled into the conjunctival sac and applied to the skin sutures. A loop suture is passed through the edge of the lower lid over a peg, the lid is drawn up over the cornea and taped to the brow.

Postoperative care: In the average case, postoperative care is rather simple. The eye is dressed daily for the first three or four days and the cornea inspected. The cornea is kept well lubricated with ointment. Generally the lid is edematous and droops, hence the Frost suture may be removed after the second or third day. If silk has been used, the sutures come out on the sixth day. If the cornea is clear the eye is left open and 1 per cent methyl cellulose drops or a bland ointment is exhibited every four hours. The cornea is watched closely for signs of keratitis.

It is remarkable how few corneas give trouble. In most cases the immediate postoperative period is passed without signs of irritation and the cornea accepts its newly exposed status without incident. Medication is gradually tapered off and then discontinued.

Comment: When initially resecting the skin triangles to each side of the skin strap it is best to err on the side of conservatism. If the triangles are too small a little more skin may always be resected to correct the overlap. However, if too much is resected the lid will be narrowed and the lid fold will be practically nonexistent. The vertical skin scars are somewhat slow in fading out but ultimately do. The author's procedure (fig. 216) gives a much better lid fold than this procedure.

Reese Orbicularis Sling—Modified

In 1924 Reese improved Darier's original orbicularis strip procedure. This operation has more or less gone out of style but may still be useful in selected cases. The technic has been modified here further by using longer and thicker pedicles thus reducing recurrences. In modified form the Reese procedure seems to be the simplest and best orbicularis sling.

Procedure (fig. 218):   After suitable anesthesia, a horizontal skin incision is made 6 mm. above the lid margin from canthus to canthus. The skin is undermined upward and downward to expose a 10 mm. wide strip of orbicularis along the whole length of the lid. Horizontal incisions are made in the exposed orbicularis to form two pedicles and the flaps are dissected up leaving a 5mm. central portion undisturbed. Sutures of 5–0 silk are passed through the ends of the pedicles and the needles cut off (fig. 218*A*).

The upper lip of the skin-muscle wound is picked up and the whole central portion of the lid is undermined upward almost to the brow (fig. 218*B*). A deep bite is taken with a stout 3–0 or 4–0 double-armed silk suture in the muscle strip and tarsus where it remains attached centrally. The needles are passed up behind the orbicularis then through the muscles of the brow to emerge a couple of millimeters above the center of the brow. They are left untied (fig. 218*C*).

About 12–15 mm. medial to the emerging suture above the medial end of the brow, a Reese ptosis knife is entered. The instrument is pointed centrally at an angle of about 45° and the skin and muscle are penetrated. The knife is passed behind the orbicularis with movements from side to side to create an ample tunnel for the drawing up of the pedicle. When the fenestrated end of the knife emerges, the suture of the medial pedicle is threaded through and the pedicle is drawn up. The same procedure is carried out with the lateral pedicle (fig. 218*D*).

The central suture is now drawn up and tightened so that the lid margin lies in the desired position—usually just above the upper limbus. It rarely fails to sag a little hence overcorrection is desirable. The suture is tied over a rubber peg (fig. 218*E*). The medial muscle flap is now tautened so that the end lies in the wound. It is fixed into position by means of a subcuticular 5–0 chromic suture. The skin is closed with 5–0 silk. The lateral muscle flap is tightened and sutured similarly.

The skin incisions are closed with 5–0 interrupted silk sutures or 5–0 plain catgut sutures in the case of a child (fig. 218*F*). A Frost suture is passed through the lower lid over a peg, the lid is drawn up over the cornea and the suture is fastened to the brow with adhesive.

Comment: Formerly I used this procedure rather frequently. But after several years, too large a percentage of the lids began to droop again. Recently I have not used muscle slings.

When and if used, care must be taken to make the muscle flaps at least 8–10 mm. wide. They dry out and fray at the ends and, if too narrow, are useless as pedicles because they are too weak to bear the weight of the lid. Darier must have discovered this very early. Although Reese made his muscle pedicles 6 mm. wide, this is still not enough. They should also be made long enough so that they do not have to be pulled too

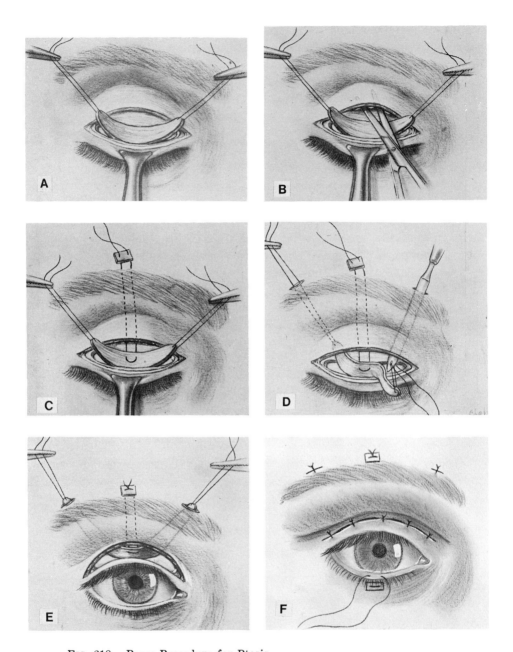

FIG. 218.   Reese Procedure for Ptosis.
A. The skin is incised and undermined upward and downward and two flaps of
    orbicularis muscle are raised.
B. The skin and muscle above are undermined.
C. The central suture is placed.
D. The lateral flaps are drawn up.
E. The brow sutures are tied.
F. The lid incision is closed.

hard to emerge above the brow. Wisely, Reese used a stout central suture to increase the effect of the sling.

Overcorrection is mandatory and the lid should be pulled up until further tension would cause tenting. Postoperative lagophthalmos is of rather short duration—much less so than with skin or fascia flaps; probably because the lid sags sooner.

Complications of Frontalis Sling Surgery

The frontalis sling procedure has advantages and disadvantages vis-a-vis levator surgery. The main advantage is that it is a much simpler technic. The main disadvantage is that it substitutes other physiologic defects for the ptosis. Levator resection at best results in a normal eyelid. Frontalis sling repair at best results in a raised lid which is far from normal.

Some of the postoperative complications of frontalis sling repair— and this applies to any of the acceptable technics—are inherent in this modality and are unavoidable. It makes no difference whether skin, orbicularis, fascia, muscle tendon, metal wires or other alloplastic material is used for the sling; the inherent complications are irremediable. Other complications, however, are avoidable as experience is gained. I have encountered enough of these to be able to discuss them with feeling and some authority.

Unavoidable (Intrinsic) Complications

The complications which must follow frontalis sling surgery are:
PTOSIS ON LOOKING UP. In the normal eye the width of the palpebral fissure increases on looking up and decreases on looking down. With a frontalis sling the reverse is true. Since at best, frontalis action is a poor replacement for levator action, upward movement of lid and globe are not synchronous. In the average case with normal superior rectus action, globe elevation is much superior to lid elevation hence the globe moves up behind the poorer moving lid in upward gaze. A mechanical ptosis results.

LID LAG ON LOOKING DOWN. Since the upper lid is fastened to the brow it cannot follow the full movement of the globe in downward gaze. The result is an obvious lid lag which is a cosmetic blemish but not a serious pathologic defect. This defect is much more apparent in monocular cases and is one of the cosmetic (not functional) objections to unilateral sling surgery. As a matter of fact, Beard has argued for a *bilateral* sling operation in *monocular* congenital ptosis where public appearance is important. He feels, and justly so, that such a procedure gives two abnormal eyelids which, however, are presentable in appearance and move synchronously, and that the postoperative state is more pleasing cosmetically than "the result obtained by unilateral maximum levator resection or unilateral brow suspension." However true, the necessity for such a drastic move must be overwhelming indeed and must override all normal considerations. No one should undertake lightly the conversion of a normal lid into a cripple.

Cosmetically, lid lag is the most serious of the unavoidable postoperative complications. It is sometimes possible to teach a patient to bend the head instead of turning the eyes when looking down. It is not easy to break a longstanding habit. But in the case of a strongly motivated person, such as a public performer, it may be possible. If so, it will take a good deal of the curse off a frontalis sling operation and make it far more acceptable.

LAGOPHTHALMOS OR FAILURE TO CLOSE THE EYES IN SLEEP.   (Not to be confused with lid lag.) The average patient with a frontalis sling has little difficulty with voluntary lid closure. This is especially true when autogenous fascia is used. However, most patients have some degree of lagophthalmos in sleep. The eye may roll up sufficiently for corneal coverage but exposure of the lower sclera is common. However, I have rarely experienced any difficulty as a result of this somnific lagophthalmos.

ARCHING AND WRINKLING OF THE BROW.   Elevation of the lid is of course attained by upward arching and wrinkling of the brow to a greater or lesser extent. The physiologic defect here is a double one for even with sufficient elevation the resultant lid movement is not normal. The action of the levator has been wrongly compared to that of a window blind. It is not. The levator because of its origin pulls the lid *up and back* thus deepening the physiologic lid fold; the frontalis simply pulls the lid straight up. Hence, it is one of the important unavoidable defects of frontalis sling action. On the other hand, in the straight-ahead position the cosmetic effect is usually good. Winking and blinking are also impeded by the sling.

Avoidable Complications

The avoidable complications are those which can usually be eliminated by experience and the employment of proper materials and technics.

UNDERCORRECTION.   This is the most common postoperative complication. It is usually due to failure to pull the lid up sufficiently high. It is also caused by not allowing for a certain amount of subsequent sag of the lid which always occurs. There is a fairly generalized belief that healing causes some cicatrization and consequent raising of the lid. I have never seen this happen. Usually there is a tendency to subsequent droop, hence the precautions taken in the technic to prevent this.

Another important cause of undercorrection is misjudging the position of the globe and raising the lid margin to the upper limbus of a globe which is too low. Since the operation is frequently done under general anesthesia this is not a difficult mistake to make. Use of too easily absorbable material is another cause. Some loosening of the knot when nonabsorbable material is used is a rarer complication. The undercorrection may be so slight as to be cosmetically acceptable. If too much occurs, the only recourse is reoperation.

Experience has shown that the best results are obtained when the lid is raised to a point beyond which subsequent tightening of the sling results in notching. Thus, one can avoid dependence on the untrustworthy position of the globe. This has never produced an overcorrection in my hands and has given me the most consistently good results.

OVERCORRECTION. This is not as common as undercorrection. It results from tightening the sling too much due to overestimation of subsequent lid droop. Another cause is adapting the margin of the ptotic lid to a globe which has rolled up too high. Correction of this defect is not simple and may be more difficult than the original operation since one must isolate and loosen the sling if possible. The sling is not always identifiable and then one must loosen the subcuticular tissues sufficiently to allow the lid to drop down. As in the case of levator overcorrection, this is not always an easy matter. Overcorrection is best avoided by following the suggestion for height adjustment already given.

NOTCHING OR TENTING. This always means overcorrection. If a single sling is used this should be taken care of on the operating table by loosening the sling knot until the notch disappears. If two or three vertical fascial strips are used, tenting is caused by one being pulled up too high. This should be immediately released to regularize the lid curve. Correcting a notch postoperatively may be as difficult as repair of total overcorrection. Curiously enough a certain percentage of notches tend to straighten out in time and may disappear. However, this takes a long time, or the notch may never straighten out completely.

TRUE LAGOPHTHALMOS. Inability to close the eye voluntarily can also be due to overcorrection. This happens more commonly with the use of wires and sutures than with the use of autogenous fascia. If it persists, reoperation will have to be done. (Incidentally, this points up one of the important objections to levator surgery in the presence of an inactive levator. The question is often asked, "Since the lid must be hung up anyway, why not do it by means of a shortened levator?" The answer is that if an inactive levator is shortened enough to correct ptosis, voluntary closure is abolished and lagophthalmos results—the same as in overcorrection with a frontalis sling.)

RECURRENCE. This is always possible. Suture knots can and do come completely untied, necessitating reoperation. The use of absorbable materials, such as collagen and preserved fascia, has given me a high recurrence rate. It dropped to almost nil when I went back to autogenous fascia. The type of technic used has had little effect on my recurrence rate.

Rupture of the sling with recurrence, especially if a silk suture is used, is rare but has occurred. An uncommon cause of recurrence is when the fascial sling taken is too short and two lengths have to be sewed together. The suture may give way and the sling along with it. It is wiser to go back and take a fascial strip of adequate length. I know because it happened to me.

ECTROPION.   A pulling away of the lid margin from contact with the globe is rare. It most commonly occurs in cases in which the eye is deep-set and the plane of the frontalis is a good deal anterior to the lid and globe. Here also, too much tightening of the sling will result in the lid standing away from the globe even though it is in normal position otherwise. Unless this is severe, it is not too obvious a defect and usually only of slight cosmetic importance.

EXPOSURE KERATITIS.   This is remarkably rare. One would expect corneas which are uncovered for the first time after many years to be highly susceptible to the hazards of exposure and infection. This has not been my experience. It has been many years since I have encountered an exposure keratitis after ptosis surgery. However, once it occurs, it requires long and careful nursing with proper medication and protection of the cornea day and night. It can be troublesome indeed. Therefore the rare cases which show vertical muscle palsies or absence of Bell's phenomenon should not have frontalis sling surgery. This is asking for trouble.

CHRONIC EDEMA.   Edema of the lid was seen most frequently when I was using wire for the sling. This sometimes proved so intractable that the sling had to be undone and the wire removed. While this did not occur often it was enough of a nuisance to cause me to abandon all kinds of wire for slings.

INFECTION.   Acute primary infection is rare and I do not recall a case. However, secondary or delayed infection with some of the newer allopathic materials has been reported. Almost every conceivable material has been used in frontails sling surgery. Many, such as gold chain, kangaroo tendon and others, have long been abandoned and fortunately are one with Nineveh and Tyre. Newer materials, such as methyl methacrylate, Supramid, Silastic and other allopaths, have recently come to the fore. I have tried most of them and have abandoned them. Secondary infections with these may be low grade but are sometimes so persistent as to require removal of the sling.

At first glance it would seem that the complications already listed are similar to those encountered with levator surgery. Certainly overzealous-

ness will give overcorrection and carelessness undercorrection with both
modalities. And infection, that handmaiden of misfortune, may affect
any ptosis operation. The differences, however, are as basic as the
variance in the technics. In levator surgery almost all complications are
preventable; in frontalis sling surgery mechanical ptosis, lid lag and
lagophthalmos are inevitable. Indeed, unless they are produced the operation is a failure. Because of this inevitability of some of the complications I have, over the years, tried and discarded many technics and
materials and have thus at least reduced the preventable complications.

Use of the Superior Rectus

Use of the lifting power of the superior rectus to replace an inactive
levator was suggested first by Motais and then by Parinaud in 1897. This
modality is now falling into disuse and it is not hard to understand why.

The Motais technic uses a thin tongue of muscle fashioned from the
central third of the superior rectus, which is sutured to the tarsus. The
modifications which followed—notably those by Shoemaker and Kirby—
do not change this essentially. It has two serious faults: 1. The thin
friable muscle strip often pulls away from its insertion to the tarsus.
Resuturing it may or may not help and frequent manipulation does not
do the integrity of the anemic muscle strip much good. 2. In many of
the cases in which the muscle strip remains firmly attached to the tarsus,
notching of the upper lid occurs due to the narrow point of attachment.

In the Parinaud technic, with its numerous modifications, in which
there is a broad adhesion between the intact superior rectus and the
tarsus, the superior rectus may also pull away from its tarsal attachment,
but this happens relatively less frequently and there is less tendency
toward central notch formation. Hence any technic which creates a
strong broad adhesion between the superior rectus and the tarsus would
seem preferable.

But other objections remain and are inherent in all procedures
which transfer the function of the levator to the superior rectus, whether
the full superior rectus or only a strip of it is used:

1. Hypotropia and diplopia develop in well over half of the cases
due to the drag of the lid on the eyeball. For this reason Spaeth states
that superior rectus surgery is only indicated in bilateral congenital
ptosis and there is a good deal to be said for this opinion. While the
hypotropia and diplopia are sometimes overcome, or vision is sufficiently
suppressed by patients to attain a modicum of comfort, others find the
condition unbearable and the operation must be undone. Obviously the
ideal case for monocular superior rectus surgery is the one in which an
amblyopia or amaurosis exists, or in which there is at least complete
absence of the fusion faculty to facilitate suppression.

2. Lagophthalmos, with exposure of the cornea especially during sleep, is a common concomitant of superior rectus surgery since the lid margin is located permanently at the upper limbus and moves with the eyeball. The patient must be tided over the first three or four weeks or even longer by frequent instillations of mineral oil, methyl cellulose or other medicaments during the day, and patching at night since Bell's phenomenon does not help much here. Keratitis is not common but is more frequent than in frontalis surgery.

3. Interference with normal winking and blinking is another result and may also lead to drying out of the cornea.

The advantages of this procedure are that in successful cases the upper lid is in normal position and moves synchronously with the globe. Another advantage is that a good lid fold with natural curvature is created if notching is avoided.

Trainor Technic (Modified)

In the rare cases when superior rectus surgery seems desirable the simple technic described by Trainor in 1935 has been found useful. This is a slight modification of the operation described by Nida in 1928. Trainor fuses the upper lid to the superior rectus by means of a strip of tarsus taken from the upper tarsal border which is slipped under the superior rectus muscle. The rationale is similar to the Jameson procedure reported in 1937.

Procedure (fig. 219): Several drops of 0.5 per cent tetracaine are instilled into the conjunctival sac. The upper lid is everted and a solution of 2 per cent procaine with epinephrine is used to balloon out the retrotarsal fold of conjunctiva. A few drops are also injected into the superior rectus muscle. A strip of tarsoconjunctiva 3 mm. wide is fashioned at the upper border of the tarsus by making two horizontal incisions opposite the insertion of the superior rectus muscle and freeing the strip at one end (fig. 219A). This is undermined leaving the other end attached. The strip of tarsoconjunctiva should not be more than one and one half times as long as the width of the superior rectus muscle with their centers coinciding.

A speculum is slipped under the lids and the eye is rotated downward by means of a 4–0 silk suture passed through the limbus at 12 o'clock or some similar device. The insertion of the superior rectus is exposed and the conjunctiva cleared away from the tendon in order to permit the tarsoconjunctival strip to be slipped under it (fig. 219B).

The speculum is removed and a small mosquito clamp is passed under the superior rectus muscle toward the attached end of the tarsal strip. The free end of the strip is grasped (fig. 219C), pulled under the muscle and sutured firmly into its original position so that the surfaces

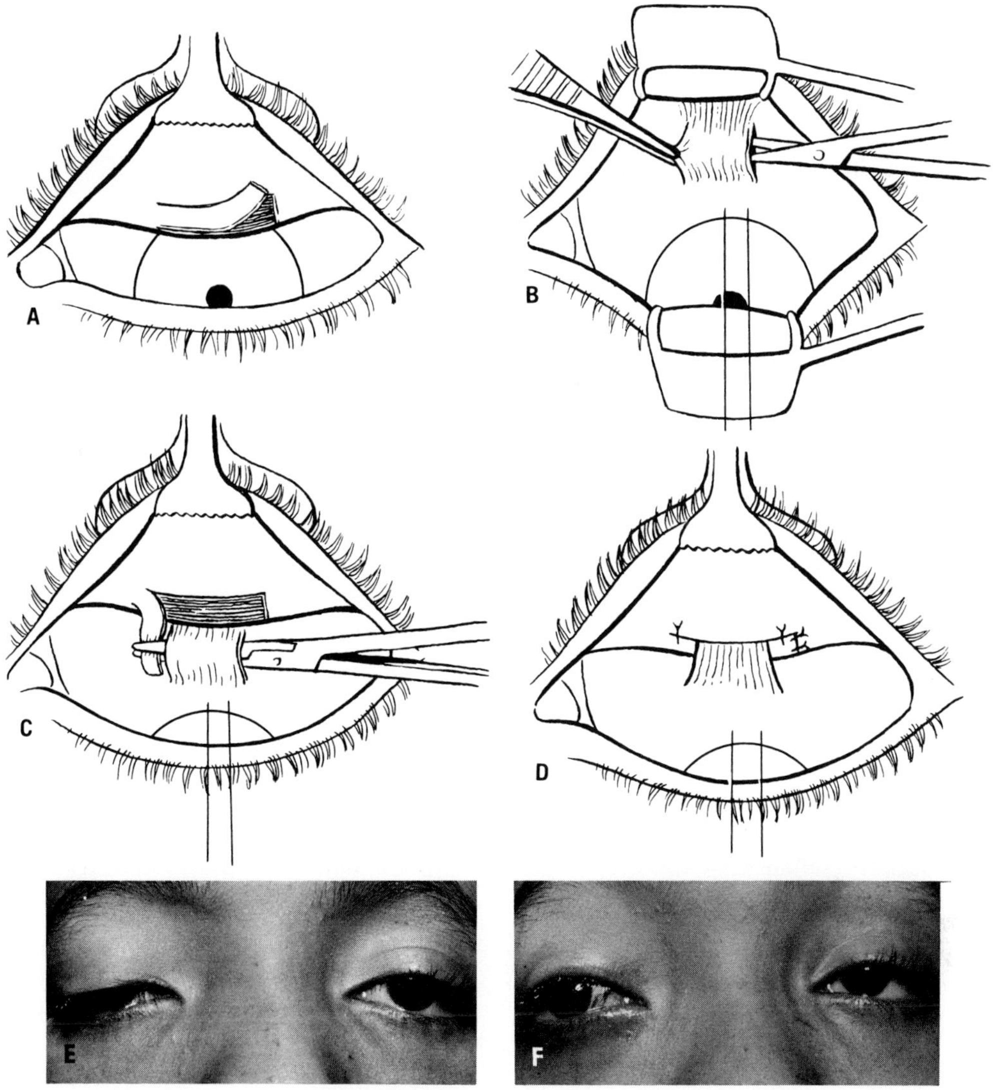

FIG. 219.   Trainor Procedure for Ptosis.
A.   The lid is everted and a narrow horizontal flap of tarsoconjunctiva is **raised** at the attached tarsal border.
B.   The superior rectus muscle is exposed.
C.   The tarsal flap is drawn under the rectus muscle.
D.   The flap is centered and sutured into position.
E. and F.   A case of complete congenital ptosis before and after repair.

coincide and the strip is in its normal position when the lid is reinverted (fig. 219D). Figures 219E and F show a case of complete congenital ptosis before and after correction.

It is necessary to adjust the lid so that the hammock is swung in the exact center else the lid will sag to one side and will heal in poor position. This is difficult to adjust later without unfastening the strip and doing the operation over. If necessary, additional sutures should be added between the strip and muscle at each end to assure that the strip stays in good position. The conjunctiva around the superior rectus muscle need not be sutured.

Comment: The chief complication is entropion which may develop during the first postoperative week. The reason for this is not obvious but it is probably due to a relative shortening of the tarsoconjunctival lamina by the incision and displacement of part of the tarsus. Adhesive strips or eversion of the cilia with collodion may be tried but experience has shown that unless the response to these conservative measures occurs rapidly it is useless to wait. One must then resect a horizontal strip of skin and muscle from the upper lid in order to counteract the entropion. This is usually quite successful since it restores the widths of the two lid laminae relative to each other.

A second possible complication is a sagging of the whole upper lid as a result of too loose a tarsal sling. This happens when the tarsal strap is cut too long allowing for a lax hammock which the weight of the lid drags down. In this case the strip must be exposed and sutured to the tarsus and to the ends of the superior rectus muscle to take up the slack.

The tarsal sutures to each side of the superior rectus muscle should be fairly close to the muscle otherwise the tarsal strip will bend and sag and the lid will come down too low as indicated; on the other hand, they must clear the muscle enough so that when the lid is reinverted it does so without difficulty. If the tarsal strip is too narrow, and in the rare instances when this operation is done in an elderly individual with a thinned, atonic tarsus, the strip may tear. In this case another type of procedure must be done.

This is a simple procedure which also offers the advantage of easy reversibility if necessary. It is worth trying in the rare cases where superior rectus surgery is indicated.

COMPLICATED CONGENITAL PTOSIS

About 20–25 per cent of all congenital ptosis cases are complicated by ophthalmoplegias or other congenital anomalies.

Ptosis with Ophthalmoplegia

This is the largest group in this category. The most common muscle involvement is the superior rectus which has a common embryonic origin with the levator (Chap. 1). However, all types and varieties of extraocular muscle involvement may appear including complete third nerve palsy. As a general rule, it is best to attempt to get orthophoria first, especially in vertical deviations, before the ptosis is corrected. This will help to gauge the relative position of the lids for the ptosis repair.

Ptosis with Other Anomalies

A smaller group of congenital ptosis cases, probably less than 3 per cent—are complicated by such anomalies as epicanthus, phimosis and telecanthus (widening of the medial intercanthal distance). The mongoloid syndrome is the most common and frequently shows all of these anomalies. The best procedure here is to repair all other anomalies first and the ptosis last. These procedures are described in Chapter 18. The ptosis is frequently complete and some type of frontalis suspension is usually required.

Synkinetic (Paradoxical) Ptosis

This is a small group of complicated congenital ptoses including synkinetic, periodic and intermittent cases all of which are uncommon. The best known is the pterygoid-levator synkinesis (Marcus Gunn syndrome). In this condition there is a ptosis of the lid when at rest and a retraction above the level of the opposite lid when the mouth is opened. In many cases the lid also retracts when the jaw is moved away from the ptotic lid and droops when moved toward it. It is always unilateral. The jaw-winking tends to grow less as Gunn himself pointed out in his original article, hence repair should be postponed as long as possible.

There are other rare forms such as reverse jaw-winking (the phenomenon of Marin Amat) in which the upper lid droops with movements of mastication. Raising and lowering of the upper lid on horizontal movement of the opposite lid and raising of the upper lid of one eye on downward movement of the other eye also occur.

COMPLICATED ACQUIRED PTOSIS

Traumatic Ptosis

Such cases are due to direct or indirect injury to the levator or its nerve connections by cuts, concussion and hemorrhage involving the nerve or nerve centers. Operative trauma due to removal of orbital tumors, surgery of the superior rectus and even cataract extraction have been known to produce ptosis.

The one important thing to remember about acquired ptoses—and this is especially true of the traumatic type—is that they are easily subject to overcorrection. Hence levator resection, which is the usual operation in these cases, should be done very conservatively with some undercorrection. This is a place where the Fasanella and Servat procedure may be used to good advantage.

Although these ptoses rarely require anything but levator surgery they are placed in this complicated category because they are frequently self-correcting and therefore require special handling. They have been

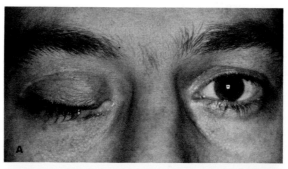

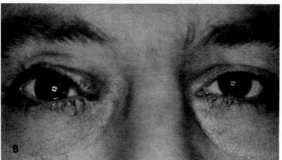

FIG. 220.   Traumatic Ptosis Repair.
A.   Traumatic ptosis of right upper lid.
B.   Repair by anterior levator resection.

known to start improving sometime after the injury and have sometimes gone on to complete recovery. Hence no repair of traumtic ptosis should be done for at least a year or until six months have elapsed with no obvious improvement. Figures 220*A* and *B* show the result of an 8 mm. levator resection of what appears to be a complete ptosis. This was a traumatic ptosis due to injury with a pitchfork. Fortunately the eye escaped uninjured.

Senile Ptosis

This type of ptosis is a phenomenon of the aging process probably due to loss of general muscle tonus including the levators. It is almost always bilateral (fig. 221*A*) and may be of any degree though not always identical in both eyes. It may be a manifestation of localized congenital weakness which manifests itself in early and adult life by a drooping of the lid when the patient is tired at the end of the day. Later it becomes a frank ptosis.

Here also, as in all acquired ptoses, overcorrection is easy and should be guarded against by aiming for some undercorrection (fig. 221*B*).

Myogenic and Neurogenic Ptosis

Acquired myogenic ptosis is rare. A typical example is myasthenia gravis which is characterized by muscular weakness and fatiguability due

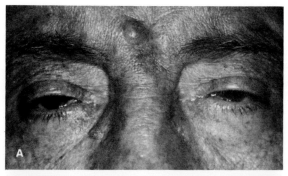

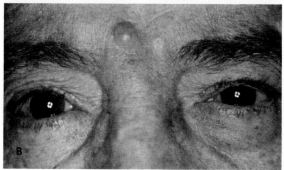

Fɪɢ. 221.   Senile Ptosis Repair.
A.   Bilateral senile ptosis.
B.   Repair by levator resection.

to failure in transmission of nerve impulses across the myoneural junction. Frenkel found that ocular signs are present in 55 per cent of all
cases of myasthenia gravis of which ptosis is the most common. As is
well known it is improved by Tensilon (edrophonium chloride) and
prostigmine (neostygmine bromide).

Hereditary myogenic ptosis is typified by progressive external
ocular myopathy (progressive external ophthalmoplegia). This is a
diagnosis, sometimes missed. The condition is characterized by bilateral
ptosis with or without ophthalmoplegia of one, some or all the extraocular muscles of one or both eyes. It may appear early in childhood but
most commonly the onset is in the second decade of life. In at least
half the cases a familial history of one or more members having the same
disease is ascertainable. The pattern of inheritance is autosomal and
dominant. Histologic and electromyographic evidence points over-
whelmingly to muscular dystrophy as the cause of progressive external
ocular myopathy.

Such eyes and their corneae seem to be especially vulnerable to
exposure hence even when there is a good Bell's phenomenon the patient
should be warned that complete surgical repair of the ptosis will not be
done.

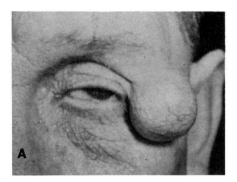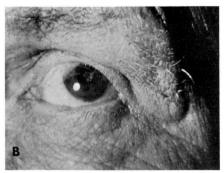

Fig. 222.   Pseudoptosis due to Plexiform Neuroma.
A.   Upper lid pulled down by weight of tumor.
B.   Tumor resected and lid in normal position.

PSEUDOPTOSIS

The conditions described under this heading are those in which the ptosis is not the result of levator malfunction and in which the ptosis may be correctible by removal of the causative factor.

Pseudoptosis Due to Globe Displacement

Backward displacement of the globe decreases support to the upper lid and may be due to long-standing anophthalmos, enophthalmos, microphthalmos and phthisis bulbi. In long-existing cases there is a paresis of the levator due to nonuse and an actual levator resection may have to be done.

Pseudotosis Due to Lid Displacement

Inflammations, tumors or scar tissue may produce a mechanical ptosis. The ptosis of trachoma is much less common than it used to be and requires a tarsal resection and mucosal grafting to prevent entropion of the upper lid. Mechanical ptosis due to weighing down by tumors or binding down by scar tissue must be corrected by surgery. (Figs. 222*A* and *B* show a lid pulled down by plexiform neuroma and the correction.)

CONDITIONS SIMULATING PTOSIS

Dermachalasis and Blepharochalasis

Dermachalasis (Senile Skin Atrophy; Baggy Lids) is a condition which may be mistaken for ptosis. Blepharochalasis is an inflammatory condition of the lids which is sometimes mistaken for ptosis. Both conditions are discused in Chapter 19.

Oriental Palpebral Fissure

The Oriental palpebral fissure is narrower than that of the white and black races and the upper lid rarely has a furrow; hence the lid fold usually hangs down to or over the lid margin. Such a lid gives the appearance of ptosis because of its pudgy appearance and the absence of a fold. The handling of this condition is discussed in the chapter on Congenital Anomalies (Chapter 18).

REFERENCES

ANGELUCCI, A.: Levator resection. Thirteenth Int. Cong. Med., Paris, 1900.

BEARD, C.: Ptosis with jaw-winking. Am. J. Ophth. *59*:252, 1965.

BERKE, R. N.: Congenital ptosis: Classification of two hundred cases. Arch. Ophth. *41*:188, 1949.

————: An operation for ptosis utilizing the superior rectus muscle. Arch. Ophth. *42*:685, 1949.

————: A simplified Blaskovics operation for blepharoptosis. Arch. Ophth. *48*:460, 1952.

————: Results of resection of the levator muscle through a skin incision in congenital ptosis. Arch. Ophth. *61*:177, 1959.

————: The surgical treatment of jaw-winking ptosis. Trans. Ophth. Soc. Austr. *25*:69, 1966.

————, and WADSWORTH, J. A. C.: Histology of levator muscle in congenital and acquired ptosis. Arch. Ophth. *53*:413, 1955.

BISHOP, J.: Cited by Beard, C. H., Ophthalmic Surgery, ed. 2. Philadelphia, P. Blakiston's Son & Co., 1914, p. 234.

BLASKOVICS, L.: A new operation for ptosis with shortening of the levator and tarsus. Arch. Ophth. *52*:563, 1923.

————: Treatment of ptosis. Arch. Ophth., *1*:672, 1929.

BODIAN, M.: Repair of ptosis using human sclera. Am. J. Ophth. *65*:352, 1968.

BOWMAN, W. P.: Report of the chief operations performed at the Royal London Ophthalmic Hospital for the quarter ending Sept., 1857. Ophth. Hosp. Rep. and J. Royal Lond. Ophth. Hosp. 1857–1859, vol. 1, p. 34.

CALLAHAN, A.: Levator recession with reattachment to the tarsus with collagen film. Arch. Ophth. *73*:800, 1965.

CARBAJAL, V. M.: Surgery of ptosis associated with jaw-winking. Am. J. Ophth., *47*:352, 1959.

CRAWFORD, J. S.: Repair of ptosis using frontalis muscle and fascia lata. Trans. Amer. Acad. Ophthal. Otolaryng. *60*:672, 1956.

DARIER, A.: Operation du ptosis complet par autoplastie du greffe musculaire. Ann. d'ocul. *118*:93, 1897.

DERBY, G. S.: Correction of ptosis by fascia lata hammock. Am. J. Ophth. *11*:352, 1928.

DICKEY, C. A.: A superior rectus fascia lata sling in correction of ptosis. Am. J. Ophth. *19*:660, 1936.

DIMITRY, T. J.: Hereditary ptosis. Am. J. Ophth. *4*:655, 1921.

DRANSART, H. N.: Deep palpebrofrontal ligatures for ptosis. Ann. d'ocul. *84*:88, 1880.

ETZINE, S.: Congenital ptosis with paradoxic eyelid movements. Am. J. Ophth. *61*:793, 1966.

EVERBUSH, O.: Zur operation der congenitalen Blepharoptosis. Klin. Monatsbl. Augenh. *21*:100, 1883.

FALLS, H. F., SLOAN, D. B., Jr., and BRYSON, J. M.: Clinical use of cobalt irradiated fascia lata. Am. J. Ophth., *64*:426 (Pt. 1), 1967.

FASANELLA, R. M., and SERVANT, J.: Levator resection for minimal ptosis. Another simplified operation. Arch. Ophth. *65*:493, 1961.

FERGUS, F.: An easy operation for congenital ptosis. Brit. Med. J., *1*:762, 1901.

Fox, S. A.: Ptosis with elephantiasis and ectropion. Am. J. Ophth. *33*:1144, 1950.
_____: Postoperative complications of levator surgery. Arch. Ophth. *65*:345, 1961.
_____: Complications of frontalis sling surgery. Am. J. Ophth. *63*:758, 1967.
_____: A new frontalis skin sling. Am. J. Ophth., *65*:359, 1968.
_____: Congenital ptosis: Levator resection. J. Ped. Ophth. *1*:26, 1964.
_____: Congenital ptosis: Frontalis sling. J. Ped. Ophth. *3*:25, 1966.
Frenkel, M.: Myasthenia gravis: Current trends. Am. J. Ophth. *61*:522, 1966.
Friedenwald, J. S., and Guyton, J. S.: A simple ptosis operation. Am. J. Ophth. *31*:411, 1948.
Frost, A. D.: Supportive suture in ptosis surgery. Am. J. Ophth. *17*:1633, 1934.
Gifford, S. R., and Puntenny, I.: Modification of the Dickey operation for ptosis. Arch. Ophth. *28*:814, 1942.
von Graefe, F. W. E. A.: Cited by Beard, C. H., op. cit., p. 231.
de Grandemont, G.: Nouvelle operation du ptosis congenital. Bull. et. mem. Soc. franc. d'opht. *9*:80, 1891.
Greeves, R. A.: Operation for relief of congenital ptosis. Proc. Roy. Soc. Med. *26*:1478, 1933.
Gunn, R. M.: Congenital ptosis with peculiar associated movements of the affected lids. Trans. Ophth. Soc. U. K. *3*:283, 1883.
Henderson, J. W.: Tarsal-periosteal-frontalis sutures for the correction of palpebral ptosis. Trans. A.A.O.O., *61*:701, 1957.
Hess, C.: Eine operation methode gegen ptosis. Arch. f. Augenh. *28*:22, 1893–1894.
Hildreth, R. H.: Insertion of levator palpebrae muscle. Am. J. Ophth. *24*:749, 1941.
Hunt, R. T.: On the treatment of ptosis by operation. London Med. Gaz. *7*:361, 1831.
Iliff, C. E.: A simplified ptosis operation. Am. J. Ophth. *37*:529, 1954.
_____: Surgical management of ptosis. Ethicon. Somerville. 1963.
_____, et al.: Symposium: Ptosis complications. Tr. A.A.O.O. *63*:663, 1959.
Jameson, R. C.: Surgical management of ptosis with special reference to use of the superior rectus muscle. Arch. Ophth. *18*:547, 1937.
Johnson, C. C.: Blepharoptosis. Am. J. Ophth. *38*:129, 1954.
_____: Blepharoptosis. Arch. Ophth. *66*:793, 1961.
_____: Blepharoptosis. Arch. Ophth. *67*:18, 1962.
Jones, L. T.: Anatomy of the upper eyelid. Am. J. Ophth. *57*:943, 1964.
Kestenbaum, A.: Panel discussion: Ocular physiology in clinical practice. Am. J. Ophth. *51*:161, 1961.
Kirby, D. B.: A modified Motais operation for blepharoptosis. Arch. Ophth. *57*:327, 1928.
Koster, W.: Cited by Spaeth, E. B., Principles and Practice of Ophthalmic Surgery. Philadelphia, Lea & Febiger, 1944, p. 388.
Lancaster, W. B.: Discussion of the Reese operation. Arch. Ophth. *53*:26, 1924.
de Lapersonne, F.: Sur quelques modifications dans les operations du ptosis. Arch. d'opht. *1*:497, 1903.
Leahy, B. D.: Simplified ptosis surgery. Arch. Ophth. *50*:588, 1953.
Machek, P.: An operation for ptosis with the formation of a fold in the upper lid. Arch. Ophth. *44*:539, 1915.
Marin, Amat, M.: Sur le syndrome ou phenomena de Marcus Gunn. Ann. d'ocul. *156*: 513, 1919.
McCord, C. D.: Correction of minimal blepharoptosis. Am. J. Ophth. *67*:957, 1969.
Millard, D. R., Jr.: Oriental peregrinations. Plast. & Recons. Surg. *16*:319, 1955.
Motais, M.: Operation du ptosis par la greffe tarsienne d'une languette du tendon du muscle droit superieur. Ann. d'ocul. *118*:5, 1897.
_____: Etat actuel de la methode operatoire du ptosis par la suppleance du muscle droit superieur. Bull. Acad. de med. (Paris) *49*:430, 1903.

NIDA, M.: Ptose congenital opére par un noveau procédé. Bull. Soc. Ophthal. (Paris) *10*:566, 1928.

PAGENSTECHER, A.: Cited by Fuchs, E., Textbook of Ophthalmology. Philadelphia, J. B. Lippincott Co., 1917, p. 964.

PANAS, P.: Blepharopexie. Maladies des yeux. *11*:140, 1894.

PARINAUD, H.: Nouveau procédé operatoire du ptosis. Ann. d'ocul. *118*:13, 1897.

PANG, H. G.: Surgical formation of upper lid fold. Arch. Ophth. *65*:783, 1961.

PAYR, E.: Plastik Mittels frier Faszien Transplantation bei Ptosis. Deutsch. Med. Wchnschr. *35*:822, 1909.

PERETZ, W. L.: Tarsal sling surgery for ptosis. Am. J. Ophth. *56*:278, 1963.

REESE, R. G.: An operation for blepharoptosis with the formation of a fold in the lid. Arch. Ophth. *53*:26, 1924.

ROBERTS, J. B.: A new "muscle substitution" operation for congenital palpebral ptosis. Ophth. Record. *25*:397, 1916.

RYCROFT, P. V.: The complications and results of ptosis surgery. Trans. Ophth. Soc. U. K. *87*:291, 1967.

SAYOC, B. T.: An improved ptosis operation. Am. J. Ophth. *48*:392, 1959.

SCHIMEK, R. A., and CUSACK, P. L.: Evaluation of a modified Blaskovics operation (Iliff technique) for blepharoptosis. Am. J. Ophth. *46*:819, 1958.

SCHULTZ, R. O., and BURIAN, H. M.: Bilateral jaw winking reflex associated with multiple congenital anomalies. Arch. Ophth. *64*:946, 1960.

SHOEMAKER, W. T.: Observations on the Motais operation for ptosis. Ann. Ophth. *61*:608, 1907.

SIMPSON, D. G.: Marcus Gunn phenomenon following squint and ptosis surgery. Arch. Ophth. *56*:743, 1956.

SNELLEN, H.: Levator tendon shortening for ptosis. Heidelberg, Report German Ophth. Soc., 1883.

SPAETH, E. B.: Blepharoptosis congenital and acquired. Tr. A.A.O.O. Mar.-Apr., 1946, p. 147.

SWAN, K. C., and KEIZER, J. P.: Levator advancement and resection without tarsectomy for blepharoptosis. Am. J. Ophth. *45*:229 (Pt. 2), 1958.

TAGGART, H. J.: Modification of Motais operation. Trans. Ophth. Soc. U. K. *53*:327, 1928.

TANSLEY, J. O.: A congenital ptosis case and operation. Tr. Am. Ophth. Soc. *7* (Part 2):427, 1894–1896.

TILLETT, C. W., and TILLETT, G. M.: Silicone sling in correction of ptosis. Am. J. Ophth. *62*: 521, 1966.

TRAINOR, M. E.: Operation for lid ptosis. Trans. Sec. Ophth. A.M.A. 1935, p. 93.

WARTENBERG, R.: Inverted Marcus Gunn phenomenon. Arch. Neur. Psych. *60*:584, 1948.

WHEELER, J. M.: Correction of ptosis by attachment of strips of orbicularis muscle to superior rectus. Trans. Sec. Ophth. A.M.A. 1938, p. 130.

WHITNALL, S. E: On a ligament acting as a check to the action of the levator palpebrae superiors. J. Anat. & Phys. *45*:131, 1911.

WIENER, M.: Surgical correction of ocular disfigurement. Surg. Gyn. & Obst. *58*:390, 1934.

WILDER, W. H.: Operation for ptosis. Annal. Ophth. & Oto. *7*:39, 1898.

YOUNG, G.: An operation for congenital ptosis. Brit. J. Ophth. *8*:212, 1924.

CHAPTER 18

Congenital Anomalies

MANY OF THE LESIONS discussed in previous chapters such as coloboma, ectropion, entropion and blepharophimosis have their replicas in the rare forms of developmental abnormalities. In addition there are congenital deformities of lid fissure, size, fold, margin, pigmentation, etc., ad. inf. Although all are rare, when taken in the aggregate congenital anomalies of the ocular adnexa are not uncommon. Such drugs as thalidomide, the maladministration of oxygen and diseases such as small-pox have not tended to reduce the incidence of congenital anomalies. As a matter of fact, it has been estimated that one person in 20 to 25 is born with a significant genetic defect, i.e., about 3 to 4 million of the estimated 80,000,000 born each year. This has become especially true in recent years with the death rate of the newborn steadily dropping due to advances in modern medicine and therapeutics. As a result many more congenital anomalies are being perpetuated than in former years.

Although many syndromes of abnormalities have been known for many years, it was only in 1959 that their relationship to chromosomal aberrations became recognized. For instance, it is now known that the 13–15 autosomal trisomy syndrome is the most important in ocular pathology. The science of genetics in the past few years has made tremendous strides and more chromosomes are beginning to yield their secrets. It is far from a forlorn hope that in the not so distant future these studies will help predict congenital anomalies and thus help in their prevention.

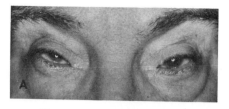 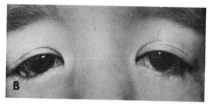

FIG. 223.   Palpebral Fissure Obliquity.

A. Mongoloid hyperobliquity.   *B.*   Antimongoloid obliquity.

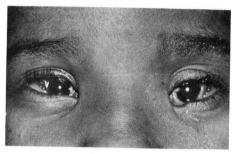

FIG. 224.   Bilateral Multiple Palpebral Fissure Anomalies.

ANOMALIES OF PALPEBRAL FISSURE OBLIQUITY

The normal Caucasian palpebral fissure slants slightly upward from the medial canthus with the lateral canthus being 1 to 2 mm. higher. The Mongolian fissure usually shows an exaggeration of this obliquity so that there appears to be a more definite upward and outward slant.

Anomalies of the palpebral fissure among Caucasians include mongoloid obliquity, i.e., an exaggeration of the acute slant upward and outward (fig. 223*A*) and antimongoloid obliquity with the fissure slanting downward and outward (fig. 223*B*). The causes of both these anomalies are obscure. They have been variously attributed to absence or malformation of the lateral canthal ligaments, as well as to malformation and malposition of the orbital bones.

Such cases are rare and are frequently associated with other anomalies. Thus the patient pictured in figure 223*A* also had blepharophimosis and microphthalmos. The patient pictured in figure 223*B* also had epiblepharon (fig. 237*A*) which was repaired but the antimongoloid obliquity was not a sufficient cosmetic blemish to warrant surgery. The patient pictured in figure 224 had not only hypermongoloid obliquity but phimosis, esotropia, entropion, colobomata and lacrimal stenosis. Thus where there is one anomaly, others may not be far behind.

DISPLACEMENT OF THE CANTHI—EURYBLEPHARON

Congenital lateral displacement of the medial canthi (telecanthus) occurs rarely as an isolated phenomenon. It is seen much more commonly

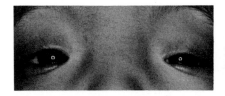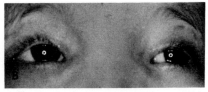

FIG. 225. Typical Mongoloid Syndrome.

A. Lateral displacement of medial canthi (telecanthus), epicanthus inversus, ptosis and blepharophimosis.

B. After correction. Note shortening of intercanthal space and exposure of caruncles.

as part of a mongoloid syndrome which includes ptosis, blepharophimosis and epicanthus inversus. While some cosmetic improvement may be obtained by a shortening of the medial canthal ligaments and repair of the other anomalies, it is almost impossible to restore these patients to normalcy. Figure 225B shows the child pictured in 225A after ptosis surgery, lateral canthoplasty, shortening of the internal canthal ligaments and epicanthus repair.

Congenital lateral displacement of the lateral canthi is even more rare than displacement of the medial canthi and only few cases have been reported. The condition was first described by Denig in 1894. The child pictured in figure 226A shows this condition with the right lateral canthus displaced outward much more than the left. It appears almost as if the skin of a normal outer canthus has been pulled outward strongly thus exposing the conjunctiva. Repair, when necessary, is usually accomplished by a lateral canthoplasty.

Euryblepharon is a related congenital syndrome first described by Desmarres in 1854 of which lateral canthal displacement is probably only a part. It is a symmetrical enlargement of the palpebral fissure with large eyelids (megaloblepharon) and, usually, some lateral ectropion.

A typical example of this is pictured in figure 226B. Repair (fig. 226C) was accomplished in two stages. In the first, lateral canthoplasties (fig. 121) were done to shorten the palpebral fissures. In the second stage the size of all four lids was reduced by resecting full thickness wedges of tissue apex up. It is difficult to eradicate all stigmata of the syndrome but certainly a great deal can be done to improve the apparance of the child.

Reports of the repair of such conditions appear occasionally. Most are rather complicated and include formation of new canthi by means of fashioning and crossing tarsal strips or sectioning and crossing the lateral canthal ligaments. In using these methods one must be careful not to cause a permanent surgical narrowing of the palpebral fissure. Wheeler reported correction of a case of congenital absence of the lateral canthal ligaments by anchoring strips of the orbicularis to the

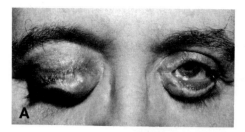 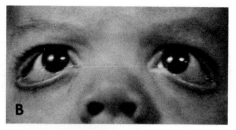

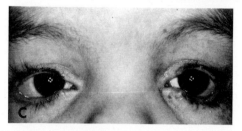

FIG. 226.   Megaloblepharon and Euryblepharon.
A.   Congenital megaloblepharon.
B. and C.   Euryblepharon before and after correction.

orbital margin (fig. 227). It may also be accomplished by replacement of the canthal ligament by substituting fibrous tissue in the area or by pedicle flaps from the upper lid. Upward and downward displacement of both medial and lateral canthi on the other hand is not unusual following trauma and repair of these conditions is accomplished relatively easily as shown in Chapters 9 and 10.

ANKYLOBLEPHARON

Congenital ankyloblepharon (*ankylē* = noose; *blepharon* = eyelid) is a fusion of a portion of the lid margins with a consequent shortening of the palpebral fissure. Two distinct types of this rare congenital malformation have been described: (1) the simple type in which the lid margins are fused directly to each other and (2) ankyloblepharon filiforme adnatum (fig. 228) in which the lid margins are connected by bands of extensible tissue which interfere with the opening and closing of the lids. Both types are presumed to be primary growth aberrations due to failure of epithelium to cover the marginal mesoderm and permitting its fusion in the two lids.

Simple Ankyloblepharon

The most common point of fusion is the outer canthus; more rarely it is the medial canthus which is involved. As usual, this anomaly rarely occurs by itself but frequently accompanies anophthalmos, microphthalmos, ptosis, etc. The ankyloblepharon here is repaired by simple lateral canthoplasty (fig. 124).

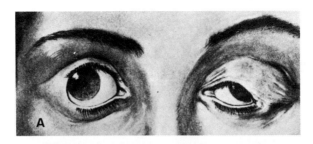

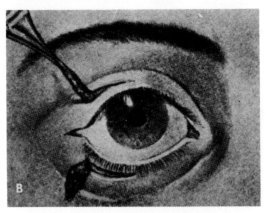

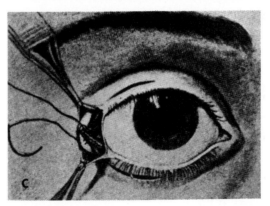

FIG. 227.   Congenital Absence of Lateral Canthi (Wheeler).
A.   Preoperative appearance.
B.   Flaps of orbicularis are dissected up.
C.   The flaps are sutured to the periosteum.

Ankyloblepharon Filiforme Adnatum

This form of ankyloblepharon (fig. 228) is even rarer than the simple type. The name was proposed by von Hasner who reported the first case in 1881. The lid margins are not fused but are usually connected by a single unilateral band or tissue which may occur anywhere in the lid fissure. However, bilateral and multiple unilateral bands have also been reported quite recently (Rogers; Khanna). The bands have varied any-

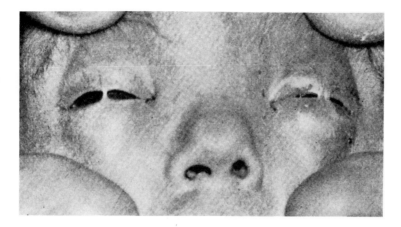

Fɪɢ. 228.   Ankyloblepharon Filiforme Adnatum. (Rogers, W. J.: Courtesy
Archives of Ophthalmology).

where from 0.2 to 5 mm. in width and 1.0 to 10.0 mm. in length. They
are characteristically so elastic as to be stretchable to almost double their
length. The area of attachment is between the ciliary line and the tarsal
gland openings. Other accompanying anomalies may be harelip and
cleft palate.

Treatment is quite simple. All reports agree that excision of the
bands is all that is necessary. The fine remnants disappear without
leaving a trace.

Blepharophimosis

Congenital blepharophimosis (other forms are described in the
following chapter) is an uncommon condition characterized by a diminution in the size of the palpebral fissure. The lids and their margins are
normally differentiated, hence it differs from ankyloblepharon in which
there is a fusion of the lid margins. It may occur rarely by itself and is
transmitted as a dominant characteristic by either male or female (Duke-
Elder). More commonly it is associated with other congenital anomalies,
especially epicanthus and ptosis as noted above (figs. 223, 225 and 229).

Congenital blepharophimosis is sometimes confused with epicanthus.
However, though they are often synchronous they are never synonymous.
As in senile epicanthus (q.v.) the epicanthal fold hides some of the lid
fissure but does not shorten it. In blepharophimosis, on the other hand,
there is an actual physical diminution in the dimensions of the fissure.
The fissure in the adult usually measures somewhere from 25 to 28 mm.
in length and 8 to 10 mm. in width. In the infant it is considerably
shorter but not much narrower. In the cases pictured in figure 223 the
fissure measured 18 by 5 mm. and in figure 224 the length of the fissure
was only 20 mm.

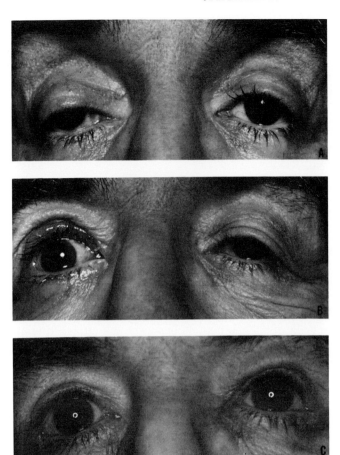

FIG. 229.   Complicated Ptosis.
A.   Bilateral congenital blepharophimosis with ptosis.
B.   Note the shortness of the palpebral fissures.
C.   Appearance after repair.

Probably the simplest and most frequently used procedure for the correction of congenital blepharophimosis is von Ammon's lateral canthoplasty (fig. 124). Most commonly this is done in conjunction with a ptosis repair or an epicanthus repair.

EPICANTHUS

Congenital epicanthus is a fold of skin which juts out on the side of the dorsum of the nose and projects over the inner angle of the eye so as to cover part or all of the canthus. It is always bilateral, although one side may be more developed than the other.

Epicanthus is a permanent feature of all members of the Mongolian race. It is also quite common in mild form in a large percentage of Caucasian babies but fades out early in life as the child grows older and the bridge of the nose develops. Hence it should not be operated on until the age of 10 and then only if it has remained stationary for several years. At one time it was attributed to excess skin covering the inner canthus. However, it is now known to be caused by a tautening due to the pull of too little vertical skin.

It is often found with a flattened nasal root. When present with blepharophimosis, as it frequently is, the appearance is that of a pair of palpebral fissures which are too wide apart because of the epicanthal folds covering the medial canthi.

Congenital epicanthus was first reported by Schön in 1828. Since then four types have been described. Von Ammon named the condition and described the first three types:

1. *Epicanthus supraciliaris:* when the epicanthal fold has its origin from the region of the eyebrow.

2. *Epicanthus palpebralis:* when it arises from the upper lid above the tarsus.

3. *Epicanthus tarsalis:* when the epicanthus stems from the superior tarsal fold (fig. 230*G*). This is normally seen in Orientals but like epiblepharon is anomalous in Caucasians.

4. *Epicanthus inversus* (fig. 225*A*) was the first described in detail by Braun in 1922, although it had been noted earlier by others. This is substantially different from other epicanthi in that the fold arises in the skin of the lower lid and fades as it approaches the upper lid. Ptosis, phimosis, superior rectus weakness and an abnormally long distance between the medial canthi are also practically the rule as concomitant conditions.

The older procedures for repair of congenital epicanthus usually depended on skin excision or realignment based on the theory that too much was present. Thus, Von Ammon excised a spindle of skin over the root of the nose. Arlt excised semilunar skin segments, including the epicanthi and Berger excised arrowhead segments. Beard advised paraffin injections to "build up the bridge of the nose" although he later conceded that "the mass of paraffin that is put into the tissues has a treacherous way of sometimes changing its form and its location." Verwey straddled the epicanthus with a horizontal >— the single leg pointing toward the nose. He then undermined the triangle of skin between the two lateral legs and pulled it medially thus converting the Y to a V.

Such procedures may be of some value in mild forms of epicanthus but are valueless in severe epicanthus because, as noted above, it is due to an actual shortage of vertical skin between the canthus and the nose which pulls the skin fold over the canthal angle. Rogman in 1904 was apparently the first to appreciate this and to point out that the proper procedure for repair of congenital epicanthus was not resection but realignment of the canthal skin. All present operative procedures are based on his original technic. A method based on Blair's double Z plasty technic will give good results.

Double Z Plasty (Blair)

Procedure (fig. 230): Six millimeters nasal to the canthus a 15 mm. slightly curved vertical skin incision with concavity toward the canthus is made. From the center of this an 8 mm. horizontal incision directed nasally is made. From the ends of the curved incision, two additional incisions are made upward and downward toward the lower and upper lid margins respectively, terminating almost at the lid margins at a point about 4 mm. lateral to the canthus (fig. 230A). The resulting flaps are undermined and transposed—first the two upper (figs. 230B, C and D), then the two lower—and sewed into position with interrupted 5–0 silk sutures (figs. 230E and F).

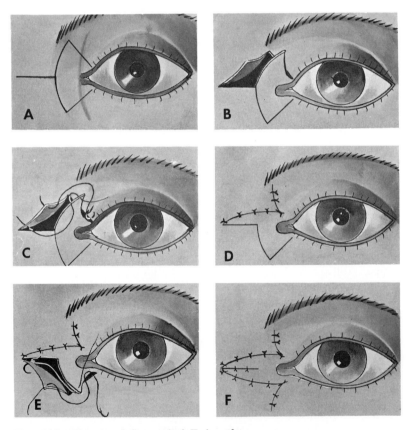

Fig. 230.   Repair of Congenital Epicanthus.
  A.   Skin incisions.
  B.   The upper flaps are dissected up.
  C.   The sutures are placed.
  D.   The flaps are transposed and sutured into position.
  E.   and F.   The lower flaps are raised, transposed and sutured into position similarly.

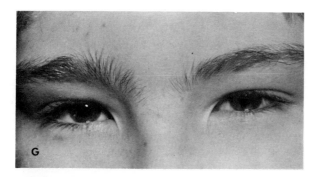

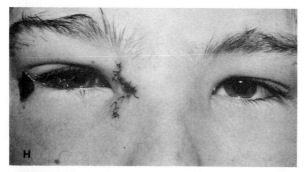

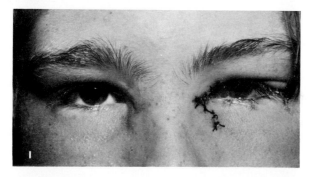

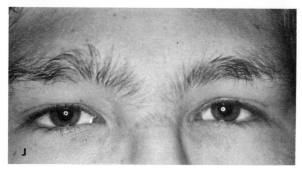

FIG. 230 (*Continued*)

G. A case of bilateral congenital epicanthus.

H. and *I.* After repair and before removal of sutures.

J. Final result.

(After Blair, Brown and Hamm.)

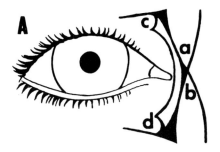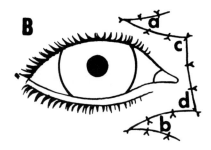

FIG. 231.   Double Z Plasty Repair of Epicanthus—Spaeth.
A.   Flaps *a* and *b* are marked out and flaps *c* and *d* are outlined and elevated.
B.   Flaps *a* and *c* are undermined, transposed and sutured into position. The
     lower flaps *b* and *d* are similarly transposed and sutured.

A firm dressing is applied. This is changed in 48 hours and daily
thereafter with the sutures being removed on the fifth or sixth day.
Figure 230*G* shows a bilateral epicanthus and figures 230*H, I* and *J* show
steps in the repair and the final result.

Comment: For some reason scar formation and discoloration is
quite severe here. Ultimately the scars do fade out almost completely but
it may take as long as six months. In the author's experience massage has
not served to hasten absorption of the scars.

Double Z Plasty (Spaeth)

Another procedure which gives good results is Spaeth's double Z
plasty. He divides the epicanthal fold into two skin triangles which are
moved into the upper and lower lids, smoothing out the fold and relieving
the vertical tension.

Procedure (fig. 231):   The epicanthal fold is put on vertical stretch
by an assistant and a curved line is marked out with an antiseptic dye
parallel with and slightly medial to the curve of the fold. This line is
convex toward the nose and extends above and below the fold. Two lines
are now drawn from the approximate center of this first line. One is
directed up and medially forming flap a; the other is directed down and
medially forming flap b. When completed, a figure much like an X is
formed.

From the upper and lower ends of the first incision two additional
lines are now drawn *laterally:* The upper line is directed down and
laterally toward the upper lid margin forming flap c; the lower line is
directed toward the lower lid margin forming flap d. These lines will be
almost horizontal or will bend acutely toward the lid margins depending
on the degree of epicanthus. The less the epicanthus the more acute the
angulation and vice versa (fig. 231*A*). The marked-out lines are incised
through skin and muscle. The upper flaps a and c are undermined,
transposed and sutured into position. The lower flaps b and d are trans-

posed and sutured similarly (fig. 231*B*). Since the flaps are not always of equal size the undermining in the lid may have to be extensive to avoid kinking. Also, the flaps may have to be trimmed to fit snugly.

Postoperative care is the same as described for the previous procedure.

Comment: Epicanthi vary in degree and position. Hence in marking out the incision lines it might be wiser to incise flaps c and d first, dissect them up then pull each over toward the nose and estimate where and how large flaps a and b should be. They may have to be trimmed later as in all cases of epicanthus.

Since human skin is variable this also will affect flap transposition so that they may not fit exactly into their beds; they may be slightly short or too long. In the former case additional careful dissection and undermining will help to prevent retraction. It might also be wise to anchor the skin sutures into the subjacent muscle. If too long, the flaps can be trimmed to fit.

Mustardé has also devised a procedure for the repair of epicanthus. It is effective but requires more incisions and hence leaves more scars than the technics described above. Voeresmarthy has suggested elimination of the epicanthus by shortening the medial palpebral ligament.

Epicanthus, especially the Mongoloid type, is frequently accompanied by blepharophimosis, telecanthus and ptosis. The latter was discussed in Chapter 17. Blepharophimosis is corrected by lateral canthoplasty as shown above. Roveda uses the Blair canthoplasty at the lateral canthus and a modification of the Verwey epicanthus technic for the correction of epicanthus combined with blepharophimosis.

TELECANTHUS

Telecanthus is a name given by Mustardé to a widening of the medial intercanthal distance. This condition is not as rare as might be expected; it is however, most common as part of the Mongoloid syndrome (fig. 225*A*). It is improved by a tucking of the medial canthal ligaments as shown in figure 110. Some freeing of the surrounding orbital fascia may also be necessary. This repair will always help and though there will not be complete restoration to normal, the improvement can be appreciable (fig. 225*B*).

THE ORIENTAL LID

A large percentage of Oriental eyelids have no folds. These are the "single eyelids" as distinguished from the "double eyelids" which have a distinguishable lid fold Since the palpebral fissure is narrower, the lid often gives the appearance of ptosis although this is normal in Oriental races (fig. 233*A*).

The Oriental eyelid owes its typical appearance to a lower point of union of the septum orbitale with the levator and to a more abundant fat content. There is a thin layer of subcutaneous fatty tissue as well as a significant amount of preseptal and pretarsal fat and, occasionally, hypertrophy of the orbicularis. Hence to "occidentalize" such a lid, subcutane-

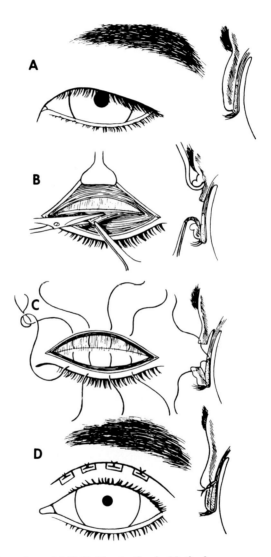

FIG. 232.   Creation of Lid Fold—Author's Method.

A.   Oriental eye with lid fold down at margin.

B.   An incision is made through skin and muscle below the upper tarsal border. The skin-muscle lamina is dissected upward and downward. Fat and hypertrophied orbicularis fibers, if present, are resected.

C.   Four equally spaced sutures are passed through the lower skin lip, the upper tarsal border and the upper skin lip. Additional skin sutures are placed for complete closure.

D.   On closure the lid furrow is at the upper tarsal border.

ous fat and hypertrophied orbicularis may have to be excised. In addition, a moderate amount of supraorbital fat must be resected if presenting. Requests for creating a lid fold and Westernizing such lids are not infrequent.

Lid Fold Procedure—Author's Technic

Procedure (fig. 232): An Ehrhardt clamp is inserted and the lid drawn down so that the skin is tautened. Just below the upper tarsal border an incision is made through skin and muscle following the curve of the border. The upper and lower lips of the wound are dissected up and down for good tarsal exposure. The upper lid dissection should go high enough to expose the upper tarsal border fully.

If fat presents this should be resected forthwith. This will reduce the fatty appearance of the supratarsal portion of the lid. If the orbicularis fibers are hypertrophied these should also be resected (fig. 232*B*).

Four double-armed 5–0 silk sutures, equally spaced, are then inserted as follows: The needles are passed through the lower lip of the wound, through the upper tarsal border and then through the upper lip of the wound. The sutures are tied over very small rubber pegs. Two are placed 3 mm. to each side of midline and two additional sutures 5 mm. nearer each canthus. Thus there will be four approximately equally spaced such sutures. Additional skin sutures are added for good closure (fig. 232*C*). The lid furrow is now at the upper tarsal border (fig. 232*D*).

The eye is patched lightly and the patch removed on the second postoperative day. Dark glasses may be worn thereafter until the operative reaction has subsided. The sutures are removed on the fifth or sixth day.

Comment: Both lids may be done at once unless there is objection from the patient. Reaction is usually slight and the result is permanent. I have found it unnecessary to advance the levator even slightly or to indulge in any other fancy maneuvering with sutures. Tautening the lower lip of the skin wound by fastening it to the tarsus and thus creating a lid furrow has been enough to create an occidental lid fold since loose upper lid skin is anchored to the furrow at the upper tarsal border (figs. 233*A* and *B*).

If on closure it appears that there is too much loose skin giving too much lid fold, some but not too much of the skin should be excised. In operating on the second eye, the same amount of skin should be resected so that the folds will be equal.

Creation of Occidental Lid Fold—Pang

A simple and ingenious method for creating a lid fold in an oriental eyelid has been devised by Pang who makes no skin incision.

Procedure (fig. 234): After suitable preparation, a fold is pushed up in the lid skin with a spatula and the deepest part of the fold is marked

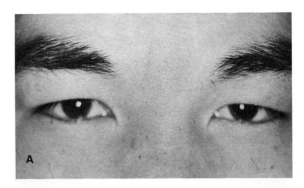

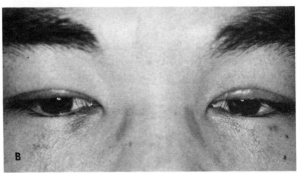

FIG. 233.   Creation of Occidental Lid Fold—Author.
A.   Oriental lids.   *B.*   After correction.

off with an antiseptic dye (fig. 234*A*). The lid is anesthetized on skin and conjunctival surfaces over the superior tarsal border. The anesthesia is kept to a minimum so as not to distort the tissues.

Three double-armed 4–0 silk sutures are inserted as follows: One needle of the central suture goes through the skin where marked with the dye then upward through orbicularis, levator and conjunctiva to emerge 2 mm. *above* its point of entrance (fig. 234*B*). The needle is reinserted in the conjunctiva and traces the same course backward to emerge on the skin surface 3 or 4 mm. lateral to its mate (fig. 234*D*). The other two sutures are similarly inserted medially and laterally and are tied over rubber pegs (fig. 234*C*). As the sutures are tied the skin is pulled up and a fold is created (fig. 234*E*). The eye is dressed daily and the sutures are removed in 10 to 12 days.

Comment: Both eyes are done at one sitting. Since the conjunctival loop part of the suture is higher than the point of exit on the skin, a fold is formed as the suture is tied and the skin is pulled up. The sutures are left in for a longer time than usual for fibrous bands to form. However, with no incision, the only doubtful feature of this procedure is maintenance and longevity of the fold. As a matter of fact, Pang himself points out that since the procedure does not require a skin incision it "may be repeated many times."

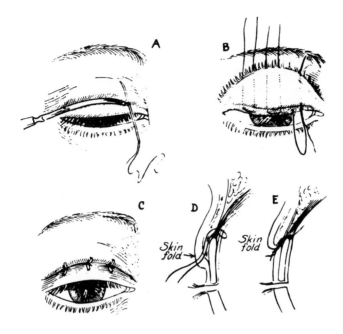

FIG. 234.   Creation of Occidental Lid Fold—Pang.

A.   The lid is indented to make a fold at the upper tarsal border.

B. and *C.*   Three double-armed sutures, equally spaced, are passed upward and backward to emerge on the conjunctival surface. They then retrace their course and are tied.

D.   Lateral view showing route of the sutures from skin to conjunctiva and back.

E.   Lateral view of skin fold after sutures are tied.

Making a fold in an oriental or traumatized lid requires no elaborate surgery; it may require something more than subcutaneous sutures. A permanent surgical furrow created at the upper tarsal border gives the fold a better chance to endure.

Millard resects a 5 mm. skin strip at the upper tarsal border and thins out the subcutaneous tissue and orbicularis muscle fibers in the exposed wound. When the orbicularis is incised the fat which herniates through is resected. At the same operation a modified Z is done at the medial canthus which stretches the skin and tends to do away with the epicanthus.

Incidentally this is now a frequent operation in Japan as an office procedure. The lid is everted, the tissue above the upper tarsal border is grasped, fat and muscle are removed and the lid sutured.

CONGENITAL ECTROPION

Primary congenital ectropion is even more rare than congenital entropion and rarely appears by itself. Figure 235 shows such a case combined with epicanthus. Figures 226*A* and *B* illustrate other cases of

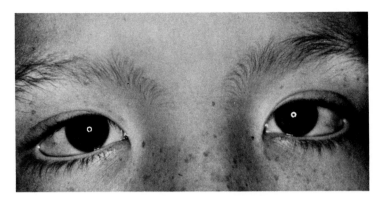

FIG. 235.   Congenital Ectropion with Epicanthus.

congenital ectropion as part of other syndromes. Repair is described
under figure 226.

It may be wise not to hurry surgery as a few reports indicate that
there is a tendency to spontaneous reinversion of the ectropion in the
rare cases when it appears alone.

CONGENITAL ENTROPION

Primary entropion is an uncommon congenital anomaly. It is much
rarer than the secondary type of congenital entropion which is mechanical
and usually due to lack of support to the lid margin by a small or absent
globe. The importance of this anomaly is in the injury which might be
caused to the cornea by the inversion of the margin and lashes.

It is not always easy to distinguish clinically between congenital
entropion and epiblepharon when the skin fold of epiblepharon pushes
the cilia against the globe. The main difference is the position of the
lid margin which in true entropion is inverted along its entire length
(fig. 236 E), not unlike senile entropion. In epiblepharon, on the other
hand, it is the skin of the lid which impinges on the margin and pushes
the cilia against the globe, especially in downward gaze (fig. 237).
Another clinical difference is that epiblepharon occurs relatively more
commonly and may disappear by the end of the first two years but not
always. It therefore may not require surgery. This is not true of congenital entropion which becomes aggravated with growth and always
requires surgical intervention. For this reason, if the cornea can be kept
intact, it is always best to watch the newborn infant for several months,
and preferably to the end of the first year, before undertaking surgery.

Congenital entropion usually involves both lower lids and is commonly due to hypertrophy of the marginal orbicularis fibers although
deficiency of the tarsal plate has also been reported. The usual indicated
procedure is that of Celsus, i.e., resection of enough skin and muscle to
cause eversion of the lid to a normal position.

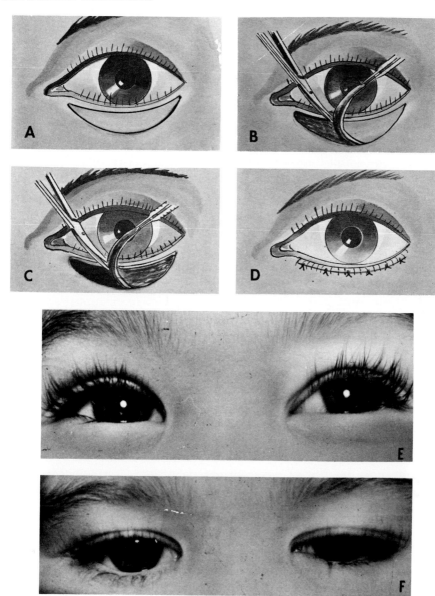

Fig. 236.   Repair of Congenital Entropion by the Celsus Technic.
A. and B.   A skin spindle is marked off on the lower lid and resected.
C.   The exposed muscle is resected.
D.   The wound is closed.
E. and F.   A case of bilateral congenital entropion before and after correction.

Procedure (fig. 236):   The skin of the lid is pinched up between the fingers and the amount necessary to remove in order to correct the entropion is estimated and marked out with an antiseptic dye in the form of a spindle (fig. 236 A). The skin is incised and resected (fig. 236B). Usually it is necessary to resect a strip of the hypertrophied muscle as well (fig. 236C). The wound is closed with 5–0 interrupted silk sutures (fig. 236*D*). Figures 236*E* and *F* illustrate a case of bilateral congenital entropion before and after repair.

EPIBLEPHARON

Epiblepharon is a congenital anomaly marked by an enlarged pretarsal skin fold which may extend over the lid margin and press the cilia against the globe. It was first described by von Ammon in 1841. In the upper lid (epiblepharon superior) it is characteristic of the Mongolian races but it is a Caucasian anomaly (fig. 237*A*). It is seen more frequently in the lower lid in white races (fig. 237*B*).

Curiously the frequent impingement of the lashes on the cornea may have little clinical effect and signs and symptoms such as injection of the globe and lacrimation may be absent. This may be due to an acquired tolerance. However, in other cases epiphora and conjunctival injection may occur in the early months of life.

Epiblepharon of the lower lid has a tendency to disappear spontaneously, usually during the first year. Hence if the eye condition warrants it, surgery should be postponed. If persistent, the state of the eye will decide what course is to be followed and later surgery may be done for cosmetic reasons only. Repair is easily accomplished by the simple excision of the skin fold.

DISTICHIASIS

Distichiasis (*di* = two; stichos = row) is a congenital anomaly in which an accessory row of lashes occurs along the posterior border of the lid margin in the position of the meibomian glands. Like most of the other conditions mentioned in this chapter, distichiasis is rare and one can span an ophthalmologic lifetime without seeing a case.

Distichiasis is something of an ophthalmologic changeling: it is often misspelled, viz., districhiasis, dystichiasis, dystrichiasis. There seems to

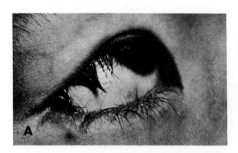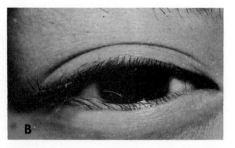

FIG. 237. Congenital Epiblepharon.
A. Epiblepharon superior—right upper lid (with epicanthus).
B. Epiblepharon inferior—right lower lid.

be some doubt as to its gender : it is *le* distichiasis and *der* distichiasis in French and German, but in Latin it becomes distichiasis congenit*a* ver*a*. It is constantly coupled with trichiasis as if the two were fraternal twins instead of being distant cousins.

Whatever distichiasis is, it is not trichiasis. In trichiasis the *normal* lashes have become distorted and misdirected so as to cause conjunctival and corneal irritation; frequently this is due to cicatrization of the lid border. In distichiasis it is an *accessory row* of lashes on the posterior border of an otherwise normal lid margin which is the cause of the trouble.

The clinical characteristics of distichiasis are replacement of the normal meibomian gland openings by lashes which are thinner, shorter and lighter in color than the normal cilia. The number may vary from 4 to 20 and they may be present in all four lids in varying numbers although they are usually more profuse in the lower lids than in the upper. Kuhnt considered distichiasis to be a heterologous developmental anomaly in which the meibomian glands are replaced by cilia. Others such as Begle and Erdmann believed that it is a sign of atavism in which the cilia are the product of the same anlage but in which differentiation has failed to take place. A strong hereditary factor has been noted in many reports and distichiasis is apparently a dominant hereditary characteristic since transmission is direct without sex predilection. Curiously, few concomitant congenital anomalies have been reported, but in rare cases congenital ectropion, ptosis and maxillofacial dysostosis occur simultaneously.

Ocular irritation is not as constant a factor as one would think. This is believed due to the shortness of these accessory lashes—lanugolike is a frequent descriptive adjective. On the other hand, distichiasis can cause great discomfort and require surgery.

The treatment of distichiasis has not been completely satisfactory probably due to the fact that few authors have had enough cases to work out a satisfactory technic of repair. Epilation, electrolysis and resection of the offending cilia-bearing tarsal strip with the grafting of mucous membrane or tarsoconjunctiva are the three methods of repair usually suggested.

A case of lower lid distichiasis (fig. 238*A*) was repaired satisfactorily by the author with the following technic :

Procedure (fig. 238): After suitable instillation and infiltration anesthesia the lid is split and the dissection is carried downward to attain complete separation of the two laminae. A vertical incision is made through the tarsoconjunctival lamina close to each canthus thus creating a sliding flap of tarsoconjunctiva. The upper 3 mm. of this flap containing the offending accessory cilia are resected (fig. 238*B*). After making sure that the flap is completely mobile, it is pulled up so that its cut edge

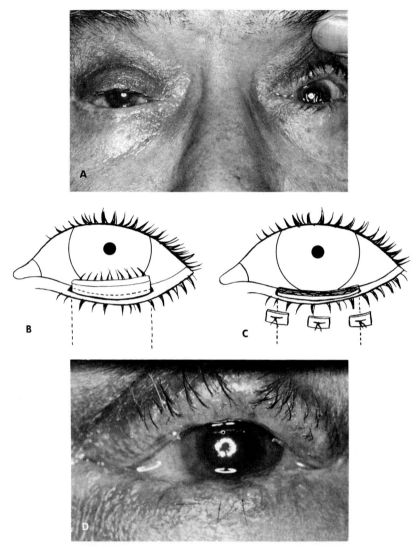

FIG. 238.   Correction of Distichiasis.

A. Distichiasis of left lower lid. Note accessory row of lashes against the cornea.

B. The lid is split in the gray line, the tarsoconjunctiva is mobilized, pulled up
    and offending lashes resected.

C. The tarsoconjunctival lamina is pulled up slightly above the skin-muscle
    lamina and sutured into position by three 4–0 double-armed silk sutures
    passed through both laminae from behind forward and tied over pegs. Two
    similar sutures are passed through to straddle each vertical incision and are
    also tied over pegs.

D. Final result.

is slightly higher than the anterior skin-muscle edge to counteract subsequent retraction, and the two vertical conjunctival incisions are closed
with interrupted 6–0 chromic catgut sutures.

Three double-armed 4–0 silk sutures are passed through both laminae
from the conjunctival surface forward about 2 mm. below the margin and

tied over a peg. One of these double-armed sutures is centrally placed. Each of the side sutures is so located as to straddle the medial and lateral incisions in the tarsoconjunctiva (fig. 238C).

A firm dressing is applied and changed at two day intervals. Sutures are removed on the tenth day. (The final result is shown in figure 238D).

Comment: As mentioned above, another method of repair is to graft a strip of tarsoconjunctiva taken from the upper border of the upper lid tarsus to fill in the dehiscence caused by resection of the upper tarso-conjunctival strip. However, this is not always available as some of these cases have had previous conjunctival disease. In a case seen by the author, Stevens-Johnson disease had made tarsoconjunctiva unavailable. Since both upper and lower lids were involved, tarsoconjunctival flaps were fashioned in both lids and the repair carried out according to the above technic. The raw tarsconjunctival edges of the upper and lower lids were then sutured to each other. This worked quite well.

Overcorrection by pulling the tarsoconjunctival flap beyond the skin-muscle lamina is important to allow for retraction and because there is always a tendency in these lids to become entropic on account of the loss of tarsoconjunctiva. If this does occur a Panas (fig. 200) or Graefe procedure (fig. 201) is enough to restore the balance.

Scheie and Albert believe that distichiasis can also be acquired in long-standing inflammation and hyperemia of the lids and conjunctiva especially in association with the late changes in Stevens-Johnson disease. There is a good deal in this theory. How else does one explain the sudden appearance of discomfort in an elderly individual who has never had corneal irritation and who shows fine, unpigmented lashes appearing from the area of the meibomian glands? It can only be assumed that these are of recent origin. Scheie and Albert also suggest the use of the operating microscope for these fine lanugolike cilia. This is an excellent idea.

Other Types of Displaced Cilia

While distichiasis is the most common of the rare anomalies other types of displaced lashes have been reported. Figure 239 shows a cluster of displaced cilia well above their normal position in the ciliary margin. This is a rare anomaly indeed. It is a minor cosmetic blemish which is readily remedied by extirpation of the cilia with their roots.

EPITARSUS

Epitarsus, sometimes called congenital pterygium, is a conjunctival anomaly consisting of a fold of conjunctiva between the fornix and the tarsus. Most commonly it is seen in the upper lid and is usually sufficiently free to allow a probe to pass through.

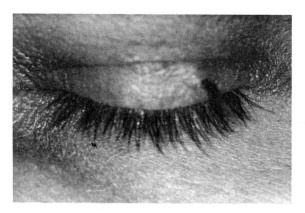

FIG. 239.   Rare Congenital Upward Displacement of Cilia Cluster—Left
Upper Lid.

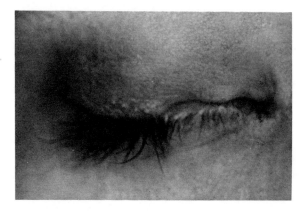

FIG. 240.   Congenital Coloboma Right Upper Lid.

Originally thought to be a congenital anomaly, it is probably not a developmental malformation but due to neglected acute conjunctivitis of the membranous type usually occurring in the young. Since it rarely interferes with the movement of the eyeball, surgery is not required.

COLOBOMATA

Congenital colobomata are most commonly situated on the inner half of the upper lid; the next favored site of predilection is the outer half of the lower lid. Usually only one occurs; however, multiple colobomata have been reported in all four lids. The coloboma is typically triangular with the base at the margin but quadrangular and rounded colobomata are not rare (fig. 240). The etiology of these lid defects has never been properly explained; however, they are not hereditary as Thylmann showed in 1919.

The repair of congenital lid colobomata does not vary from the colobomata of traumatic and neoplastic origin previously discussed.

DERMOID CYSTS

Dermoid cyst (epidermoid cyst, oil cyst) is a congenital lesion arising from primitive ectoderm at the site of closure of the fetal cleft. It may occur in the orbit, the brow, the lid, diploë of the skull or the paranasal sinuses. However, it is most commonly seen—and felt—under the skin at the outer angle of the superior orbital margin (fig. 241A). The upper inner orbital angle is the next most common site (fig. 241B).

The cyst is usually round or oval and about the size of a small cherry when first seen. Although it may not enlarge sufficiently to be noticed until after the age of twenty, it not uncommonly appears before the age of five. On palpation it may feel soft like a fatty tumor. Just as often it is hard and solid due to distention of the cyst wall. The cyst may contain nothing but a white sebaceouslike material composed of desquamated epithelial products. Or it may contain hair, oily material from sebaceous glands, brownish hemorrhagic fluid and cholesterin crystals.

Dermoid cysts which are large and deep require careful x-ray study. They may involve the cranial fossae and require neurosurgical attention. However, most are quite superficial and can be easily resected through an anterior skin approach. Care should be taken to excise the whole cyst

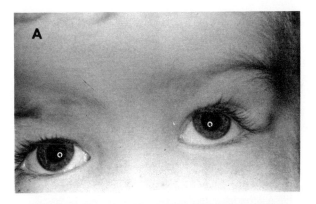

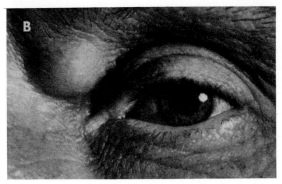

FIG. 241. Congenital Dermoids.
A. Above lateral canthus.   B. Above medial canthus.

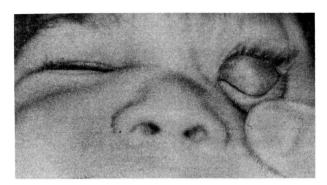

FIG. 242.   Congenital Cyst of Conjunctiva.

wall. Reese points out that remnants of epithelium which are left behind
may become necrotic and act as a foreign body giving rise to an apparent
clinical recurrence of the cyst.

CONJUNCTIVAL ANOMALIES

In congenital conjunctival ectropion, another unusual condition, the
conjunctiva extends for some distance around the outer surface of the lid
margin. It is due to a shortening of the lid skin; grafting is usually
required here.

Congenital conjunctival cysts are rarely reported. Figure 242 presents a cyst in an eleven month old baby. The cyst was present at birth
and filled the whole lower cul-de-sac. At operation it was found to have a
very thin wall subconjunctivally and to be filled with a clear, viscous,
slightly straw-colored fluid. Resection effected a complete cure.

REFERENCES

VON AMMON, F. A.: Klinische Darstellungen der angeborenen Krankheiten des
    Auges und der Augenlider. Berlin, G. Reimer, 1841, p. 6.
BERGER, E.: Epicanthus. Arch. d'Ophthal. 18:453, 1898.
BLAIR, V. P. et al.: Surgery of the inner canthus and related structures. Am. J.
    Ophth. 15:498, 1932.
BRAUN, C.: Eine besondered Form der Epikanthus mit Kongenitalis Ptosis. Klin.
    Mbl. Augenheilk. 68:100, 1922.
DE VOE, A. G., and HORWICH, H.: Congenital entropion and tetrastichiasis of upper
    lids, palpebral hyperpigmentation and mental deficiency. Arch. Ophth. 52:865,
    1954.
DIEFFENBACH, J. F.: Die operative Chirurgie. Leipzig, F. A. Brockhaus, 1845, p. 470.
DUKE-ELDER, S.: System of Ophthalmology. St. Louis, The C. V. Mosby Co., 1963,
    Vol. 3, Pt. 2.
EDMUND, J.: Blepharophimosis congenita. Acta Genet. Statist. Med. 7:279, 1957.
FOX, S. A.: Ptosis with elephantiasis and ectropion. Am. J. Ophth. 33:1144, 1950.
————: Primary congenital entropion. Arch. d'ophth. 56:839, 1956.
————: Distichiasis. Am. J. Ophth. 53:14, 1962.
VON HASNER: Ankyloblepharon filiforme adnatum. Ztschr. Augenh. 2:429, 1881.

HUGHES, W. L.: Surgical treatment of congenital phimosis. Arch. Ophth. *54*:586, 1955.

JOHNSON, C. C.: Operation for epicanthus and blepharophimosis. Am. J. Ophth. *41*:71, 1956.

KHANNA, V. N.: Ankyloblepharon filiforme adnatum. Am. J. Opthth. *43*:774, 1957.

LEBLOND, E.: Etiologie de l'entropion congenital. Arch. d'Ophthal. *27*:782, 1907.

LEJEUNE, J., GAUTIER, M., and TURPIN, R.: Les chromosomes humains en culture de tissues. Compt. Rend. Acad. Soc. *248*:602, 1959.

LEVITT, J. M.: Epiblepharon and congenital entropion. Am. J. Ophth. *44*:112, 1957.

LONG, J. C., and BLANDFORD, S. E.: Ankyloblepharon filiforme adnatum with cleft lip and palate. Am. J. Ophth. *53*:126, 1962.

MILLARD, D. R.: The oriental eye and its surgical revision. Am. J. Ophth. *57*:646, 1964.

OSTRIKER, P. J., and LASKY, M. A.: Congenital eversion of the upper eyelids. Am. J. Ophth. *37*:779, 1954.

PANG, H. G.: Surgical formation of upper lid fold. Arch. Ophth. *63*:783, 1961.

ROBBINS, J., FISHMAN, R., MEDENIS, R., and ROSENTHAL, I.: Congenital microphthalmos. Am. J. Ophth. *55*:901, 1963.

ROGERS, W. J.: Ankyloblepharon filiforme adnatum. Arch. Ophth. *65*: 114, 1961.

ROGMAN, J.: Nouveau procede operatoire pour corriger l'epicanthus. Ann. d'ocul. *131*:464, 1904.

ROVEDA, J. M.: Epicanthus et blepharophimosis. Ann. d'ocul. *20*:551, 1967.

SAYOC, B. T.: Anatomic considerations in the plastic construction of a palpebral fold in the upper eyelid. Am. J. Ophth. *63*:155, 1967.

SCHEIE, H. G., and ALBERT, D. M.: Distichiasis and trichiasis; origin and management. Am. J. Ophth. *61*:718, 1966.

SCHWARTZ, O., and JAMPEL, R. S.: Congenital blepharophimosis associated with a unique generalized myopathy. Arch. Ophth. *68*:52, 1962.

SINGH, S.: Epitarsus and allied postinflammatory conjunctival adhesions. Arch. Ophth. *63*:503, 1960.

SMILLIE, J. W.: External ankyloblepharon with pseudoexotropia. Am. J. Ophth. *43*:460, 1957.

SPAETH, E. B.: Further considerations of the surgical correction of blepharophimosis (epicanthus). Am. J. Ophth. *41*:61, 1956.

UCHIDA, J. C.: A surgical procedure for blepharoptosis vera and for pseudo-blepharoptosis orientalis. B. J. Plast. Surg. *15*:271, 1962.

VERWEY, A.: Over het maskergelaat en zijn behandeling. Net. tij. v. gen. *45*:1596, 1909.

VOERESMARTHY, D.: Elimination of a congenital epicanthus by shortening of medial palpebral ligament. Klin. Monatsbl. Augenh. *151*:66, 1967.

WAARDENBERG, P. F., FRANCESCHETTI, A., and KLEIN, D.: Genetics in Ophthalmology. Springfield, Ill., Charles C Thomas, 1961.

WHEELER, J. M.: The use of the orbicularis palpebrarum muscle in surgery of the eyelids. Am. J. Surg. *42*:7, 1938.

CHAPTER 19

Miscellaneous Acquired Anomalies

ATROPHY OF LID SKIN
  DERMACHALASIS
  BLEPHAROCHALASIS

FAT HERNIA

ELEPHANTIASIS NOSTRAS

ANKYLOBLEPHARON

BLEPHAROPHIMOSIS

LAGOPHTHALMOS
  PARALYTIC
  CICATRICIAL
  MECHANICAL

PTOSIS OF LOWER LID

BLEPHAROSPASM

ATROPHY OF LID SKIN

THERE ARE TWO IMPORTANT TYPES of lid skin atrophy which require plastic repair: dermachalasis and blepharochalasis.

Dermachalasis (Senile Lid Skin Atrophy, "Baggy" Lids, "Puffs")

Dermachalasis (*derma* = skin; *chalasis* = relaxation) or senile atrophy of the lid is a common condition which usually appears after the age of fifty but which may develop in younger individuals. It affects both upper and lower lids and is due to relaxation and thinning of the skin, loss of muscle tonus and loosening of the fibrous connections between the skin and fascia orbitalis. In addition there is frequently a herniation of orbital fat through a weakened fascia orbitalis especially nasally. In the later stages the skin of the upper lid becomes so stretched as to hang over the free lid border like an apron and may overlie the medial canthi (fig. 243*A*). In the lower lid fascial relaxation causes bagginess and the typical sac-like bulging due to fat herniation (fig. 245*A*).

Blepharochalasis

Blepharochalasis (blepharo = lid; chalasis = relaxation) is a rare condition usually of the upper lids, appearing in younger individuals. More rarely the lower lids may also be involved (fig. 243*B*). Well over half the reported cases have been in patients under the age of twenty. The sexes are equally affected as are the lids although a few unilateral cases have been reported. The condition usually starts at puberty with intermittent painless edema and redness of the lids; it is aggravated by crying and menstruation. Repeated attacks result in loss of elasticity, subcutaneous atrophy and capillary proliferation. Ultimately the skin of the lid becomes permanently stretched, hangs down over the lid margin and

424

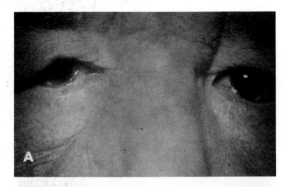
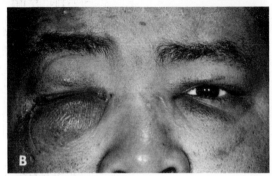

FIG. 243.   Lid Skin Atrophy.
A.   Dermachalasis (senile lid skin atrophy; baggy lids.)
B.   Blepharochalasis.

may interfere with vision as in dermachalasis. There may be so much stretching of the lid tissues that orbital fat and even the lacrimal gland prolapse downward. Ordinary lid skin atrophy occurs much later in life.

Repair of Upper Lid Skin Atrophy

The only treatment for both these conditions, i.e., dermachalasis and blepharochalasis, is surgical. This means excision of the redundant skin and resection of prolapsed orbital fat if present. Both these conditions, especially the baggy lower lids, are cosmetic repairs. However, man's urge to improve his appearance or correct a deformity goes back as far as history and will not be denied.

Procedure (fig. 244): The skin fold is picked up loosely and the amount to be resected marked off with an applicator dipped in sterile dye solution. It will be found that the marked-off area usually tapers to a point medially, but is rounded laterally because there is greater redundancy of skin at the temporal side of the lid (fig. 244*A*). It is important to mark off the area before injection because it is difficult to gauge the amount to be resected afterward. The lower line of incision should be in the lid furrow at the upper border of the tarsus in order to preserve a good fold and hide the incision scar.

The area is injected with a solution of 1 or 2 per cent procaine with epinephrine 1:50,000. An Ehrhardt clamp may be inserted under the lid which is put on stretch and the skin to be resected incised with a knife along the line previously drawn. The skin is undermined and resected. The wound is closed with 6–0 braided silk sutures placed close to the edge and the eye is patched (fig. 244E). The eyes are dressed on the second and fourth day and the sutures are removed on the fifth day. Result of repair is shown in figures 244F and G.

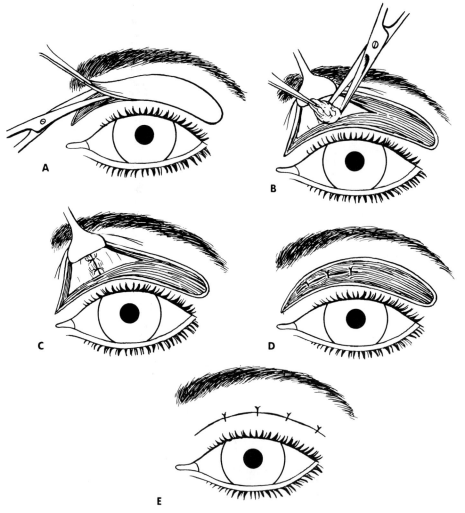

Fig. 244.   Repair of Upper Lid Dermachalasis.
A. Lines of skin incision. The outlined skin is resected.
B. In case of fat bulges the orbicularis fibers are separated horizontally and a vertical incision is made in the orbital fascia to expose the fat which is resected.
C. The fascia is closed vertically.
D. The orbicularis fibers are closed separately.
E. The skin wound is sutured with interrupted 5–0 silk sutures.

When orbital fat is also to be resected, it is done before the skin wound is closed. Usually the fat bulge presents nasally. The orbicularis fibers are separated horizontally by blunt dissection and the orbital fascia is exposed. There should be enough exposure to permit incision of the fascia vertically for about 15 mm. The prolapsed fat is resected and the orbital fascia resutured with 6–0 chromic catgut (figs. 244*B* and *C*). With the patient lying flat there is a tendency for the fat to fall back into the orbit. Hence when the patient is in the supine position, gentle pressure should be made backward on the globe and all the presenting fat resected. Unless this is done, the fat bulge will reappear again when the patient resumes the erect position. The orbicularis is closed horizontally as it was opened (fig. 244*D*). The skin is, of course, sutured as shown in Figure 244*E*. A firm supportive dressing is applied.

Comment: Experience has shown that in skin redundancy of the upper lid, the tendency is to remove too little rather than too much. A good rule is to leave just enough skin so that the patient can close his eyes without tension. Taking more than this will obliterate the lid fold; taking much less will result in undercorrection. This may sound drastic, but after a half dozen of these have been done, the truth of the above statement will become apparent.

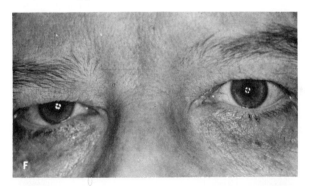

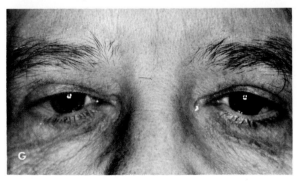

Fig. 244 (*Continued*)

F. Bilateral lid skin atrophy.

G. Result of repair.

Repair of Lower Lid Skin Atrophy

Dermachalasis of the lower lid is probably even more common than that of the upper lid (fig. 245*A*). Here also it may be due entirely to simple skin redundancy or there may be relaxation of orbital fascia with herniation of orbital fat in addition. It has been shown that lower lid fat usually herniates through in two bundles, a larger medial clump and a smaller lateral one. On the whole, surgery of lower lid dermachalasis requires more care as the lid may have to be tautened both vertically and horizontally. Since the lower lid is much narrower than the upper, over-correction with consequent ectropion is not difficult to attain hence circumspection in skin resection must be used.

Procedure (fig. 245): After suitable cleansing, the patient is asked to look up thus tautening lower lid skin. Whatever loose skin remains is then pinched horizontally, the amount to be resected without causing ectropion is estimated and marked off on the lid with methylene blue or gentian violet. The line of highest incision is placed close to the ciliary margin where it will be least conspicuous. The skin is pinched up vertically below the external commissure and the amount to be resected (if any) again marked off. Anesthetic solution with epinephrine is then injected subcutaneously. If simple skin resection is planned, it should be done cautiously—a thin strip at a time—watching the effect to assure that no ectropion results (fig. 245*B*).

If orbital fat is also to be resected, the skin-muscle lamina is dissected down to the lower orbital rim thus exposing the fascia and two vertical incisions are made in the fascia medially and laterally (fig. 245*C*). The eye is pressed back gently into the socket and all presenting fat is resected medially and laterally without pulling on it. Hemostasis is carefully made to assure that no bleeding points remain. The fascia is closed vertically with 6–0 chromic catgut as in the upper lid (fig. 245*D*); the skin muscle lamina with 5–0 interrupted silk sutures (fig. 245*C*). In closing, only enough undermining is done to bring the wound lips together snugly (fig. 245*E*). The eye is patched and dressings changed every other day. Sutures are removed on the fifth day. The patch is left off soon thereafter. Figure 245*F* shows the final result.

Comment: At the risk of repetition let it be said again that greater care is needed for lower lid than upper lid dermachalasis. Both skin and fat should be resected cautiously. It is better to do a secondary repair for undercorrection than to have an overcorrection. Replacing bulges with ectropion or hollows makes few friends. Also the orbital fascia should not be tautened too much as this also may give ectropion.

The lower lid may remain red and discolored for several weeks following repair unless all bleeders are well tied off or the cautery used to assure *complete* hemostasis before the skin incision is closed.

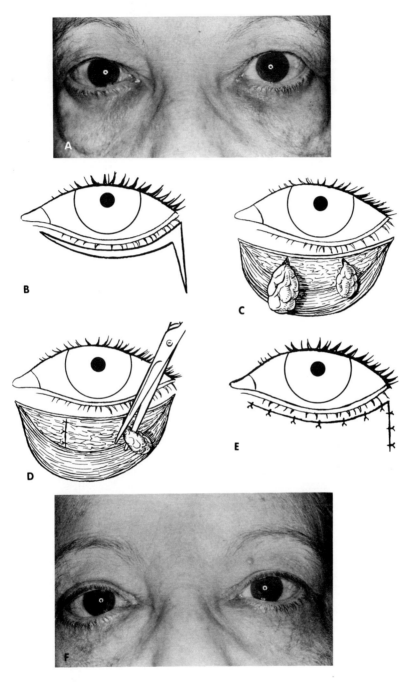

FIG. 245. Repair of Lower Lid Dermachalasis.
A. Bilateral lower lid "bags."
B. Skin incisions.
C. Exposure of orbital fat bulges (if any) through orbital fascia.
D. Fat is resected and fascia closed.
E. Skin is pulled up, excess resected and skin sutured.
F. Appearance after repair.

Incidentally, repair of "baggy" lids is not always an innocuous procedure. A recent report by Hartman, Morax and Vergez describes four cases of unilateral blindness following such a repair. The authors postulate a reflex vascular spasm due to pulling on the orbital fat and do not believe the retrobulbar injection was a cause. In all cases some pallor of the disc was apparently due to vascular changes at the posterior pole. Two of the cases recovered completely; the other two had considerable visual loss.

Fat Hernia

Fat hernia has already been mentioned in relation to dermachalasis, blepharochalasis and the aging process. However, it sometimes occurs as a primary entity in younger individuals, especially in the lower lid and may protrude through a weakened area in the orbital fascia or inclosed in what appears to be a separate fibrous pouch. Such conditions as myxedema and systemic pathology such as allergy, anemia and kidney disease must be ruled out. Resection and repair is the same as described above. Fat hernia of the conjunctiva is discussed in Chapter 12.

Elephantiasis Nostras

Elephantiasis nostras (solid edema) is a hypertrophy of the lid tissues due to recurrent inflammation. This is a rather unusual condition characterized by a solid edema in which the tissues are of the consistency of rubber which do not pit. There is neither pain nor tenderness. A curious characteristic is that the swelling is confined to the tissues outside the orbital margin. This is especially noticeable in the lower lid (right lower lid in fig. 250C).

It is most commonly due to chronic edema or recurrent erysipelas. The pathologic changes are infiltrates of the chronic inflammatory type through the derma, subcutaneous tissues and even the orbicularis muscle. The blood vessels may show endothelial proliferation and thrombosis.

Procedure: The area to be resected is bunched up in the fingers and marked off with an antiseptic dye. If possible, the figure should assume the approximate shape of the horizontal spindle. The area is anesthetized and the skin resected. A tough, glistening white subcutaneous tissue will next be encountered which should all be excised. The skin is then readjusted, excess is resected and the wound closed with 5–0 interrupted silk sutures.

Comment: The original skin resection should not be overgenerous below the lower lid in order to avoid overcorrection. After the subcutaneous tissue has been resected, if excess skin remains, it may be excised.

ANKYLOBLEPHARON

Ankyloblepharon, usually traumatic, was discussed in Chapter 7 and seen in figure 86. It differs from phimosis in that the lids retain their identity (figs. 247 and 248) in which no lid structure is visible in the affected areas. Treatment of ankyloblepharon was also discussed in Chapter 7.

BLEPHAROPHIMOSIS

Blepharophimosis (*blepharon* = lid; *phimosis* = contraction) is a rare condition characterized by a diminution in both dimensions of the palpebral fissure without involvement of the lid margins. Several types have been described which may be classified as follows:

Congenital (Discussed in the previous chapter.)

Acquired

    Senile

    Spastic

    Inflammatory

    Traumatic

Senile Blepharophimosis

This is a rare anomaly first described by Elschnig in which the medial or temporal skin at the canthus rides over and covers the canthal angle. It is due to the greater tonus of the orbicularis which has overcome the support given to the canthus by the lax senile orbital fascia and is similar to the clinical entity which has been called external blepharo-

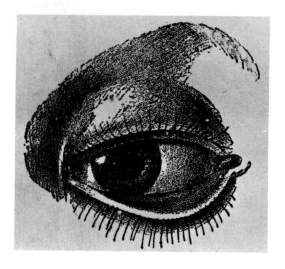

FIG. 246. "External Blepharophimosis" of Fuchs. Note resemblance to epicanthus.

phimosis by Fuchs (fig. 246). Actually this is not a true blepharophimosis since the skin merely overrides the lid fissure whose dimensions
are not shortened. A more apt name for the condition which may occur
laterally or medially is senile epicanthus (see figs. 111A and B), previously seen. Treatment consists in the resection of the excess skin.

Spastic Blepharophimosis

This is a similar pseudocondition described by Dimmer in 1911. It is
caused by continued and protracted blepharospasm causing a stretching
of the skin tissues. This may be medial or lateral and the treatment here
also is the resection of excess skin.

Inflammatory Blepharophimosis

Blepharophimosis may also be caused by severe, longstanding conjunctival inflammation such as pemphigus, trachoma, Stevens-Johnson
disease, ulcerative blepharitis, etc. (fig. 247A). This produces a small
palpebral fissure due to conjunctival shrinkage and may be accompanied
by lateral epicanthus, entropion or both. In modern days with our more
effective medicaments it has become a rare clinical entity. Repair consists in the creation of a new conjunctival fornix or sac to restore freedom of movement to the globe (fig. 247B). No surgery is undertaken
until all inflammation has disappeared.

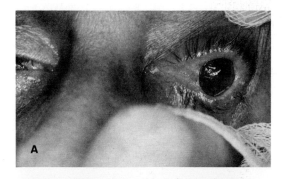

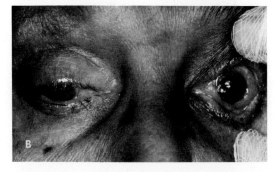

FIG. 247. Inflammatory Blepharophimosis.
A. Obliteration of medial fornix due to pemphigus.
B. After repair by mucous membrane graft.

Traumatic Blepharophimosis

Another type of blepharophimosis, rarely mentioned, is due to loss of support of the medial or lateral canthal ligament caused by trauma or surgical repair of neoplasm. This allows the involved canthus to move medially or laterally and shorten the palpebral fissure. A typical case is shown in figure 248*A* due to trauma at the lateral canthus with avulsion of the lateral canthal ligament, medial displacement of the canthus and shortening of the whole palpebral fissure. Repair here is surgical and means the creation of a new lateral canthal ligament to pull the lateral canthus outward into its proper position.

Procedure (fig. 248):   A vertical incision is made through skin and muscle just temporal to the lateral orbital margin and parallel with it. The tissues are undermined medially to uncover the lateral third of the orbit and hemostasis is attained by pressure and ligature.

Where there has been trauma or previous surgery with resultant scarring the lateral canthal ligament may be absent or difficult to identify. However, there is always so much scar tissue in the area that a strip of it can be fashioned to serve as the equivalent of a ligament as in this case. (Failing this, a strip of fascia may be used but this is rarely necessary.)

The lateral canthal ligament or its substitute is freed from the fibrous tissue of the area by wide dissection (fig. 248*B*). In addition the adjacent orbital fascia must be sufficiently incised so that the ligament can be drawn laterally with ease. The ersatz ligament is pulled over and sutured to the orbital tubercle behind the orbital rim with 4–0 chromic catgut (fig. 248*C*). This also draws the outer canthus laterally. Care is taken that the point of suture is at the same height as the lateral canthal ligament of the other eye. The muscle is closed with plain catgut and the skin with 4–0 interrupted sutures. The sutures are removed on the sixth day. The final result (fig. 248*D*) is seen several weeks later.

Comment: At the end of the operation the fissure is narrowed due to the strong pull on the lids laterally. After two or three weeks, however, the fissure gradually widens and adjusts to a more normal appearance.

The same procedure is used no matter what the trauma. Analogous repairs at both canthi, though somewhat more complicated, are shown in figures 128 and 129.

Blepharophimosis is also possible at the medial or lateral canthus due to surgical trauma. Figure 249*A* illustrates a surgical blepharophimosis due to the removal of a tumor of the right lower lid. The surgery apparently had been quite extensive. Repair was accomplished here by a medial canthotomy and suture of skin to conjunctiva in each lid essentially as in figure 86.

Procedure (fig. 249):   A medial canthotomy is made as far nasally as possible. Excess fibrous tissue, if any, is resected between the skin and

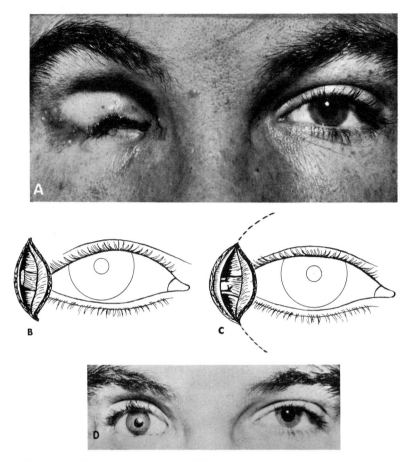

FIG. 248. Traumatic Blepharophimosis.
A. Blepharophimosis due to avulsion of lateral canthal ligament.
B. The lateral half of the orbit is exposed and the canthal ligament or its equivalent dissected up. The orbital fascia is incised for greater mobility.
C. The ligament is sutured to the periosteum in the area of the lateral orbital tubercle.
D. Result of repair.

conjunctiva and the skin is sutured to the conjunctiva in each lid with 5–0 silk interrupted sutures. The palpebral fissure is filled with ointment and a patch applied. The eye is dressed daily and any tendency to adhesion between the lids is discouraged by separation with a glass rod. Sutures are removed on the sixth day.

Comment: The initial incision is made as far medially as possible because no matter how one tries there will be some readhesion of the lids at the nasal canthus. Sometimes it is wise to interpose a piece of rubber dam the first few days to prevent this. The final result is seen in figure 249*B*.

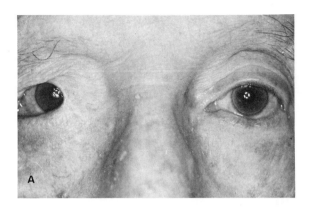

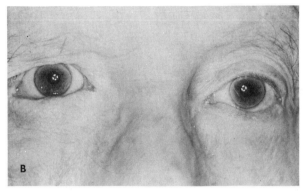

FIG. 249. Medial Blepharophimosis Repair.
A. Medial blepharophimosis as a result of tumor excision.
B. Result of repair.

LAGOPHTHALMOS

Lagophthalmos (*lagos* = hare which, it is believed, sleeps with its eyes open) is a condition in which it is difficult or impossible to close the eyes completely. In mild cases it is possible to squeeze the eye shut but in the more severe cases the eye is permanently open. In almost all cases the eye is open in sleep to a greater or lesser degree. The seriousness of this affection lies in the corneal exposure which may give rise to keratitis ēlagophthalmo, corneal ulceration and permanent visual loss. The most common clinical types follow.

Upper Lid Retraction—Paralytic Lagophthalmos

Paralytic lagophthalmos is usually due to peripheral lesions of the facial nerve with paralysis of the orbicularis. It is commonly accompanied by ectropion or, at least relaxation of the lower lid with consequent epiphora. It may also be due to lid retraction as in Graves' disease or in the Claude Bernard syndrome. The severe tearing and corneal exposure due to lagophthalmos cause organic and psychic trauma frequently calling for definitive surgery.

The permanent repair of the lagophthalmos of exophthalmos or of facial nerve palsy should not be undertaken unless these conditions are completely stationary and have been so for some time. If the exophthalmos is progressive, some decompression procedure of the orbit is indicated. There are many good procedures for this including a recent one by J. P. Smith. If the lagophthalmos is temporary and improvement may be expected, it may suffice to unite the lids by means of one or two temporary tarsorrhaphies until function of the orbicularis returns. Or a lateral tarsorrhaphy of the Wheeler or Elschnig type (Chapter 10) which allows for preservation of the lashes, may be done and later undone.

In stationary cases which are severe and offer no hope of subsequent improvement, the Fuchs type of lateral tarsorrhaphy may be used. All these lateral tarsorrhaphies tend to narrow the palpebral fissure and therefore enhance the appearance of the patient as well as protect the cornea.

Levator Recession—(Modified)

In the more advanced nonprogressive cases a levator recession is of value. This lowers the lid to its normal position over the eyeball. The procedure was introduced by Blaskovics in 1923, modified by Goldstein in 1934 and is shown in figure 214. It may be done by the skin or conjunctival routes. The former is the simpler and is commonly used by the author.

The procedure causes relaxation of the eyelid so that it tends to resume its normal position and ride lower on the cornea. This helps cover the cornea when the eye is closed. If performed by the conjunctival route, the preliminary steps are the same as outlined for a ptosis procedure. Once the levator tendon has been dissected free, it is recessed as described. Figures 250C and D show the result of levator recession in a case of nonprogressive paralytic lagophthalmos of the right upper lid (figs. 250A and D).

Lower Lid Retraction—Paralytic Lagophthalmos

As in the case of the upper lid, mild cases of lower lid lagophthalmos may be treated by temporary paracentral tarsorrhaphies if improvement is expected. This, however, is rare. Usually such cases are due to permanent paralysis of the orbicularis and permanent definitive treatment is required.

Some cases may be so severe as to require a lid shortening procedure. If there is an accompanying frank ectropion, the type of repair will depend on the severity of the ectropion and some ectropion type of procedure described in Chapter 15 may be put to good use. Thus severe

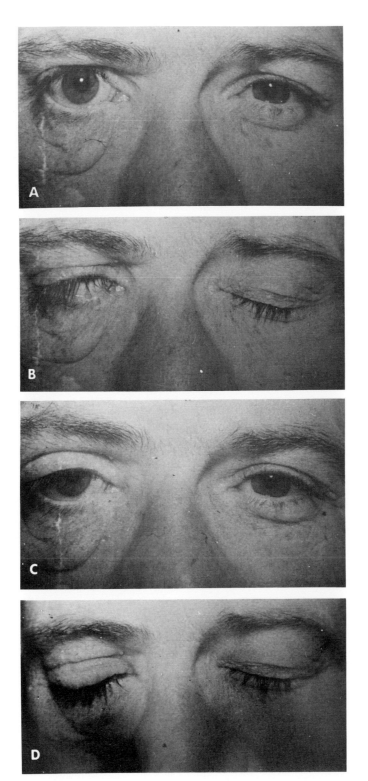

Fig. 250. Correction of Paralytic Lagophthalmos by Levator Recession.
A. and B. Lagophthalmos of right upper lid with the eye open and closed.
C. and D. Result of levator recession.

paralytic ectropion is the ideal place for the Kuhnt-Szymanowski operation which will bring the lid back up against the globe (cf. fig. 179). If
less severe, one of the other procedures for lid shortening may serve.

Beard has pointed out that a certain percentage of facial palsy cases
are not benefited by nerve crossing, nerve grafting or facial suspension
with fascia or nonabsorbable sutures. These require relief of the lagophthalmos and he has suggested an ingenious "triple threat" procedure.

Procedure (fig. 251):   If the ectropion of the lower lid is severe, it
is corrected by some ectropion procedure (see Chapter 15). If not severe,
a Fuchs lateral tarsorrhaphy is done as described in figure 119. If nasal
lagophthalmos or ectropion persists, closure at the medial canthus is also
indicated. Such procedures have been described in figures 108 and 171.

In severe facial palsy the brow on the affected side also droops.
Beard recommends suture of the brow to the periosteum for permanent

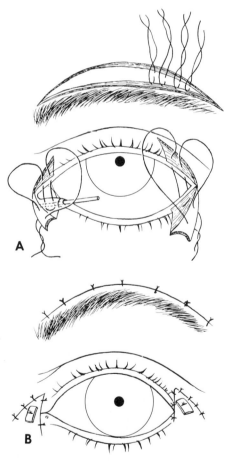

Fig. 251.   Repair of Lower Lid Paralytic Lagophthalmos (Beard).
A. The lower lid ectropion is corrected by means of medial and lateral cantho-
plasties. The drooping brow is sutured to periosteum.
B. Appearance on closure.

results. A deep incision is made just above the brow and 4–0 Supramid interrupted buried sutures are used to fasten the brow to the periosteum of the frontal bone (fig. 251A). The sutures are in the depths of the incision just above the hairline of the brow. The muscle layer is closed with 4–0 plain catgut and the skin with 4–0 dermalon (fig. 251B). Previous excision of skin above the brow has been discontinued in order to leave excess skin above the brow to give some semblance of wrinkling.

Comment: As Beard suggests, none of these procedures gives ideal results to sufferers from facial palsy but they help—sometimes considerably.

Gay, Salmon and Welkstein have suggested topical sympatholytic therapy for pathologic lid retraction. They use bethanidine and guanethidine sulfate for endocrine lid retraction with N. VII palsies and orbital myositis. There were no serious systemic reactions but all patients developed Horner's syndrome. J. W. Henderson severs the smooth muscle attachment to the tarsus for mild upper lid cases. For greater effect the tarsal attachments of the striate muscle are cut. In the lower lid the musculofascial attachments along the inferior border of the tarsal plate are cut. He reports favorable results in the majority of cases.

An ingenious steel spring prosthesis to help close the eye in facial paralysis has not fulfilled the promise originally held out for it.

Cicatricial Lagophthalmos—Lower Lid

Cicatricial lagophthalmos is the lagophthalmos of trauma and, more rarely, of disease. The problem is usually one of reconstruction and lost tissue replacement. Cicatricial ectropion and lagophthalmos are frequently coexistent. Hence, what has been said elsewhere (Chapter 15) about cicatricial ectropion and lagophthalmos applies here just as well and often poses the same problem.

Figure 252A shows such a case. While the ectropion here does not seem to be severe, the scarring was so extensive as to prevent closure (fig. 252B). Scarring of the upper lid also helped in the lagophthalmos.

The procedure of repair here (fig. 252C) was essentially the same as described in Procedure 185. The final result (figs. 252D and E) shows the ability of closure restored.

Cicatricial Lagophthalmos—Upper Lid

A not infrequent type of upper lid cicatricial lagophthalmos is seen in figure 253A in which the lid margin is normal but so much upper lid skin has been lost that the eye cannot be closed. This is best repaired by a free lid skin graft from the contralateral upper lid.

Procedure (fig. 253): A horizontal incision is made 6 mm. from the margin of the right upper lid. The skin is undermined upward and the lid is mobilized so that it can be brought down to its normal position. Two

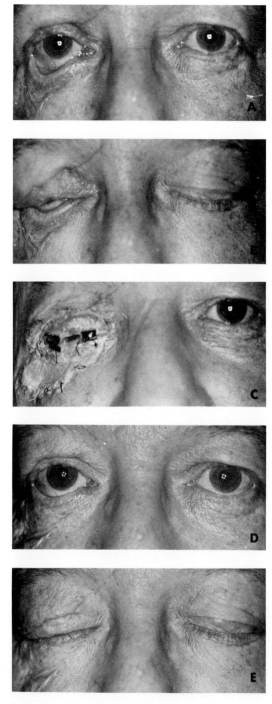

FIG. 252.   Repair of Cicatricial Lagophthalmos—Lower Lid.
A. and B. Traumatic cicatricial lagophthalmos of the right eye.
C.   Appearance six days after repair with split skin graft.
D.   Appearance after complete repair.
E.   Ability to close lids is restored.

surgical tarsorrhaphies are prepared (fig. 253*B*). A spindle-shaped skin graft is taken from the contralateral upper lid and sewed into position in the right upper lid. The left upper lid wound is closed with interrupted 5–0 silk (fig. 253*C*).

A firm pressure dressing is applied to the right eye. This is changed in five days and reapplied for three more days. All sutures are removed at this time. The tarsorrhaphies are opened six weeks later. The final

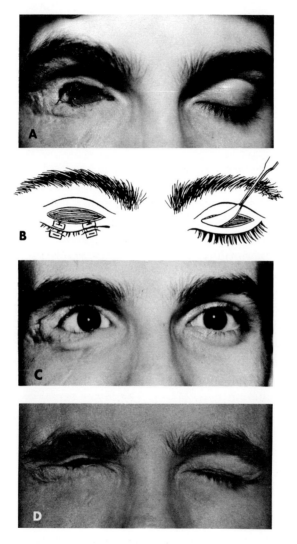

FIG. 253.   Repair of Cicatricial Lagophthalmos—Upper Lid.
A.   Inability to close right eye due to loss of upper lid skin tissue.
B.   The right upper lid is mobilized by free dissection and tarsorrhaphies are made. A free skin graft is taken from the left upper lid for implantation in the right upper lid.
C.   Appearance after six weeks with prosthesis in place.
D.   Ability to close the eye is restored.

result is shown in figure 253*D* with the ability to close the eye restored.

Comment: A split skin graft was used in the preceding procedure because two lids were involved. Since a larger graft was necessary it was easier to use epidermis. With only one lid involved here, use of whole skin would have been the simpler technic.

Mechanical Lagophthalmos

Mechanical lagophthalmos is not common. The chief causes are exophthalmos, buphthalmos and high axial myopia. Another type of mechanical lagophthalmos may be due to forward displacement of the globe by orbital tumors, cysts, hemorrhages, etc. with consequent prevention of lid closure. Many of these conditions are not amenable to lid surgery.

PTOSIS OF LOWER LID

Vertical shortening of the lower lid is rare but troublesome to correct. Obear and Smith point out that in such cases the lower lid margin is more deeply curved exposing the sclera below the limbus and giving an appearance of pseudoexophthalmos and pseudoectropion. The etiology may be orbital fracture, operation on the inferior rectus muscle or foreshortening of the conjunctival fornix after enucleation. The diagnosis is easily made by inspection and measurement noting the widened affected palpebral fissure. Repair by transplanting tarsus from the upper to the lower lid helps to narrow the interpalpebral space, increase lower lid support and elevate the supratarsal fold.

Procedure (fig. 254): The lower lid is everted and a horizontal incision 2 or 3 mm. from the lid border is made through the tarsoconjunctiva. The incision runs 3 mm. medial to the lateral canthus to 3 mm. lateral to the punctum (fig. 254*A*). The lower tarsal edge is undermined on the anterior tarsal surface to widen the wound gap. A tarsal graft from the same (or contralateral) upper lid about 3 mm. from the lid margin (fig. 254*B*) is taken. The width of the tarsoconjunctival strip is 4 to 5 mm. The graft is dissected up and sewed into the lower lid wound with interrupted 6–0 chromic sutures (fig. 254*C*). The upper lid wound is closed with through and through interrupted 5–0 silk sutures tied on the skin surface (fig. 254*D*). The lids are splinted together by an intermarginal suture with the prosthesis in place if the socket is anophthalmic. A pressure dressing is applied. The intermarginal suture is removed in 6 or 7 days and the upper lid sutures in 2 weeks. If anophthalmic, the patient may require a new prosthesis.

Comment: This procedure may also be helpful in lower lid entropion which sometimes develops in long-standing anophthalmic sockets.

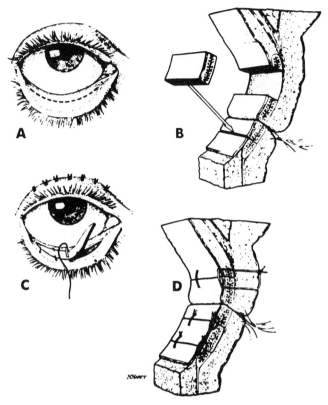

FIG. 254. Elevation of Ptotic Lower Lid—Obear and Smith.

A. The tarsus is incised and the lower tarsal edge undermined to cause it to retract.

B. A tarsal graft from the ipsilateral upper lid is taken.

C. The graft is bedded into the lower lid.

D. The upper lid dehiscence is closed.

(Courtesy American Journal of Ophthalmology.)

BLEPHAROSPASM

In a counsel of desperation Gerold in 1843 suggested treating intractable blepharospasm by "neglecting the spasm and carving a hole in the upper lid opposite the pupil through which the unfortunate patient could peep." Our mastery of this mysterious and dreadful affliction has not improved materially since Gerold's day.

Blepharospasm is an involuntary, persistent and forcible contraction of the orbicularis muscle causing firm closure of the eye and lasting from a fraction of a second to hours. It has been classified in many ways. However, two main categories suffice for clinical purposes: (1) symptomatic and (2) essential.

Symptomatic blepharospasm includes reflex spasm of the orbicularis due to corneal, conjunctival and lid irritation as well as retinal stimulation due to bright light. A rarer subsidiary type is the tonic spasm of the orbicularis found in postencephalitic parkinsonism and similar affections.

Essential blepharospasm has no connection with the eye itself, and there is no obvious organic cause. It is usually bilateral and may be clonic or tonic, usually the latter. It may vary in severity from occasional involuntary blinking to almost complete and permanent forceful closure of the eyes. The severe cases are crippling and disabling. In some cases the patient is blind to all intents and purposes and cannot fend for himself. This is the type of blepharospasm discussed here.

The etiology is unknown. Cortical and peripheral nerve lesions, psychogenic, psychosomatic, hysterical, senile and arteriosclerotic causes have been blamed. None has been proved but the psychogenic factor is certainly important.

In what must be a prize example of understatement, Duke-Elder says, "The treatment of blepharospasm, at any rate in its more severe degrees, is somewhat unsatisfactory." He does add that it is "always difficult and frequently disappointing." Actually, the difficulty of treating essential blepharospasm is as great as the mystery of its etiology.

That there is no dependable, accepted treatment is proved by the myriad types of therapy suggested. The reports cited here are only a few of the many to be found in the literature. Alcohol injection (Fumagalli, Benedict) has probably been the most popular and frequently used procedure. Henderson, who has studied the subject at length, has shown that even a long series of alcohol injections is effective for only six to nine months at best. Neurotomy or neurectomy (Talko, Gurdijian and Williams; Dvorak and Nemec), electrocoagulation (Safar and Spitzmuller), canthotomy (Pochisov) myectomy plus neurectomy (Friede, Callahan), galvanic current stimulation (Yealland), psychotherapy, hypnotism, shock treatment, hormones, antispasmodic drugs, sedatives, tranquilizers and crutch glasses have all been tried. The effectiveness of all these has been something less than conspicuous. Forcible attempts at opening the eyes simply increase the spasm. I know of no one who has used Gerold's heroic and despairing suggestion, but the temptation has sometimes been strong.

In 1951 I reported a case of postencephalitic blepahrospasm due to Parkinson's disease. The patient was so blinded by the blepharospasm that he had to be led around. It was controlled by resection of the orbicularis of both upper lids leaving only the pretarsal fibers intact. Eight months after operation the blepharospasm was still controlled. When seen five years later, some blepharospasm had returned but the patient could get around by himself and was gainfully employed.

This technic has not been as effective in the treatment of essential blepharospasm. Better results have been obtained with the resection of the upper and lower orbicularis muscle sparing only the pretarsal fibers.

In recalcitrant cases the effect has been further enhanced by a frontalis sling.

Operative Technic

Procedure (fig. 255): A skin incision is made 3 mm. below the margin of the lower lid from canthus to canthus and the skin is undermined downward to expose the whole lower orbicularis muscle. Starting at the attached tarsal border, all the orbicularis fibers extending down to its lower border, running medially to the nasocanthal angle and laterally to the insertion at the raphé, are resected. This leaves only the pretarsal fibers intact (fig. 255). All bleeding points are clamped and tied.

A skin incision is now made in the upper lid over the attached tarsal border and is curved downward at each canthus to meet the ends of the previously made lower lid skin incision. The skin is undermined upward until the hair follicles appear beneath the brow. Medially and laterally full exposure is obtained as in the lower lid. The whole expanse of exposed upper lid orbicularis is resected (fig. 255). Again, all bleeding points are clamped and tied.

When the whole operative site is dry, the skin incisions are closed with interrupted 5–0 silk sutures and a firm pressure dressing is applied.

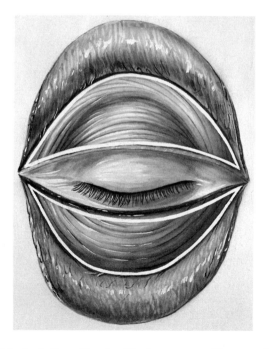

FIG. 255. Orbicularis Resection for Blepharospasm. Upper and lower lid skin is dissected upward and downward to expose the orbicularis. The whole muscle except the pretarsal fibers is resected (areas enclosed by white lines).

The pressure is left on for three days. Sutures are removed on the fifth or sixth day.

In resecting the orbicularis, the skin incisions are made over the attached tarsal border in the upper lid and just below the border in the lower lid, respectively, because scars in these sites are least conspicuous. The lid fold covers the incision in the upper lid and the cilia mask the incision in the lower lid.

There are no specific contraindications to this surgery. General restrictions are those which forbid any surgery in any individual. Unless all bleeding is meticulously stopped and pressure applied postoperatively, edema and discoloration may persist sometimes for two or three months. However, it always disappears ultimately.

It is my custom to do the lids of each eye separately. The second eye may be done any time after removal of the dressing from the first eye. There is no contraindication to operating on both eyes at once, if for example, the patient is from out of town and time is important. However, I think it is better psychology to leave one eye free at all times.

When the improvement is not sufficient or if there is recurrence, the addition of a frontalis sling to each upper lid has helped materially. It is immaterial what technic is used to insert the frontalis sling; any of the standard procedures will do. However, I believe that the material used for the sling is important. I have come to prefer autogenous fascia as the most likely to maintain its effectiveness and the least likely to give postoperative complications.

Comment: Urist reported use of the frontalis sling in milder cases of blepharospasm. I have found this modality more useful as an adjuvant to orbicularis resection. As stated, I prefer to use autogenous fascia even though it means an extra step and a longer operation. Collagen and preserved fascia have given me too many recurrences. Metal wires have caused intractable edema in a high percentage of cases. Other alloplastic sutures may cause delayed infection or may ultimately break. I have found autogenous fascia, therefore, to be the most desirable.

Use of the frontalis sling in these cases is not as drastic as it sounds. Since the levator in the patients I have seen is intact, wrinkling and contraction of the brow is not necessary for opening the eye. The sling here merely acts as a brake to forced closure and no ill effects result except the slight lagophthalmos in sleep. This is a small price for these desperate people to pay.

The literature attests to the fact that neurotomy or neurectomy, or both, has never been completely successful, else it would not be constantly rediscovered. For best results one must use a nerve stimulator for identification and get every branch of the nerve supplying both lids as far medially as the nose. This is a long and tedious process. Blind resection of the branches will leave some twigs intact—frequently important ones. Or it will destroy branches beyond the involved area and give unwanted paralyses. Also, there is the constant expectation of nerve regeneration which makes this an untrustworthy modality.

There are few definite conclusions to be drawn from any suggested treatment of essential blepharospasm. In my experience, orbicularis resection as described gives results at least as good as any reported in the literature. There is no embarrassment of normal closure. This may seem impossible with so much muscle resected, but I have seen this result too often not to be certain. The trouble is that some patients still continue to close their eyes altogether too well. The addition of a frontalis sling buttresses the effect of orbicularis resection when needed. Also, the hope that something can be done and the actual surgery may be a powerful psychic adjuvant in all these cases.

Reports of final results are of no great value when a condition may change overnight. The word "cure" should be used cautiously in conjunction with blepharospasm. Amelioration of symptoms is possible, as is restoration of the patient's confidence. But given a seemingly identical pair of cases, one may go on apparently indefinitely after operation with regression of symptoms. The other may show recurrence in three months. And the affects of an intractable blepharospasm may be substantially moderated in one case and unchanged in another. My own experience and the warily worded reports in the literature offer no balm to the seeker after a sure cure.

Although the definitive etiology is unknown, men who have studied the subject agree that a strong psychogenic element is present in essential blepharospasm. It may even be the only cause. Hence, surgical treatment of its organic manifestations is at best an indirect modality. Until we learn more about the etiology of this dread disease, no method of treatment will be wholly satisfactory.

Irvine, Daroff, Sanders and Hoyt have described an unusual type of familial reflex blepharospasm which is commonly psychogenic. It was an heredofamilial disorder in a father and two children. Goldstein and Cogan have reported an apraxia of lid opening which may be confused with ptosis or blepharospasm. Actually, it is an impairment of the lid opening function without paralysis or blepharospasm. It is a nonparalytic motor abnormality in which there is only momentary difficulty in lid opening.

Ptosis of the Globe—Enophthalmos Supratarsal Depression

These acquired conditions are mainly the result of orbital fractures and will be discussed in Chapter 21.

REFERENCES

BEARD, C.: Canthoplasty and brow elevation for facial palsy. Arch. Ophth. *71*:386, 1964.

BENEDICT, W. L.: Treatment of blepharospasm. Trans. Am. Ophth. Soc. *39*:227, 1941.

BONIUK, M., and ZIMMERMAN, L. E.: Tumors of the eyelids. Arch. Ophth. *69*:698, 1963.

CALLAHAN, A.: Intractable blepharospasm. Am. J. Ophth. *60*:788, 1965.

DVORAK, M., and NEMEC, J.: Beitrag zur Neurochirurgischen Therapie der hartnackigen Blepharospasmus. Ophthalmologica *148*:130, 1964.

FOX, S. A.: Relief of intractable blepharospasm. Am. J. Ophth. *34*:1351, 1951.

————: Essential idiopathic blepharospasm. Arch. Ophth. *76*:318, 1966

FRIEDE, R.: The surgical treatment of blepharospasm. Klin. Monatsbl. Augenh. *133*:270, 1958.

FUCHS, E.: Textbook of Ophthalmology, ed. 5. Philadelphia, J. B. Lippincott Co., 1917, p. 953.

FUMAGALLI, A.: La injesioni sottocutanee de alcool nella cura de blepharospasmo e del'entropion spastico. Ann. Ottal. *38*:163, 1909.

GAY, A. J., SALMON, M. L., and WELKSTEIN, M. A.: Topical sympatholytic therapy for pathologic lid retraction. Arch. Ophth. *77*:341, 1966.

GEROLD, J. H.: Quoted by Duke-Elder, S., Textbook of Ophthalmology, vol. 5. St. Louis, C. V. Mosby Co., 1952, p. 5162.

GOLDSTEIN, I.: Recession of levator muscle for lagophthalmos and exophthalmic goitre. Arch. Ophth. *11*:389, 1934.

GOLDSTEIN, J. E. and COGAN, D. G.: Apraxia of lid opening. Arch. Ophth. (Chicago) *73*:155, 1965.

GURDIJIAN, E. S., and WILLIAMS, H. W.: The surgical treatment of intractable blepharospasm. J.A.M.A. *91*:2053, 1928.

HARTMAN, E., MORAX, F. V., and VERGEZ, A. Serious visual complications of surgery of "baggy lids." Ann. d'ocul. *195*:142, 1962.

HENDERSON, J. W.: Essential blepharospasm. Trans. Am. Ophth. Soc. *54*:453, 1956.

————: Relief of eyelid retraction. Arch. Ophth. *74*:205, 1965.

IRVINE, A. R., DAROFF, R. B., SANDERS, M.D., and HOYT, W. F.: Familial reflex blepharospasm. Am. J. Ophth. *65*:889, 1968.

NAFFZIGER, H. G., and JONES, O. W.: Surgical treatment of progressive exophthalmos following thyroidectomy. J.A.M.A. *99*:638, 1932.

NEMETH, L.: Blepharophimosis and its operation. Am. J. Ophth. *49*:1357, 1960.

OBEAR, M., and SMITH, B.: Tarsal grafting to elevate the lower lid margin. Am. J. Ophth. *59*:1088, 1965.

POCHISOV, N.: Operation bei spastichem Lidumschlag, Vestn Oftal *6*:131, 1935.

SAFAR, K., and SPITZMULLER, W.: Elektrokoagulation als neues Behandlugfahreh gegen schweren Blepharospasmus, Ztschr. Augenheilk *76*:337, 1932.

SFORZOLINI, G. S.: Operation for blepharospasm. Brit. J. Ophth. *48*:165, 1964.

TALKO, J.: Klinische Krampfe der Augenlider: Neurotomie der Supraorbitalnerven. Klin. Mbl. Augenheilk *8*:129, 1870.

URIST, M. J.: Bilateral blepharospasm. Arch. Ophth. *58*:520, 1957.

VANNAS, S.: A method for correction of the retracted upper eyelid. Acta. Ophth. *36*:444, 1957.

YEALLAND, L. R.: Hysterical disorders of vision with special reference to the phenomenon of the contraction of the antagonists. Brit. J. Ophth. *2*:545, 1918.

CHAPTER 20

Socket Repairs

FORNIX REFORMATION

FORNIX RECONSTRUCTION

SOCKET RECONSTRUCTION
WITH MUCOUS MEMBRANE
WITH EPIDERMIS

THE INFERIOR FORNIX of the anophthalmic socket is of greater importance than the superior in the satisfactory fitting of a prosthesis.
The upper fornix need only be of sufficient depth to prevent the artificial
eye from slipping out from under the upper lid. The lower fornix, however, does most of the weight bearing and must be deep enough to
supply firm anchorage for the prosthesis in the usual upright position of
the head. This is why, in socket reconstruction, the dissection is carried
well below the lower orbital rim to provide a sufficiently deep lower
gutter. The gradual abandonment of the integrated implant has re-
affirmed the importance of the lower fornix in the proper fitting of an
artificial eye.

When a socket has been badly traumatized, enucleation should be
done carefully and tears in Tenon's capsule repaired. Also a well-fitting
conformer should be inserted to minimize post-traumatic contraction as
much as possible. Otherwise there may be a tendency for the orbital
contents to prolapse forward with a shallowing or obliteration of the
lower fornix making retention of a prosthesis impossible. Figure 256
illustrates the extreme of such a case. This is not postoperative chemosis
but an irreducible prolapse of orbital contents three months after enucleation.

REFORMATION OF FORNIX

A more common type of prolapse is seen in the socket of old enucleations, especially if there has been no implant into Tenon's capsule (fig.
257A). Here the lower fornix is shallowed and converted into a downward sloping shelf which pushes the lower lid down and out and prevents retention of a prosthesis. The repair of these conditions is accomplished as outlined below:

Procedure (fig. 257): The conjunctiva of the fundus of the socket
is incised horizontally from lateral to medial canthus and undermined
to the upper and lower lid edges. The lower conjunctiva is pulled out of
the way and all fibrous tissue and prolapsed fat resected.

449

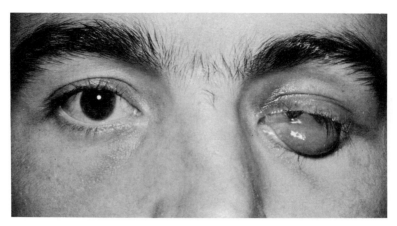

FIG. 256. Prolapse of Contents of Left Lower Fornix. (Fox, S. A.: Courtesy American Journal of Ophthalmology.)

The inferior fornix is recreated by blunt dissection close to the lid wall and carried down to the periosteum below the orbital rim, as is done for socket reconstruction (fig. 257B). The conjunctival incision is closed with a running 5–0 silk suture (fig. 257C). Three double-armed 4–0 silk sutures on large cutting needles, spaced equidistantly, are then passed from within outward through the floor of the newly created cul-de-sac. The needles are carried close to the periosteum below the lower orbital rim and brought out on the skin surface where they are tied over pegs (figs. 257E and F).

An alternative and perhaps better technic is to pass the three double-armed sutures equidistantly through a length of stiff plastic tubing which has been cut to fit snugly into the lower fornix (fig. 257D). As the sutures are tied the tubing is drawn down and exerts an even pressure along the whole floor of the fornix. A conformer is inserted to assure healing of all the tissues in proper position and a firm pressure dressing is applied for three days. On the sixth day the sutures are removed, the socket cleaned, the conformer reinserted and the eye patched daily thereafter until all reaction has subsided. A permanent prosthesis may be inserted any time after the second week (fig. 257G).

Comment: The problem of repair here is not difficult. No conjunctiva need be grafted since none has been lost. It is simply a matter of reforming the inferior fornix by reshuffling the orbital contents and assuring that they heal in proper position.

If there is not much shelving of the lower fornix and little adventitious tissue is to be resected, a simpler type of repair may be used. This is done by means of a vertical conjunctival incision close to the lateral canthus which is large enough to allow a scissors to be entered so that the whole conjunctival sac may be undermined (fig. 258). The incision is then closed and the lower fornix recreated as in the previous procedure. The disadvantage of this procedure is that it does not permit the

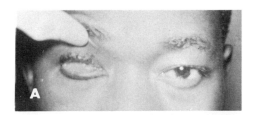

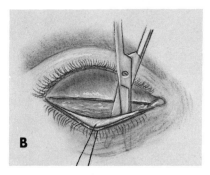

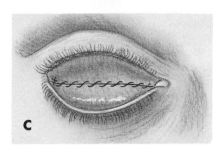

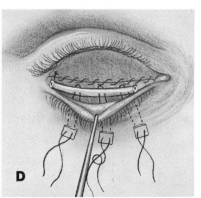

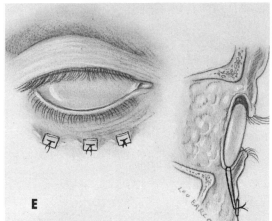

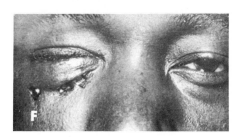

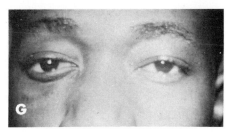

FIG. 257. Repair of Prolapsed Lower Fornix.

A. A case of prolapse and shelving of right lower fornix.

B. The conjunctiva of the fundus is incised horizontally from lateral to medial canthus and completely undermined to the lid margins in order to mobilize it. The dissection is carried down into the depths of the lower fornix below the orbital rim.

C. The conjunctival wound is sutured.

D. Three double-armed sutures are passed through a length of plastic tubing which is drawn into the lower fornix as the sutures are passed through the depth of the fornix to the orbital rim to emerge on the skin surface.

E. The sutures are tied over pegs.

F. Appearance before removal of the sutures.

G. Result with prosthesis in place.

(Fox, S. A.: Courtesy American Journal of Ophthalmology.)

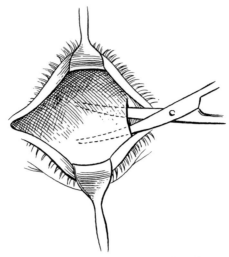

FIG. 258.   Technic for Repair of Lower Fornix by Means of Simple Undermining. Sutures Are Used to Recreate the Lower Fornix As in Figure 257.

resection of prolapsed fat or fibrous tissue from the lower fornix if any exists. On the other hand it is a simpler technic which requires less conjunctival incision and suturing and hence offers less potential conjunctival loss in cases where the lower fornix can be recreated without tissue resection.

Fornix Reconstruction

The ideal lining for a socket is mucous membrane. Where there is a slight deficiency in the existing conjunctiva due to minor contraction, excision of the scar and readjustment by means of a V-Y or Z plasty may be all that is required. Occasionally small conjunctival grafts from the normal fellow eye may suffice. If larger grafts are needed, buccal mucous membrane—labial, malar or both—may be used to reform a fornix.

If part of the socket such as a fornix has been destroyed by trauma, infection, chemical burns, etc., reconstruction with a buccal mucous membrane autograft is the best method. The lower and medial fornices are most commonly affected in trauma. The technic of repair of the lower fornix follows:

Procedure (fig. 259): A stout double-armed suture is passed through the central edge of the lower lid to serve as a retractor and give good exposure. An incision is made through the tissue of the lower fornix from one canthus to the other. This is placed close to the lid wall in order to preserve as much of the conjunctiva as possible. The dissection is carried down to the lower orbital rim and somewhat beyond in front of the periosteum. The caruncle should also be preserved for cosmetic reasons, if possible (fig. 259A).

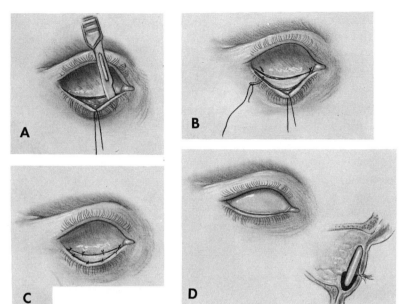

FIG. 259. Reconstruction of an Absent Lower Fornix by Mucous
Membrane Graft.
A. The conjunctiva is incised and the fornix deepened as in figure 257.
B. and C. A mucous membrane graft is obtained and sewed into place.
D. A conformer is inserted (not too tightly) and a pressure dressing is applied.

All fibrous tissue should be resected. Mucous membrane is obtained from the lower lip or cheek as outlined in Chapter 3 and sewed into position with interrupted sutures to cover the raw surface in the cul-de-sac (figs. 259B and C). A conformer is inserted to fill the socket (fig. 259D) and a pressure dressing is applied for five days. On the fifth day the dressings are removed, secretions carefully sponged off and the pressure dressing replaced for three more days without disturbing the conformer. On the eighth day the conformer is taken out and the sutures removed. "Take" is usually complete at this time. A conformer must be kept in the socket for at least three more weeks to counteract contraction. A light dressing, such as a patch, suffices until all reaction has subsided and healing is complete. A permanent prosthesis may be inserted three weeks after operation.

Comment: When the globe is present, it is, of course, not possible to use an ordinary conformer in the socket. Many types of special conformers made of cardboard, plastic material, glass and metal which do not rest on the cornea have been suggested. The author has simply used three double-armed sutures passed through the fundus of the cul-de-sac or through a length of plastic tubing as described above (fig. 257). This has been found just as effective as any type of skeleton conformer which attempts to protect the cornea and often does not. A pressure dressing here too is required.

The conformer inserted at the end of operation should fit snugly but must not be so large that it has to be forced in as this will stretch the wound and may rupture the sutures. Such accidents always make for a smaller fornix, for every time that the conjunctiva is sutured, no matter how carefully, it is shortened and hence the socket dimensions diminished. It may be better to put in an easily fitting conformer first then, after the wound is healed, the size of the conformer is gradually increased as the conjunctiva and socket stretch.

Mucous membrane shrinks—sometimes a great deal. To counteract this all fibrous tissue is resected, a generous graft is taken and the conformer is kept in the socket until all signs of contraction have disappeared. This is usually after the fourth week.

This method applies to all four fornices. Figure 260 is a rather unusual case which shows the result of grafting buccal mucous membrane

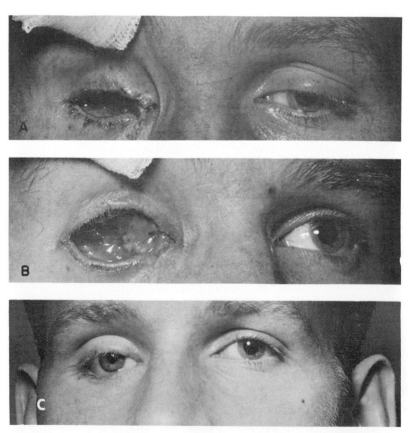

FIG. 260.   Reconstruction of a Medial Fornix by Mucous Membrane
Graft.
A.   Appearance before repair.
B.   Appearance after repair with mucous membrane graft by technic described in figure 259.
C.   Result with prothesis in place.

to form an absent medial fornix which prevented the insertion of a prosthesis. The technic used here differed in no way from that described above. It should be unnecessary to repeat that if the eye is present nothing but mucous membrane should be considered. Epidermis would set up an intractable keratitis.

SOCKET RECONSTRUCTION

The generally contracted socket, as well as the obliteration of the fornices by scar and granulation tissue, is most commonly due to trauma. Occasionally severe infections such as panophthalmitis and orbital cellulitis and too free use of x-rays (fig. 263) are etiologic factors. Where most of the socket has been obliterated, one must resort either to multiple membrane grafts or to an epidermic graft. The better and more natural of the two is, of course, mucous membrane and although it takes longer and requires more surgery, it is the more desirable. Enough mucous membrane is usually not available from the lower lip and malar mucous membrane will have to be taken unless the loss is not great.

Socket Reconstruction with Mucous Membrane

Procedure (fig. 261): An incision is made in the fundus of the remaining socket (fig. 261A) from canthus to canthus and lining of the socket undermined to the lid margins. If the remnants of the remaining conjunctiva are healthy, they should be preserved as every millimeter is precious. As much buccal and malar mucous membrane as needed is then taken, as described in Chapter 3, and sutured into the socket. The first strip is sutured into the lower fornix, the next into the upper fornix and the last into the fundus where the strips of mucous membrane are sutured to each other (fig. 261B). A conformer which fits snugly but not too tightly (it may extrude) is fitted into the socket to supply counterpressure to the pressure bandage. It should be possible for the lids to close fairly well over the conformer, if not, the conformer is too large. A pressure dressing is applied for six days, removed, the socket cleaned carefully and reapplied for three more days. By then "take" should be good (fig. 261C). The conformer is removed, cleaned and reinserted.

Mucous membrane will contract if permitted and the conformer should be kept in at least six weeks to overcome this as much as possible. A prosthesis is then inserted.

Comment: The patient is given an antiseptic mouth wash the first week to use after meals. The mucous membrane regenerates quickly and I have never attempted to close the wound with sutures. The main postoperative complication is shrinkage of the grafted mucous membrane. Hence the conformer should always be in place. In some cases the con-

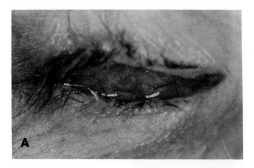
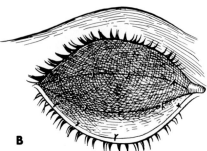
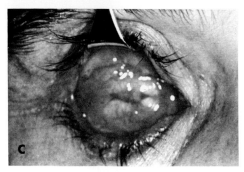

FIG. 261.   Reconstruction of Socket with Buccal and Malar Mucous
Membrane.
A.   Contracted socket.
B.   Reconstruction with mucous membrane from three separate areas.
C.   Final result.

former may have to be changed for a smaller one during the early stages.
After several weeks the conformer is gradually enlarged again.

Smith repairs the socket much as described above but uses a wire
suture to hold the conformer against the lower orbital rim to assure
against its extrusion.

Socket Reconstruction with Epidermis

Almost 50 years ago Wheeler presented an excellent method of total
or subtotal reconstruction of an obliterated socket with epidermis.
Briefly, the technic consisted of dissecting the contracted socket lining
away from the lids. The dissection was carried down below the lower
orbital rim to the periosteum, behind the canthi medially and laterally,
and as far as the orbital rim above. A form or stent of dental compound
was molded to fit the socket. An epidermic graft was then taken, preferably from the upper outer aspect of the thigh, wrapped around the
stent, epithelial side inward, placed in the socket and a firm pressure
dressing applied.

After using this method for some time, it was noted that the stents
tended to be the same shape and, in most cases, approximately the same
size, i.e., about 30 by 40 by 3 mm. It seemed obvious then, that if an

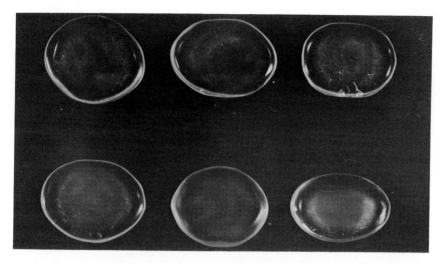

FIG. 262. Acrylic Stents Used in Socket Reconstruction. (Fox, S. A.: Courtesy American Journal of Ophthalmology.)

acrylic form of the proper size and shape were available, it would do away with the awkward, time consuming, dental compound molding technic. Accordingly, a series of these acrylic forms was made, the largest measured 32 by 42 mm., the smallest 22 by 38 mm. (fig. 262). They are 1.5 mm. to 2 mm. thick. The one most frequently used measures 28 by 38 mm., which is slightly smaller than that suggested by Wheeler. Experience has proved the value of these forms. They are kept sterile by immersion in 1:1000 Zephiran solution.

Preoperative preparation of the site includes several minimum requirements. These are:

1. The eradication of all infectious foci from the surrounding area such as chronic sac infections, fistulae, infections of the socket itself, blepharitis, skin affections of the lids, etc. A preoperative course of antibiotics continued for three or four days postoperatively is recommended, especially where the socket has been chronically infected for a long time.

2. If surgery of the lids is required, this should be completed before socket surgery is undertaken.

3. If the orbit is not intact, this should be repaired first.

Procedure (fig. 263): The lids are dissected up from the socket contents if adherent. Only skin and orbicularis should be included in the dissection. However, if the tarsus is intact, it may also be preserved. Every attempt should be made to save as much of the lid edges as possible, for these will contribute greatly to a final good cosmetic result. This is not always possible in cases of severe trauma. The dissection is carried downward beyond the orbital rim to the periosteum, laterally and medially behind the canthi and above to the orbital roof. If necessary,

an external canthotomy is performed to facilitate exposure and mobility
of the lids.

The next step is to resect all fibrous and granulation tissue. Fibrous
tissue over nonmovable surfaces—especially if old and no longer subject
to contraction—may sometimes be left in situ, but here it should be
removed. An epidermal graft will shrink somewhat in any case, but if
it is placed on a bed from which all fibrous tissue has been resected, the
shrinkage is minimal and need not be feared.

On the other hand, failure to remove such tissue may allow enough

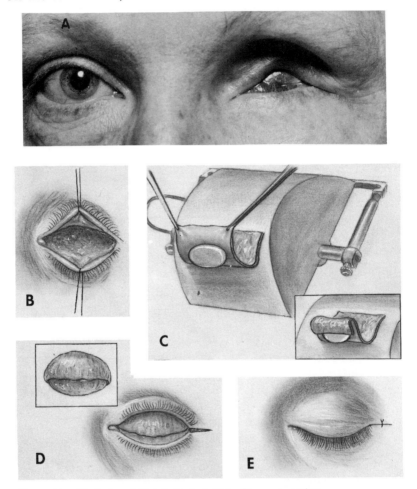

FIG. 263.   Technic of Total Socket Skin Reconstruction.
A.   Total absence of socket following x-ray therapy.
B.   The lids are dissected up, the upper and lower fornices deepened and all
      remnants of conjunctiva are resected.
C.   A split skin graft is taken with the Padgett dermatome and wrapped around
      a conformer, raw surface outward (see text).
D. and E.   A canthotomy is performed (if desired) and the graft, wrapped
      around the conformer, is inserted. The canthotomy incision is sutured. A
      firm pressure dressing is applied.

shrinkage so as to negate the whole operation. An acrylic conformer that will fit snugly into the socket and fill out its dimensions is then chosen. The socket is now ready for the graft (fig. 263B).

The donor site chosen (the inside of the arm, the upper outer aspect of the thigh or the lower abdominal wall) is previously prepared by an assistant by thorough cleaning, sterilization and draping. The exact area from which the graft is to be taken is measured and marked out with some antiseptic dye such as gentian violet and a piece of epidermis is cut with the dermatome as described in Chapter 3, figure 25.

The dermatome is placed on a prepared sterile flat surface. The corners of the graft are grasped in small forceps, the previously chosen acrylic form is placed on the epithelial side of the graft (fig. 263C) which is wrapped around the entire form, raw surface outward. This should be done without stretching the graft to avoid later shrinkage. The graft is inserted into the socket with the overlapped portion facing anteriorly (figs. 263D and E). It is unnecessary to suture the lids together if a conformer of the proper size has been chosen. A patch, several gauze fluffs and a firm pressure bandage complete the dressing.

No oiled silk or similar material that prevents absorption should be used as part of the dressing. Since no skin sutures that may become adherent to the gauze are present, there is no need for this. Furthermore, damming up of secretions may prevent a take. The donor site is covered

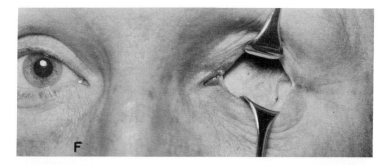

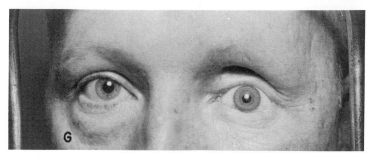

Fig. 263 (Continued)

F.   Appearance of socket after repair (note sparing of caruncle).

G.   Result with prosthesis in place. (See text for use of newer dermatomes.)

with nonadherent plastic mesh and a layer of plain gauze and bandaged. When this is removed after 10 or 12 days, the site is usually found to be completely re-epithelialized if the graft has not been too thick.

The eye dressing is removed on the sixth day, excess graft, if any, between the lids removed, the surface sponged with warm saline to clean away secretions and the pressure dressing reapplied for four more days. By this time the graft has taken completely (fig. 263F). The conformer may be removed, the socket irrigated and all excess tissue cleaned away. The inside of the socket is coated with a thin layer of sterile ointment and a skeleton conformer (fig. 18) is inserted. This permits adequate drainage and need not be removed for some time. Daily cleansing is then carried out for some two weeks when the socket should be ready for a prosthesis (fig. 263G).

Comment: If discharge from the socket is anticipated, the first dressing may be done a day or two sooner for inspection and cleansing. As long as the conformer is left undisturbed this may be done with impunity. If the tarsi are intact, it may be advantageous to leave them as this reduces the tendency toward postoperative entropion in these cases.

Unless a piece of epidermis is large enough to overlap the whole conformer, it is hard to handle and one is not quite sure of its staying in place. Consequently enough epidermis is taken to cover the conformer completely whether the socket reconstruction is total or subtotal. Since epidermis can easily be spared one need not hesitate to take a little too much. Too little may necessitate further surgery. If this technic is followed a "take" is practically assured.

The substitution of the acrylic conformer for the dental compound does much to simplify the procedure. Molding of the dental compound, mud-pie fashion, is an irksome and wearisome business. The water in which the stent is fashioned must be the right temperature—about 120° F. If hotter than this, the stuff sticks to the gloves like glue; if colder, it cannot be molded easily. A previously prepared conformer of the proper size and shape does away with all this.

An ingenious rubber conformer has been devised by Hughes. At the operating table this is cut to pattern to fit the socket and used in the same fashion as the acrylic conformer. The rubber has the advantage of elasticity so that it is fitted into the socket easily after it has been covered with epidermis; it is also removed just as easily. The procedure is otherwise the same as described above. Use of the dermatome instead of the skin knife also adds to the smoothness of the procedure. The modern electric dermatomes such as the Padgett and Brown make the taking of epidermis even easier now than formerly.

Many donor sites offer themselves: the anterior abdominal wall, the outer and inner thigh (if hairless) or inside of the arm. The last is preferable because the site is easily accessible and causes the patient less inconvenience during convalescence than would the taking of a graft from the thigh or abdomen. Of course, the left arm is usually used unless there is some contraindication such as left-handedness.

Like mucous membrane, epidermis will shrink, though not as much, if care is taken to keep the conformer in. Mustardé has invented an external fixation device which is fixed to a headcap of plaster. It has steel rods fixed to the conformer to keep it firmly in place. I have not yet found a need for it.

Aftercare of Reconstructed Socket

The matter of hygienic care of the socket after this type of operation is important. Much has been said and written concerning the difficulty of keeping such a socket clean of debris, infection and odor. Presumably this is especially true of those sockets containing a lining of epidermis. It has been observed that when there is free drainage of tears, the socket usually stays normally clean. When lacrimal drainage is obstructed, it is a good deal harder to avoid infection.

This is true of all empty sockets, grafted or ungrafted. An empty socket does not have the benefit of a normal tear conducting mechanism, which is the cleaning agent of the eye. When the lower punctum is absent, as it is in many traumatic cases, this is especialy true. Tears, mucus and debris tend to collect and stagnate. Low grade infections are easily set up and are hard to eradicate. If epidermic grafts are too thick—and this is more true of those taken with a knife—sebaceous material and epithelial debris will aggravate the condition. Use of the dermatome which permits the taking of a thin, uniform graft, tends to obviate this to some extent.

It is also true that a socket completely lined with epidermis has no tears and is therefore dry. The prosthesis also appears dull as a consequence. Occasional minimal lubrication with a bland ointment goes far toward enhancing the appearance of such a prosthesis. In time the epidermal surface becomes smooth and shiny with little or no exfoliation of epithelium and the dryness is controlled by regular lubrication.

The patient must be instructed in the proper toilet of the socket by careful cleansing and irrigation. This is a requisite in all cases. When infection has set in, treatment is difficult and unrewarding. The old-fashioned 2 or 5 per cent silver nitrate solution, firmly applied each day to the socket with an applicator, has been found to be as effective as anything to control odor and infection. It works well on both mucous membrane and epidermis. Sulfa drops are used as an adjuvant.

REFERENCES

BENOIT, M.: Restauration de la cavité orbitaire par autoplasties chez les blessés de guerre. Paris, Thesis, 1920.

CLAY, G. E., and BAIRD, J. M.: Restoration of orbit and repair of conjunctival defects with graft from prepuce and labia minora. Tr. Sect. Ophth. A.M.A. 1936, p. 252.

CRUISE, R. R.: Operation for contracted sockets. Tr. Ophth. Soc. U. K. *39*:126, 1919.

DE VOE, A. G.: Experiences with the surgery of the anophthalmic orbit. Am. J. Ophth. *28*:136, 1945.

DIMITRY, J. J.: The socket after enucleation and the artificial eye. Arch. Ophth. *31*:18, 1944.

FOX, S. A.: Some methods of lid repair and reconstruction. III. Socket reconstruction wth epidermis. Am. J. Ophth. *30*:190, 1947.

————: Some methods of lid repair and reconstruction. VI. Reformation of the inferior fornix. Am. J. Ophth. *31*:1441, 1948.

GREEAR, J. N.: The use of buccal mucosa in restoration of the orbital socket. Am. J. Ophth. *31*:445, 1948.

GUYTON, J. S.: Enucleation and allied procedures: A review and description of a new operation. Tr. Am. Ophth. Soc. *46*:472, 1948.

HERZENDERFER, A.: Plastic surgery of the orbit. Ophthalmologica *139*:115, 1960.

HUGHES, W. L.: Socket reconstruction. A new form and method of handling the skin graft. Arch. Ophth. *26*:965, 1941.

LAGROT, F., PY, N., ALCAYDE, M., and LAVERGNE, E.: Restoration of orbital sockets and conjunctival cul-de-sacs. Arch. d'opht. *17*:769, 1957.

MUSTARDE, J. C.: Repair of contracted socket. *In* Plastic and Reconstructive Surgery of the Eye and Adnexa. Troutman, Converse, and Smith, (Eds.) : Washington, D.C., Butterworth's, 1962, p. 148.

SHERMAN, A. E.: The retracted eye socket. Am. J. Ophth. *35*:89, 1952.

SMITH, B.: Reconstruction of the eye socket. Arch. Ophth. *71*:517, 1964.

STRAMPELLI, B.: A technique for restoration of the conjunctival cul-de-sac. Boll. ocul. *37*:682, 1958.

WEEKS, J. E.: Operation for contracted socket. Brit. M. J. *2*:398, 1913.

WHEELER, J. M.: Restoration of the obliterated eye socket. Am. J. Ophth. *4*:481, 1921.

CHAPTER 21

Bony Orbit Repairs and Late Complications

BLOWOUT FRACTURES
EARLY DIAGNOSTIC SIGNS
MATERIALS FOR REPAIR
SURGICAL REPAIR
EARLY POSTOPERATIVE COMPLICATIONS

LATE COMPLICATIONS
ENOPHTHALMOS
SUPRATARSAL DEPRESSION

STALLARD HAS STATED, "Fractures of the orbit have become more frequent chiefly because of the misbehavior of selfish fools in automobiles and an ever increasing corps of scurvy knaves who inflict facial assaults with blunt weapons when robbing." This may not be the whole story but there is little with which to disagree. Fractures of the orbit are fractures of violence due to, civil or military, accidental or intentional trauma.

"BLOWOUT" FRACTURES

The most vulnerable of the orbital bones is the floor and this is the most common fracture, the so-called "blowout" fracture. As far back as 1944, King and Ford described the etiology and pathology of what we now know as the blowout fracture. Smith and his co-workers, as a result of experimental work, have shown that the blowout fracture is caused by a sudden increase in intraorbital pressure due to a blow which displaces the orbital contents backward. In this type of injury the orbital rim remains intact but the orbital floor is fractured to greater or lesser extent with a downward herniation of the contents into the antrum. The result is ptosis of the globe, diplopia, restriction of vertical movements of the globe, pseudoptosis, enophthalmos and supratarsal depression. In addition, there may be lid abrasion, laceration, ecchymosis and emphysema due to fracture into the nasal sinuses.

Frequently such patients are first seen in a state of shock when the primary treatment is directed toward the patient himself and not the globe. However, as soon as the patient can stand it, preferably within the first week after trauma, surgical exploration of the orbit should be undertaken. Stereoscopic x-rays are indispensable and may show an orbital floor fracture immediately. On the other hand, early x-rays may show nothing except clouding of the maxillary and ethmoid sinuses. However, in the presence of diplopia, pseudoptosis and impedance of vertical

463

ocular movement, fracture should be suspected and surgical exploration done.

Early Diagnostic Signs

A history of injury with an obvious vertical muscle imbalance and a positive muscle traction test (resistance to upward rotation of the globe) is enough to give a diagnosis of orbital floor fracture according to Cole and Smith even without positive x-ray findings. However, the diagnosis is not always clear-cut and may be masked by facial edema or the symptoms may be so mild that fracture is not suspected.

There may be other early signs which help make the diagnosis. Since most cases are not surgical emergencies, examination should be complete and unhurried: Ptosis of the globe and enophthalmos where present after injury are always indicative of orbital floor pathology. In case of doubt, exophthalmometry helps. Infraorbital anesthesia due to injury to the infraorbital nerve fibers, downward displacement of the lateral canthus, ptosis and flatness of the cheek with facial asymmetry, is always suggestive of possible bony orbital damage. Other signs such as malocclusion, trismus and unilateral nasal bleeding are somewhat farther afield but all merit investigation. In fact, a complete eye examination is always in order because an appreciable percentage of such cases show serious ocular injuries including hyphema, corneal laceration and even rupture of the globe.

X-rays play an important part in the diagnosis and sometimes clinch it. Zizmor et al. have pointed out that the early diagnosis of blowout fracture established by x-ray and its interpretation is important before surgery. The main x-ray signs are: (1) fragmentation of the bone of the orbital floor, (2) depression of bony fragments and (3) prolapse of orbital soft tissues into the upper half of the maxillary sinus. On the other hand they may reveal nothing at first. X-rays should be taken in the Waters and Caldwell view in lateral projection. Linear tomograms may help. However, even if all these are negative other signs should be looked for.

It has been pointed out that orbitography is not an innocuous procedure. It is contraindicated in orbital infection, allergy to contrast media and perforations of the globe. Orbitography runs the same risks as any orbital injection: perforation of the globe, retrobulbar hemorrhage, retinal artery spasm and the possibility of intravenous injection of the contrast solution.

Milauskas and Fueger believe the patient should first be tested for allergy to the contrast medium and that the test be done by someone familiar with the anatomy of the orbit. Plain orbital films are taken first for contrast.

The contrast medium they use is intended primarily to show orbital floor fractures and consists of 3.5 cc. of 50 per cent Hypaque, 3.0 cc. of 2 per cent xylocaine and 0.5 cc. of Wydase. The needle is first advanced slowly along the orbital floor with small amounts of xylocaine being injected. After obtaining akinesia the needle is slightly withdrawn again, the syringe is changed to one containing contrast medium and about 6 to 7 cc. injected straight ahead, medially and laterally along the orbital floor.

Four views are taken: The first shows the orbital floor in profile with the patient's head in the standard posteroanterior position and the central ray directed 30 degrees caudad. The second shows the anterolateral segment of the floor and maxillary sinuses with the head rotated 20 degrees and the central ray 35 degrees caudad. The third is a Water's view to show the anterior-inferior orbital rim. The fourth is a lateral view showing the facial bones in a second plane. (This paper of Milauskas and Fueger should be read in full for details.)

If clinical signs are minimal, most authors feel that it is wise to observe the patient seven to ten days. Many patients having slight diplopia will improve spontaneously. But if enophthalmos, impaired motility, diplopia, a positive direction test and positive x-ray findings point to damage of the orbital floor, then surgery should be undertaken especially if the condition tends to worsen. I have seen cases with apparently minimal trauma and few other early signs whose x-rays showed a tremendous fracture with prolapse of orbital contents into the maxillary sinus. Such cases will never improve spontaneously.

If done early, before there is a loss of orbital fat due to atrophy and traumatic inflammation and before there is permanent injury to the inferior oblique and rectus muscles from fibrosis, a good result is usually obtained. When the muscles are freed and the globe and orbital fat raised back to normal position, the enophthalmos and the supratarsal depression are reduced. For the orbit is a truncated cone of hard, unyielding bone lying on its side with its apex pointing backward and its only opening pointing forward. When its contents are restored, they must go forward for there is no other place for them to go. Hence both the enophthalmos and supratarsal depression are improved.

However, after some time has elapsed and atrophy and fibrosis take their toll, improvement is still possible but it is more difficult to attain and the result will not be as good.

Materials Used

Various materials for repairing the orbital floor and raising the globe have been used. Among them are cartilage, bone, plastic plates, polyvinyl plastic sponge, fascia and muscle. Bone obtained from the iliac crest is good. Preserved cartilage and plates of methyl methacrylate resin (fig. 265) are also good for this purpose.

More recently such materials as Silastic, polyethylene, Supramid, dacron surfaced silastic, processed bovine bone, Teflon and Marlex have been used. Rapidly polymerizing acrylic (cranioplast) has also been suggested for fashioning the needed plate at the operating table.

Repair of Orbital Floor

Figure 264A is a case of ptosis of the left globe with supratarsal depression and enophthalmos due to fracture of the orbital floor. Repair was accomplished by the use of a plate placed under the periosteum of the orbital floor to bridge the break and push the eye upward.

Procedure (fig. 264): A horizontal skin incision is made in the lower lid 1 or 2 mm. above the lower orbital rim parallel with the orbital rim and running from canthus to canthus (fig. 264B). The lower lip of the wound is undermined downward to expose the orbicularis muscle. A similar horizontal incision is made in the muscle just below the orbital rim and the periosteum is exposed along the whole lower orbital margin (fig. 264C).

The periosteum is incised and undermined as far back into the orbit as necessary to allow exploration of the orbital floor (fig. 264D). The fracture is located, bone fragments, if loose, removed and orbital fat and muscles gently freed if they are caught in the fracture line. A wedge-shaped piece of methyl methacrylate or its equivalent cut to pattern is then inserted under the periosteum (fig. 264E). This is inserted apex backward so that the base lies at the orbital margin. The anterior edge of the plate must not jut out beyond the orbital rim and obliterate the lower fornix. In case of anophthalmos, care must be taken that the base is not too thick or it will interfere with the proper fitting of a prosthesis.

The plate is pushed back far enough so that the height of the globe is the same as that of the fellow eye or even a little higher. If insufficient, an additional thin plate may be added. After the plate has been wedged into position firmly, the periosteum is closed with 4–0 chromic catgut

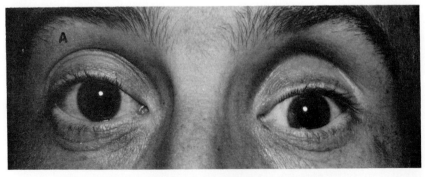

FIG. 264.   Repair of Ptosis of the Globe.
A. A case of ptosis of the left globe due to fracture of the orbital floor.

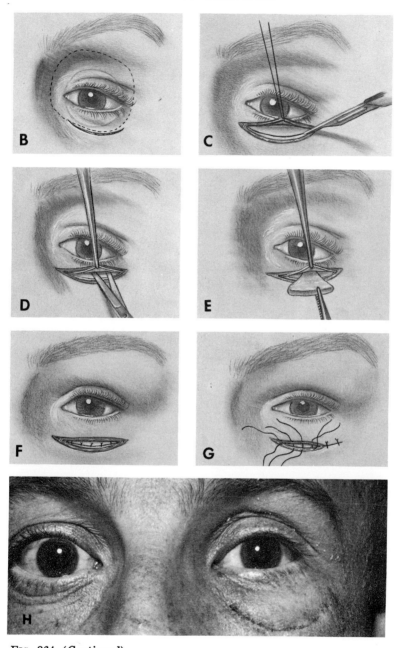

FIG. 264 (*Continued*)

B. The skin and muscle are incised. (Dotted line, margins of bony orbit.)
C. The periosteum is exposed and incised.
D. The periosteum is undermined.
E. A plate is inserted and the ptosed globe is elevated.
F. The periosteum is closed.
G. The skin is sutured.
H. Final result.

(Fox, S. A.: Courtesy Archives of Ophthalmology.)

sutures. The orbicularis is closed with plain catgut (fig. 264*F*) and the skin is closed with a running silk suture (fig. 264*G*). A firm pressure dressing is applied and kept on for 5 days. The eye is dressed daily until the reaction has subsided. The sutures are removed on the sixth day.

Comment: By this procedure the eye and orbital contents are pushed up, the supratarsal depression is done away with as much as possible and the lid fold is restored (fig. 264*H*). Instead of a plastic plate, bone may also be used as an autograft, homograft or even heterograft (see Chapter 3).

Other technics of repair have been suggested. Cunningham and Marden believe that with the Caldwell-Luc approach and antral packing no bone graft is necessary. Abrahams and Dodd suggest a double approach: subperiosteal and a Caldwell-Luc through the maxillary sinus. But the direct infraorbital approach described above has been found to be the simplest and best in these cases.

If plastic plates are used they may be prepared previously. They should be triangular, measuring about 18 to 20 mm. along the base and a bit longer at the sides. The thickness should be anywhere from 3 to 6 mm., thinning out to about 2 mm. at the apex and base (fig. 265). It is wise to have several plates of methyl methacrylate resin made up in varying sizes and thicknesses. These are kept in 1:1000 Zephiran solution. At the operating table it is a simple matter to choose the one which gives the right elevation of the globe. A sufficient number of these have been used successfully by the author so that they can be recommended. No reaction to the resin has been noted. The advantage of using a plastic plate instead of a bone autograft is that the patient is spared an additional operation and hence scarring and pain; also there is no absorption to be concerned about.

Use of prepared plastic plates has been found more convenient and less time-consuming than molding the newer plastic powder at the operating table. As time goes on, however, this opinion may be changed.

Postoperative Complications

Other problems frequently arise in connection with orbital injuries. Edema of the lower lid sometimes persists for months but gradually disappears. Placing the skin and muscle incisions at different sites as described above helps diminish this. Postoperative hemorrhage, tissue reaction to the implant and chronic infection are rare. Migration or extrusion of the implant happens more often and, to counteract this, some surgeons wire the plate to the orbital floor. Also strabismus, ptosis, epiphora and canthal deformities may have to be dealt with. Tears through the canaliculi are not unusual. The handling of these injuries are discussed in Chapters 9 and 23.

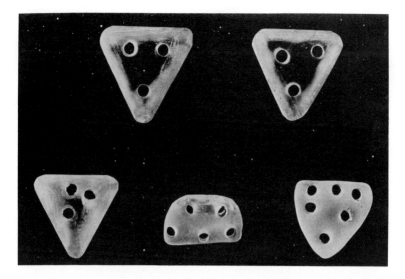

FIG. 265.   Methyl methacrylate plates for propping up the globe.

Other fractures occur. Fractures of the orbital floor may occur without blowout. Fractures of the orbital rim and roof require assistance from the rhinologist and maxillofacial surgeon. Fractures of the medial wall are extremely rare but have been reported. They have been described with the retraction syndrome, enophthalmos and in conjunction with a fine orbital floor fracture and entrapment of the medial rectus muscle. Even in these rare cases the clinical signs were most important though x-ray evidence was equivocal. It is the *clinical* evidence of muscle involvement which warrants surgical interference. Supraorbital and other facial bones are the responsibility of the maxillofacial surgeon also. Only if the lacrimal system is involved does it become an ophthalmic problem in these cases.

Repairs of the orbital floor are practically the same whether early or late once the primary effects of the trauma have subsided. But in late repairs there often remain other problems once the ptosis of the globe has been repaired. These are primarily enophthalmos and supratarsal depression.

LATE COMPLICATIONS

Enophthalmos

Enophthalmos may be congenital or acquired as in Horner's syndrome and such unusual diseases as progressive lipodystrophy. All these are rare.

Traumatic enophthalmos is most commonly caused by a fracture of the orbital floor as noted above. It is often accompanied by supratarsal depression and pseudoptosis. Pseudoptosis is due to the enophthalmos which reduces the support of the globe to the upper lid. The enophthalmos is probably due to multiple causes such as loss of orbital contents into the maxillary sinus with consequent increase in the orbital space or the inferior rectus may be caught in the fracture and immobilize the retro-placement of the globe. In delayed cases there is actual atrophy of the orbital fat. Early repair may be of great value if not much of the orbital contents have been displaced into the maxillary sinus and before atrophy has taken place. As shown above (fig. 264), repair of the orbital floor will often raise the eyeball and push it forward, fill out the supratarsal depression and furnish support for the upper lid.

If there is much loss of retrobulbar tissue with the passage of time due to inflammation or atrophy or both, or if much of the orbital contents have been lost into the antrum, then late repair of the orbital floor by bone graft or plastic plate will raise the globe but the enophthalmos will be little improved because there is not enough orbital tissue behind the eye to push it forward. Indeed, if the globe is pushed up too high behind the upper lid in an effort to reduce the enophthalmos, pseudoptosis will be increased and nothing will be gained but a cosmetic condition worse than the original one. Figure 266 illustrates such a case. This patient, hurt in an automobile accident, suffered injuries to the globe and orbit. The globe was ptosed, shrunken and enophthalmic. Enucleation was refused when first seen. A bone graft repair of the floor had already been done and, in an attempt to push the eye forward, it had been pushed up behind the upper lid (fig. 266A), with a resultant pseudoptosis. Since the eye was sightless, a cosmetic repair was simply effected by a deeply curved shell placed in front of the shrunken globe (fig. 266B). Sometimes the best surgery is no surgery at all.

However, if the eye has retained useful vision or if a prosthesis cannot be used for some reason, the enophthalmos may sometimes be improved by repairing the orbital floor. Then if the enophthalmos still persists a strip of fascia may be pushed backward toward the socket apex under the eye. This is done carefully and slowly until enough content is added to the depleted socket to fill out the orbit and bring the eye forward. By this method some improvement is usual but complete repair cannot be expected in neglected cases.

Recently other methods of correcting this deformity have been re-ported. Stone has suggested the implantation of pyrex glass beads. Smith, Obear and Leone have also suggested glass bead inplantation for the enophthalmos of anophthalmos. Shannon and Coyle have reported a good result in remolding a depressed orbital floor and maxilla by rubber silicone injection of medical silastic 382 with stannous octoate. A soft material is formed after injection. Hill and Radford have injected a mixture of Silastic RTV-S-5392 and stannous octoate into the anoph-

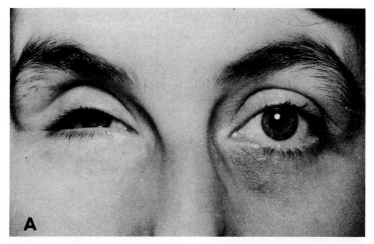

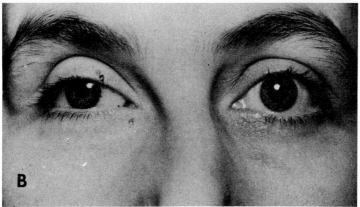

Fig. 266. Use of Shell Prosthesis.
A. Phthisis of the right eye, enophthalmos and pseudoptosis of the upper lid.
B. Simple repair with covering shell prosthesis.

thalmic socket in cases of advancing enophthalmos. However, this procedure is not without complications. To avoid them the authors suggest the following procedure:

1. Give repeated injections of 1 cc. rather than all at once.

2. Make injection through the lateral palpebral ligament rather than through the orbital septum.

3. Inject air as the needle is withdrawn to prevent tracking the silicone mixture.

4. Exert pressure over the site until the material is vulcanized.

5. Check set-up time of the exact sterile mixture in the operating room.

Supratarsal (Retrotarsal) Depression

Supratarsal (retrotarsal) depression or upper tarsal sulcus is a deep indentation of the upper lid above the tarsus due to loss of support

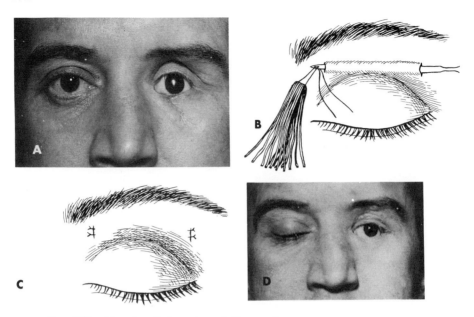

F<small>IG</small>. 267. Repair of Supratarsal Depression.
A. A supratarsal depression of left upper lid.
B. A subcutaneous tunnel is prepared and the fascial strips are drawn through.
C. The skin incisions are tightly closed.
D. Result of repair.

behind it. It is often seen in cases of orbital floor fracture and in old enucleations (fig. 267A). As shown above, atrophy and loss of orbital contents because of breaks in the orbital floor is the cause. In the case of old enucleations, especially those in which there has been no implant into Tenon's capsule, the cause is loss of the support of the bulb as well as downward displacement and/or atrophy of the retrobulbar contents. Here the prosthesis sags downward and backward, the upper lid lacks support and supratarsal depression results.

As with enophthalmos, the early traumatic cases in which loss of orbital contents has not been severe may be corrected along with the ptosis of the globe by repair of the fracture of the orbital floor. However, in those cases in which there is no ptosis of the globe and in late cases in which repair of the orbital floor does not reduce the enophthalmos and supratarsal depression, separate repair will have to be made. This has been attained by the implantation of fascia, cartilage chips, fat, muscle, skin, thin plastic plates or surgical sponge. On the whole, fascia is probably as good as anything. Fat and skin should be avoided because of the great shrinkage. Fascia also shrinks but not enough to mar the usual good result obtained.

Procedure (fig. 267): Starting at the temporal end of the eyebrow a 15 mm. downward incision, slanting outward slightly, is made. A similar incision slanting medially is made at the nasal end of the eyebrow. A long narrow blunt-pointed scissors is entered under the muscle at the temporal incision and a tunnel is fashioned immediately under the brow from one incision to the other.

A long strip of fascia about 20 cm. long and 0.5 cm. wide is taken from the thigh (see Chapter 3) by an assistant and kept in a gauze sponge moistened with warm saline until ready for use. The fascial strip is cut in half and each half is doubled over to make two double strips 5 cm. long and 0.5 cm. wide. A suture is passed through each doubled end. Each strip is shredded lengthwise with scissors or knife. A blunt-pointed Reese knife is passed through the temporal end of the tunnel to emerge at the nasal end where each suture is threaded through the instrument and the fascial strips pulled through, adjusted and centered. There should be an appreciable overcorrection so that the lid bulges out (fig. 267B).

The ends of the fascia are tucked in or resected if too abundant. The wound is closed at both ends with a couple of 4–0 plain catgut sutures and the skin is closed with 5–0 silk sutures (fig. 267C). Good closure should be obtained so that both the muscle and skin wound lips are tightly closed and the fascia sealed in well. A firm supportive dressing is applied. This is changed daily after the third day and the skin sutures are removed on the fifth postoperative day. Figure 267D shows the result of this procedure which is usually quite adequate.

Comment: If plastic material such as Silastic is used it should be one of the softer kind which can be easily cut to pattern at the operating table. This has proved inert and gives no tissue reaction. It has served well in many cases and spares the patient the taking of autogenous fascia. This type of "banana" implant suggested by Bartlett and others is well worth considering.

REFERENCES

ABRAHAMS, I. W.: Repair of orbital floor defects with premolded plastic implant. Arch. Ophth. 75:510, 1966.

ABRAHAMS, I. W., and DODD, R. W.: Orbital floor fractures. Arch. Ophth. 68:159, 1962.

BALLEN, P. H.: Rapidly polymerizing acrylic in reconstruction of the orbit. Am. J. Ophth. 56:378, 1963.

BARCLAY, T. L.: Diplopia in association with fractures involving the zygomatic bone. Brit. J. Plast. Surg. 11:147, 1958.

BARTLETT, R. E.: Plastic surgery for the enucleation patient. Am. J. Ophth. 61:68, 1966.

BENNETT, J. E., and ARMSTRONG, J. R.: Repair of bony orbit with methyl methacrylate. Am. J. Ophth. 53:285, 1962.

BROWNING, C. W.: Alloplast materials in orbital repair. Am. J. Ophth. 63:955, 1967.

BROWNING, C. W., and WALKER, R. V. The use of alloplastics in 45 cases of orbital floor reconstruction. Am. J. Ophth. 60:684, 1965.

COLE, H. G., and SMITH, B.: Eye muscle imbalance complicating orbital floor fractures. Am. J. Ophth. 55:930, 1963.

CONVERSE, J. M.: Blowout fracture of the orbit. Plast. Reconstr. Surg. *29*:408, 1962.

CONVERSE, J. M., and SMITH, B. C.: Enophthalmos and diplopia in fractures of the orbital floor. Brit. J. Plast. Surg. *41*:265, 1957.

CONVERSE, J. M., COLE, G., and SMITH, B.: Late treatment of blow-out fracture of the floor of the orbit. Plastic & Recon. Surg. *28*:183, 1961.

CONVERSE, J. M. et al.: Orbital blowout fractures. Ten year survey. Plast. Reconstr. Surg. *39*:20, 1967.

CUNNINGHAM, J. D., and MARDEN, P. A.: Blowout fracture of the orbital floor. Arch. Ophth. *68*:492, 1962.

DEVOE, A. G.: Fractures of the orbital floor. Trans. Am. Ophth. Soc. *54*:502, 1956.

DUKE-ELDER, S.: Textbook of Ophthalmology. St. Louis, C. V. Mosby Co., vol. 5, p. 5195.

EDWARDS, W. C., and REDLEY, R. W.: Blowout fracture of medial orbital wall. Am. J. Ophth. *65*:248, 1968.

ERDBRINK, W. L.: Blow-out fracture of the orbit. Am. J. Ophth. *49*:1037, 1960.

FISCHBEIN, F. I., and LESKO, W. S.: Blowout fracture of the medial orbital wall. Arch. Ophth. *81*:162, 1969.

FOX, S. A.: Use of preserved cartilage in plastic surgery of the eye. Arch. Ophth. *38*: 182, 1947.

HILL, J. C., and RADFORD, C. J.: Treatment of advancing enophthalmos in the ocular prosthetic patient. Am. J. Ophth. *60*:487, 1965.

KING, E. F., and FORD, E.: Fractures of the orbit. Tr. Ophth. Soc. U. K. *64*:134, 1944.

LA GRANGE, F.: Fractures of the Orbit. London, University of London Press, 1918.

MILAUSKAS, A. T., and FUEGER, G. F.: Serious ocular complications associated with blowout fractures of the orbit. Am. J. Ophth. *62*:670, 1966.

MILLER, G. R., and GLASER, J. S.: The retraction syndrome and trauma. Arch. Ophth. *76*:662, 1966.

MOWLEM, R.: Bone and cartilage transplants. Brit. J. Surg. *29*:182, 1941.

SHANNON, G. M., and COYLE, J. J.: Rubber silicone injections. Arch. Ophth. *74*:811, 1965.

SMITH, B., OBEAR, M., and LEONE, C. R., JR.: The correction of enophthalmos associated with anophthalmos by glass bead implantation. Am. J. Ophth. *64*:1088, 1967.

STONE, W., JR., and FASANELLA, R. M.: Complications of Eye Surgery. Philadelphia, Saunders, 1965, p. 397.

VANNAS, S.: On the use of rib cartilage for the correction of cosmetic defects. Acta Ophth. *24*:225, 1946.

WOLTER, J. R., and PFISTER, R. R.: Polyethylene in reconstruction. Am. J. Ophth. *52*:672, 1961.

ZIZMOR, J., SMITH, B., FASANO, C., and CONVERSE, J. M.: Roentgen diagnosis of blowout fracture of the orbit. Trans. Am. Acad. Ophth. Oto. *66*:802, 1962.

CHAPTER 22

Enucleation and Allied Procedures

THE NEED for emptying the globe, Tenon's capsule or the orbit of their contents occurs often enough in connection with plastic surgery of the ocular adnexa to warrant discussion here.

While the indication for exenteration of the orbit is usually clear cut and, indeed, mandatory, the choice between enucleation and evisceration is not always easy to make. The dilemma is greater and the decision more critical in the young than in the aged, in the female than in the male, in the socially active than in the recluse. Economic and social stress as well as widespread accounts of medical "miracles" have caused the public to expect a great deal from the surgeon medically and cosmetically—sometimes more than he can possibly or safely deliver. Youth, sex, economic requirement and other considerations are all important, but they must not be allowed to sway the surgeon's judgment or to override his minimum requirements of safety.

Hence the decision as to type of procedure deserves deliberate and adequate general discussion with the patient or family or both before it is undertaken. In this way there will be no misunderstanding about what is to be done, why it is being done and what to expect as a result.

ENUCLEATION

Enucleation (enucleatio bulbi; excision of the globe) is the surgical procedure in which the globe is separated from all its attachments and removed from the orbit.

Historical Summary

As near as can be ascertained Lange in 1555 was the first to report an attempt at enucleation or extirpation as it was then called. No details of the operative technic were given. In 1583 Bartisch of Saxony gave the first description of globe extirpation: He passed a heavy suture through the eyeball, pulled it upward, and then proceeded to slash away at its attachments with a sharp spoonlike instrument until it was free. This was such a brutal operation that Bartolini (as reported by Guthrie in 1823) tried to modify it by using hooks to pull out a cancerous eye. This milder procedure was followed three days later by the death of the patient in convulsions.

As time passed minor "improvements" in technic began to appear. Thus in 1646 Fabrici de Hilden separated the conjunctiva from the bulb first and then used a double-edged knife instead of a spoon to separate the globe from its attachments. In 1790 Louis substituted a curved scissors for the knife. None of the many minor technical modifications did much to relieve the severity of the operation for in 1830 MacKenzie reported that a woman who needed an enucleation was first bled until she was unconscious and then the eyeball was rapidly resected before recovery.

It can thus be readily understood why enucleation was an exceedingly rare procedure until the middle of the nineteenth century, being limited almost entirely to large cancerous growths. Then in 1841 O'Ferrall in Ireland and Bonnet in France simultaneously proposed an enucleation technic very much like that used today. As in so many instances this was arrived at almost accidentally. O'Ferrall was confronted with a globe completely proptosed by an orbital tumor. He discovered how simple it was to remove the globe by severing the muscles, the conjunctival and fascial attachments and the optic nerve and reported on the ease and safety of the procedure. After this the scope of the enucleation operation widened slowly to include all conditions which give a blind, painful, unsightly and otherwise useless eye. Although the technic has been modified and refined considerably since then, it remains substantially the operation reported in 1841.

Indications

The most important indications for enucleation are: (1) intraocular malignancies, (2) eyes mangled by injury, (3) penetrating wounds with intraocular inflammation and loss of vision which are likely to initiate a sympathetic ophthalmia and (4) blind, painful and disfigured eyes. To this might be added, (5) blind, painless and disfigured eyes which are unsightly and which impair a patient's economic usefulness.

In the presence of an intraocular tumor, enucleation is a life-saving measure; the probability of sympathetic ophthalmia makes enucleation compulsory. In the assured absence of these two imperative indications, one may weigh the choice between enucleation and evisceration.

Anesthesia

General or local anesthesia may be used, but the former is preferable. If local anesthesia is used the patient should be well sedated preoperatively. Retrobulbar injection consists of about 2.5 cc. of 1 per cent xylocaine with adrenalin into the region of the ciliary ganglion and another 2.5 cc. into the apex of the orbit with a longer 5 cm. needle. In addition the conjunctiva is ballooned up with the same solution all around the cornea and into the fornices.

Operative Technic

A speculum is inserted into the conjunctival sac and a canthotomy performed if the eye is large, distended by tumor or otherwise swollen. This helps to make access to the eye easier for the neurotomy. The conjunctiva is circumcised close to the limbus and undermined into the fornices. This is done by starting the incision at 12 o'clock then down each side of the cornea to 6 o'clock. The four rectus muscles are picked up on a muscle hook one by one as in any muscle procedure and cut close to the sclera at their insertions with a minimum of surgery and without freeing their fascial attachments.

Some prefer to take a small scleral stump when the muscle is separated from the globe. This prevents the end of the muscle from fraying and makes suturing together of the muscles easier. An exception to this is made in the case of the lateral rectus by leaving a 4 mm. stump of tendon attached to the globe which may be grasped by a small hemostat to facilitate subsequent manipulation. (Alternatively a deep bite is taken in the muscle stump with a stout silk suture. This is especially valuable in eyes which have been long inflamed and whose muscles are friable.)

The speculum is then removed, placed under the conjunctiva, pressed back to proptose the globe between its arms and locked into position. The oblique muscles are identified and also cut close to their insertions and all tissues adhering to the sclera are separated. A muscle hook is passed all around to make sure that the globe is free of all connections.

The stump of the lateral rectus is picked up in a hemostat by an assistant and the globe is pulled forward and adducted strongly to give good exposure for the nerve section. The closed enucleation scissors is slipped in temporally close to the eyeball, then pressed downward and medially until the optic nerve is encountered. The blades are opened and pushed forward to straddle the nerve. The eye is pulled forward by the assistant, the scissors is pressed backward and the optic nerve cut across as far behind the globe as possible.

The surgeon should be certain of the position of his enucleation scissors astride the nerve. Should adjacent orbital tissues be cut instead

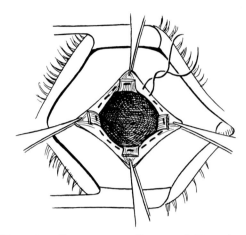

FIG. 268.   Purse-string Closure of Tenon's Capsule.

of the nerve, unusual hemorrhage will well up and obliterate the field and
thus obscure the position of the optic nerve. The loose eye is pulled forward, any remaining strands of attachment are severed and the eye
freed and wrapped in a moist sponge preparatory to being sent to the
laboratory for pathologic examination.

An alternative method of enucleation to be recommended is the use
of a tonsil snare instead of an enucleation scissors. The author has used
this often with satisfaction since there seems to be less bleeding when the
nerve and its vessels are crushed with a wire snare rather than cut
cleanly across with the scissors. When the snare is used it is passed over
the bulb inside Tenon's capsule after the muscles are cut. Care is taken
that no tissue except the optic nerve is caught in the snare. The eye is
grasped, pulled forward and enucleated.

A useful maneuver is to pick up the nerve in a hemostat before
enucleation and crush it several millimeters behind the globe. This is
allowed to remain in place several minutes and is effective in reducing
the gush of hemorrhage after neurotomy.

The cut edge of Tenon's capsule is caught up in three or four hemostats placed equidistantly and drawn apart to allow the insertion of long
gauze strips which fill up the cavity and with which digital pressure is
exerted backward to stop the bleeding. The old method of using hot packs
for hemostasis and incidentally parboiling the tissues of the orbit is
avoided. The use of pressure and some patience is all that is needed in
most cases. Rarely are hemostatics necessary.

Once hemostasis has been achieved, closure of Tenon's capsule is
begun and here there are a number of alternatives. Perhaps the oldest
and simplest method is the use of a purse-string suture (fig. 268).
(Another method of closure is pictured in figure 269.) The hemostats
attached to Tenon's capsule are held up and spread to facilitate insertion

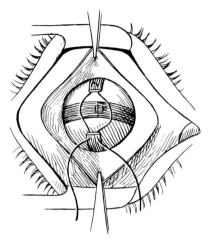

FIG. 269. Suturing of Recti Muscles.

of the suture. A 4–0 chromic purse string suture is passed about 3 mm. below the cut edge of Tenon's capsule all around, the four recti muscles being included in the suture (fig. 268). The hemostats are removed and, unless there is some definite contraindication, an implant is customarily inserted. In general the contraindications to an implant are few. Recent inflammation, fear of neoplasm or a Tenon's capsule so lacerated that it will not hold an acrylic ball may all dispose a surgeon to leave an empty socket. Again, enucleations done under emergency conditions, as near the battlefield in wartime, may not allow sufficient time for the surgical niceties. Many delayed balls have been implanted as a consequence.

The implant may range from the old-fashioned ordinary hollow glass sphere to the highly complicated creations to which the recti are attached for better motility. If an ordinary plastic sphere is used— usually about 18 mm. in diameter—this is most easily inserted with an introducer (fig. 274D). Care should be taken that the implant lies deep in the orbit and is not too superficially placed. In the latter case it is pushed down gently with the forefinger into its normally deeper position. After this the purse string is pulled taut and tied. This should cover the implant easily without tension. If the purse string does not give sufficient closure, accessory sutures must be used to close Tenon's capsule completely. The conjunctiva is now closed with a running suture of 5–0 silk or 6–0 chromic catgut if preferred.

Toilet of the socket is made. A well fitting, not too tight, conformer is inserted and a pressure bandage with head roll applied for five days. This is then removed, the socket cleaned, the conformer reinserted and the eye patched daily until ready for the temporary prosthesis which, in the usual case, is from two to three weeks after operation. The conformer must be retained until the socket is ready for a temporary prosthesis which can usually be worn in about two or three weeks.

Immediate Complications

Conjunctival adhesions form readily in an eye which has been inflamed for a long time, for the conjunctiva is atrophic and friable making undermining difficult and buttonholing a possibility, if not a probability. Careful dissection is advised.

In operating on a severely traumatized lacerated and soft eye it is not always easy to identify the tissue planes. It helps, after the conjunctiva has been undermined, to identify and isolate the rectus muscles on muscle hooks or sutures, lift them up and thus expose the mangled globe. If there are only one or two lacerations they may be sutured and the globe injected with saline to facilitate handling. If the globe is too macerated for that, stout sutures are passed through the sclera near the limbus at 3 and 9 o'clock and passed to an assistant who pulls the eye forward so that the surgeon can proceed with the operation. Sometimes the eye is so soft and wrinkled that care must be taken not to cut through sclera when the muscle tendons are cut. In cutting the optic nerve the presence of a large posterior staphyloma or a very soft globe may cause the scissors to cut through the posterior sclera leaving the optic nerve behind. It may be identified after hemostasis, grasped with a fixation forceps and resected; this is not always easy.

Secondary hemorrhage may occur if the dressing is not carefully applied or if it is removed too soon. This is not common if the above routine is followed. If the secondary hemorrhage is slight the dressings may be removed and a firmer bandage reapplied. If severe, one must remove the dressing, evacuate dammed up blood if present and reapply a firm pressure dressing. Under such conditions loss of the implant is not uncommon.

Reaction to operative insult in enucleation is much less severe than in the case of evisceration but occasionally extensive ecchymotic swelling of the lids is seen with much chemosis of the conjunctiva which pushes out between the lids. There is no specific treatment, but the exposed conjunctiva is treated with daily liberal application of antibiotic-cum-steroid ointments and moderate pressure over the socket. In rare cases the chemosis is so great and the conjunctiva so tense that the circulation of the area is threatened. Under those conditions it is wise to make a series of radial cuts in the conjunctiva to evacuate some of the serosanguinous subconjunctival fluid and thus relieve the pressure. Hot packs and antibiotics are also in order.

The socket must be dressed daily and lubricated constantly to prevent symblepharon and loss of cul-de-sac. The conjunctiva must be gotten back under the lids as soon as there is enough shrinkage. The writer has seen such cases which have required mucous membrane grafts later, although there was no sign of infection. Fortunately, such postoperative complications are rare, but when they do occur it usually takes a long time for the socket to recover sufficiently to accept a prosthesis.

Infection is fortunately uncommon. If it occurs the implant may not only be extruded but there is a frequent shrinkage of the whole socket due to fibrosis so that on recovery it has to be relined partially or completely before a prosthesis is accepted.

Late Complications

Loss of the implant has been rare in the author's experience. However, when it happens one must attempt to reimplant the ball using a smaller size. If one has used one of the integrated types of implant, it is better to revert to a simple ball on reimplantation. Isolation of the recti a second time is difficult technically and the final movement of the prosthesis is probably no better on reimplantation, hence this is usually not attempted.

In the presence of a clean socket, secondary implant should be done at once before conjunctival shrinkage sets in. As it is, conjunctiva—and hence some depth of socket—is lost with every reimplantation. In the presence of infection no surgery should be attempted until complete subsidence of the infection and for several months thereafter when all the fibrous contraction will have been completed. It may then be found that socket reconstruction is in order. Or enough socket may be left to contain a prosthesis without an implant, although this is rare.

Iliff has suggested a novel and ingenious approach to replacement of the extruded implant. He makes an incision below the outer brow to penetrate the socket and reinsert an implant. He thus avoids infected conjunctiva and facilitates removal of scar tissue.

Atrophy of orbital contents is the price paid by every socket for loss of its eyeball. This may be so slight as to be inconspicuous cosmetically. Or it may lead to a grim, inevitable chain of cosmetic blemishes including supratarsal depression, pseudoptosis, migration of the implant, loss of motility and even enophthalmos.

Supratarsal depression may develop ultimately, despite the best fitting implant. If sufficiently severe it may be repaired as described in Chapter 21.

Pseudoptosis is not uncommon with or without an implant and is due to loss of support supplied to the lid by the globe. In the early stages this may be counteracted by a more convex, better fitting prosthesis. Later, the pseudoptosis may be converted into a frank acquired ptosis requiring levator resection. Here the rules about operating on acquired ptosis must be kept in mind (Chapter 17).

Migration of the implant may be due to tears in Tenon's capsule, to improper fixation of the implant or for no apparent reason. Reimplantation is the only cure (fig. 270).

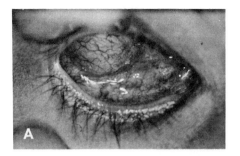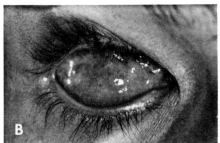

Fig. 270. Migration of Implant.
A. Implant in upper outer angle of socket.
B. After reimplantation.

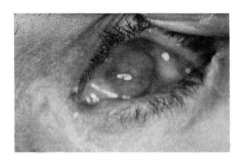

Fig. 271. Conjunctival Cyst of Left Socket.

Impairment of motility is usually due to migration of the implant. Even with reimplantation some of this is permanently lost.

Enophthalmos, i.e., retroplacement of the prosthesis, can sometimes be repaired by repositioning. If no implant has been used a secondary implant procedure may correct the defect (fig. 274).

A rare late complication is the development of a conjunctival cyst due to irritation from a poorly fitting prosthesis (fig. 271).

Ptosis occasionally develops which is sometimes amenable to 1 per cent phenylnephrine hydrochloride. If long lasting, a levator resection may have to be done.

Comment: As indicated, the above procedure is perhaps the simplest of many alternative enucleation technics with many variations. Some surgeons, for instance, prefer to enucleate the eye from the nasal side and it is true that the optic nerve, due to its course lateromedially from before backward, is more easily picked up medially. However, the freedom allowed by the open temporal side of the orbit with no interference from the jutting nose makes up for the closer medial approach. With the help of a canthotomy when necessary, no difficulty in finding and straddling the nerve is experienced.

Again, many surgeons prefer to isolate the four rectus muscles, then suture lateral to medial and inferior to superior over the implant before closing Tenon's capsule (fig. 269). Isolation of the muscles in this fashion is, of course, necessary when integrated implants are used. (See discussion of Implants below.)

However, it must be confessed that, to this day, the author is not convinced that suturing the recti together instead of simple purse-string closure gives sufficiently better movement to warrant the additional time and effort involved. On the other hand, the technic of rectus suture is not so laborious that it may not be continued by those who prefer it and are convinced of its effectiveness. The even simpler crossed mattress suture (fig. 274C) may also be used instead of the purse string.

Retention of the implant in the author's experience has not been a problem. The important factors here are: (1) complete hemostasis, (2) use of an implant which is not too big (usually about 18 mm.), (3) good closure of Tenon's capsule, (4) insertion of a conformer into the conjunctival sac at the end of the operation and (5) a firm pressure dressing which is not removed for five days and which assures healing of tissues in proper position.

IMPLANTS

In 1885 Mules first suggested using a glass ball in the scleral cup after evisceration. In 1886 Adams Frost reported the implantation of a ball into Tenon's capsule after enucleation and suturing the horizontal and vertical recti separately over it. Shortly thereafter Lang proposed an almost identical procedure but included the capsule of Tenon in the sutures. Hence the Frost-Lang technic of implantation into Tenon's capsule after enucleation.

Since the days of Mules and Frost-Lang it has been generally agreed by ophthalmologists that when an eye has been eviscerated or enucleated, the socket, for both physiologic and cosmetic reasons, should have some sort of an implant into Tenon's capsule or the scleral cup unless there is a definite contraindication. The implant, whether primary or secondary, is important for several reasons: (1) It fills out the socket and obviates "enophthalmos," i.e., retroplacement of the prosthesis. (2) It aids movement of the prosthesis. (3) It prevents or at least minifies supratarsal depression and pseudoptosis of the upper lid. (4) If a sufficiently large implant is used, secondary retraction of the socket is less likely to occur.

Enucleation causes a loss of 25 to 30 per cent of the total orbital volume of 6.5 to 7.0 cc. This is not entirely replaced by an 18 mm. ball implant and prosthesis. Furthermore, although this is not unanimous, is seems to be a common opinion that the size of the orbit tends to diminish after enucleation and that this diminution is lessened by the presence of an implant in the socket. Reports of studies of the amount of loss vary from "not of cosmetic importance" to as much as 20 per cent.

Many materials of various shapes and sizes have been and are being used for this purpose, including gold, silver, aluminum, lead, zinc, tantalum, platinum, celluloid, sponge, cotton, asbestos, glass, wool, rubber, silk, catgut, peat, agar-agar, paraffin, bone, fat, cartilage, plastics and many others. In recent years the advent of the inert resin polymers has made plastic conformers, implants and prostheses, very popular and deservedly so. They are now available in many shapes and all sizes.

In 1941 Ruedemann conceived the brilliant idea of the integrated implant, i.e., an implant to which the rectus muscles are attached. He reported it in 1945. In 1946 Cutler presented a somewhat different type of integrated implant. A host of modifications followed such as those of Nocito, Guyton, Stone, Allen, Troutman, Arruga and many, many others. Some of these were exposed implants, i.e., they protruded through the conjunctiva and required a coupling pin or some similar device to which the prosthesis could be attached. Others were buried under the conjunctiva; one, Troutman's, was magnetic.

It is impossible to enumerate let alone describe here all the various types of integrated and semi-integrated implants. In general all of them, exposed and buried, may be divided into two large groups:

1. Those whose upper surface is covered with an inert metallic mesh, such as tantalum, to which the four rectus muscles are attached. 2. A tunneled implant containing openings through which the muscles are passed and sewn together.

On the whole experience with exposed integrated implants has not been a happy one; in fact they have generally fallen into more and more disuse recently. A large proportion of them have eroded through and have either been extruded or have required removal. A few still in place are accompanied by so much discharge despite all sorts of treatment that it is impossible to keep the socket clean for any length of time. Most of the panaceas offered in the literature to keep such a socket free of discharge have proved ineffective in the author's hands, and, as far as ascertainable, in the hands of most other ophthalmic surgeons.

As a result, the exposed integrated implant despite its undisputed cosmetic advantages of movement has been abandoned. As a matter of fact the author has begun to feel that perhaps too much has been made of the motility factor. It would seem far better to have a prosthesis with an excursion of 35° to 40°, a clean socket and less chance of extrusion than to have an excursion of 50° to 60° with a constantly discharging socket and almost certain ultimate extrusion. In the author's experience the vast majority of patients are quite content with *some* excursion and learn to accommodate themselves to the loss of complete excursion nicely.

The buried implant as devised by Allen, Ellis, Troutman and others seems to meet some of these objections. If the movement is not quite as free as with the semiburied implants, it is quite adequate cosmetically

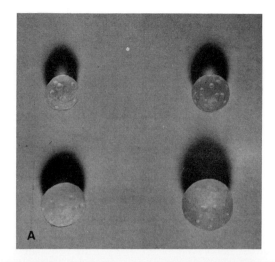

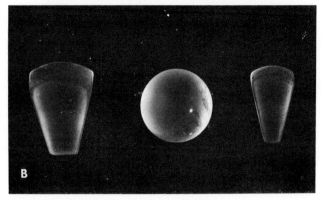

FIG. 272. Acrylic Implants.
A. Pitted acrylic ball implants.
B. Smooth cone and ball acrylic implants.

and the disadvantages of profuse discharge and, probably, ultimate extrusion are reduced to a minimum.

At this writing the feeling of most surgeons is that there is little to choose in motility between the ball implant and the buried integrated implant and the pendulum seems to be swinging away from the integrated implant altogether although buried integrated implants are still in use to lesser degree.

For some years now the writer has used with satisfaction a plain acrylic ball in cases of enucleation and secondary implant into Tenon's capsule (fig. 272*A*). It is an unpolished, pitted ball to which tissues adhere readily and hence is not prone to frequent displacement. Another worthwhile shape is shown in figure 272*B*.

Strampelli and Valvo have reported a rather curious biologic method for an integrated prosthesis. A tube of buccal mucosa is formed into which the pedicle of an attached mushroom-shaped prosthesis is inserted.

The covered pedicle is then fastened to an opening in the scleral cup after evisceration. The authors report using it with satisfaction in nearly 1000 cases.

EVISCERATION

Evisceration (eviseratio bulbi) is the complete removal of the ocular contents through an opening in the cornea or sclera.

Historical Summary

As in the case of enucleation, the first evisceration seems to have been performed somewhat accidentally by Beer in 1817 as the result of an expulsive choroidal hemorrhage during an operation for iridectomy. It was subsequently used rather sparsely and remained something of a curiosity with a number of weird modifications being reported. These included removal of the iris and lens only (Chevallereau), removal of the cornea, iris and lens (Critchett), amputation of the anterior half of the sclera (Lagrange), and removal of the posterior half of the sclera (Nicati), to mention but a few. Finally in 1884 the evisceration procedure was legitimized when both Graefe and Mules pointed out its undoubted value in minimizing the danger of meningitis. Mules' operation of evisceration with glass ball implantation in 1885 proved something of a milestone in ophthalmic surgery and—with minor modifications—has remained the classic evisceration procedure to this day.

Indications

Time was when the only primary indication for evisceration of the globe in ophthalmic surgery was an acute intraocular inflammation with irreparable destruction of vision or panophthalmitis. The reason for evacuating the scleral contents rather than enucleating the eyeball was to avoid the spread of infection along the optic nerve and its sheath when the optic nerve is cut. Evisceration was rarely done under other circumstances because the fear of sympathetic ophthalmia was omnipresent and omnipotent. In recent years with the advent of the steroids and the fear of sympathetic ophthalmia dispelled to a large extent, there has been a reawakening of interest in evisceration as a surgical technic in blind, scarred, traumatized and phthisical eyes. The cosmetic advantage in movement gained by retaining the scleral cup with its muscular attachments is undeniable. When the scleral cup is filled with an implant of plastic or metal the advantage is even further enhanced.

However, even with the bugaboo of sympathetic ophthalmia laid to rest there is always the possibility, even though remote, that an unsuspected malignancy may be overlooked. This should always be borne in mind and the surgeon must weigh carefully this possibility against the improvement in appearance and movement to be gained. Certainly evacuation of the scleral cup should be done with meticulous care and the contents warrant routine pathologic study even though no malignancy is suspected.

Hence the general indications for evisceration now are most blind eyes which are deemed safe for scleral implant. This includes a globe macerated by trauma, an eye blinded by absolute glaucoma, uveitis and buphthalmos, unsightly eyes due to much corneal scarring, etc. If some of these indications seem to coincide with indications for enucleation it should also be remembered that no evisceration should be done (1) in the presence of phthisis bulbi, (2) if thorough pathologic examination of the ocular contents is desired or (3) if there is any question of tumor involvement. No implants should be used in the presence of inflammation, acute or chronic.

Anesthesia

The operation may be done under local or general anesthesia. However, the latter is preferable and always used by the author. Not only is the painful eye more difficult to anesthetize by local injection, but there is always danger of a backward spread of contaminated material in an infected eye.

Operative Technic

Procedure (fig. 273):   While the fundamental technic of evisceration is standard there are some variations. Some surgeons prefer to save the cornea, others do not; some empty the scleral cup anteriorly, others make a meridional scleral incision at various distances behind the limbus and scoop out the contents that way. Some prefer an implant into the scleral cup, others are content with the motion and support furnished to a prosthesis by the collapsed scleral stump. While retention of the cornea gives a larger cup and permits the introduction of a larger implant, it makes for a small opening into the globe and hence for greater difficulty in evacuating the contents and in examining the inside of the globe to ascertain that every shred has been removed. For this reason the corneal resection technic is preferred by the author. In the absence of any inflammation in eyes which have been traumatized there can be no objection to an implant into the scleral cup if it is decided to use the evisceration operation.

In the case of a quiet uninfected eye, the conjunctiva is picked up close to the limbus at 12 o'clock. By undermining and cutting, an incision is carried down each side of the limbus to 6 o'clock completing the circumcision. Care is taken to cut as close to the limbus as possible so that

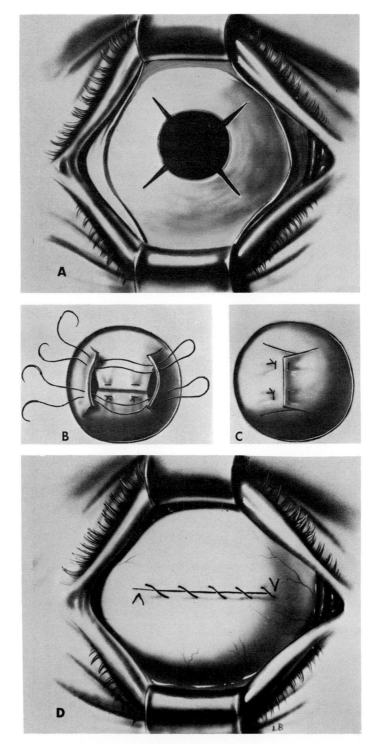

FIG. 273. Technic of Eviseration.
A. The scleral cup is emptied and four radial incisions are made.
B. and C. Horizontal and vertical flaps are sutured.
D. The conjunctiva is closed with a runnnig suture.

no conjunctiva is sacrificed. The conjunctiva is then undermined for about 10 mm. all around without injury to the extraocular muscles. (For some reason the inferior rectus is most likely to be cut accidentally.) An incision is made with a Graefe knife or other suitable instrument through the upper half of the limbus as for a cataract extraction. Resection of the cornea is completed with scissors and the cornea discarded. Some surgeons make their incision through the sclera just anterior to the insertions of the muscle tendons. However, no advantage is seen in discarding so much valuable sclera and diminishing the size of the scleral cup that much.

While an assistant retracts the lips of the scleral cup to give good exposure, an evisceration spoon or scoop is inserted between the sclera and the uveal tract and the intraocular contents thoroughly scooped out. If any uveal shreds remain they must be curetted out or wiped out with a tightly wound gauze sponge. The inside of the cup is irrigated with a suitable sterile solution and inspected under good illumination to assure complete evacuation of all uveal remnants.

Four radial incisions about 5 mm. long are made in the edge of the scleral cup between the recti muscle insertions in the four quadrants (fig. 273A), a plastic ball—usually no more than 16 mm. in diameter—is inserted and the scleral cavity closed. This is done by first suturing the upper and lower flaps horizontally by means of two double-armed 3 or 4–0 chromic catgut sutures, then the two vertical flaps are similarly sutured (figs. 273B and C). The conjunctival sac is closed with a horizontal running suture of 6–0 silk (fig. 273D). The ball implant should be of such size as to allow closure of the scleral flaps without tension. The slightest strain in closure is an invitation to extrusion when postoperative chemosis sets in. A conformer which does not fit too snugly is inserted into the conjunctival sac and a firm pressure dressing with head roll is applied. This is untouched for five days when the pressure dressing is removed. The socket is cleansed, the conformer reinserted and a simple patch applied until healing is complete and the socket is ready for a prosthesis.

In the presence of a frank infection the procedure is much simpler. No attempt is made to undermine the conjunctiva nor to insert an implant. The cornea is resected and the contents of the sclera evacuated as described above. The inside of the sclera is thoroughly cleansed and irrigated with an antiseptic solution and swabbed out. Antibiotic ointment is instilled and the eye lightly bandaged in order not to dam up secretions. The eye is dressed twice daily, the socket irrigated and antibiotic ointment instilled. This routine is continued until all discharge has ceased in about five or six days. In about 10 to 14 days the scleral cup has shrunken sufficiently for the conjunctiva to heal over. The socket is ready for a temporary prosthesis in three or four weeks.

Postoperative Course and Complications

The reaction to evisceration is much more stormy than to enuclea-tion. Pain and discomfort during the first two or three days may be severe. Chemosis sometimes takes two or three weeks to subside. Plenty of sedation should be exhibited to keep the patient comfortable and bed rest the first 24 to 48 hours is advisable. In general the postoperative course is longer than with enucleation.

Where no ball has been implanted, the sclera ultimately shrinks to a small stump which, however, has fair movement and offers a satisfactory base for a prosthesis.

Comment: Evisceration gives a better cosmetic result than enuclea-tion for several reasons. First, the contents of the socket are much less disturbed. Second, the socket is fuller with the scleral bulb-cum-implant in place. Third, since the ocular muscle attachments are left uncut, motility is better than with the best integrated implant.

On the other hand, the disadvantage of evisceration is the greater difficulty of getting a good pathologic report of the contents. Scrapings of the uveal tract are more difficult to fix and study microscopically. How-ever, it can be done. The danger of sympathetic ophthalmia has already been discussed.

The choice of enucleation or evisceration is a frequent one in ophthalmology; the former is the safer procedure, the latter the more rewarding cosmetically. This may be an oversimplification, but not too much. In recent years improvement in prostheses has tended to improve cosmetic results in enucleation. On the other hand, improvement in therapeutic modalities has lessened the dangers of evisceration. The author does not presume to make a choice for others, but he opts for enucleation in most instances.

DELAYED IMPLANTS INTO TENON'S CAPSULE

Delayed or secondary implant into Tenon's capsule is rather uncom-mon. However, when enucleation is done under emergency conditions or in isolated communities where ball implants are not available, secondary implants may be done later. The reasons are always cosmetic: to enhance movement of the prosthesis, to counteract a pseudoptosis, to fill out a supratarsal depression, to modify retroplacement of the prosthesis or to replace a displaced implant.

Anesthesia must be ample if done under local since the socket usually contains much fibrous tissue to which the anesthetic does not always penetrate completely.

Procedure (fig. 274):   The conjunctiva, which is usually found to be

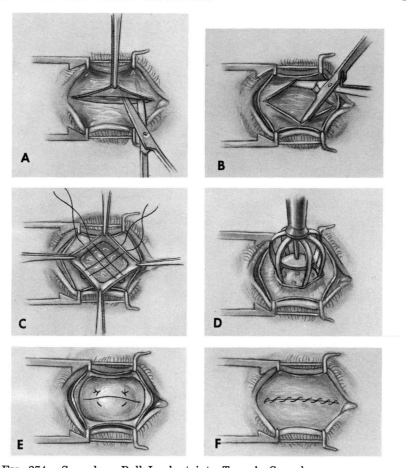

FIG. 274. Secondary Ball Implant into Tenon's Capsule.

A. The conjunctiva is incised horizontally and undermined upward and downward.
B. Tenon's capsule is opened and deepened with forceps.
C. Two crossing mattress sutures are placed in Tenon's capsule.
D. A plastic ball is inserted.
E. Tenon's capsule is closed.
F. The conjunctiva is closed.

quite thick due to previous surgery, is incised horizontally in midline and undermined to expose Tenon's capsule (fig. 274A). An opening is made into the capsule and enlarged with scissors to obtain good exposure. A large Kelly clamp is inserted and opened gently so that the capsule is stretched and the opening deepened. This is important, for the implant must have adequate room in the capsule without pressure being used to keep it in place (fig. 274B).

The edge of Tenon's capsule is grasped by four mosquito clamps opposite the approximate insertions of the rectus muscles. Two double-armed mattress sutures of 4–0 chromic catgut are passed about 3 mm.

from the cut edge of the capsule from below upward diagonally as follows: from the angle between the lateral and inferior recti to the angle between the medial and superior recti; and from the angle between the medial and inferior recti to the angle between the lateral and superior recti (fig. 274C).

A 16 or 18 mm. plastic ball is inserted into Tenon's capsule by means of an introducer and the sutures are firmly tied (figs. 274D andE). The conjunctiva is closed in the horizontal meridian by a 5–0 silk running suture knotted at both ends (fig. 274F). A slightly curved plastic conformer with the concavity inward is inserted and a pressure bandage applied.

The patient is kept in bed for 24 hours. The bandage is not removed until the fifth postoperative day. The socket is cleaned, the conformer reinserted and a simple patch reapplied for two or three more days. A conformer is worn in the socket until a permanent prosthesis is obtained two or three weeks later.

Comment: With this procedure, extrusion of the implant is rare. Retention is accomplished by (1) sufficient dissection to give the implant ample room, (2) the use of the conformer in the socket in conjunction with (3) a firm pressure dressing which is undisturbed for five days. The probabilities are that the kind of suture or type and shape of implant used do not make much difference in the retention of the implant.

RETROBULBAR ALCOHOL INJECTION

Injection of alcohol into the region of the ciliary ganglion may be done in those rare cases of blind, painful eyes in which more extensive surgery is contraindicated or refused. This is a simple procedure but not without possible complications.

The conjunctiva is anesthetized by instillation of several drops of 0.5 per cent proparacaine and a retrobulbar injection of 2 cc. procaine-epinephrine solution or its equivalent is made into the region of the ciliary ganglion as for a cataract extraction. The syringe is removed leaving the needle in situ. Three minutes later 2 cc. of an 80 per cent solution of alcohol is injected through the same needle.

The postoperative effect ranges from slight to severe with pain, chemosis, ptosis and extraocular muscle palsies sometimes appearing. Usually all these subside leaving a normal appearing eye. Occasionally the muscle paresis and ptosis persist. In the case of a blind painful eye in an old person who cannot or will not be subjected to major surgery this procedure may have to be considered.

It is occasionally necessary to repeat the alcohol injection after several months if the affect wears off.

Opticociliary Neurotomy and Neurectomy

Opticociliary neurotomy and neurectomy are old operations in which the optic and posterior ciliary nerves are cut without enucleating the globe. In earlier days it was apparently used by such men as Arlt, Müller, von Graefe and Schoeler as a neurotomy. It was Schweigger who introduced neurectomy by resecting a piece of the optic nerve. Later Meyer, Herman Knapp, Pagenstecher, De Wecker and many others used it to a considerable extent.

Theoretically it should be a very useful procedure since it is not difficult technically and has a lot to offer cosmetically; and the patient ends up with his own eye which, unless completely unacceptable cosmetically (in which case this operation would not be done) is a good deal better than any artificial eye. This procedure is now so rarely used—perhaps justly so—that it has been forgotten by most older ophthalmologists; young ophthalmologists have probably never heard of it.

As in the case of retrobulbar alcohol injection, the main indication is as a substitute for enucleation in a blind, painful eye which is still fairly normal in appearance and hence worth saving; i.e., such eyes as are seen occasionally in absolute glaucoma. The contraindications are many: (1) intraocular inflammation, (2) unsuspected intraocular tumor, (3) possible sympathetic ophthalmia and (4) the profuse hemorrhage which follows section of the nerve and which is sometimes difficult to control with the globe in place, etc. In rare instances the hemorrhage is so intractable as to impose enucleation of the globe immediately or a couple of days later.

Procedure: The conjunctiva is incised and the lateral rectus muscle exposed and cut from its insertion, a suture is passed through it and it is retracted. A stout suture is passed through the stump of the muscle, the eye is strongly adducted and the conjunctiva and Tenon's capsule are opened sufficiently to give exposure of the optic nerve which is severed. If a neurectomy is preferred a hemostat is clamped on the optic nerve and a 5 mm. section of the nerve is resected flush with the scleral surface. A gush of blood follows which requires removal of the speculum and digital pressure to attain hemostasis. A good deal of patience is sometimes required here. When the bleeding has stopped, the speculum is replaced. The eye is rotated nasally again ad maximum and all the ciliary nerves passing into the sclera in the neighborhood of the optic nerve are cut to prevent transmission of pain sensation. The lateral rectus is resutured to its stump and the conjunctiva closed, although it might be wise to leave a drain in place. A firm pressure dressing is advised.

Postoperatively there is some exophthalmos which may persist, but which ultimately recedes. There is also corneal anesthesia which gradually disappears. The tension remains normal or is slightly higher.

There is complete freedom from pain if all the ciliary nerves are cut.

Comment: Obviously this is not an operation to be undertaken lightly or frequently, yet it requires less manipulation than an enucleation or an evisceration. Also it is alluring cosmetically since it retains the patient's eye; and with the section of all the ciliary nerves it also gives complete freedom from pain. Why has it fallen into disuse?

The difficulty of controlling hemorrhage in some cases is probably one reason, although this may be minified to some extent by crushing the nerve first with a hemostat as described under enucleation. Some have reported return of pain due to regeneration of the ciliary nerves. Also there is mention in the old records of corneal necrosis and bulbar atrophy. On the other hand Meller states that neither neuropathic keratitis nor atrophy of the eyeball develop. Externally since the eye retains its vascular connections there may be nothing to show that the eye is blind; movement is normal.

I have not used this procedure in recent years.

EXENTERATION

Exenteration of the orbit, i.e., emptying the orbit of the periorbita and its contents is a mutilating operation which is always approached by the surgeon with hestitancy and some distaste. Fortunately it does not have to be done very often. Where it is indicated however, usually for malignancy, there should be no delay since it is a life saving procedure and procrastination can cause such irreparable damage as mestases or dangerous local extensions.

Indications

As noted, the indications for exenteration are orbital malignancies originating in the lids, lacrimal gland, eye or orbit itself whose spread can only be prevented by surgery. This includes such conditions as malignant melanosis, melanomas not limited to the globe, carcinomas, sarcomas except lymphosarcomas (which are quite radiosensitive), diffuse mixed tumors of the lacrimal gland, epitheliomas which have invaded deep into the orbit and malignancies of the bulb which have penetrated into the orbit.

Metastatic malignancies from primary foci elsewhere rarely justify exenteration and usually call only for palliation and control of pain. Also a tumor which has invaded the sinuses extensively as well as the orbit is no longer a purely ophthalmologic problem.

Operative Technic

Operative technic varies with the surgeon and there is no agreement as to how much of the lids to save or, indeed, whether they should be saved at all. Certainly where the lids are involved in the neoplasm there can be no argument about their resection. As in all surgery for malignancy the rule is to resect as much tissue as is deemed necessary for the safety of the patient. Details of repair are secondary.

The technic of complete exenteration with removal of periorbita with all its contents and resection of both lids is as follows. (It is always best to use general anesthesia in these cases.)

Procedure: A canthotomy is made at the lateral canthus and the lid margins are sutured together. The orbital margins are palpated and outlined with an antiseptic dye. Enough skin should be left so that retraction after section will not leave the orbital margin bare. The incision is made along the lower orbital rim down to periosteum, continued upward laterally and medially and finally along the upper orbital rim (fig. 275A). Incisions made in this order avoid interference by bleeding from above as much as possible. Bleeding may be controlled by ligature and diathermy coagulation or actual cautery.

Next the periosteum is incised around the orbital rim in similar fashion. It is closely adherent here, but once inside the orbit it is easily stripped away from the bony walls by means of a periosteal elevator. Adhesions at the medial and lateral canthal ligaments, the origin of the inferior oblique muscle and the pulley of the superior oblique are cut with blunt pointed scissors. Care is taken also not to penetrate the lamina papyracea of the ethmoid and, sometimes, the roof of the orbit which may be quite thin.

If there is any malignant involvement or chance of involvement of

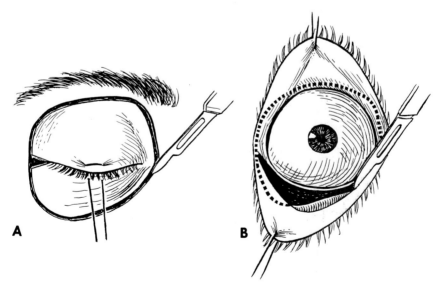

FIG. 275. Lid Incisions for Exenteration.
A. Through and through incision at orbital rim for total resection of lids.
B. Conjunctival incision at orbital rim sparing the lids. Dotted line marks orbital outline.

the lacrimal sac, this is undermined with the periosteum and the duct tied off. The ethmoidal arteries and the branches of the lacrimal arteries are tied off or closed with cautery.

When the whole periosteum has been freed from the orbital walls it remains attached at the apex by the muscles attached to the annulus of Zinn and by the nerves and vessels passing through the optic foramen and the upper and lower orbital fissures. Bleeding is again controlled by diathermy or cautery. A long blunt-pointed scissors is passed close to the bone along the orbital wall at the upper outer angle and the external and inferior muscles and the structures passing through both orbital fissures are cut. If the medial muscles and optic nerve remain intact, the periorbita are shifted laterally and the section completed from the medial side. The entire orbital contents are thus mobilized and removed.

Bleeding is usually profuse and is controlled by tamponade with dry gauze and digital pressure. This may take five to ten minutes. All oozing points are controlled by diathermy and the apex is inspected again. It must be cleaned of any possible malignant tissue by actual cautery or fulguration. If vessels protrude at the apex they are tied off, if possible, and cauterized to prevent further bleeding.

The bared walls of the orbit are inspected and whatever tags and fragments of tissue remain adherent are cleaned off. The walls are also inspected for possible malignant invasion and this is chipped away as completely as possible, care being taken to stay in uninvolved bone so as to avoid spread of malignant material. The orbit is packed with dry gauze if it is to be grafted at once or with petrolated gauze followed by a pressure bandage if it is to be grafted later or not at all.

At this point it must be decided whether the socket should be grafted with split skin at once or whether granulations should be allowed to form for about two weeks before grafting or whether granulations should be allowed to fill the orbit before a socket is grafted. This latter takes much longer (fig. 276B). If bleeding or ooze is uncontrolled, it is wise to wait some time to make sure that the graft is not destroyed by a hemorrhage under it. However, if the socket is dry and clean the patient can be spared additional surgical delay by immediate grafting.

A split skin graft about 4 inches square and 0.06 inches thick is taken with the dermatome from that part of the upper thigh which is freest of hair—usually the inner aspect in the male. By means of several stitches the graft is shaped into a rough cone raw side outward, pushed into the orbit and the outer edges sewed to the skin all around the orbital rim thus keeping the graft in proper position. A tampon of nonadherent gauze is packed into the orbit so that the graft is adherent to the orbital wall all around. Or the graft may be molded around the tampon first and then packed into the orbit. A pressure bandage is applied.

This is removed in four or five days, but the orbital packing is kept in a full ten days. At this time it is removed slowly and carefully so as not to disturb the graft. The skin sutures at the orbital rim are removed. All loose necrotic pieces of overlapping graft are snipped away without disturbing healthy tissue. The graft is cleaned gently with a moist sponge soaked in antibiotic solution, antibiotic ointment is instilled and a patch applied. The patch is changed as often as necessary to keep it clean, but the inside of the orbit is allowed to heal without too much manipulation. Crusts usually form which are not removed until the end of the third week. Then they are moistened and gently picked off. The only dressing necessary at this point is a patch.

If thought necessary, radiation therapy is begun during the fourth week after which a plastic prosthetic device is fitted into the orbital cavity or to a spectacle frame in front of the cavity.

Alternative Procedures

In many cases the lids are not involved in the orbital neoplasm and this offers the opportunity for surgical variations to those surgeons who believe that it is worthwhile to save the lids. These alternatives vary all the way from saving the whole full thickness lid to saving only the lid *skin* up to the ciliary margin.

If both lids are uninvolved and are to be saved they are everted strongly after canthotomy and the conjunctiva incised all around at the orbital rim down to periosteum. Then the periosteum is incised and exenteration as outlined above is carried out (fig. 275B).

Reese prefers to split both lids so that only the lash line and skin are anterior and the rest of the lid layers posterior. The dissection is carried in this plane to the orbital rim all around. Here the periosteum is incised and the periorbita with contents cleaned out as usual. Thus only the lid skin and lashes are saved.

Another procedure is to make the incision in the *tarsoconjunctiva* about 3 mm. from the ciliary margin. This saves not only all the skin-muscle but also the whole lid margin. The chances of preserving viable cilia are much enhanced if this is done (fig. 276A).

Still another method used is to incise the skin of both lids horizontally about 3 mm. back of the lash line (fig. 276B). These are undermined to the orbital rim and exenteration then carried out. Thus most of the lid skin is saved and tucked into the orbit over the split skin graft at the end of the operation. Another variation includes skin and muscle instead of only skin in the above incision.

There is no point in saving the whole lid or only the lid skin with its margin, unless they are preserved so as to be of some ultimate cosmetic usefulness. For if the preserved lids are left alone they are soon retracted back into the orbit by the healing process and an ugly inversion

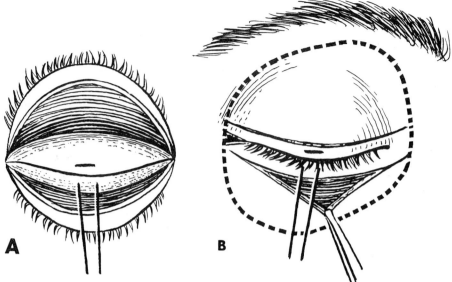

FIG. 276. Lid Incisions for Exenteration.
A. Tarsoconjunctival incision sparing the cilia and skin-muscle lamina.
B. Lid incision which saves the skin only. Dotted line marks orbital outline.

results. Later the lids can be dissected out again and some sort of socket reconstructed, but the result is never as good as when a primary procedure is used.

Reese has handled this ingeniously in cases in which there is no bony extension of the malignancy and which require no postoperative radiation therapy. He preserves the skin including the lashes of the lids. Then after exenteration of the orbit the temporalis muscle including its deep fascia is mobilized from the temporal fossa down to its insertion into the mandible. An opening is made in the lateral wall of the orbit and a 20 mm. gold sphere is placed in the apex of the orbit to help fill it. The temporalis muscle-cum-fascia is pulled through the orbital wall opening and used to fill out the rest of the orbit. The lids are sutured at the margin and a pressure dressing applied. Later the socket is reconstructed with a split skin graft and a prosthesis worn.

If the malignancy does not involve the conjunctiva this can also be preserved by circumcision at the limbus. Then after the temporalis muscle has filled out the orbital cavity, the cut edges of the conjunctiva are sutured to each other, a conformer inserted and a pressure dressing applied. The socket is then treated as after an enucleation.

Reese reports that some of the complications after this procedure of temporalis transplant are: (1) Recurrence of the malignancy unnoted until late, sometimes too late, perhaps. (2) Temporary difficulty with jaw movement. (3) Some sinking in of the temple on the involved side. (4) Paresthesias around the skin of the orbit are also not infrequent due to severance of the supraorbital and infraorbital nerves.

If time is not a factor, the simplest procedure of all is to do no grafting but to allow the orbit to fill in with granulation tissue for about two-thirds or three-fourths of its depth. This usually takes two or three months. But it may take ten or twelve months (fig. 277). During this time the socket is kept clean by irrigation and changing of the gauze dressing every few days. A patch is used externally. The patient need not be confined but is allowed to resume his normal activities and may even go back to his job. On the other hand, a split skin graft gives an earlier dry field although the surface may continue to shed for some time.

When the orbit has granulated in sufficiently, a new socket is created by an epidermal graft as outlined in Chapter 20. For this purpose it is best to use the technic shown in figure 275B for preservation of the lids.

Comment: There is this to be said for those who prefer to do complete lid resection in exenteration of the orbit: It is a moot point whether the final cosmetic result of saving the lids and their margins and recreating a socket for the reception of an artificial eye is worth all the time and labor involved. Plastic prosthetic devices are now being made which fit into the orbital cavity or which are attached to a spectacle frame and close the opening into the socket. Their resemblance to the eye and its adnexa is so lifelike that no surgeon however painstaking and skillful can hope to equal them. On the other hand, it has been argued that retention of the patient's own lids and socket is to be preferred from a psychological standpoint. Despite this, unless the patient himself insists on it—some do—he would be much better off economically and cosmetically to choose an artificial prosthesis in most cases. Many patients undergo a number of surgical procedures and then end up with something so unlifelike that a black patch is far more decorative.

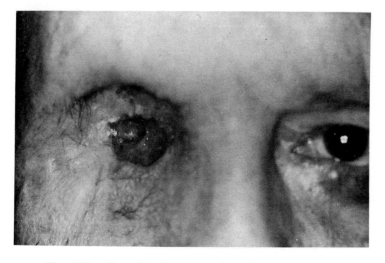

Fig. 277. Granulated Socket after Twelve Months.

ABLATION OF THE SOCKET

In 1872 Streatfeild suggested ablation of the socket in some cases of enucleation. This was revived by Green in 1882 and by Alt in 1903. Naquin reported on it in 1961 and Rycroft in 1962.

Ablation of the socket is attained by extirpation of the conjunctiva, tarsi and lid margins after enucleation. Rycroft also suggested extirpation of the lacrimal gland to prevent fistula formation. A sphere may be implanted into the muscle cone and the cut lid margins sutured to each other horizontally.

The main indications for this somewhat unusual procedure are (1) objection by the patient to an artificial eye and (2) inability to wear a prosthesis due to age, mental disability or lid abnormality.

Obviously such an operation will not be done very often but in the few cases where it is indicated it may not be as objectionable as might at first appear. As mentioned above, modern progress in prosthetics can offer alternatives which equal a plastic eye cosmetically.

REFERENCES

ALLEN, J. H.: A buried muscle cone implant. Arch. Ophth. 43:879, 1950.
ALT, A.: Removal of the eyeball together with the tarsi, conjunctival sac and lid margins. Am. J. Ophth. 20:69, 1903.
ANDREW, E.: Enucleation of the eyeball with obliteration of the conjunctival sac. Brit. M. J., p. 1155, 1885.
ARRUGA, H.: Improvement in the technique of evisceroenucleation with introduction of an orbital implant. Arch. Soc. oftal. hispano-am. 20:1049, 1960.
BARTLETT, R. E.: Plastic surgery for the enucleation patient. Am. J. Ophth. 61:68, 1966.
———, and LEWIS, F.: Evaluation of enucleations and eviscerations. Am. J. Ophth. 58:835, 1964.
BELLIZZI, A. M.: Technique of epithelialization of the orbit in exenterated patients: Critical study of 55 cases. Rev. brasil oftal. 17:301, 1958.
BERENS, C., and BREAKY, A. S.: Evisceration utilizing an intrascleral implant. Brit. J. Ophth. 44:665, 1960.
BURCH, F. E.: Evisceration of the globe with scleral implant and preservation of the cornea. Tr. Am. Ophth. Soc. 34:272, 1939.
CUTLER, N. L.: A universal type integrated implant. 32:253, 1949.
ELLIS, O. H. A new orbital implant. Am. J. Ophth. 32:990, 1949.
FOX, S. A.: Implantation into Tenon's capsule. Am. J. Ophth. 29:1571, 1946.
GREEN, J.: An operation for the removal of the eyeball together with the entire conjunctival sac and the lid margins. Am. J. Ophth. 1:65, 1884.
HAVRE, D. C.: Obtaining long section of optic nerve at enucleation. Am. J. Ophth. 60:272, 1965.
HOWARD, G. M., KINDER, R. S., and MACMILLAN, A. S., JR.: Orbital growth after unilateral enucleation in childhood. Arch. Ophth. 73:80, 1965.
HUGHES, W. L.: Evisceration. Arch. Ophth. 63:36, 1960.
ILIFF, C. E.: Tumors of the orbit. Tr. Am. Ophth. Soc. 55:505, 1958.
———: The extruded implant. Arch. Ophth. 78:742, 1967.
KENNEDY, R. E.: The effect of early enucleation on orbit. Am. J. Ophth. 62:277, 1965.

MARIN AMAT, M.: Capsuloscleral implants. Arch. Soc. oftal. hispano-am. *17*:625, 1957.

McCLAREN, L. R.: Primary skin grafting after exenteration of the orbit. Brit. J. Plast. Surg. *11*:57, 1958.

MELLER, J.: Ophthalmic Surgery. New York, Blakiston, 1953, p. 197.

NAQUIN, H. A.: Exenteration. Arch. Ophth. *51*:850, 1954.

_____: Extirpation of conjunctiva, tarsi, and lid margins following enucleation of the eye. Am. J. Ophth. *51*:227, 1961.

PRINCE, J. H.: Ocular Prostheses. Baltimore, Williams and Wilkins Co., 1946.

REESE, A. B.: Exenteration of the orbit with transplantation of the temporalis muscle. Am. J. Ophth. *45*:386, 1958.

REESE, A. B., and JONES, I. S.: Exenteration of the orbit and repair by transplantation of the temporalis muscle. Am. J. Ophth. *51*:217, 1961.

RICHARDS, P. D.: Microscopic findings in scleral shell after evisceration. Arch. Ophth. *66*:108, 1961.

RUEDEMANN, A. D.: Plastic eye implant. Am. J. Ophth. *29*:947, 1946.

_____: Evisceration with retention of the cornea. Am. J. Ophth. *45*:433, 1958.

RUEDEMANN, A. D., JR.: Modified Burch type of evisceration with scleral implant. Am. J. Ophth. *49*:41, 1960.

_____: Use of silicone implant for evisceration and enucleation. Am. J. Ophth. *54*:868, 1962.

RYCROFT, B. W.: An operation for the treatment of severe contraction of the socket. Brit. J. Ophth. *46*:21, 1962.

SOUDERS, B. F., and FORESTNER, H. J.: Plastic ocular prostheses in unusual socket. Tr. Am. Acad. Ophth. & Otol. *51*:46, 1946.

STRAMPELLI, B., and VALVO, A.: Durable mobility of ocular prostheses. Am. J. Ophth. *62*:643, 1966.

STREATFEILD, J. E.: On the preservation or destruction of the conjunctiva in cases of extirpation of the globe. Lancet., p. 821, 1872.

TROUTMAN, R. C.: A magnetic implant. Arch. Ophth. *43*:1123, 1950.

VEIRS, E. R.: Evisceration. Arch. Ophth. *65*:621, 1961.

CHAPTER 23

Affections of the Lacrimal System

THE TEARS, formed by the lacrimal gland, pass through ductules opening into the temporal half of the fornix conjunctivae. They are spilled over the open globe into the conjunctival sac and are directed by the normal blinking process into the lacus lacrimalis. From here they are sucked up by the puncta (mostly the lower, since man is an upright animal) into the canaliculi, the lacrimal sac, the nasolacrimal duct and finally end up in the inferior meatus (Chapter 1).

Viewed with a coldly scientific eye this is not a very efficient mechanism. The conduction of the tears over the open eyeball to the puncta depends on lids of the proper shape, in the proper position, which are functioning properly. The openings and ducts of the system from the puncta onward are small and narrow. Much can go awry and frequently does with this tear conducting system, a system which any self-respecting engineering student would indignantly disown.

Tears may be underproduced and overproduced. They may be produced in normal quantities and the passages blocked by inflammation, trauma, neoplasm or a lid which is out of position or distorted. Overproduction may be brought on by ocular inflammatory disease, a speck of dirt, a whiff of smoke, a medicinal drop or nothing more concrete than a surge of emotion. In all these circumstances the conducting system immediately proves inadequate and tears spill over onto the cheek which reacts by becoming red and inflamed. It is indeed remarkable that so small a percentage of the population has tearing problems. Yet, in the aggregate, there are enough to keep the ophthalmologist constantly aware of the inadequacies of the lacrimal system.

HISTORICAL SUMMARY

Epiphora and lacrimation probably began with the first man and have never ceased. At least records of attempts to treat lacrimal affections go back to ancient times. It would seem that Celsus—probably the greatest innovator and most quoted surgeon the world will ever know—excised the diseased sac down to the bone and then cauterized the fossa with red hot irons. In the second century A.D. Archigenes destroyed the sac with caustics and then bored holes into the nose for drainage. Early in the eighteenth century Woolhouse (1724) revised the operation into a complete dacryocystectomy instead of incising the sac and letting it drain into the nose. Berlin repopularized the operation of dacryocystectomy in 1868 and so it has remained to this day.

As far back as 1716 Anel first did probing and syringing of the sac. But it was not until 1857 that the immortal Bowman introduced graduated lacrimal probes and also slit the canaliculus to facilitate probing. From then until the beginning of the twentieth century probing, slitting the canaliculus and dacryocystectomy were the accepted methods of handling lacrimal obstruction.

Although man's ingenuity was able to conceive the principle of the dacryocystorhinostomy almost 2,000 years ago and perhaps earlier, it was not until the beginning of the twentieth century that the conquest of sepsis and the refinements of surgical technic permitted perfection of the operation. When they did come, changes came rapidly. In 1904 Toti reported his procedure for external dacryocystorhinostomy. He made a hole in the sac and a hole in the nose and approximated the two with a tight pressure bandage. This operation did not have many followers among ophthalmologists because the early technic was difficult and—more to the point—the results were not very good. In 1910 West and in 1911 Polyak reported a method of dacryocystorhinostomy by the nasal route and in 1911 Forsmark also reported his method for transplanting the sac into the nose. Now events moved even faster. Blaskovics in 1912 excised part of the sac wall and planted it into the nose and in 1914 Kuhnt was probably the first to suture flaps of nasal mucosa to the periosteum of the bony opening in an effort to limit troublesome granulations.

Ohm in 1920 was the first to suture the margins of the nasal mucosa to the sac. This was improved in 1921 by Dupuy-Dutemps and Bourguet who, using the external route, placed their incisions in such a way as to cover the bony margins and decrease interference from granulations. In the same year Mosher modified the Toti technic into a combined external-intranasal approach.

Compared to surgery of the tear-conducting mechanism, the surgery of the tear-forming system is quite recent. Over 100 years ago (1843) Bernard removed the orbital lobe of the lacrimal gland; De Wecker excised the palpebral lobe in 1888. This technic was perfected in 1911. Jameson reported his "graded" operation for section of the lacrimal ductules in 1937. Other methods for shutting off the tear supply from the ductules by diathermy (Strebel), x-ray (Hensen and Lorey) and alcohol injection (Tikhomirov) have been reported but have found little favor.

PRELIMINARY EXAMINATION

Epiphora

Chronic lacrimation, overproduction of tears due to hypersecretion by the lacrimal gland, is unusual. On the other hand epiphora, tearing due to obstruction or malposition somewhere in the lacrimal passages, is common. Lacrimation, aside from psychic or emotional causes, is usually due to reflex irritative stimulation. This is most commonly seen as a concomitant of ocular affections of the lids, conjunctiva, cornea, uvea, etc., i.e., in many types of diseases or injuries of the eye. Among these are blepharitis, trichiasis, entropion, ectropion, keratitis, corneal erosion, corneal ulcers, scleritis, etc. Nasal conditions such as chronic sinusitis, polyps, etc. also may cause tearing. Obstruction of the punctum by cilia is not uncommonly seen. To this may be added all kinds of irritative phenomena such as smoke, dust, bright lights, etc. These all have to be excluded by the examiner.

Excessive tearing can be very annoying; sufficiently so to warrant some kind of surgery if palliative measures fail. The surgeon must be certain that such reparable causes as large refractive errors and chronic infections of the nose and sinuses are not present. A thorough rhinologic examination is indicated as to the condition of the nasal mucosa and the patency of the nasolacrimal duct into the lower meatus. If these are all normal, a systematic examination of the tear-conducting mechanism must be undertaken. This should be thorough. Finding an obstructed lower canaliculus after an uncomplicated dacryocystorhinostomy operation could be a nerve-shattering experience.

External examination of the lid margins for trichiasis, malformations, entropion and early senile or mild cicatricial ectropion is in order; all these can produce tearing.

The conjunctival sac should be inspected for infection and sources of irritation. Atresia, spasm, eversion, slitting or abnormal position of the lower punctum should be looked for. The slit lamp will be found to be of great help here if the punctum is not easily visible. (It should be remembered that the normal position of the punctum is against the globe and if it is visible it is out of position.)

Investigation of lacrimal channel patency is then done. The fluorescine dye test is easily accomplished. Two drops of 2 per cent fluorescine solution a few minutes apart may be instilled into the conjunctival sac and the patient asked to blink several times. A minute or two later the patient is asked to blow his nose or spit into a gauze sponge or the nasal inferior meatus is wiped with a cotton applicator. Appearance of the yellow dye proves canalicular patency which may or may not be complete. If the dye comes through easily and quickly, then overproduction of tears should be suspected. If it takes longer than a few minutes, then there may be partial obstruction due to narrowing of the duct by swollen mucosa, tumor, a blocked inferior meatus, etc.

If no dye comes through then the sac should be irrigated with saline. If the dye has to be forced through into the nose then partial obstruction exists in the nasolacrimal duct. If the irrigating fluid comes through clear then the dye obviously did not pass through the puncta and canaliculi into the sac and there is, most commonly, obstruction in the canaliculi, even though the saline could be forced through into the nose.

Campbell, Smith, Richman and Anderson recommend a simple test for lacrimal obstruction: Four drops of fluorescine are allowed to pool in the lacus and the patient is told to blink forcibly several times. Excess fluid is wiped away. The sac is massaged briefly and gently. At 2, 4 and 6 minutes oral and nasal secretions are collected on tissue paper and examined. This test is statistically reliable and more comfortable than irrigation through the puncta.

S. T. Cohen has constructed a fine 0.5 mm. lacrimal probe with a cold fiber-optics light source which is easily visible in the lacrimal system and is of help in locating obstructions and in surgery.

Syringing with normal saline or boric solution will be easy with no obstruction present or will require some pressure if there is constriction. The solution will flow back if the lower canaliculus is completely obstructed. If the flow back is through the upper canaliculus then the opening into the sac or nasolacrimal duct, i.e., the common punctum, is closed. If the obstruction is in the nasolacrimal duct, which is the most common site, the sac itself will be seen or felt to dilate with the solution and pressure on it will cause a retrograde flow through the puncta. Chronic dacryocystitis may show a visably distended sac (mucocele or dacryops) which causes purulent material to regurgitate into the conjunctival sac on pressure.

An x-ray investigation with the instillation of a radiopaque material will dissolve all doubts as to the point of obstruction. I used radiopaque material to diagnose lacrimal stenosis as far back as 1947. Many authors have confirmed its value since. Figures 278A and B show points of obstruction of the tear-conducting mechanisms.

To sum up, tearing may be due to an overproduction of tears which

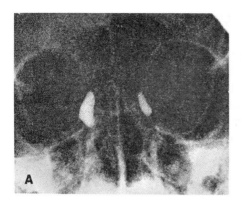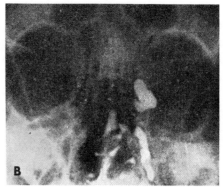

FIG. 278.   Outline of Lacrimal Sac and Duct with Radiopaque Material.
A.   Bilateral chronic dacryocystitis. Larger right sac has been involved for six
months; left small sac three weeks.
B.   Traumatic chronic dacryocystitis 9½ months after injury. Note distension
and convolution of sac. Patency maintained for a while as shown by free
passage of Lipiodol into nose. Surgery finally became necessary on closure.

is rare or to an obstruction in the tear-conduction mechanism anywhere
from the punctum to the inferior turbinate. To help the patient means
reducing the production of tears or reopening obstructed passages. Procedures to meet most of the commonly encountered contingencies are
discussed below.

Underproduction of Tears

Lack of tear production is usually due to keratoconjunctivitis sicca
(Sjögrens disease) although xerosis of the conjunctiva should not be
overlooked. All such eyes should be subjected to the simple Schirmer test
as follows:

A piece of No. 41 Whitman filter paper, 5 mm. wide and 35 mm. long
is folded 5 mm. from one end. The folded end is inserted into the
unanesthetized eye between the palpebral and bulbar conjunctiva at the
junction of the middle and lateral third of the lower lid. This is done
bilaterally and the patient is asked not to close his eyes (fig. 279).

If less than 15 mm. of the free portion of the filter paper near the
lid margin is moistened in five minutes, there is a deficiency of tear
production. While the Schirmer test is not 100 per cent trustworthy, it is
still valuable because it provides an indication of excessive secretion or
the lack or absence of tear secretion. Symptomatic treatment should not
depend on it and it should also be remembered that tearing *normally
decreases with age.*

Jones has pointed out that it is possible to have pseudoepiphora, i.e.,
a complaint of tearing, when there is hyposecretion of the basic tear
secretory glands. Such patients usually complain of burning and tearing
when the eyes are actually dry and require treatment.

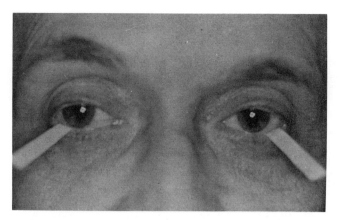

FIG. 279. Sjögren's Test for Tear Production.

Such eyes call for local medical care such as artificial tears, methyl cellulose drops and bland ointments. Scleral contact lenses may help also. However, general medical and nasal conditions should not be overlooked. Sealing of the lacrimal puncta (discussed below) should be tried although this is not a panacea. Neither is transplantation of the parotid duct which is heroic treatment probably best reserved for conjunctival xerosis.

SURGERY OF THE TEAR-PRODUCING MECHANISM

Indications for operation on the lacrimal gland and ductules are fewer than in former days. Perfection of dacryocystorhinostomy technics and the gradual abandonment of the once popular dacryocystectomy have reduced the need. However, in the absence of all signs of disease of the ocular adnexa and in all cases where the surgeon has exhausted his ingenuity in reopening obstructions of the tear-conducting channels, there is no recourse save to attempt to diminish the production and flow of tears. Palliative measures such as astringent drops will have been tried with the usual lack of success. There are patients who seem to withstand constant tearing with much greater equanimity than others. Some, however, will demand and require assistance and the surgeon must be prepared to render it.

Section of the Lacrimal Ductules (Jameson)

This procedure, proposed by Jameson in 1937, has fallen into disuse in recent years probably because its results have been disappointing. However, it still has its protagonists and has proved effective in some cases.

Procedure: After instillation of several drops of 0.5 per cent tetracaine or proparacaine the outer half of the conjunctival sac is anesthetized by subconjunctival injection of 1 per cent lidocaine or procaine with adrenalin. A horizontal conjunctival incision is made about 5 mm. below the everted upper tarsal border from the outer canthus to the beginning of the bulbar conjunctiva as seen in figure 280*A* but somewhat lower.

A blunt-pointed Stevens scissors is introduced subconjunctivally and all the conjunctiva of the external fornix from the upper tarsal border down to *below* the external commissure is undermined. The dissection at the lateral canthus should come close to the lower lid border temporally in order to include one or two of the largest ductules which open into the lower cul-de-sac. Bleeding is minimal and when it ceases the conjunctiva is closed with 6–0 interrupted silk or catgut sutures. A firm dressing is applied for two days then a patch until healing is complete.

Comment: Jameson's instructions call for the conjunctival incision to be made *below* the external commissure. However, it is simpler to make the incision higher and to undermine both lips of the conjunctival wound upward and downward. The dissection should be just beneath the conjunctiva so that the points of the scissors are always visible. In this way injury to the levator or the fascia with release of orbital fat will be avoided. The surgery is simple and the healing prompt although the conjunctiva may remain injected for some time. Jameson originally used no closing sutures. However, there seems to be nothing gained from leaving the wound open; sutures hasten healing.

Resection of the Palpebral Lobe of the Lacrimal Gland

Many years ago Wheeler pointed out the advantage of resecting the palpebral lobe of the lacrimal gland and advised it as an adjunct to all cases of lacrimal sac extirpation. He stated, "Excessive dryness of the eye does not occur following this operation and the results are eminently satisfactory."

Despite the perfection of the operative technic by Axenfeld in 1910 this procedure is not used much now and yet it is of value in cases of epiphora in which obstruction cannot be relieved or where more elaborate surgery such as dacryocystorhinostomy is contraindicated in the old and infirm. In fact the results are sometimes better with this relatively simple operation than with some of the more complicated procedures devised by brilliant technicians.

Procedure (fig. 280):   Anesthesia is obtained by conjunctival instillation of 0.5 per cent tetracaine and infiltration of the lateral half of the conjunctival sac with 1 per cent procaine or lidocaine with epinephrine. The area is massaged until the anesthesia is well absorbed.

The lid is everted on an Ehrhardt clamp and the eye rotated down and in. The accessory lobe of the gland usually presents immediately as a bulge beneath the conjunctiva just below the outer edge of the tarsus. If

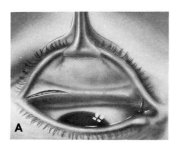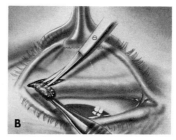

FIG. 280.   Resection of Palpebral Lobe of Lacrimal Gland.
A.   The conjunctiva is incised below the attached tarsal border.
B.   The presenting portion of the gland is resected and the conjunctiva sutured.

not, a blunt instrument pressing behind the everted lid brings it into view.

An incision is made in the conjunctiva from the outer canthus to the upper corneal limbus as in the previous procedure (fig. 280A). As the conjunctiva is undermined upward the palpebral lobe of the lacrimal gland comes into view and the conjunctiva is dissected away from its capsule. The gland is grasped and carefully separated from its surroundings without injury to the levator or fascia. The palpebral portion of the lacrimal gland is a lobulated structure and varies in size. It may be large and compact or may present many small discrete lobules. In any case it is not a difficult dissection and can be easily accomplished (fig. 280B).

After the gland lobules are excised, the lips of the conjunctival wound are spread and the conjunctiva is undermined upward and downward to include the whole lateral half of the conjunctival sac as for the Jameson procedure. By this means all the openings of the lacrimal ductules are sectioned including those that lie in the lower lateral fornix.

The wound is re-examined to make sure that no remnants of the gland are left behind and closure made with a few 6–0 chromic catgut sutures. The conjunctival sac is irrigated and a firm pressure dressing applied for 48 hours. The eye will remain injected for a couple of weeks.

Comment: It has been stated that removal of the entire palpebral lobe of the lacrimal gland destroys the two to six main secretory ductules from the main gland and hence the entire secretory function of both glands is inactivated. Nothing of the sort happens. As a matter of fact, the main postoperative complication is that tearing is not sufficiently reduced.

Neither section of the lacrimal ductules by itself as suggested by Jameson, nor extirpation of the palpebral portion of the lacrimal gland which really combines both operations, will cause complete cessation of lacrimation. However, the operation is usually effective in reducing tearing to bearable proportions which is a relief to the patient.

Other complications with this procedure are ordinarily slight. Injury to the levator is rare and hemorrhage is not too difficult to control unless one is lavish with one's dissection. A dry eye following this procedure has never been seen by the author.

Surgery of the Orbital Lobe of the Lacrimal Gland

INDICATIONS: Incision of the orbital lobe of the lacrimal gland is sometimes necessary for drainage of an abscess or for pathologic diagnosis. Total resection may be necessary for such conditions as neoplasm, cyst and persistent fistula.

Preliminary signs such as fullness of the upper lid fold, a palpable mass in the lacrimal gland region, diplopia, exophthalmos, limitation of eye motion, etc. all point to the need for immediate investigation for neoplasm. And here one must stand ready to carry the surgery farther and deeper if the diagnosis of malignancy is established.

The most common of all neoplasms is the mixed tumor of the lacrimal gland; carcinomas are much less common. Both require wide and deep investigation of the orbit and resection of bone if involvement is found. The less malignant tumors of the lacrimal gland such as lymphoma and lymphosarcoma require diagnosis and irradiation not resection. True mixed tumors, cysts, etc. should be excised intact.

Reese has suggested the following action based on the biopsy report: If the diagnosis is mixed tumor, a Krönlein procedure is done and the whole tumor extirpated. In case of a carcinoma, extirpation should be immediate or within a few days. If the report shows a lymphosarcoma closure, then irradiation is the procedure of choice. In the presence of a chronic granuloma the wound is closed since these lesions ultimately resolve spontaneously. Reese states that only about half the neoplastic lesions require extirpation. In the case of epithelial tumors with bone involvement Reese and Jones report that exenteration with bone resection of all the involved bone offers encouragement.

Removal of the gland does not always give a dry eye. The basic tear glands, such as Wolfring's and Krause's glands and the mucin secreting glands of the conjunctiva continue to keep the eye sufficiently moist in most cases.

RESECTION OF THE ORBITAL LOBE OF THE LACRIMAL GLAND. *Procedure (fig. 281):* Excision of the orbital lobe of the lacrimal gland can be carried out under local anesthesia if desired and indicated. The retrotarsal fold of the conjunctiva of the upper cul-de-sac is infiltrated with procaine or lidocaine 2 per cent with epinephrine. The outer two-thirds of the lid is then infiltrated deeply close to the upper orbital rim from the lateral canthal angle then inward beyond the center of the

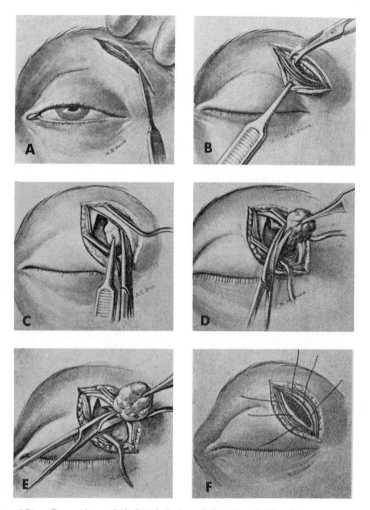

FIG. 281. Resection of Orbital Lobe of Lacrimal Gland.
A. Preliminary skin incision.
B. Separation of the muscle fibers by blunt dissection.
C. The fascia is incised, the gland exposed and the anterior surface freed.
D. The posterior surface is freed.
E. The gland is cut free from its posterior attachments.
F. The fascia is closed separately. Skin sutures follow.

brow. The area is massaged gently to assure spread of the anesthetic and absorption by the tissues.

The outer half of the brow is pulled slightly upward so that the lower brow edge lies somewhat above the bony orbital margin and an incision is made below the hair line through skin and subcutaneous tissue down to but not including the orbicularis fibers. The incision should start just lateral to the middle of the brow and follow the curve of the orbital rim outward for 2.5 cm. (fig. 281A). The brow is allowed to slip back to its normal position and the wound lips retracted. All bleeding points are stopped by pressure or ligature. The fibers of the exposed orbicularis are separated by blunt dissection to expose the subjacent fascia orbitalis as it joins the orbital periosteum along the whole length of the wound. The lips of the orbicularis wound are retracted to give good exposure. The septum orbitale is picked up with sharp forceps close to the orbital rim, nicked with blunt pointed scissors and the incision completed along the whole length of the wound. With care the levator and other tissues lying beneath the orbital fascia need not be endangered (fig. 281B).

The lower lip of the fascia is retracted bringing into view a thin layer of orbital fat and the anterior edge of the lacrimal gland lying immediately behind. This is a small flattened lobulated mass, yellowish pink and somewhat darker in color than the orbital fat. Varying pathologies will of course distort the gland both in size, shape and appearance.

The anterior edge of the lobe which is quite thin is grasped with forceps and pulled forward gently. By blunt dissection the upper surface is freed from its connections to the bone starting at the medial end and working laterally (fig. 281C). It is then pulled forward, raised slightly and, starting medially again, the lower surface is gently separated from its fascial attachments all the way to its lateral pole (fig. 281D). As it is freed it is pulled forward and the posterior margin, which is thicker than the anterior, is pulled forward and cut free from its attachment to the lacrimal nerve, vessels and palpebral lobe (fig. 281E). This is followed by a gush of blood which is stemmed with gauze sponges and pressure. If necessary, bleeding points should be tied to assure a dry field. This permits a careful inspection of the wound to see that no remnants have been left behind and obviates secondary hemorrhage which makes for slow healing and possible ptosis.

When the wound is dry and ready for closure the fascia orbitalis is closed separately with interrupted 4–0 chromic catgut sutures (fig. 281F). The orbicularis muscle fibers usually fall together nicely; if not, they are also caught up with a few sutures. The skin is closed with 4–0 silk sutures either subcuticularly or by interrupted skin sutures. A firm pressure dressing is applied and left in place for three or four days unless complications develop. Skin sutures are removed on the fifth or sixth day.

Comment: Although the rule in the surgery of neoplasms is never to open an encapsulated tumor, it is sometimes justified, as Reese points out, when life is at stake. When biopsy reveals a nonmalignant condition one either proceeds as above or, as in the case of lymphosarcoma, one closes and irradiates. Malignancy calls for a wider orbitotomy, bone inspection and resection, if necessary, and whatever else the exigency of the case requires for the benefit of the patient.

In dissecting out the gland its relationship to the surrounding structures should be borne in mind to avoid complications. (See Chapter 1 for anatomy of the gland.) Medially the orbital lobe of the gland lies on the levator aponeurosis which indents it and divides into two lobes—the palpebral portion lying under the aponeurosis. Posteriorly the gland lies on the fascial expansion between the superior and lateral recti which separates it from Tenon's capsule.

Several operative complications are possible. Too long an incision gives a longer than necessary scar. Too deep an incision involves the levator and may give ptosis. If this is seen in time immediate suture may repair the damage. Too rough a dissection will cause unnecessary bleeding hard to control. Penetration of the conjunctiva—especially laterally—is not difficult and should be repaired with plain catgut at once. Hemorrhage is always annoying—even more so than in enucleations and fraught with the grave consequences of permanent ptosis. Hence bleeding should be carefully and methodically controlled before closure.

ALCOHOL INJECTION: Injection of alcohol into the orbital lobe of the lacrimal gland has sometimes been suggested as a cure for epiphora and lacrimation. While this is a comparatively simple procedure, it is far from innocuous and a stormy postinjection course is not uncommon. Extreme pain with some proptosis and even ptosis ensues. All however usually recede. The patient must be adequately sedated until symptoms disappear.

Surgery of the Tear-Conducting Mechanism

Affections of the tear conducting system offer, in the main, problems of obstruction, i.e., atresia, malposition, strictures and scarring. It is amazing how much trouble a system measuring something less than 1.5 inches in its whole length can cause. These troubles vary both quantitatively and qualitatively.

The Puncta

The punctum is a tiny opening, slightly oval, situated on the papilla lacrimalis which lies at the junction of the ciliary and lacrimal portions of the lid border. Both upper and lower puncta are normally turned in against the globe. Since man in the waking state is usually perpendicular, it is the lower punctum which is most important.

The punctum may be spastic, everted, dilated, atresic or absent. If inspection does not disclose it easily, investigation with the slit lamp usually helps. Due to spasm or inflammation it may appear as a tiny stenosed dimple. Once the opening is found simple repeated dilations may be enough to restore its function.

CONTRACTED PUNCTUM—"SNIP" PROCEDURES: If the punctum does

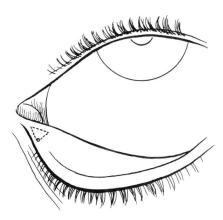

FIG. 282. Three Snip Procedure. Vertical and horizontal incisions are made in the canaliculus and the resultant triangular flap is resected (see text).

not respond to simple dilation a short vertical snip of the posterior wall of the vertical canaliculus with a sharp pointed scissors has been advised by Jones as effective. This slitting of the canaliculus must be minimal or its tear-absorbing function will be destroyed. Sometimes this also is not enough and if occlusion recurs the "three snip" procedure introduced by Hoffman in 1904 may be tried.

THREE SNIP PROCEDURE FOR PUNCTAL ATRESIA. *Procedure (fig. 282):* This is done under simple instillation anesthesia supplemented by a few drops of lidocaine 1 per cent with epinephrine injected into the punctum and canaliculus. The punctum is well dilated, a short fine pointed scissors is inserted vertically down to the ampulla so that the posterior conjunctiva is between the blades, and the conjunctiva is cut. A thin bladed scissors or a fine canaliculus knife is then inserted into the canaliculus with the blade facing slightly backward toward the globe and a 3 mm. horizontal incision is made. The resultant triangular flap is picked up with a fine toothed forceps, put on stretch and cut off at the base. Bleeding is stopped in a few minutes and a patch applied.

Comment: No "snip" procedure, however minor, is indicated unless repeated dilations of the punctum have proven ineffective. And even here the three snip procedure may result in eventual conjunctival contraction which may require further slitting.

It is claimed that the one snip procedure preserves the capillary attraction of the canaliculus while the three snip does not. However, once the vertical canaliculus is cut, it would not seem to matter whether its integrity is destroyed by one snip or three snips. Hughes and Maris use a 1.5 Holth punch to make an opening in cases of stenosed canaliculi. Since they get good results with their procedure one wonders how important capillary attraction is in these cases.

INDWELLING SUTURE FOR ATRESIA OF PUNCTUM. An alternative pro-

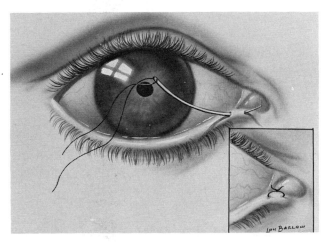

Fig. 283.   Indwelling Suture for Punctal Atresia. A heavy suture threaded on a blunt round needle is passed into the canaliculus and brought out more medially. The suture is pulled through and tied. (See inset.)

cedure for an absent or closed punctum with a normal canaliculus is the insertion of an indwelling suture for several weeks.

Procedure (fig. 283):   Thorough slit lamp inspection usually reveals the previous site of the punctum. The area may have to be perforated with a needle after anesthesia and then dilated with a punctum dilator. When entrance into the canaliculus has been obtained, the canaliculus and sac are irrigated to assure patency of the rest of the tear-conducting channels. Once this is ascertained a heavy 3–0 silk suture is threaded on a straight round blunt pointed needle which is inserted through the dilated punctum into the canaliculus for about 4 mm. The point of the needle is tilted upward and cut down upon. The suture is drawn out through this opening, the needle removed and the suture tied securely.

If the punctum cannot be located, a vertical incision is made medially over the canaliculus. The canalicular lumen is then located and a fine lacrimal probe is passed laterally until the area of the punctum is found.

The suture is left in position for at least four weeks before it is removed. During the last two weeks it is moved back and forth daily in order to assure epithelialization and permanency of the enlarged punctum. The medial stab wound usually closes over by itself or is sutured on removal of the suture. This procedure also is not a panacea but it is quite simple to do and successful sufficiently often to warrant a trial.

Comment: In all cases where the punctal end of the canaliculus has been destroyed by trauma or excision of a tumor, Callahan suggests slitting the medial remnant of the canaliculus and uniting the cut mucosal edges to the conjunctiva above and below. He states that this is sometimes successful in maintaining an opening into the canaliculus.

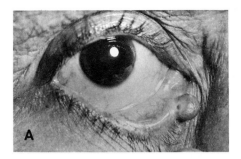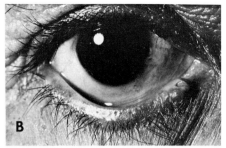

FIG. 284.   Repair of Benign Punctal Tumor.
A. Benign tumor surrounding punctum.
B. After repair.

EVERSION OF LOWER PUNCTUM.   Eversion of the punctum is commonly due to an early ectropion. In the early cases a localized cautery puncture beneath the punctum or a simple conjunctivoplasty (see Chapter 15, figs. 169 and 170) may suffice. If due to a cicatricial ectropion then plastic repair of the lid must be done.

REPAIR OF ENLARGED PUNCTUM.   Epiphora may be due to destruction of punctal efficiency by too vigorous probing or slitting of the canaliculus. Repair is sometimes possible by decreasing the size of the punctum surgically as reported by Hallum. After suitable anesthesia of the area the point of a Graefe knife is introduced into the punctum and the edges freshened laterally leaving the medial angle untouched. The freshened conjunctival edges are closed with interrupted 6–0 silk sutures. Epiphora may not be completely relieved but improvement may be expected.

SURGICAL OCCULUSION OF PUNCTUM.   In keratitis, sicca occlusion of the puncta and canaliculi is sometimes done. This is discussed below in canalicular surgery. However, sometimes the puncta alone can be sealed off as suggested by Barbera; this allows for an evaluation of the occlusion.

TUMORS OF THE PUNCTUM.   Neoplasms around the punctal area are far from rare. An example of this was shown in Chapter 9, figure 116. Some may be small and benign (fig. 284A). In such a case the patient is fortunate and simple surgery will leave him an intact punctum (fig. 284B).

However, the basal cell carcinoma shown in the right lower lid of figure 285A involved the whole punctal area and required the same type of repair (fig. 285B) as described in figure 116 which is a good deal more complicated. Healing resulted in an excellent cosmetic result (fig. 285C) and—fortunately—a good, large punctum (fig. 285D). This patient was more fortunate than the one pictured in figure 116.

The Canaliculi

Obstruction of the canaliculus is the most challenging and at the

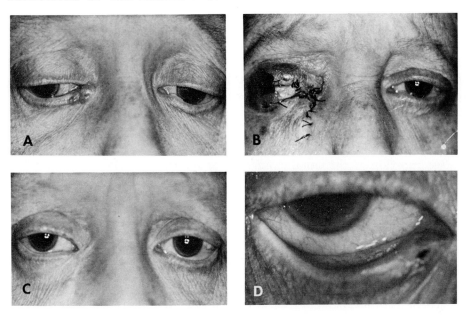

FIG. 285.   Repair of Malignant Punctal Tumor.
A.   Malignancy around right lower punctum.
B.   Repair according to technic described in figure 116.
C.   Result of repair.
D.   Note large reconstructed punctum.

same time the most frustrating of all lacrimal system lesions. Here, even more than in operations on the sac and duct, failure frequently dogs the surgeon.

The canaliculus is about one cm. long, the first 2 mm. of which comprise the vertical portion. Every millimeter of this crooked little tube is subject to inflammation and acute and chronic cystic dilatation, narrowing and obstruction by dacryoliths, actinomyces, sporotrichosis, traumatic scarring and congenital malformation. Occlusion of the upper canaliculus is not as important because most of the tear draining from the eye is done by the lower canaliculus. But when the latter is obstructed tearing is certain.

Early and mild obstruction may be helped by a few careful probings with No. 1 or 2 probes. Success is rare because adhesions heal again promptly.

Mild obstruction of the canaliculus by dacryoliths (usually due to actinomyces) and other fungi can sometimes be treated by astringent medication, irrigation, careful probing and mechanical expression. If the inflammation is mild and easily responsive to medication the patient is fortunate. Cystic dilatation may also be a medically responsive problem. If necessary, the canaliculus can be opened and cleaned out (see below). However, obstruction of the lower canaliculus by traumatic scarring or persistent low-grade inflammation frequently baffles the

ingenuity of the ophthalmic surgeon. Until quite recently indwelling
plastic tubes left in the canaliculi for weeks and months after penetration
of the obstruction seemed to be the answer. Many of these procedures
were ingeniously contrived and beautifully executed. Later returns, however, made a mirage of success. The constriction and obstruction gradually and implacably returned.

If the cicatricial obstruction of the canaliculus is complete, Veirs
recommends reconstruction with mucous membrane. Involvement of the
medial portion of the canaliculus and/or the common punctum calls for
the use of the Veirs rod or more recent Silastic tube as described below.
Obstruction of the lateral half of the canaliculus should be corrected by
Jones' conjunctivodacryocystorhinostomy as described below.

REPAIR OF EARLY CANALICULAR TEARS. Avulsion of the lower lid
from the medial canthus is one of the most common forms of lid trauma.
Inevitably, of course, this means destruction of the lower canaliculus. If
the ends can be found and repaired at once the chances for success are
not bad. However, not all cases are seen at once and, unfortunately,
hemorrhage and edema will often obscure the canalicular break.

As the lower canaliculus progresses from the punctum toward the
medial canthus it lies at first close to the lid margin on the conjunctival
surface. More medially it sinks deeper into the tissues until it pierces the
lacrimal fascia. Hence the end of a probe inserted into the canaliculus disappears from view after it has traveled 4 or 5 mm. If the break is close to
the punctum the two ends can be found easily. But the more medial to
the punctum the injury lies, the more difficult it becomes to find the
nasal end of the break.

If the ends of a freshly torn lid are examined closely the canalicular
ends can sometimes actually be seen. It is then relatively easy to thread
them together by suture or plastic tube and complete the repair. However,
more often the injury is seen too late for this. Even here if the torn
ends of the lid are held together evenly by an assistant, it is surprising
how often a section of plastic tubing or a probe through the lower punctum
will find the medial end of the break. Such a case is pictured in figure
286A. This should always be tried several times before hope is given up.
Veirs feels that waiting a day or two makes the ends easier to find because the canalicular lining turns a paler color than the surrounding
conjunctiva.

REPAIR OF TORN CANALICULUS. *Procedure (fig. 286):* The ends of
the canaliculus are found and brought together and the probe is passed
through into the lacrimal sac (fig. 286A). A length of fine, soft polyethylene tubing is attached to the probe. The probe in the end of the sac is
held by an assistant and the end is easily palpated. A small incision is
made with a knife through all the tissues down to the probe which is
drawn out with the tubing and brought out from the sac. The ends of

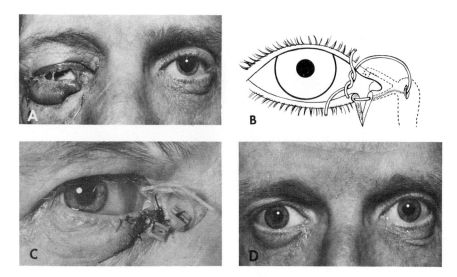

Fig. 286.   Canalicular Repair with Polyethylene Tube.
A.   Avulsion of right lower lid with tear through the canaliculus.
B.   A polyethylene tube is threaded through the tear and brought out from the sac through a cut in the overlying tissues.
C.   The lid is repaired (see figure 113).
D.   Final result.

the tube are tied together and pulled to one side so that they do not irritate the eye (fig. 286B). The tissues of the lid around the break are repaired on the skin, margin and conjunctival surfaces and the repair completed as seen in Chapter 9, figure 113. Figure 286C shows the completion of the procedure and figure 286D the final result.

This is a modification of the Selinger technic which I have used occasionally for the last ten years with satisfactory results.

Comment: Many schemes have been devised for finding and fitting together the ends of a torn canaliculus. Some are a little hare brained. However, all must be at the disposal of the surgeon because the canalicular ends are sometimes difficult indeed to find. A few are listed below:

a.   An easily visible fluid such as boiled milk may be injected through the upper canaliculus in the hope that it will emerge through the lower and thus disclose the point of the break.

b.   Morrison suggests closing off the ipsilateral nostril, dropping some fluid into the eye and injecting air through the upper canaliculus which may then be seen emerging as bubbles from the medial torn end of the lower canaliculus.

c.   A bent probe (see figure 287) or needle may be passed through the upper canaliculus then through the common canaliculus and out through the medial torn end of the lower canaliculus. (This is easier said than done.) A heavy suture is fastened to this and drawn through.

d.   Cutting down on the sac and retrograde passing of a length of

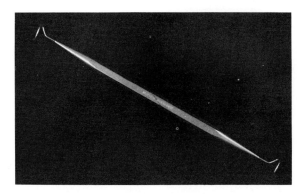

FIG. 287.   Worst's   Pigtail   Probe.

tubing through it into the lower canaliculus may have to be done when all other methods fail.

"PIGTAIL" PROBE REPAIR (WORST).   Recently Worst has reported use of a "pigtail" probe (fig. 287) one end wound clockwise and the other counterclockwise which facilitates finding the torn canalicular ends.

Procedure (fig. 288): The clockwise end of the probe is passed gently through the upper canaliculus. It is manipulated through the common punctum into the lower canaliculus and then through the medial end of the break. A suture is fastened to the end of the probe which is then pulled backward and out through the upper punctum. The medial end of the suture is drawn out the temporal end of canaliculus and lower punctum by means of the counterclockwise end of the probe. (If desired, a very fine soft length of plastic cannular tubing is attached to the suture and the tubing is drawn through the canaliculi and both puncta.) The suture ends are tied to prevent slippage (fig. 288*B*).

The break in the lid is repaired on skin, margin and conjunctival surfaces as described in figure 113. The ends of the suture are fastened to the brow or cheek (fig. 288*C*). The suture must be left in position at least three weeks before removal. During the last week it may be moved gently back and forth to try to maintain patency of the canaliculus. The final result is seen in figure 288*D*.

VEIRS CANALICULAR MALLEABLE ROD REPAIR.   Good results in canalicular repair may be obtained with the Veirs malleable rod especially if used in freshly severed canalicular tears.

Procedure (fig. 289): The slightly tapered end of the rod* is pushed through the lateral, then the medial ends of the torn canalicular break (fig. 289*A*). It is pushed in until only the silk suture at its other end extends through the punctum. A needle is threaded on to the suture and a bite is taken in the skin near the punctum to anchor the rod firmly in place (fig. 289*B*). The rod is kept in 10 to 14 days.

---

* Ethicon No. 703 on 4–0 silk.

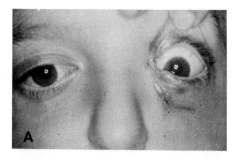
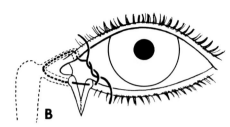
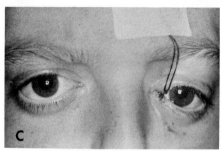
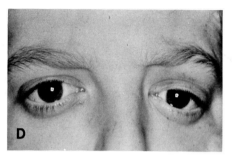

FIG. 288. Lower Canalicular Repair by Suture Passed through the Upper
Canaliculus.

A. Preoperative appearance.
B. The suture is threaded through and tied.
C. Completion of repair.
D. Final result.

OTHER METHODS OF CANALICULAR REPAIR. The literature is replete
with methods for the repair of torn canaliculi. Jones threads a dermal
suture through the canaliculus, sac and duct which emerges in the nose.
The canalicular ends are sutured under an operating microscope. The
lids are sutured as desired. The ends of the dermal suture are taped above
the brow. Sisler uses No. 90 polyethylene tubing with a Worst pigtail
probe. Griffith reports 62 per cent success with a polyethylene tube brought
out through the nose much as in the Jones method. Picó prefers the Veirs
malleable rod and reports 8 out of 9 successes with it. These are but a few
of the many reports and shows the variance in the methods used. All are
doomed to failure unless *used early enough.*

OLD CANALICULAR TEARS. The above method may suffice in fresh
injuries. Almost nothing suffices in old injuries. The author has found
no stratagem worth recommending once the canaliculus is invaded by
scar tissue. Even if the broken ends are found, cleaned and carefully
sutured, the lumen at the point of the break always tends to contract and
is a constant source of trouble—even after tubing has been kept in the
canaliculus for many weeks. Hence the importance of starting the
repair on such cases as soon as possible.

Olson and Young suggest using a 3 inch segment of a vein taken
from the patient's hand or forearm for canalicular reconstruction. They

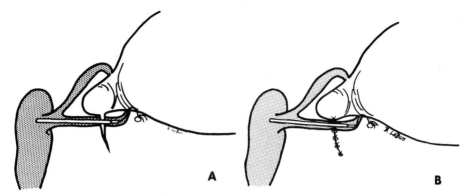

FIG. 289.   Use of Veir's Malleable Rod for Canalicular Repairs.
A.   The rod is pushed in to bridge the canalicular break.
B.   The break is repaired and the attached suture anchors the rod firmly in place.
(Veirs, E. R.: Courtesy Transactions American Acad. Ophth. & Oto.)

state that they have obtained a functional punctum and canaliculus with this method.

STRICTURES OF THE CANALICULUS.   Success in relieving this condition is something less than spectacular. The favorite procedure is to thread polyethylene tubing into the canaliculus through the upper punctum and have it in for a year in some cases. Others draw the tubing out through the nares. Veirs canalicular rods are probably simpler and just as effective. My success with polyethylene has been less than satisfactory.

SLITTING THE CANALICULUS FOR OBSTRUCTION.   This procedure is rarely carried out in the lower lid now as it has been found ineffective in curing epiphora. The exceptions as mentioned above are (1) the case of a tiny spastic punctum where a single vertical or medial *short* snip or the "three snip" procedure are used. (2) The removal of dacryoliths and the clearing out of other fungus infections such as streptothrix. In the latter case the canaliculus is opened horizontally nasal to the punctum, cleaned out, swabbed with KI solution and resutured. KI drops are then used for several weeks postoperatively.

There is some indication for slitting the upper canaliculus, however, and that is, if it becomes necessary in probing for congenital stenosis of the nasolacrimal sac and duct. This prevents traumatic enlargement of the lower punctum which occurs so easily not only in infants but in adults as well.

SURGICAL CLOSURE OF PUNCTUM AND CANALICULUS.   The indication for purposive closure of the lower punctum and canaliculus is hyposecretion of tears. The most common condition causing hyposecretion is keratoconjunctivitis sicca. Other rarer conditions are acute affections of the lacrimal gland such as Mikulicz's disease, hypothyroidism, lacrimal gland resection and obstruction of the tubules due to an overwhelming and devastating conjunctivitis such as xerosis. It should also be borne in mind that lacrimal secretion decreases with old age and diminution of the tear supply may have a slight or severe affect on the well-being of the eye depending on the amount of tear secretion left. Symptoms may vary from a mild irritative conjunctivitis to a severe keratitis which puts the cornea in jeopardy.

If the condition is mild, palliative drops of methyl cellulose, Locke's solution, tear substitutes or estrogens may help. However, severe cases of keratoconjunctivitis may call for closure of the lower punctum and canaliculus to conserve whatever small supply of tears is formed.

Procedure: The punctum and canaliculus are anesthetized with 0.5 per cent tetracaine instillation and infiltration of 2 per cent lidocaine. The punctum is dilated sufficiently to permit introduction of a *cold* thin curved electrode into the canaliculus for about 3 mm. The lid is everted slightly so that the exact position of the electrode may be seen and adjusted under direct inspection. The coagulating current is then turned on slightly for a second or two to a dull glow. Too much current must not be used to prevent injury to surrounding tissue.

A tight suture is passed around the canaliculus about 2 mm. medial to the punctum following coagulation. The upper punctum and canaliculus are similarly treated. Despite the apparent inevitability of closure with such treatment, stubborn canaliculi have been known to resist closure. In such cases the treatment is repeated. Even with complete closure this type of repair is not a panacea and medical care often has to be continued.

The Common Punctum

As in the canaliculus, stenosis, partial or total, of the common punctum is not uncommon. It may be partial or complete and due to infectious or traumatic causes. Recently Veirs has reported a simple technic for correcting stenosis of the ampullary portion of the common canaliculi with a canalicular steel rod.

Procedure (fig. 290): After suitable local infiltration anesthesia, a lacrimal probe is passed through the upper canaliculus and then through the stenosed common canaliculus into the lacrimal sac (fig. 290*A*). The probe is withdrawn and the patency assured by saline lavage through both upper and lower canaliculi.

A stainless steel rod with a 4–0 silk suture swaged on one end is passed through the upper canaliculus as far as the medial wall of the sac. The proximal end of the rod is within the upper canaliculus and only the suture protrudes from the upper punctum. The rod is anchored by suturing the protruding suture to the skin adjacent to the punctum (fig. 290*B*). The rod should remain in position two or three months.

Some inflammation may occur around the suture in which case the suture is cut close to the punctum and the knot removed. The rod usually

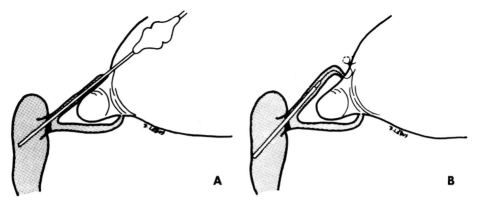

FIG. 290.   Veir's Rod for Stenosed Common Punctum.
A.   A probe is forced through the stenosed common punctum into the sac from
the upper canaliculus.
B.   A stainless steel rod is inserted and left in 2 to 3 months.
(Veirs, E. R.: Courtesy Archives of Ophthalmology.)

remains in position but it may dislodge. An alternative is to knot the
suture close to the rod to prevent the rod slipping into the sac. Veirs
has had good results with this technic and feels that it may relieve more
extensive stenosis but the rate of correction may not be as high as when
the common punctum alone is obstructed.

Comment: Various methods of doing this repair have been reported. Beard has pointed out that probing of the common punctum and
canaliculus is rarely successful. After opening the sac he passes a
probe into the canaliculus until there is tenting of the common punctum
into the sac. An incision is then made over the area of tenting until the
probe is exposed. All the tissue about the tip is resected and the canalicular mucosa is anastomosed to the sac with 6–0 chromic sutures. This is
not unlike the Arruga procedure.

The Nasolacrimal Sac and Duct

PROBING OF THE NASOLACRIMAL DUCT IN INFANTS.   The one com-
pelling indication for probing of the lacrimal sac and nasolacrimal duct
is congenital stenosis. If done early enough—before the age of two
months, if possible—it is usually successful after one or (occasionally)
two probings. The obstruction in these cases is a membrane across the
nasolacrimal duct lumen which, once pierced, remains perforated and
ends the tearing. One should not wait beyond two months to do this.
Success may be obtained several months later but the chances are less.

The indication for probing in an infant is epiphora usually accompanied by a mucopurulent discharge which does not respond to medication, massage or irrigation.

Conservative treatment such as astringent and antibiotic drops
should be tried first. The mother should be instructed how to keep the

sac clean if infected and how to massage the area at least 3 to 4 times a day. If tearing persists, probing is done next.

There is some difference of opinion as to whether the procedure should be done in the hospital under general anesthesia or in the office under local. This will depend to a large extent on the individual surgeon and the assistance which he commands in the office for keeping a squirming infant sufficiently immobile to perform the delicate probing. It has been done successfully both ways.

In the younger infants the pain threshold is so low that instillation of a few drops of proparacaine 0.5 per cent into the conjunctival sac is usually enough.

Procedure: The lower canaliculus is irrigated first to assure its patentcy and also to clean as much of the pus as possible out of the sac. Sometimes purulent material becomes inspissated and several irrigations are required to clean the sac out completely. When clear, solution is seen to regurgitate one then proceeds with the probing.

The best instrument is a thin lacrimal needle (23 or 24 gauge) on a 2 cc. syringe containing 10 per cent sodium sulfacetamide solution. It also helps to have the needle somewhat curved forward so as to avoid interference from the brow. If the lower punctum has been frequently dilated for previous irrigations and treatments, it is better to use the upper punctum to avoid permanent injury to the lower.

The punctum is well dilated and the lacrimal needle passed into the canaliculus first vertically then horizontally until the bony wall of the nose is reached. The cannula is turned vertically again and, hugging the bony wall, is pushed downward and slightly backward into the sac and on into the nasolacrimal duct and inferior meatus. Sometimes the perforation of the membranous obstruction can be felt but not always. The lacrimal needle is left in position a little while to contain bleeding and then slowly withdrawn. A few drops of the sulfacetamide solution are injected as the needle is withdrawn. After several days the sac is irrigated to assure patency. If the sac remains closed, a second probing may be done as soon as the effects of the first have worn off. If the duct still remains closed, a rhinostomy is in order.

PROBING THE ADULT NASOLACRIMAL DUCT. Probing the adult obstructed nasolacrimal duct is a much more thankless proposition and is rarely successful unless done shortly after the obstruction begins. This is rare as patients usually seek help only after the tearing has continued for some time and the obstruction has existed long beyond the time when it will respond to conservative treatment. If there is no improvement in the epiphora after two or three probings, dacryocystorhinostomy should be advised. It goes without saying that acute infection is a contraindication to any probing.

ACUTE DACRYOCYSTITIS. Acute infections of the lacrimal sac are not uncommon. The part of the sac *below* the medial canthal ligament is covered only by skin and orbicularis fibers and hence little resistance is offered to the distensions and swellings of infection and inflammation. The clinical picture is typical and cannot be mistaken: a red swollen area *below* the medial canthus in the nasocanthal angle. Incision and drainage is easily accomplished.

Procedure: Anesthesia is general for children. A little local ethyl chloride usually suffices for the adult. The eye should be closed and covered. Incision is made with a scalpel as for a dacryocystectomy below the canthal ligament. The incision is deep enough to enter the abscess cavity and long enough to reach the lower part of the sac. The purulent material is evacuated, a drain is inserted, a moist dressing is applied and covered with a loose bandage. The dressings are changed daily and the drain shortened and finally removed on the fourth or fifth day. Healing is usually spontaneous but recurrences are not infrequent. Chronic dacryocystitis may persist or a fistula may form unless further corrective surgery is done.

LACRIMAL SAC FISTULA.   Fistulae of the lacrimal sac are the product of recurrent dacryocystitis—chronic or acute. In rare instances they may be congenital. In attempting surgical correction the surgeon should be prepared to do a dacryocystectomy or a rhinostomy depending on the condition of the lacrimal sac. Rarely is the opening of the fistula into the sac so small or the condition of the sac so good that excision of the fistulous tract may be done leaving normally functioning lacrimal drainage.

In congenital fistulae it is sometimes possible to resect the whole tract, cauterize it and attain closure with normal sac drainage. Following repeated dacryocystitis this is rare.

DACRYOCYSTECTOMY.   The most common seat of obstruction of the tear-conducting apparatus is at the junction of the nasolacrimal sac and duct. Having found the lower punctum and canaliculus patent and in good working order (patency of the upper punctum and canaliculus alone is not enough) and having established the point of obstruction to the sac or duct, the surgeon must decide on whether to do a dacryocystectomy or dacryocystorhinostomy.

Today the indications for dacryocystectomy are few. Generally they are limited to (1) the rare case of malignancy or tuberculosis or syphilis of the sac, (2) patients with gross nasal conditions such as ozena, lupus, bony malformations, etc., (3) cases where there has been so much chronic infection of the sac that it will stand no surgery, in which case a conjunctivorhinostomy may be tried, (4) cases of chronic dacryocystitis where all other surgery has failed.

Procedure (fig. 291):   The lacrimal sac is cleansed thoroughly of all mucoid and purulent material by irrigation and the area is anesthetized. The author prefers local anesthesia. However, general anes-

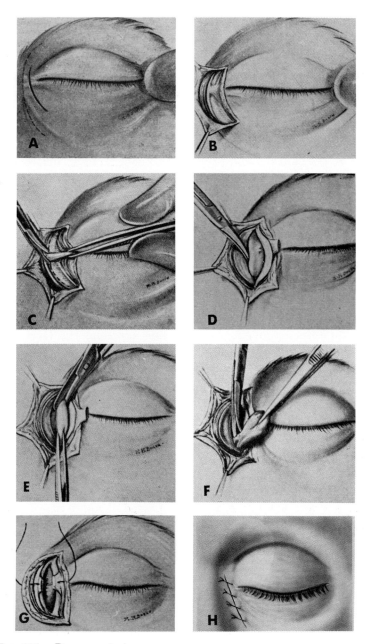

Fig. 291. Dacryocystectomy.

A. Skin incision.

B. and *C.* The canthal ligament is exposed and cut.

D., E. and *F.* The sac is freed and resected. The medial canthal ligament is sutured.

H. Skin closure.

thesia is a must in children and is not contraindicated if preferred by adults, although the anesthetist with all his paraphernalia can be a nuisance in this area.

Anesthesia is attained by conjunctival instillation and infiltration. The whole area over the lacrimal crest is infiltrated with 2 per cent lidocaine to which epinephrine has been added. A deep injection above the canthal ligament over the dome of the lacrimal sac is also made. Some surgeons prefer to inject the supraorbital, supratrochlear and infra-orbital nerves. The area is massaged gently for a few minutes to assure good absorption of the anesthesia.

A skin incision is made 3 mm. medial to the medial canthus starting 3 mm. above the canthus and proceeding about 2 cm. below. The incision follows the curve of the anterior lacrimal crest (fig. 291A). The skin is undermined, a lacrimal retractor is inserted and the muscle split by blunt dissection along the line just below the attachment of the medial canthal ligament. The speculum is reinserted so as to be inside the muscle layer. This exerts pressure on the muscle fibers and lessens bleeding. The nasal attachment of the canthal ligament is freely exposed (fig. 291B), grasped with forceps and cut close to its insertion to the bone (fig. 291C). A blunt pointed Stevens scissors is inserted into the lacrimal fascia above and the fascia cut the whole length of the skin incision following the curve of the anterior lacrimal crest, thus exposing the lacrimal sac.

The sac is freed by blunt dissection from the nasal wall of the fossa from dome to neck (fig. 291D). The orbital fascia is held up and out and the sac is freed on the orbital side (fig. 291E). The canaliculi are cut, the dome of the sac is grasped and pulled forward and the sac is freed posteriorly all the way down into the duct, the attachment to which is now cut (fig. 291F). The wound is thoroughly irrigated and the walls of the lacrimal fossa are curetted to get all the remnants of the sac, if any. It may be swabbed with iodine if there has been much infection. The wound is then inspected to assure that no pockets of pus or remnants of the sac are left behind. A probe is passed through the nasolacrimal duct into the nose to assure an open channel for drainage.

The ends of the medial canthal ligament are sutured with 4–0 chromic catgut (fig. 291G). The edges of the orbicularis are also sutured with a few interrupted catgut sutures if they do not fall together easily. If the wound has been infected a small rubber drain is inserted into the depths of the lower end of the incision. The skin is closed with inter-rupted 5–0 silk sutures inserted somewhat obliquely from below upward and medially (fig. 291H).

If a drain has been used the wound is dressed lightly and redressed daily and the drain removed on the fourth or fifth day. If no drain has been inserted the dressing is left in place for two days then repatched daily and the skin sutures removed on the fifth or sixth day.

Comment: Some prefer a straight skin incision instead of one which follows the curve of the anterior lacrimal crest. However, the latter has not been found to produce undue scarring as claimed. In fact after several weeks the skin scar is usually indistinguishable from its surroundings.

Also some surgeons prefer to make the original incision right down to periosteum. There is no objection to this. An experienced surgeon who knows his anatomy will have no difficulty with either incision.

Complications of a dacryocystectomy operation are due mainly to lack of recognition of landmarks or rough handling of tissues. During the operation cutting of the angular vessels will cause profuse hemorrhage, interfere with the procedure and delay the operation. The angular vessels cross the canthal ligament. With care they may be recognized and pushed out of the way laterally. Incision too far medially fails to expose the sac and leaves a bad skin scar. Some prefer an incision 11 mm. nasal to the canthus. This is a somewhat more conspicuous position than 3 mm. medial to the canthus. If the sac is very friable and not removed en masse—pieces may be left behind which give rise to recurrences and fistula formation. Care must be taken in freeing the sac not to break through the lacrimal bone and cause possible osteomyelitis or an ethmoidal sinusitis.

In the dissection of the lateral wall of the sac orbital fascia may be cut and fat extruded. When this happens it is best to sew the cut up at once to prevent herniation of more orbital fat. Failure to find the sac is experienced by young surgeons. Injecting saline through the canaliculus may dilate it and help in its location. A probe passed through the lower canaliculus into the sac and left in place is always a trustworthy guide. Injection of dye preoperatively is not advised as the sac may be ruptured and the dye may stain all the surrounding tissues making it even more difficult to identify the sac. Hematoma postoperatively is not common but chronic dacryocystitis is, if all the remnants of the sac have not been removed.

Epiphora to a greater or less degree continues in a majority of cases. Theoretically this should give patients a lot of trouble. Actually some are fairly comfortable as every eye surgeon will attest. The reason is probably twofold. The tear secretion of the normal eye is reduced in older people and at best half of this is disposed of by evaporation. This leaves little to trouble the patient especially in summer unless the eye is infected or otherwise irritated. When the tear sac, which is the source of irritation is removed, epiphora diminishes. Also, in most cases the patient has had epiphora for a long time and has learned to cope with it hence, to this extent, he is no worse off than he was before.

If tumor is suspected or encountered—and this is the most important indication for this operation—then the periosteum as well as the sac is removed in toto. Bony involvement, if obvious or even suspected, means removal of bone. This is a good place for the use of Mohs' paste to assure complete tumor removal before closure (see Chapter 26).

Dacryocystectomy had its heyday twenty-five years ago; it is an uncommon operation today.

DACRYOCYSTORHINOSTOMY.   As indicated above, the idea for dacryocystorhinostomy is almost as old as the history of man. But it is only in the last few decades that it has become a workable concept. In fact, the technic, substantially as it is used today, was established within a period of less than twenty years dating from Toti (1904) to Dupuy-Dutemps (1921).

The indications for dacryocystorhinostomy are long-standing incurable epiphora in healthy individuals of any age who have not had prolonged chronic dacryocystitis, although even here the operation is indicated. For if the sac is found unusable, a canaliculorhinostomy may then be done without having sacrificed anything. Patients with mucocele offer a good prognosis.

Procedure (fig. 292):   Anesthesia is the same as described above for dacryocystectomy with the addition of a spray of 5 per cent cocaine into the nostril plus a tampon of cocaine with adrenalin into the middle meatus as high as it will go. This is removed before the bone trephine is used. The preliminaries including irrigation of the sac, etc., are the same as for dacryocystectomy.

The skin and fascia incisions are made as for dacryocystectomy, i.e., 3 mm. medial to the canthus. The skin is undermined to expose the orbicularis to the nose. The muscle is split down to periosteum—the split being carried downward on a line with the medial canthal ligament. The medial canthal ligament is cut at its insertion giving free exposure to the whole sac. The periosteum is cut and then carefully undermined laterally with a periosteal elevator down to the anterior lacrimal crest leaving bare bone. The dissection is carried up and down and laterally so that sac and periosteum are freed as far laterally as the posterior lacrimal crest so that the whole lacrimal fossa is clean (fig. 292A). The angular vessels should not be injured because they pass just anterior to the lacrimal crest. However, they may be tied off if cut.

The lacrimal sac after exposure and mobilization is pulled laterally out of harm's way with a smooth retractor thus exposing the lacrimal fossa. The 10 mm. Iliff trephine of the Stryker saw is so placed as to straddle the lower anterior lacrimal crest about one third anteriorly and two thirds posteriorly and the bone cut away. The trephine is directed slightly backward and medially to avoid the ethmoid cells. The trephine generates heat and should be irrigated with cold saline during the cutting process. Usually the bone plus comes away cleanly. The opening into the nose is enlarged with rongeur still more to the posterior lacrimal crest and to reach down to the junction of the sac and duct so that no pocket is left below for the collection of mucopurulent material. The edges of the window are smoothed (fig. 292B).

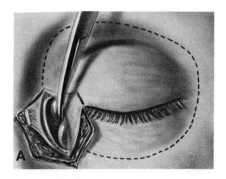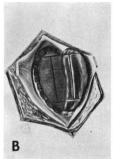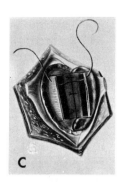
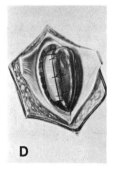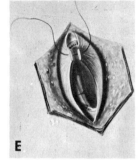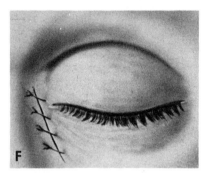

FIG. 292. Dacryocystorhinostomy.
A. The sac is exposed as in the previous procedure and retracted laterally.
B. The nasal mucosa is exposed by trephine and rongeur. Capital I incisions
   are made in the sac and nasal mucosa to create two flaps.
C. The posterior flaps are sutured.
D. The anterior flaps are sutured.
E. The ends of the canthal ligament are brought together and sutured.
F. Skin closure.

When completed the bony window should measure 1.5 by 2 cm. with
the long diameter vertical and should include all the bone between the
anterior and posterior lacrimal crests including the anterior crest. It cannot be emphasized too strongly that the success of the operation depends
to a large extent on a large enough opening. If an ethmoid cell is
encountered it may be cut away but there should be adequate nasal
drainage to avoid postoperative infection. Bleeding from the bone is
usually not severe, and controllable by bone wax if necessary.

A probe is slipped through the lower canaliculus into the lacrimal
sac and the medial wall identified. With this as a landmark a vertical
incision is made in the medial wall of the sac from the fundus to its
juncture with the duct. At each end of the vertical incision horizontal
incisions are made so that the total incision is I-shaped thus creating an
anterior and posterior flap. A similar incision is made in the exposed
nasal mucosa again creating two rectangular flaps (fig. 292B). The two
posterior flaps are sutured together with three 5–0 or 6–0 chromic catgut
sutures (fig. 292C). These fall together easily but the suturing takes

place in a small deep hole and requires careful maneuvering with good assistance and lighting. Small half-curved, quarter-inch needles may be used or the special dacryocystorhinostomy needles now obtainable. The anterior flaps are sutured in similar fashion (fig. 292D).

The wound is cleaned and irrigated. The orbicularis muscle is closed with several catgut sutures including one which unites the canthal ligament (fig. 292E). Skin closure is as for dacryocystectomy (fig. 292F). A firm dressing is applied without too much pressure. If bleeding continues from the nose the nostril is packed—not too tightly—for 48 hours. The wound is dressed daily and the eye cleansed. Skin sutures are removed on the fifth day. Some surgeons begin irrigation of the sac at once; others when the sutures are removed, others after the second postoperative week. Irrigation is done daily for a week then at longer intervals until no longer required.

An alternative procedure and one which is simpler yet apparently just as effective is to make an anterior flap only of sac and nasal mucosa instead of anterior and posterior flaps. In this technic the vertical incision in the sac is made in the medioposterior aspect of the sac. The horizontal incisions are then made laterally from the upper and lower end of this incision. In the mucosa the vertical incision is made close to the posterior edge of the bony window and the horizontal incisions from the upper and lower ends of the incision. In this way two large flaps are created which are sutured anteriorly.

Comment: The technic just described is subject to variations. Some prefer an anterior flap only (as I do); others a posterior flap. Still others use no flaps but simply make large openings in the juxtaposed sac and nasal mucosa as Toti did in his original operation. Many of these variations make a virtue of necessity because the tissues are frequently so devitalized and so friable that little can be done with them except resect them and leave a wide opening. This is not surprising when one considers that the main causes of lacrimal sac obstruction are ascending inflammations from the nasal and sinus mucosa.

When confronted with mucosal tissue which is too friable to handle and which will not retain a suture the mucosa presenting in the bony nasal opening should be completely resected if enough is not available for an anterior flap. Usually the tissue of the sac is in sufficiently good condition to permit suture of one of the lips of the incised sac to the periosteum bordering the bony opening into the nose. If the opening is large enough to withstand subsequent closure by granulation tissue the operation can be successful. In fact this seems to be the major requirement of all dacryocystorhinostomy surgery, viz., an opening big enough in size and low enough in position so that it will not close or become obstructed by material collecting in the lower portion which has nowhere to go. It would seem as if the flaps—anterior, posterior or both—are a secondary consideration and are not of primary importance.

The most immediate complication during operation is hemorrhage which is difficult to control after closure. Hence all bleeding is controlled before closure. Alger's method of placing one deep suture above the upper punctum and another deep in the lower angle of the orbit to emerge on the nose may be of help here. Other later and rarer complications are scarring due to a poorly placed incision and inadvertent injury to the puncta, canaliculi, etc.

The next common complication is stricture of the common punctum and the neighboring canaliculus. Many stratagems are used by surgeons to prevent strictures and keep openings from closing. Iliff leaves a catheter in the sac running out through the nose to avoid the rhinostomy sutures. Picó uses a silk suture from the punctum through the nose which is tied at both ends and moved at each dressing to dislodge any granulations or blood clots present in the bony opening. Jones uses a dermal knotted suture in cases of closure of the common punctum after dacryocystorhinostomy. Veirs makes a passage through the closed area and pulls through a wick of 3 or 4 strands of No. 3 Dermaline from the lower punctum into the nose. This is anchored to the lid and left in position 10 to 14 days. Mirabile and Tucker use a silicone sponge implant between the flaps which is extended down through the nose. This is kept in for 6 weeks.

The most depressing late complication is, of course, closure of the opening by granulation tissue with resumption of tearing. This usually occurs within two months after operation. Irrigation and probing are rarely helpful once this has occurred. Reoperation is the only recourse—with enlargement of the bony opening. By this time the mucosa is still harder to suture and failures are more frequent. Recurrence of infection is another late complication.

Success with the dacryocystorhinostomy procedure varies from 70 per cent to almost 100 per cent depending on the reporter and, probably, on how long a time after operation the report covers. In general the final fate of the procedure is evident within two or three months after operation.

CONJUNCTIVODACRYOCYSTORHINOSTOMY (JONES). This operation is indicated and should be tried in closure of the medial 3 or 4 mm. of both ipsilateral upper and lower canaliculi whether congenital, traumatic or due to disease. Other indications are complete closure and absence or lack of function of the ipsilateral canaliculi. The operative technique as described by Jones follows:

Procedure (fig. 293): The preliminary steps for the conjunctivo-dacryocystorhinostomy (C-D-C-R) are the same as for the dacryocysto-

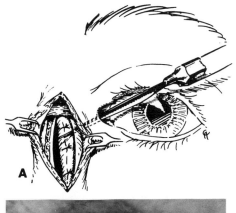
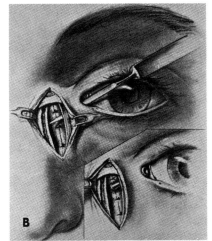
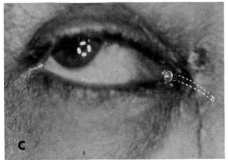
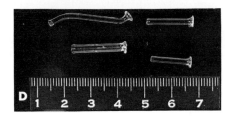

FIG. 293. Conjunctivodacryocystorhinostomy (Jones).
A. Hypodermic needle creates a track which is followed by a narrow Graefe knife.
B. Needle is withdrawn, knife enlarges the passage and polyethylene tube is placed in position (inset).
C. Result with pyrex tube in place. (Flange of tube lies inside lids.)
D. Jones Pyrex tubes. (Courtesy Dr. Alston Callahan).
(Jones, L. T.: Courtesy American Journal of Ophthalmology.)

rhinostomy. This is carried out as described above until the posterior flaps have been sutured. Jones prefers local anesthesia where at all possible and he makes his skin incision 11 mm. nasal to the canthus. In exposing the sac he cautions against cutting the medial canthal ligament because of its importance as a landmark. He also prefers to stand at the side of the patient for a better view of the tissues under the canthal ligament.

After the posterior flaps of sac and nasal mucosa have been united the caruncle is resected taking care not to cut away any excess conjunctiva. A 23 gauge hypodermic needle is bent into a mild curve with the point of the needle on the inside of the curve. With the needle held with its convexity pointing backward, the point is entered in the conjunctiva 2 mm. from the canthal angle and directed in a plane which will cause it to enter into the lacrimal sac just below the canthal angle and behind the anterior flap.

When the needle is in place a narrow Graefe knife follows the course of the needle and also enters the sac (fig. 293A) after which the needle is withdrawn. The knife is used to enlarge the passage somewhat to permit the entrance of a No. 240 polyethylene flanged tube threaded on a lacrimal probe. Using the Graefe knife as a sort of groove director the 16–18 mm. polyethylene tube with pointed ends is slid into the sac. The tube is fastened into position to keep it from pulling out by means of a 4–0 silk suture passed through its flange and then through the adjacent skin of the lid (fig. 293B inset). (The flange of the tube can be made simply by flaming it at very short intervals in a match flame. It should not be held in the flame too long or it will burn.) The Graefe knife is pulled out. The anterior flaps of sac and nasal mucosa are united. The periosteum and muscle are closed and the skin sutured as for previous operations. A pressure dressing is kept in 4 or 5 days and the eye is then patched regularly and irrigated through the tube to check on patency.

The plastic tube is replaced by a pyrex glass tube in one to four weeks after operation (fig. 293C). This should be 2.0 mm. in outside diameter with a 4 mm. collar and a 2.25 mm enlargement at the nasal end: they are custom made and vary from 10 to 16 mm. (fig. 293D). After a month or two a glass tube with a 3 mm. collar is substituted. Glass is less irritating to the tissues according to Jones, has greater capillary attraction and gets obstructed with secretions less easily.

Jones, with his skill and vast experience, maintains that these latter are simple office procedures. The inexperienced ophthalmologist may not find this tube exchange quite so easy.

Comment: This procedure is well within the competence of any ophthalmologist doing lacrimal surgery, although minutiae of technic will vary with the individual surgeon. Those who prefer general anesthesia—as I do—should not hesitate to use it. With modern hypotensive general anesthesia what it is today, bleeding is hardly more of a factor in general than in local anesthesia.

I prefer to cut the medial canthal ligament to give me better exposure—as do many others. It remains a landmark cut or uncut. I prefer to stand behind the patient and not at his side except when chiseling the bone. Although Jones uses two flaps there are many who do not (Beard uses an anterior flap only—Picó uses a posterior flap with the anterior sac flap sutured to periosteum, etc.). I prefer an anterior flap only.

I see no reason for using first a needle and then a Graefe knife to find the proper plane into the sac. It is just as easy to find the proper plane with the Graefe knife which can then be used to enlarge the opening as much as is necessary to allow passage of the tube. As a matter of fact, residents are inclined to make the passage too wide thus making it harder to retain the tube.

Complications: While the surgery is not difficult, the postoperative care is something else again. Jones states flatly that "no ophthalmologist should attempt this procedure unless he is willing to observe the intranasal end of the tube and ostium at nearly every postoperative visit or, in lieu of this, to work closely with a rhinologist." Also before operating a set of tubes and a dilator should be obtained.* The complications are manifold and Jones's instruction leaflet outlining the postoperative care accompanies each tube:

1. The patient must never blow his nose. If he does he should squeeze his lids shut or hold his finger over the tube. In case of tube obstruction a wire is reamed through the tube or saline injected.

2. If the tube comes out and the patient is seen early the passage is anesthetized and is dilated and the tube reinserted. If seen late, the passage may have to be enlarged with a Graefe knife to attain insertion.

3. A conjunctivitis or granulation may develop at the medial canthus due to a scale-like deposit around the tube. Then the tube must be removed, the scales cleaned off and the tube reinserted.

4. Notching of the lid by the tube's flange may occur. Replacement by a tube with a smaller flange or an angled tube may cure this. If the collar is submerged it may be fished out by passing a probe into the lumen and gradually easing it out by pressure.

5. Too far a protrusion externally can usually be corrected by a shortened or angled tube, removal of the upper part of the middle turbinate or a submucous resection.

6. If the plica obstructs the mouth of the tube the obstructive tissue is resected.

The patient or someone in the family should be taught to ream out the tube with wire and to irrigate it through. Above all he should be instructed to seek help immediately if the tube comes out or the eye begins to tear.

The tube starts to loosen and comes out in about a year on the average. The patient is then taught to take the pyrex tube out and leave it out for longer and longer intervals using the dilator, if necessary for reinsertion.

Anyone contemplating this surgery would be well advised to read Jones's original 1965 article for details. As stated above, it is not the surgery but the postoperative care which will be troublesome to anyone who is not a rhinologist or does not have or acquire some rhinologic know-how.

Other types of surgery have been described by Jones: canaliculorhinostomy in the absence of the lacrimal sac and conjunctivorhinostomy in the absence of both sac and canaliculi. Fortunately the need for this kind of surgery is not common.

---

* From Mr. Gunther Weiss, 2025 S. W. Briggs Court, Beaverton, Ore. 97005.

The Jones C-D-C-R in the proper hands has gotten good results and certainly should be tried where indicated, since it is one of the very few—if not the only procedure—offering hope of cure in canalicular failure.

CONJUNCTIVODACRYOCYSTORHINOSTOMY (REINECKE AND CARROLL). Recently a modification of Jones's conjunctivodacryocystorhinostomy (C-D-C-R) has been suggested by Reinecke and Carroll. They use a permanent silicone right-angled tube (fig. 294A) which needs no replacement by a pyrex tube. The indications are the same as described for the Jones C-D-C-R procedure. Here too, two technics are employed depending on the presence or absence of a previous dacryocystorhinostomy (D-C-R).

Procedure (fig. 294): If no previous D-C-R has been done the procedure is as described in Procedure 292 until the bony ostium has been made. A hypodermic needle is then passed from a point in the medial canthus lateral to the caruncle until the tip is seen in the bony nasal opening. This is followed by a cataract knife along the needle's path and the needle is withdrawn much as described by Jones. A 3 mm. stab incision is made in the sac, the knife remains in place and a No. 90 polyethylene tube is threaded on a No. 2 lacrimal probe (figs. 294B to F) is passed through the sac opening. Incisions are made in the sac and nasal mucosa, the polyethylene tube is pushed through into the nose where it is grasped with forceps and pulled out through the nares. The sac and nasal mucosa are sutured.

The silicone elbow tube is passed over the polyethylene tube and maneuvered into the nose (fig. 294G). The silicone tube is held with forceps and the polyethylene tube is drawn out completely through the nose (fig. 294H). Postoperative care consists of a supportive bandage for 24 to 48 hours when the patient is discharged and placed on topical antibiotics and steroids.

If a previous D-C-R has been done and an adequate opening exists, the silicone tube placement is a simple out-patient procedure according to the authors. Under local anesthesia a hypodermic needle is inserted from the desired point in the medial canthus through the bony ostium into the nose without a skin incision. The proper location of the needle is easily observed through the nares. The procedure of implanting the silicone tube is then carried out as described above. The patient is discharged after instillation of a few drops of antibiotic into the eye.

POSTOPERATIVE COMPLICATIONS. The authors have reported 18 cases, one bilateral. Of the 19 eyes 14 have done well. One patient had epistaxis and the tube had to be removed after 7 months but there was no further tearing. In three cases shorter Jones pyrex tubes were implanted subsequently with a cessation of epiphora. Some of these polyethylene tubes have been in place for two and a half years and have been well tolerated. This is a good record.

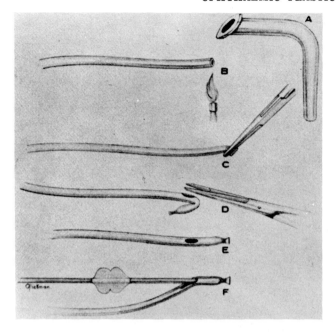

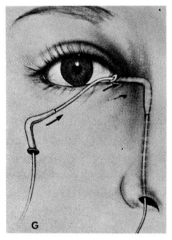
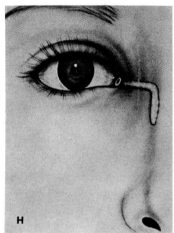

FIG. 294.   Conjunctivodacryocystorhinostomy (Reinicke and Carroll).
A.   The silicone elbow tube.
B. and C.   Heating of tip and sealing polyethylene tube.
D.   Making an opening in tube.
E. and F.   No. 2 lacrimal probe in tube.
G.   The silicone elbow tube is passed over the polyethylene tube and worked into
     position.
H.   The polyethylene tube is removed through the nostril.

  The patient is instructed to sniff a few times a day while pinching
his nostrils, this tends to keep the tube patent. No tube has slipped out
into the conjunctival sac but a few have slipped into the nose and
have had to be replaced. Apparently the silicone tube seems to be well
tolerated.

Comment: If time confirms the authors' optimism this procedure has several advantages over the Jones technic: (1) No secondary procedure is necessary for changing from a polyethylene to a pyrex tube. (2) The elbow-shaped tube decreases the chances of loss or expulsion of the tube. (3) The wider bore of the tube would seem to give less chance for obstruction. I have found it simpler to place the silicone tube first before suturing sac to nasal mucosa.

Jones has raised what seem to be some valid objections to the silicone tube. He points out that (a) it is more difficult to insert, (b) that the nasal component is a source of irritation and (c) that it has no capillary attraction: in fact, it repels the tears. He does not feel that the silicone tube can compete with the pyrex tube in most cases.

Time will furnish the answer and render its decision.

REFERENCES

ABRAHAMSON, I. A., SR., and ABRAHAMSON, I. A., JR.: Dacryocystorhinostomy with wire fistulization. Am. J. Ophth. *48*:769, 1959.

ALGER, L. J.: Hemostasis in tear-sac operations. Am. J. Ophth. *32*:845, 1949.

AMDUR, J.: Excision of palpebral lacrimal gland in epiphora. Arch. Ophth. *71*:71, 1964.

ANEL, D.: Cited by Duke-Elder, S. Textbook of Ophthalmology. St. Louis, C. V. Mosby Co., vol. 5, p. 5281.

ARRUGA, H.: Surgical treatment of lacrimation. Arch. Ophth. *19*:9, 1938.

AXENFELD, T.: Lehrbuch der Augenheilkunde (ed. 2). Jena (East Germany), Verlag von Gustav Fischer, 1910, p. 276.

BARBERRA, I. A.: A contribution to the therapy of keratoconjunctivitis sicca. Arch. Soc. oftal. hispano-am. *21*:363, 1961.

BEARD, C.: Lacrimal sac surgery. Trans. Am. Ac. Ophth. & Oto. *69*:970, 1965.

BOWMAN, W.: On the treatment of lacrymal obstruction (with lacrymal probes). Ophthalmic Hosp. Repts. and J. Roy. Lond. Ophth. Hosp. *1*:10, 1857.

BROGGI, R. J.: The treatment of congenital dacryostenosis. Arch. Ophth. *61*:30, 1959.

BURCH, M.: Roentgenography in dacryocystitis. Arch. Soc. oftal. hispano-am. *27*: 122, 1967.

CALLAHAN, A.: Reconstructive Surgery of the Eyelids and Ocular Adnexa. Birmingham, Aesculapius Publishing Co., 1966, p. 158.

CAMPBELL, H. S., SMITH, J. L., RICHMAN, S. W., and ANDERSON, W. B., JR.: A simple test for lacrimal obstruction. Am. J. Ophth. *53*:611, 1962.

CASSADY, J. V.: Dacryocystitis of infancy. Arch. Ophth. *39*:491, 1948.

COHEN, S. T.: Dacryo-transillumination. Am. J. Ophth. *63*:527, 1963.

DAYAL, Y.: External dacryocystorhinostomy. Am. J. Ophth. *51*:514, 1961.

DUPUY-DUTEMPS, and BOURGUET: Note preliminaire sur un procede de dacryocystorhinostomie. Ann. d'ocul. *157*:445, 1920.

————, and ————: Cure de la dacryocystito chronique commune et du larmoiment par la dacryocystorhimostomie plastique. Bull. Acad. méd. *86*:293, 1921.

ELLIS, P. P., BAUSOR, C., and FULMER, J. M.: Streptothrix canaliculitis. Am. J. Ophth. *52*:36, 1961.

EWING, A. E.: Roentgen ray demonstration of the lacrimal abscess cavity. Am. J. Ophth. *24*:1, 1909.

FOX, S. A.: Lipiodol studies of chronic dacryocystitis. Am. J. Ophth. *30*:878, 1947.

GRIFFITH, T. P.: Polythene tubes in canaliculus surgery. Brit. J. Ophth. *47*:203, 1963.

HALLUM, A. V.: The Dupuy-Dutemps dacryocystorhinostomy. Am. J. Ophth. *32*: 1197, 1949.

HENDERSON, J. W.: Management of obstruction of the lacrimal canaliculi with polyethylene tube. Arch. Ophth. *49*:182, 1953.

HOGAN, M. J.: Dacryocystorhinostomy. Trans. Am. Acad. Ophth. Oto. p. 600 (Jul.-Aug.) 1948.

HUGHES, W. L., and MARIS, C. S. G.: Clip procedure for stenosis and excision of the lacrimal punctum. Trans. Amer. Acad. Ophth. & Oto. *71*:653, 1967.

ILIFF, C. E.: A simplified dacryocystorhinostomy. Trans. Am. Acad. Ophth. Oto. *58*:590, 1954.

IRVINE, R. S.: Buried rubber tubes in nasolacrimal dust stenosis. Arch. Ophth. *65*:192, 1961.

JAMESON, P. C.: Subconjunctival section of the ductules of the lacrimal gland as a cure for epiphora. Arch. Ophth. *17*:207, 1937.

JONES, L. T.: The anatomical approach to problems of the eyelids and lacrimal apparatus. Arch. Ophth. *66*:111, 1961.

————: Conjunctivodacryocystorhinostomy. Am. J. Ophth. *59*:773, 1965.

————: The lacrimal secretory system and its treatment. Am. J. Ophth. *62*:47, 1966.

————: Treatment of lacrimal duct obstructions in the infant. J. Ped. Ophth. *3*:42, 1966.

JONES, L. T. and LINN, M. L.: Diagnosis of the causes of epiphora. Am. J. Ophth. *67*:751, 1969.

KUHNT, H.: Notiz zur Technik der Dacryocystorhinostomie von Toti. Zeitschr. Augenh. *31*:379, 1914.

MCPHERSON, S. D., JR., and EGLESTON, D.: Dacryocystorhinostomy. Am. J. Ophth. *47*:328, 1959.

MILDER, B., and DEMAREST, B. H.: Dacryocystography. Arch. Ophth. *51*:180, 1954.

MIRABLE, T. J., and TUCKER, C.: Dacryocystorhinostomy with silicone sponge. Arch. Ophth. *74*:235, 1965.

MORRISON, F. D.: An aid to repair of lacerated tear ducts. Arch. Ophth. *72*:341, 1964.

MOSHER, H. P.: Mosher-Toti operation on the lacrimal sac. Laryngoscope *31*:284, 1921.

MULDOON, W. E.: Restoration of patency of the nasolacrimal duct by means of a vitallium tube. Am. J. Ophth. *28*:1340, 1945.

NELSON, F.: Management of congenital occlusion of tear duct. Am. J. Ophth. *36*: 1587, 1953.

OHM, J.: Geschichtliche Bemerkung zur Verbesserung den Totischen Operation. Klin. Monatsbl. Augenh. *77*:825, 1926.

OLSON, J. R., and YOUNG, N. A.: Canaliculus reconstruction with homologous vein graft. Am. J. Ophth. *62*:676, 1966.

PILGER, I. S.: Absorable gelatin film (Gelfilm) in subconjunctival section of lacrimal ductules. Am. J. Ophth. *51*:1290, 1961.

REESE, A. B.: Treatment of lesions of lacrimal gland. Trans. Am. Acad. Ophth. Oto *62*:679, 1958.

————: Tumors of the Eye, ed. 2. New York, Harpers & Row, 1963.

REESE, A. B., and JONES, I. S.: Bone resection in the excision of epithelial tumors of the lacrimal gland. Arch. Ophth. *71*:382, 1964.

REINECKE, R. D., and CARROLL, J. M.: Silicone lacrimal tube implantation. Trans. Am. Acad. Ophth. Oto. *73*:85, 1969.

DE ROETTH, A. F. M.: Low flow of tears—the dry eye. Am. J. Ophth. *35*:782, 1952.

SELINGER, E.: Office treatment of the eye. Chicago, Yearbook Publishers, 1947, p. 63.

SISLER, H. A.: Lacrimal canalicular repair. Arch. Ophth. *79*:59, 1968.

SJÖGREN, H.: Keraconjunctivitis sicca and chronic polyarthritis. Acta Med. Scandinav. *130*:484, 1933.

TOTI, M. A.: Nuovo metdo conservatore de cura radicale delle suppurazioni croniche del sacco lacrimal (dacriocistorinostoma). Clin. med. *10*:385, 1904.

VALIERE-VIALEIX, H., ROHM, A., and CHAPUT, C.: Obliterations canaliculaires. Etiologie, diagnostic, traitement. Ann. Oculist. *194*:259, 1961.

VEIRS, E. R.: The lacrimal system: clinical application. New York, Grune & Stratton, 1955.

——————: Dacryocystography. Arch. Ophth. *55*: 410, 1955.

——————: Stenosis of the canaliculus following irradiation therapy. Am. J. Ophth. *44*:249, 1957.

——————: The lacrimal apparatus: Abnormalities and treatment of the punctum and canaliculus. Trans. Am. Acad. Ophth. Oto. *62*:684, 1958.

——————: Malleable rods for immediate repair of the traumatically severed lacrimal canaliculus. Tr. Am. Acad. Ophth. Oto. *66*:263, 1962.

——————: Stenosis of the common canaliculus. Correction with a canalicular rod. Arch. Ophth. *81*:569, 1969.

——————: Aids in restoring patency in obstructions of the lacrimal drainage system. Am. J. Ophth. *56*:977, 1963.

VISCENSIO, A. B.: Use of nylon thread and polyethylene tubing in nasolacrimal duct stenosis. Arch. Ophth. *55*:267, 1956.

WHEELER, J. M.: Removal of the lachrymal sac and accessory lachrymal gland. Internat. J. Surg. *28*:106, 1915.

WINKELMAN, J. E.: An operation for eversion of the lower lacrimal punctum. Ophthalmologica *139*:486, 1960.

WOOLHOUSE, J. T.: Definitiones Ophthalmicae, 1724, cited by Duke-Elder, S. St. Louis, C. V. Mosby Co. vol. 5, 1952.

WORST, J. G. F.: Method for reconstructing torn lacrimal canaliculus. Am. J. Ophth. *53*:520, 1962.

WRIGHT, J. C., and MEGER, G. E.: A review of the Schirmer test for tear production. Arch. Ophth. *67*: 564, 1962.

CHAPTER 24

Trauma and First-Aid

ANY DISCUSSION of an immense subject such as the emergency handling of eye injuries is bound to be more remarkable for what is omitted than for what is included. This chapter will therefore stress primarily those conditions of the ocular adnexa requiring immediate and surgical repair of one type or another. No ophthalmologist has to be told that the globe itself is the major consideration in all trumatic cases nor need he be told in a work such as this how to handle intraocular emergencies.

About 50 years ago 10 per cent of all acute eye cases admitted to the hospital were due to trauma. In recent years with the advance of industrialization this has risen to over 30 per cent. In World War II, 2.5 per cent of all casualties were eye injuries and at the present time well over half of all blind eyes in this country are due to trauma. Obviously ocular injuries are not a negligible quantity in eye care.

There is probably no organ in the body which nature has worked so hard to protect as the human eye. It lies well buried, most of it, in a depression in the skull protected by the overhanging brow above, the nose and cheek bones at the sides and below. It rests on a pad of fat on which it moves easily and which helps it to absorb shock. The lids close reflexly to protect the eye from the first sight or sound of danger. The lashes which curl upward in the upper lid and downward in the lower prevent most flying particles from getting into the eye. Secretions from glands in the lids and conjunctiva keep the eye moist and warm; tears flush out smoke, dust and foreign particles. Despite this whole complex of protective mechanisms man, ever ingenious, has managed to circumvent nature in many ways.

Over half of all eye injuries, mild and severe, are due to mobile foreign bodies of all sorts. This does not necessarily mean that all these objects are free in space. Blows by pokers, clubs, door knobs, golf clubs, broken bottles and the myriad other agents of destruction of which human invention is capable and which are attached at one end to the human fist—indeed, the human fist itself—frequently give us our worst reparative problems.

Obviously the eye is not an isolated organ floating in space but part of the general body economy. Before one treats the eye one must make sure that adequate care has been taken of the patient. This means that hemorrhage, infection, pain and shock receive first consideration before the eye examination is begun in all cases of severe general injury. This is not only good medical practice which assures the comfort and welfare of the patient, but it also obtains maximum cooperation in all necessary examinations and manipulations of the eye. If such treatment as tetanus antitoxin and gas gangrene serum is indicated it should be given at once. Antibiotics or chemotherapeutics in cases of suspected infection are also administered immediately as necessary.

Ocular Examination

Once general treatment has been rendered, ocular examination is begun as early as possible and is carried out thoroughly. Good light, proper magnification, sufficient exposure and a systematic routine are necessary to assure that nothing of importance is omitted.

The eye is thoroughly cleansed externally with soap and water. Hemorrhagic clots and all foreign matter are removed and the externa examined for fracture of the bones, emphysema and crepitation. X-rays for possible fractures of the orbital or nasal bones or unsuspected foreign bodies are taken; sometimes unexpected pathology is discovered. The lids are thoroughly examined and the ability of the levator to open and of the orbicularis to close the eye is noted. Next the conjunctival sac and the globe are examined. If edema is present the lids are pried apart, with retractors if necessary. There must be no pressure on the globe but the globe must be thoroughly inspected. The conjunctiva is examined for tears or hemorrhages. Ocular motility is checked to make sure that the extraocular musculature is unimpaired.

The condition of the cornea is noted and, if necessary, it is stained to assure its integrity. The cornea is a tough membrane, nowhere near as fragile as it appears; despite this, a metal fragment flying at high speed can penetrate deeply and sometimes all the way into the eye. The same goes for the sclera which is even easier to penetrate. The kinetic energy of a flying foreign body increases arithmetically with the mass and geometrically with the speed. Hence no matter how small, if the foreign body flies fast enough it may generate enough force to penetrate ocular tissues and lodge in the eye so that it becomes an emergency operative case.

Incidentally, one of the curiosities of eye injuries is the number of foreign bodies which penetrate the eye without the patient's knowledge. Enough of these have been seen by ophthalmologists and reported in ophthalmic literature to form a distinct clinical entity. Hence all questionable cases should be examined with as high a magnification as is available and with the slit-lamp if possible; and in case of the slightest suspicion, x-rays for intraocular foreign bodies ordered. These should be taken by a man experienced in this work.

CORNEAL FOREIGN BODY

The corneal foreign body hardly needs discussion here. However, if only because it is the most common of all eye injuries, it is included for purposes of completeness.

The so-called "cinder" is more often a particle of metal, paper, plastic, wood, dirt, sand or other debris of civilization. If it has not been in very long, a drop of tetracaine 0.5 per cent and a tightly wound moist cotton applicator suffices for its easy removal. A *moist* applicator is emphasized because, if dry, a wisp of cotton left behind can be as irritating as the original foreign body. Beginners have been known to chase an elusive foreign body across a cornea leaving a serpentine trail of epithelial abrasion behind. After a few such experiences they learn to "flip" the applicator or to use a spud or even the point of a hypo needle if nothing else is available.

The imbedded foreign body may have to be dislodged with a dull or sharp spud depending on its size, depth and duration in the cornea. The areola of pigment or "rust ring" which is a frequent companion of the neglected foreign body often requires some digging. Sometimes it is difficult to get it all out and it may be found that its complete removal is much simpler on the second day. When there has been much manipulation the aftereffects are quite painful for 12 hours thereafter. The eye should be irrigated with sterile solution, a cycloplegic instilled if ciliary irritation is expected and an anesthetic ointment applied before patching. Codeine and aspirin may also be welcomed by the patient.

Cycloplegia is *not* used routinely, especially if removal of the foreign body is simple. If cycloplegia is used it should be one of the shorter acting drugs. There seems to be no point in blurring a patient's vision for a week with atropine when healing in such cases usually takes place in 24 or 48 hours.

Foreign bodies which have penetrated deeply into the cornea to at least half or two-thirds of its depth are sometimes best removed by making a triangular corneal flap with a Ziegler discission knife.

Procedure (fig. 295): A triangular corneal flap is fashioned over the foreign body by means of two corneal incisions meeting at an apex

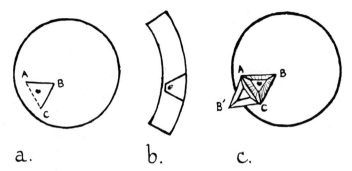

FIG. 295.   Removal of Deeply Imbedded Corneal Foreign Body.
a.   The cornea is incised along lines AB and BC.
b.   Note that the incisions are beveled toward each other.
c.   The flap AB'C is turned back to expose the foreign body.
      After extraction, the corneal flap is patted back into place.
      (Fox, S. A.:   Courtesy Archives of Ophthalmology.)

which points toward the center of the cornea. The incisions are beveled toward each other so as to approach the foreign body more closely. After sufficient depth has been attained the corneal flap is folded back on its base line, the foreign body exposed, gently freed from the surrounding stroma with the point of the knife and lifted out. If any rust stain exists it is curetted out and the corneal flap is patted back into place without sutures. The eye is then treated as for any other foreign body removal.

Two or even more foreign bodies may be present at the same time. It is embarrassing after difficult removal of a foreign body to find another in the conjunctival sac the following day—after the patient complains. Examination of the whole eye therefore should be thorough and both the loupe and slit-lamp should be used routinely here. Occasionally multiple foreign bodies of glass, plastic or metal are seen in war time and after civilian explosions. In many cases the eyes are surprisingly quiet and had best be left alone. When the eye is irritated the surgeon has the unenviable task of removing a flock of corneal bodies.

The foreign body is sometimes brittle and a small deeply imbedded piece may be left behind hence slit-lamp examination is indicated afterward to assure complete removal. Indeed the foreign body is sometimes so small that the whole operation must be done under the slit-lamp. This is simple if the uninitiated surgeon remembers, after he and the patient are settled, to hold the spud or burr in front of the objectives of the microscope, identify the instrument, and then move it slowly toward the patient's eye.

Other things may simulate the symptoms of a foreign body. If the eye is white and quiet with no foreign body present, and the patient continues to complain, one must look for a tiny scratch by staining the cornea and examining it under the slit-lamp. A loose cilia in the conjunctival sac or a tarsal "blister" on the lid margin, i.e., inspissated secretion at the opening of a meibomian gland, may also be the cause.

TRAUMA TO THE GLOBE

Fractures, emphysema and crepitation around the eyes should be looked for and x-ray examination done for fractures and unsuspected foreign bodies. The lids must be separated (by careful traction, if necessary) and the condition of the cornea and globe noted. No pressure should be applied to the globe in case of rupture. The lid margins and puncta should be investigated for trauma. The conjunctiva should be examined thoroughly for tears, foreign bodies and hemorrhages; this includes both upper and lower fornices. Ocular motility should be checked if possible.

Blows to the eye can cause anything from a mild iritis or corneal abrasion to intraocular hemorrhage, retinal detachment, choroidal tears and lens dislocation—and still leave the corneo-scleral coat intact. Hemorrhage in the anterior chamber, a flat anterior chamber, a tremulous iris, a frank corneal or scleral break with prolapse of iris and/or ciliary body is obvious and cannot be mistaken. However, there are more subtle signs to look for in case of doubt of intraocular damage or foreign body.

1. Variation in the depth of the anterior chamber.
2. A history of sudden visual disturbance.
3. A history of sudden gush of "tears" which may be due to aqueous loss.
4. Change in the shape of the pupil without materially affecting its size.
5. Sluggish reactivity of the pupil.

Most of these symptoms may appear with or without penetration of the globe. In all cases of severe undiagnosed physical trauma to the eye it is best *not to use either morphine, cycloplegics or any medication which will affect the pupil until the extent and type of injury is assessed.* In all such cases, if the patient is not in the hospital, both eyes should be patched and the patient immediately sent where definitive eye care is available. Early attention to an injured globe, in the first 24 to 48 hours, such as early suture of a corneal or scleral rupture, may mean the difference between losing and saving an eye.

The cornea needs minute inspection. In case of doubt as to injury, a drop of 2 per cent fluorescein should be instilled and irrigated out at once with sterile saline. Clean tap water will suffice if nothing else is available. Abraded and lacerated areas, no matter how minute, will show up as yellowish green stains.

Scratches of the cornea by fingernails, paper, tree branches are especially recalcitrant to treatment and, for some reason, subject to recurrence. Early treatment with cycloplegia, antibiotics and steroids is mandatory.

Ruptures of the cornea gain nothing by waiting. With the newer corneal needles the need for conjunctival flaps over corneal wounds is much less than it used to be. Suture of the cornea makes for better and quicker healing and a better visual prognosis.

More recently organic cements have been reported for treatment of corneal ruptures apparently successfully. This is an important and worthwhile step forward.

Riffenburgh has drawn attention to the fact that scleral ruptures posterior to the insertion of the recti are frequently missed despite the typical clinical picture which is commonly present: (1) There is always the history of a blow with a blunt object. (2) Frequently there are lid lacerations, hematomata and even facial fractures. (3) There is marked early chemosis usually in the area of rupture. (4) The anterior chamber is deep due to escape of intraocular contents subconjunctivally. (5) The tension is frequently as low as 2–4 mm. of Hg. (6) There is no tear or injury in the anterior eye. (7). The amount of hemorrhage varies from slight to massive. (8) The lens may be seen subconjunctivally. Recently there has been successful diagnosis of scleral rupture by ultrasound. Treatment: investigate and close the break. If it cannot be done, enucleate.

In similar fashion scleral wounds are sutured to prevent invasion of the vitreous by fibroplastic tissue. Treatment is instituted for intraocular hemorrhage and iridocyclitis. Here again, where intraocular foreign bodies are suspected, localizing x-rays are taken as soon as possible.

In the case of hyphema, bed rest with binocular patching is necessary in all but the most minimal to prevent secondary bleeding. Glaucoma should be constantly checked for and treated if found. The use of fibrinolytics has been found generally useful. Chymar and proenzyme have been found to cut total absorption time of hyphema in half. Fibrinolysin and streptokinase also promote resolution but additional irrigation has been found necessary for complete resolution of the changes associated with total hyphema.

LID REPAIRS

Owing to the looseness of the lid tissues, post-traumatic edema and hemorrhage is common and of rapid onset. If there are no breaks in skin continuity, lesser injuries are self-limiting and are probably best left alone. Cold compresses may be ordered to reduce edema and swelling. Before the lids have become thickened and unmanageable many repairs are simple which later require much more complicated surgery. However, when lids are seen after they have become swollen and edematous, it is better to wait until this has subsided. Although immediate treatment and repair of the affected parts is desirable, it is not always possible and, indeed, may not be to the best interest of the patient. Thus hemorrhage may be so great as to require absorption before a thorough inventory of the total damage can be made. Again, unless seen immediately, tissues may be so swollen and even infected that it may be more discreet to wait until some semblance of normality is restored. Repairs done under such adverse conditions often do poorly and frequently have to be done over. On the other hand once the effect of the trauma has disappeared repair should be made at once.

All wounds should be cleaned immediately, debrided and all ragged edges trimmed off. Debridement is kept to a minimum and only obviously devitalized tissue and such shreds as are manifestly unsalvageable are resected. The richness of the vascular supply, often a nuisance in lid surgery, is a great comfort here and usually makes the sacrifice of much tissue unnecessary.

Lacerations of the lid may vary from a simple extramarginal skin tear to complete lid avulsion. Repair is not difficult if anatomic fundamentals are kept in mind. The most important of these are: 1. The orbicularis fibers are always pulling horizontally and will tend to make a notch out of a marginal laceration. If neglected, the orbicularis becomes fibrosed and what could have been corrected by primary union may become a major reparative procedure. 2. A horizontal laceration through the full thickness of the upper lid my create a ptosis if the torn ends of the levator are not found and resutured. It is much easier to do it immediately than to hunt for the torn ends after cicatrization has taken place. 3. If a lid is torn away from the medial canthus it must be put back into place at once; later a normal appearing lid is a rarity and epiphora a certainty.

In extramarginal lacerations (fig. 296A) wound edges are sutured carefully. This work is often painstaking and bizarre patterns of repair not infrequent (fig. 296B); but healing is often good and worth the effort (figs. 296C and D). The secret of suturing such irregular wounds is to start closure at points which obviously fit together. Little by little other such points will appear until the whole crazy-quilt like pattern falls into place. Deep through and through extramarginal lacerations are sutured in layers and patched. If the tear is through the levator the ends must be caught up and joined to prevent ptosis. Even the best repair may result in a ptotic lid due to injury. However, if the repair is carefully made, function may ultimately return to a surprising degree even months later.

Marginal lacerations are repaired by any of the methods previously described: direct apposition, intermarginal suture, modified halving, etc.

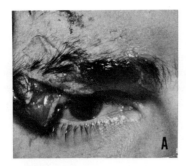
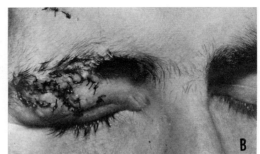
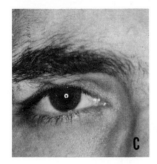
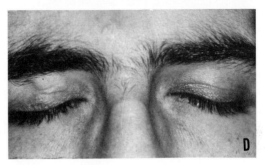

Fig. 296. Repair of Multiple Laceration.
A. Multiple extramarginal lacerations.
B. Appearance after repair.
C. and *D.* Final result with eyes open and closed.

In the larger lacerations where there has been loss of tissue, a halving repair may be needed or any of the types of repair described in Chapters 7 to 11. This will depend on the position, size and shape of the lesion (fig. 297).

In all repairs of the upper lid the normal position of the lid fold should be preserved and an effort made to have suture lines run in such a way as to retain the fold. It is more difficult to reconstruct later a lid fold which has been distorted by vertical cicatrices.

Corneal protection is of paramount importance. If the eye is proptosed by retrobulbar hemorrhage or enough lid tissue has been lost to endanger the cornea, an intermarginal suture or tarsorrhaphy is in order if this is possible. If too much tissue has been lost and a tarsorrhaphy cannot be made, other stratagems must be used. If the lower lid has been avulsed, the upper lid is brought down over the cornea and sutured to the remnant of the lower lid. If the upper lid or both lids have been lost it may be possible to mobilize the remnants of conjunctiva and suture them together as a protective flap over the cornea.

Avulsion of the lid from the medial canthus is one of the most common of lid lacerations. If the tear is through the canaliculus, as it often is and the patient is seen early enough, repair is made as shown in

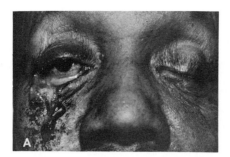
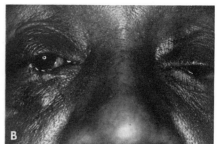

Fig. 297.   Repair of Marginal Avulsion.
A.   Avulsion of lid margin with large central tear.
B.   Result after repair.

figures 286 and 288. Suture of the laceration after the canaliculus has been repaired is described in Chapter 9. If repaired before cicatrices have formed canalicular obstruction may be avoided. Later it is almost certain.

Traumatic edema of the lid sometimes persists for months following trauma. It is probably due to obstruction of the lymph circulation. It sometimes disappears spontaneously; other times it seems to be permanent. Massage after all signs of inflammation have disappeared has been advised to counteract this; also the injection of hyalouronidase.

Tears of the conjunctiva are always amenable to repair immediately. It is an elastic membrane and though a great deal may be lost it may still be repaired by simple closure. The conjunctival sac is irrigated and cleaned of clots, the ragged edges are debrided and repair is made with 6–0 interrupted catgut or silk sutures. If done at once a good repair is almost certain.

In late cases of conjunctival injury mild symblepharon can sometimes be repaired by simple resection and closure (fig. 152) or a minor plasty. In more extensive repairs the method of Arlt is used (fig. 153). Late repairs always mean more surgery because fibrosis and scarring has set in to complicate matters; sometimes grafting of conjunctiva and mucous membrane may be necessary.

In all work done on the conjunctival sac it must be remembered that the two eyes move as a team. This is a reflex action difficult to control even with tight pressure dressings. Hence in uniocular cases, where sutures must be placed where they will appose the cornea, it might be best to use plain catgut which will soften and absorb rapidly rather than silk. Pain after lid surgery is most common when the cornea is involved and should be investigated promptly. Binocular bandaging helps control eye movements and should be used when necessary.

For all other repairs on the lids and conjunctiva the reader is referred to the various chapters on lid repairs (Chapters 5 to 13).

Burns

Burns of the eye and its adnexa may be physical, i.e., thermal or electrical, chemical or by agents of radiation.

Thermal Injuries

Physical burns are usually thermal. Flames, gasoline explosions, steam, molten metal, hot water or tar and numerous other agents may be responsible. They may be due to explosions or direct contact and all types may give any degree of burn, although the contact type is likely to be the most severe. Treatment will depend on the amount and degree of tissue involvement. First and mild second degree burns showing simple hyperemia and edema are probably best treated by moist antiseptic dressings and sedation. Intermarginal sutures or surgical tarsorrhaphy may be necessary to protect the cornea.

Aerosol spray of Providone-iodine is an antiseptic-germicide solution which has been found to facilitate the open therapy of burns providing a protective covering for denuded areas of skin. It allows a sterile crust to form and prevents destruction of the injured epithelium. Above all, such patients should be sent to a hospital immediately for adequate treatment.

Severe second degree or third degree thermal burns produce rapid coagulation necrosis. Here some surgeons prefer to cleanse the area of all dead tissue and to graft split skin at once. Others prefer to wait until all the sloughs have separated at about the end of the third week. Experience has shown that repair should be begun soon, before destruction from fibrosis has set in (fig. 298).

Chemical Injuries

Chemical burns are in a class by themselves and probably constitute the most acute of all eye emergencies. All ophthalmologists know the value of prompt and prolonged irrigation and the point will not be labored here. After the eye has been cleansed of all visible foreign material copious irrigation with quarts and quarts of water—tap water if nothing else is available—is carried out for an hour or more with rest periods in between. This has saved many an eye—but not all eyes are saved for several reasons. Some are seen too late, others show such great involvement that even heroic treatment cannot save them. Chelating agents such as EDTA (sodium ethylene dimaine tetracetate (0.137 to 1.85 per cent) are of some value in lime burns but are no panacea. Also they are quite irritating and good anesthesia is required.

The trouble is that the secondary complications of chemical burns frequently wreak more havoc than the original injuries and here the alkalis are much more serious, lethal and treacherous than the acids.

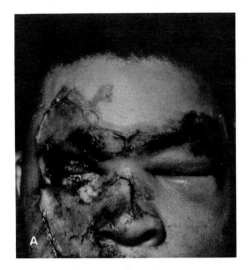
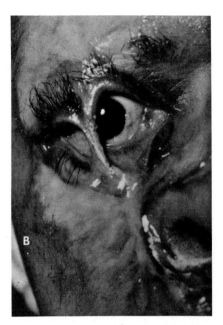

FIG. 298.   Delayed Repair of Burn.
A.   Severe third degree burn of face.
B.   Cicatrization of right upper and lower lids due to delayed repair.

Acids coagulate proteins and are rapidly neutralized and buffered by them so that they make their own tissue barriers. The clinical picture produced by weak acids is one of irritation; by strong acids corrosion. In general, penetration of tissues by strong acids is not marked and the lesion usually nonprogressive and limited to the original involved area. Its limits are demarcated and, except in overwhelming involvement, recovery may be good. Hence the prognosis may be evident soon after injury. In general, mild acid burns are treated expectantly with antibiotic and anesthetic ointments. The severe burns will probably fare best with mucous membrane grafts.

Alkali burns give an entirely different and graver picture and constitute one of the most serious—sometimes catastrophic—of eye injuries. Alkali action on proteins is the same as that of acids which is ultimate coagulation, but alkalis are proteolytic and destroy cell structures by combining with them to penetrate deeper and deeper into the tissues. Hence they spread more widely, their action is not circumscribed and it may continue for days unless prompt action is taken. Clinically an original injury with alkalis may be deceptively mild and can then destroy an eye in several days due to the progressive nature of the affect of the chemical and its tendency to late infiltration and ulceration. Alkali burns of the limbal area carry an especially poor prognosis with ischemic necrosis, rapid corneal opacification and acute iritis occurring rapidly. This is followed by a quiet stage of epithelial regeneration, vascularization of the cornea and diminution of the iritis. Ultimately a third stage ensues in which recurrent corneal ulceration, glaucoma, cataract and uveitis usually result in total blindness.

The trouble with all chemical injuries is that once they have been allowed to progress their effects are usually irreversible. Prompt action, then, is sight saving and often eye saving. Conjunctival and corneal involvement in these cases may require prompt and heroic action. Irrigation has already been discussed above. In the milder cases steroids to prevent neovascularization are valuable. In severe cases it is difficult to prevent symblepharon despite all sorts of maneuvers with glass rods and various types of conformers and daily flooding of the conjunctival sac with oils and unguents.

Devitalized conjunctiva takes on a yellowish white color and is best removed immediately after preliminary treatment. If the denuded area is large and closure is difficult, mucous membrane is grafted. This is fine if one can be sure that all the chemical has been washed out. In the case of an alkali it is hard to be certain. When the metabolism of the cornea is endangered, use of many types of materials has been advised such as rabbit peritoneum, amniotic membrane and egg membrane. However, such membranes sometimes seem to act as a closed chamber which seals in products of destruction and also as a foreign body which irritates the area.

A better procedure is the peritomy which consists of circumcising the conjunctiva all around the limbus, undermining it and allowing it to retract (fig. 299A). If it does not retract a peridectomy is done, i.e., a

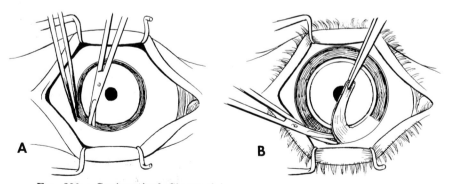

FIG. 299. Conjunctival Circumcision.
A. Peritomy. The conjunctiva is circumcised around the limbus and allowed to retract.
B. Peridectomy. A collar is resected around the limbus.

3–4 mm. collar of conjunctiva and subconjunctiva is resected all around the limbus (fig. 299*B*). This separates involved conjunctiva from the cornea and prevents the affected tissues from exerting their deleterious affects on the cornea. Mucous membrane is then grafted as required. If mucous membrane is needed in the palpebral fissure, conjunctiva from the other eye should be used or a thin sheet of buccal mucous membrane taken with the keratotome. Thick buccal mucous membrane grafts retain their pink color and are a cosmetic blemish in the palpebral fissure.

The most recent and most hopeful treatment of chemical burns according to Gould is the use of irrigation for 48 hours followed by the fitting of a flush contact lens. This allows the conjunctiva to heal normally and prevent symblepharon. The shell must be flush with the cornea and in case of change during the healing processes changes in the shell must also be made. On the other hand Horwitz reports good results with simple management consisting of debridement of dead tissue for the first 5 to 7 days plus supportive treatment with antibiotics, steroids and mydriatics; the eye is not patched.

Electrical Injuries

Lightning and naked electric wiring are the more important sources of electric burns. When severe, both affect the whole body economy tremendously hence electric burns are rarely of primary interest to the ophthalmologist alone.

The most important effect of localized external electrical burns is not unlike that seen in thermal burns and, because the body is a poor conductor, the result is immediate coagulation of proteins at the point of contact. This may or may not show definite necrosis depending on the severity of the cause as in thermal burns. However, the severity of the lesion may not be immediately apparent due to the characteristic differences between external thermal and electric burns. The electric burn does not show the typical swelling of the thermal burn. Furthermore, it is usually painless, dry, aseptic and fairly well circumscribed due to the very high temperature which is localized at the point of contact. The ultimate result is therefore a localized electrical gangrene.

In general then, depending on the severity of the lesion, electrical burns around the lids may show anything from a localized hyperemia to complete coagulation and ultimate slough of tissues. The affect on the globe may be anything from conjunctival hyperemia to complete incineration.

Treatment is expectant and symptomatic because, as stated above, the lesion is usually dry, sterile and circumscribed. However, in the case of small lesions threatened with gangrene, excision and grafting is the treatment of choice.

Radiation Injuries

Only the energy absorbed by tissues can affect them. The affects of electrical energy action on the ocular adnexa have been briefly described above. The ocular adnexa may also suffer from high frequency diathermy and electromagnetic energy, both affects also being thermal in character.

Other types of radiation burns such as those due to infrared rays are occasionally seen by ophthalmologists. In general these are (1) either flash burns in which the injury is due to the absorption of large amounts of radiant energy almost instantaneously and (2) burns of small concentration which act over comparatively long periods of time.

Flash radiation burns may be due to gunpowder explosions in a relatively confined space in which the injury is due to the dazzling flash and not to the heat generated. A more modern example is the flash of an atomic explosion. The amount of havoc caused will depend on the proximity of the individual to the source of radiation. In superficial cases only the exposed parts of the body such as the skin of the face and hands are affected. Curiously the globe itself often escapes injury because of the instantaneous response of the blink reflex and the thin film of tears over the globe. Treatment in these superficial cases is as for any mild thermal burn.

Atomic explosions also release beta rays which cause superficial burns and the more lethal penetrating gamma rays and neutrons which cause deeper lesions and much more severe damage. The more violent affects on those closer to the source of explosion are not within the scope of this volume.

The two important clinical effects of prolonged exposure to infrared rays are heat cataracts (rarely seen now) and eclipse blindness, i.e., macular lesions due to viewing a solar eclipse with the naked eye. Prophylaxis here is more important than therapy after the fact.

Eclipse Burns

The retina is highly vulnerable to the focused infrared rays of a solar eclipse. Such rays have been known to penetrate sunglasses, smoked glasses and even x-ray film with resultant visual loss. Since there are no pain fibers in the retina this occurs without alarming the patient and without his awareness until it is too late. It has often been said and truly that the safest way to observe an eclipse of the sun is not to watch it or to use the television screen.

Penner and McNair have described the progress of eclipse blindness in minute detail. The initial symptom of retinal eclipse burns are visual in about 24 hours. In the retina there are three stages to be seen: (1) First there is a central yellow spot in the foveal or parafoveal area. (2) The second stage shows an erythema of the macula surrounding the yellow

spot which is present about three weeks and fades on about the thirty-
fifth day leaving (3) an outlined circle of black pigment in the area
which is present for the 8-month duration of observation and is probably
permanent to a greater or lesser degree.

If the vision is better than 20/50 the chances of recovery to 20/20
are about 50 per cent. Pang has found the prognosis variable with the
majority of cases having visual improvement the first month and the
absolute scotoma becoming relative or small enough to permit eccentric
vision.

Retinal burns may also be due to the thermal affect of visible and
near infrared rays focused on the pigment structure behind the retina.
The normal eye can tolerate only fleeting glances at the sun. For eclipse
and sun viewing a filter which reduces solar energy 1000 times provides
a tenfold safety factor. Filters of no less than No. 4 density or shade No.
10 should be used; or photographic or x-ray film of similar density.

Ultraviolet Burns

Ultraviolet burns are in general a less serious type of radiation
injury than those caused by infrared rays because they do not penetrate
the eye. Only massive doses of ultraviolet radiation such as man is not
exposed to ordinarily, will cause intraocular damage. The most common
example of ultraviolet burn is the superficial injury suffered by exposure
of the naked eye to the rays of the sunlamp, the old fashioned Klieg
lights (now happily rare) and the acetylene torch.

Snow Blindness

Snow blindness which is neither blindness nor due to snow is also
due to ultraviolet rays reflected into the eye from wide expanses of white
snow. In all these, ultraviolet rays cause a superficial punctate keratitis
and conjunctivitis which is exceedingly painful but fortunately of short
duration. All it requires usually is an anesthetic ointment, mild cycloplegia to counteract ciliary spasm and patching of the eye for 24 to 48
hours. General sedation and analgesia may also be of help.

STRESS INJURIES

Ocular injuries due to stress occur usually as a result of anoxia or
sudden barometric decompression. In the main such injuries cause visual
disturbances such as decrease in visual acuity, peripheral field constriction, loss of discriminatory light sense and diminution or suppression of
stereopsis. Sudden decompression such as is seen in deep sea divers may
also cause subconjunctival hemorrhages, papilledema and, in severe cases,
holes of the macula. Adnexal lesions are not seen.

REFERENCES

ARTZ, C. P., and YARBROUGH, D. R. III: Present status of the treatment of burns. Bull. N.Y. Acad. Med. *43*:627, 1967.

BALLIN, P. H.: Mucous membrane grafts in chemical (lye) burns. Am. J. Ophth. *55*:302, 1963.

BUCHMANN, H. H., and FRANK, W.: Uber Kalkveratzungen und Erfahrungen in der Behundlung durch die Fruhoperation nach Passow. Klin. Montasbl. Augenh. *133*:494, 1958.

CAHN, P. H., and HOVENER, W. H.: Factors of importance in traumatic hyphema. Am. J. Ophth. *55*:591, 1963.

CALLAHAN, A., and McKERRICHER, D. E.: Molten metal burns of the inferior fornix. Am. J Ophth. *44*:178, 1957.

COLE, J. G., and BYRON, H. M.: Evaluation of 100 eyes with traumatic hyphema; intravenous urea. Arch. Ophth. *71*:35, 1964.

CZURKASZ, I.: Subconjunctival novocaine treatment of chemical burns of the eye. Arch. Ophth. *159*:560, 1958.

DOCKERY, R. W.: Role of the ophthalmologist in acute trauma. J. Kentucky M. A. *56*:449, 1958.

DUKE-ELDER, S.: Text-Book of Ophthalmology. St. Louis, C. V. Mosby, vol. 6, 1954.

FOX, S. A.: Removal of deeply imbedded foreign bodies from the cornea. Arch. Ophth. *37*:189, 1947.

FOX, S. A.: Trauma, Chap. XIV. *In* Liebman, S. D., and Gellis, S. S. (eds.): The Pediatricians Ophthalmology, St. Louis, C. V. Mosby, 1966.

GARNES, A. L., et al.: Clinical evaluation of Providone-iodine aerosol spray in surgical practice. Am. J. Surg. *97*:49, 1959.

GAT, L., and NAGY, J.: Durch Kalksalzevrursachte Binde und Hornhautlasionen bei Selbstverstummelung. Ophthalmologica *138*:406, 1959.

GEORGIDE, N. G., MATTON, G. E., and VON KESSEL, F.: Facial burns. Plast. & Reconstr. Surg. *29*:648, 1962.

GOULD, H.: Treatment of chemical burns. Highlights of Ophth. *9*:78, 1966.

HARD, D. P.: Lime burns of the external eye. Tr. Ophth. Soc. U. K. *78*:267, 1958.

HEINC, A.: Chemical burns of the eye treated with egg membrane: An experimental study. Am. J. Ophth. *48*:373, 1959.

HOLLAND, G.: Eye and lid injuries in childhood. Klin. Monatsbl. Augenh. *139*:72, 1961.

HORWITZ, I. D.: Management of alkali burns of cornea and conjunctiva. Am. J. Ophth. *61*:340, 1966.

HUGHES, W. F., et al.: Symposium on emergency treatment; management of injuries to eyes. S. Clin. North America *22*:1355, 1942.

INGRAM. H.: Injuries of the eye. Practitioner *178*:554, 1957.

LEAHY, B. D.: Thermal burns of the eye and adnexa. Am. J. Ophth. *35*:1077, 1952.

LIEBMAN, S. D., POLLEN, A., and PODOS, S. M.: Treatment of experimental total hyphema with intraocular fibrinolytic agents. Arch. Ophth. *68*:1102, 1962.

MILTHALER, B. H., and BENDER, R. F.: Tryspin in resorption of hyphema. *61*:535, 1966.

OAKS. L. W., DORMAN, J. E., and PETTY, R. W.: Tear gas burns of the eye. Arch. Ophth. *63*:698, 1960.

PANG, H. G.: Eclipse retinopathy. Am. J. Ophth. *55*:383, 1963.

PENNER, R., and McNAIR, J. N.: Eclipse blindness. Am. J. Ophth. *61*:1452, 1966.

PRIONI, P.: Treatment of acid burns of the eye. Arch. oftal. B. A. *38*:168, 1963.

RIFFENBURGH, R. S.: Contusion rupture of the sclera. Arch. Ophth. *60*:722, 1963.

ROMANES, G. J.: The treatment of eye burns. Tr. Ophth. Soc. U. Kingdom *79*:71, 1959.

RUEDEMANN, A. D.: Immediate treatment of lid lacerations. Tr. Am. Acad. Ophth. & Oto. *61*:629, 1957.

SIEGEL, R.: Buccal mucous membrane grafts in treatment of burns of the eye. Arch. Ophth. *32*:104, 1944.

WHITWELL, J.: Treatment of non-perforating ocular injuries. Tr. Ophth. Soc. U. Kingdom *79*:49, 1959.

CHAPTER 25

Radiation Therapy of Eyelid Lesions

By Joseph Newall, M.D.

MANY CONDITIONS affecting the eyelids have been treated by radiation therapy. Included have been vernal conjunctivitis, acute and chronic blepharitis, keloids, hyperkeratosis, hemangiomata and benign tumors such as neurofibroma and papilloma. The recognition of the undesirable side effects of radiation, however infrequent, and the introduction of effective alternative methods of treatment have however resulted in a reappraisal of the role of radiation therapy. In consequence, it is now generally accepted that radiation therapy has no part to play in the management of benign conditions of the lids and that its role should be confined to the treatment of malignant disease. Further discussion will therefore be restricted to this subject.

PATHOLOGY

A variety of tumors are found involving the eyelids. From the point of view of the radiation therapist, however, they may be divided into two major groups:
1. Epithelial tumors.
    a. Basal cell carcinoma and squamous cell carcinoma.
    b. Maligant Melanoma.

Director, Department of Radiotherapy, St. Vincent's Hospital and Medical Center of New York.

      c. Adenoid. Tumors arising from the hair follicles, sweat glands or meibomian glands.

   2. Malignant lymphoma.

Furthermore, these tumors may arise on the lid or may secondarily invade the lid by extension from a lesion on the adjacent face, orbit or eye.

EPITHELIAL TUMORS

General Principles of Management

Of the various forms of malignant disease which involve the eyelids only the basal cell and the squamous cell carcinoma are commonly seen.

The former accounts for about 75 per cent of all malignant eyelid tumors and the latter an additional 15 per cent. The lower eyelid is the most common site accounting for over half the lesions. The inner canthus is the site in an additional 20 to 30 per cent and about 10–15 per cent of lesions arise in the upper lid. The outer canthus is the rarest site of all accounting for no more than 5 per cent. Although clinically and histologically the basal and squamous cell carcinomata differ in no way from similar lesions arising on the skin of the face, their very special site and the consequent danger of invasion of the eye, orbit or adjacent bone and sinuses together with the importance of avoiding damage to the eye during treatment make their correct management an extremely important and special problem.

The basal cell carcinoma in particular runs a protracted course if left untreated. In neither are lymph node metastases common and distant metastases are extremely rare. The tumors therefore are seldom dangerous from the point of view of survival. They can of course be extremely disfiguring and damaging to vision. As far as their treatment is concerned both surgery and radiotherapy are probably equally effective in effecting local control of the tumor.

The decision as to which method to use must therefore depend on considerations other than survival or local control.

The principal of radiation lies in its ability to destroy malignant cells yet at the same time spare the normal tissue. This in turn depends on a greater relative radiosensitivity of the tumor cell as compared to the normal tissue cell. Although both basal and squamous cell carcinomata do normally show such radiosensitivity, it is necessary to use a high local dose. Reactions will therefore be seen in the normal tissue but these should not be gross and should be of limited duration. Because of this differential effect on the normal and the malignant cell radiotherapy should produce a superior cosmetic result. When this is important, as it certainly is in the case of the eyelid, radiation therapy should be the preferred treatment. The dangers of damage to the structures of the lids, eye and orbit all of which show a differing sensitivity to radiation (see below) have been rightly emphasized and every precaution must be taken to ensure the protection and preservation of these normal structures. It is thus imperative that the control of radiotherapy be in skilled and experienced hands. As with surgery there is no place in this field for the interested amateur. With modern technics of protection, changes in normal structures uninvolved by tumor can be kept to a minimum and the risk of damage need not be a major consideration in the choice of treatment method.

On the other hand, although small lesions of the lid margin may be excised with primary closure, generally, if more than 1.0 cm. of the lid must be removed some form of plastic repair is necessary. The consequent need for hospitalization must therefore weigh against a choice of surgery. Radiotherapy usually can be given on an out-patient basis and hospitalization is not necessary.

Proof of histology should be obtained whenever possible even though the method of treatment for the two lesions is the same.

Radiosensitivity of Structures at Risk and Their Protection

The tissues of the lid, eye and orbital contents may all be exposed to radiation. Their radiosensitivity differs and will be considered separately.

LIDS.   With the dose of radiation necessary to control these lesions, permanent loss of the eyelashes within the area treated is inevitable, as is destruction of function of the tarsal glands. These changes, however, are generally well tolerated by the patient. Some atrophy of the skin may be seen. It must be stressed that ectropion does not occur provided there has been no deep invasion of the lid by the tumor (figs. 300*A*, *B* and *C*). The conjunctiva tolerates radiation well and although a reaction to treatment similar to that in the skin develops, the only long-term reaction which may be encountered is a keratinisation of the conjunctiva which may or may not produce symptoms.

EYE.   The sensitivity of the various structures of the globe is now well recognized. The tissue at greatest risk is the lens and doses as low as 200 to 400 rads have been reported as causing cataract. It is important to separate those minor changes within the lens recognized only by the ophthalmologist from those instances where real loss of visual acuity results. Many patients however have received substantially higher doses without permanent subjective visual loss. High dose to the cornea will certainly produce ulceration and scarring. However these changes in the lens or cornea are not seen if proper precautions are taken during treatment. Protection of the tissues of the eye from the highly penetrating gamma rays of radium or radon is not possible. As a

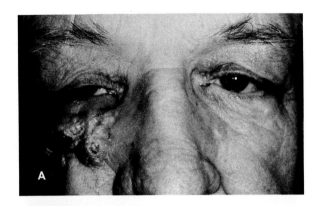

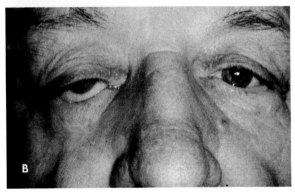

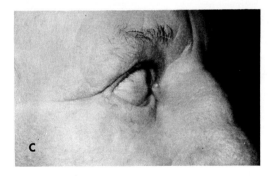

FIG. 300.
A. A 79-year-old patient with a bulky basal cell carcinoma invading the right
    lower eyelid.
B. and C. Same patient one year after treatment. (250 KV, 5000 rads in 15
    treatments over 21 days). Note the ectropion. This is inevitable when there
    is a bulky tumor with deep infiltration. It should not follow the treatment of
    small tumors confined to the lid margin.

result these latter agents are not used to treat small lesions of the lids.
A similar argument applies to the use of megavoltage external irradiation.

NASOLACRIMAL DUCT. When a tumor arises at the inner canthus irradiation of the nasolacrimal sac and duct is inevitable and a reaction within the structure causing epiphora will generally result. This may be permanent depending on the degree of scarring from tumor invasion and the development of adhesions following the reaction.

Technic of Irradiation

For small tumors of the lids and lid margins the radiation treatment of choice is external irradiation using a beam of low energy. With deeper penetration x-rays of up to 250 KV may be necessary. Megavoltage irradiation and interstitital technics using radium and similar agents should be confined to those situations where the whole orbit is to be treated and the eye sacrificed or where there is extensive bone infiltration. Even here the difficulty of protecting the opposite eye usually contraindicates radium technics.

During treatment the eye is protected by a 2 mm. lead shield curved to fit the globe (fig. 301). The shield is silverplated to filter the soft radiation from the lead and a small handle provided to facilitate insertion and removal. After preliminary anesthetization and the insertion of a few drops of a lubricant such as mineral oil the shield is inserted under sterile conditions. Great care must be taken during insertion not to injure the cornea or the conjunctiva. When an anesthetic has been used the eye must be protected until the affects have worn off. The use of antibiotics in the conjunctival sac is also desirable after use.

Care must also be taken to ensure that the noninvolved eyelid (generally the upper) is not included in the irradiation field. Although a patient will tolerate loss of lashes in one eyelid, such loss in both is disastrous.

DOSE. Although single treatments of 2250 rads are effective in curing the lesion, the cosmetic result is better if treatment is given over a more extended period, and is to be recommended. The total dose and

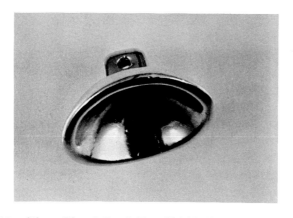

FIG. 301. Silver Plated Lead Eye Shield Used to Protect Eye.

number of fractionations will depend on the size of the fields necessary. For fields of less than 3 cm. a dose varying from 3000 rads in five fractions each of 600 rads to 4500 rads in ten fractions of 450 rads is adequate and will result in minimal permanent change other than the loss of eyelashes. For larger field sizes longer fractionation schemes should be used.

A margin of about 0.5 cm. of apparently normal tissue should be allowed around the lesion and included within the irradiated field. The exact size of this margin will depend on the appearances of the primary lesion. With larger ill-defined lesions more generous limits will be necessary.

Effects of Radiation and Their Management

IMMEDIATE EFFECTS.   Toward the end of the course of treatment, or shortly afterwards, depending on the duration, the skin within the irradiated area will become erythematous and the eyelashes will fall out. This erythema may progress to moist desquamation at the site of the tumor although not throughout the whole area. The reaction rapidly subsides and about two to three weeks after the completion of treatment the tumor will have disappeared although some crusting may remain at the primary site. It may then be a further two to three weeks before resolution is complete. Coincidentally the conjunctiva will show erythema.

As long as the area remains dry it is best to use no local medication. With the onset of moist desquamation, however, a local hydrocortisone and antibiotic ointment to the lesion and to the conjunctival sac will reduce inflammation appreciably.

LONG-TERM EFFECTS.   As has been stated loss of eyelashes within the treatment field is permanent, as is some slight atrophy of the skin within the treated area.

Particularly where there has been appreciable destruction of the lid margin by the tumor, some loss of continuity of the margin may be seen. At best this should be no more than a slight depression which causes no symptoms.

Special Situations

TUMORS OF THE INNER CANTHUS.   These tumors have a greater propensity to deep invasion and their surgical repair is more difficult. At this site in particular radiotherapy is the treatment of choice. Depending on the degree of deep invasion more penetrating irradiation may be necessary. The lacrimal duct and sac will almost inevitably lie within the treatment volume and a reaction will develop with possible late permanent epiphora. During the period of reaction careful cannulation of the duct may prevent permanent damage.

TUMORS NOT AFFECTING THE LID MARGINS. There is generally a greater laxity of skin and primary surgical closure may be more readily achieved. If this is possible then surgery is probably the treatment of choice.

RADIOTHERAPY FOLLOWING INCOMPLETE SURGERY. On occasion, patients will be referred for postoperative radiotherapy because examination of the excised specimen shows the removal to have been incomplete. Of course, when gross tumor remains radiotherapy should be given. When only microscopic evidence of disease at the periphery of the specimen is seen it is probably wise to await definite recurrence. The persistence of cells at the edges of the specimen is probably commoner than is generally realized. Einaugler and Henkind examined forty consecutive basal cell carcinomas treated by surgical excision. Of the forty, twenty had tumor cells at the margin of the specimen. However, not all of those of necessity recur. Gooding, White and Yatsuhashi, in a follow-up study of patients with basal cell carcinoma of various skin surfaces in whom marginal tumor cells were seen in the specimen, reported clinical recurrences in only 35 per cent.

RECURRENCE AFTER RADIOTHERAPY. As a general rule, in this situation and invariably where the tumors are small further radiotherapy should not be given and the tumor should be excised.

LYMPH NODE METASTASIS. Even with squamous cell carcinoma this is extremely rare and prophylactic radiotherapy or surgical dissection is not indicated. When metastases do occur surgery is the treatment of choice. The necessity for surgery need not necessarily affect the management of the primary lesion.

OTHER EPITHELIAL TUMORS. Malignant melanoma occsionally is found in the eyelid. Although infrequently, it does show some response to radiotherapy. This is unpredictable and incomplete and surgery is the treatment of choice.

The adenoid tumors are commonly stated to be radioresistant but this need not necessarily be so. In general, surgery is again the method of choice but one need not hesitate to irradiate using the same technics outlined for the basal cell and squamous cell carcinomas.

MALIGNANT LYMPHOMA

In patients with malignant lymphoma, in particular acute leukemia, bulky deposits of tumor tissue may occur in the conjunctiva and involve the lids. These tumor deposits are extremely sensitive to radiotherapy and effective control can be rapidly achieved by doses in the region of 1000 rads or less in 1 to 2 weeks (figs. 302A and B). Orthovoltage quality of radiation should be used and although an attempt can be made to protect the lens this is generally not possible. As a rule, however, this is

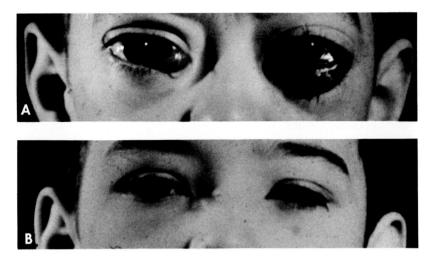

FIG. 302.   A Ten Year Old Boy with Acute Leukemic Deposits in the
Conjunctiva.
A. and *B*.   Appearance before and after treatment.

of no great importance. These patients unfortunately have a limited life
expectancy and the danger of late cataract is regrettably not a problem.
The dose given is insufficient to produce any local tissue reaction.

SUMMARY

Both radiotherapy and surgery can effectively cure basal and
squamous cell carcinoma of the lids. For tumors of the lid margin, unless
primary surgical closure is possible, radiotherapy is the treatment of
choice. It does not result in permanent change other than loss of lash.
Ectropion occurs only when there is appreciable tissue destruction
caused by the primary tumor (figs. 300*A* to *C*). With skilled radiotherapy
the structures of the eye and orbit are not at risk. Other epithelial
tumors, in particular the malignant melanoma, are probably best managed by surgery. Malignant lymphoma is satisfactorily controlled locally
by radiation.

COMMENT: A SURGICAL VIEWPOINT

BY SIDNEY A. FOX, M.D.

Dr. Newall, an expert radiotherapist, has a great deal to say above
which is logical and to the point, and I agree with most of it. Probably
no one, however, would be more surprised than he if I agreed with everything he said. My object here is not to condemn the use of irradiation

but to argue against its misuse. Irradiation and surgery should not be competing modalities but should complement each other.

There is and always has been controversy as to the best method of treating lid epitheliomas. Radiologists are certain that the ideal modality is irradiation. Opposed are those who feel that surgery is the best procedure in most cases. There are many papers in the literature to prove that both sides are right.

It occurs to me that one of the main causes of this impasse is that terms have not been properly defined and that the frames of reference vary widely. What is a cure? For a roentgenologist a cure is getting rid of the cancer. For the ophthalmic surgeon this is a preliminary step and a final cure is attained only when the patient has been restored as nearly as possible to his precancerous state.

It is this difference of definition which is probably one of the main causes of disagreement. Admittedly, if the lesion is small and away from the margin, either modality—irradiation or surgery—may be used and the lesion cured. But the larger lesions which require surgical repair after a "cure" by irradiation are the ones that always give trouble. Irradiation makes surgery long delayed and more difficult sometimes because of tissue vitiation and necrosis which may arise years later. This is why surgeons who are interested in the final appearance of their patients feel that irradiation should be used cautiously if there is any other recourse; or not at all. Reese, who has had a lifetime of experience, points out that any tumor growth can usually be arrested if a sufficient dose of x-ray radiation is given. The cost, however, can be very high and, in some cases, prohibitive.

Primary irradiation is acceptable in elderly patients with a short life expectancy. It is a must in old neglected cases where life is at stake and where surgery would obviously be too little and too late. As Dr. Newall has pointed out, it is contraindicated unless malignancy is present. In small lesions where biopsy amounts to excision, irradiation is superfluous. Bone involvement is an indication for surgery. Such lesions require so much irradiation that the bone is also destroyed; or, what is worse, bone is destroyed and not the cancer. Medial canthus lesions are amenable to both modalities and both will frequently bring on epiphora. However, the irradiated tissues of eyeglass wearers do not tolerate well the weight of the glasses. Such patients are entitled to primary surgery.

The advantage of out-patient treatment is always claimed for radiation therapy. One wonders what advantages recurrent visits to the clinic have over one hospitalization which effects both a resection and a plastic repair. The question arises especially in the larger lesions which usually need plastic repair after irradiation.

The choice of one or the other modality is often dictated—and should be—by the availability of either an ophthalmic plastic surgeon or a competent radiation therapist. In that case the choice is obviously what is available. As Dr. Newall emphasizes above, the eradication of lid tumors is not for the interested amateur but for the surgical or radiotherapy specialist.

REFERENCES

BACLESSE, F., and DOLLFUS, M. A.: Le traitement roentgentherapeutique des cancer palpebraux. J. Radiol. Electrol. *39*:832, 1958.

BROWN, J. B., and FRYER, M. P.: Carcinoma of the eyelids and canthal region. Geriatrics *12*:181, 1957.

COGAN, D. G., et al.: Symposium. Ocular effects of ionizing radiation and radiotherapy. Trans. Am. Acad. Ophth. & Oto. *63*:429, 1959.

DALLEY, V. M.: *In* R. W. Raven (ed.): Cancer, vol. 5. London, Butterworth, pp. 390–392.

EINAUGLER, R. B., and HENKIND, P.: Basal cell epithelioma of the eyelid: Apparent incomplete removal. Am. J. Ophth. *67*:413–417, 1969.

FAYOS, J. V., and WILDERMUTH, D: Carcinoma of the skin and eyelids. Arch. Ophth. *67*:298–302, 1962.

FORREST, A. W.: Tumors following radiation about the eye. Trans. Am. Acad. Ophth. & Oto. *65*:694, 1961.

FOX, S. A.: Use and misuse of irradiation in lid malignancies. Am. J. Ophth. *52*:1, 1961.

GOODING, C. A., WHITE, G., and YATSUHASHI, M.: Significance of marginal extension in excised basal cell carcinoma. New England J. Med. *273*:923–924, 1965.

LEAHY, B. D.: Beta radiation in ophthalmology. Indications, techniques and complications. Am. J. Ophth. *49*:7, 1960.

McDONALD, J. E., and WILSON, F. M.: Ocular effects of ionizing radiation and radiotherapy. Ocular therapy with beta particles. Trans. Am. Acad. Ophth. & Oto. *63*:468, 1959.

MERRIAM, G. R., JR.: Late effects of beta radiation on the eye. Arch. Ophth. *53*:708, 1955.

————: Radiotherapy in ophthalmology. N.Y. St. J. Med. *56*:3683, 1956.

MERRIAM, G. R., JR., and FOCHT, E. F.: A clinical study of radiation cataracts and the relationship to dose. Amer. J. Roentgenol. *77*:759, 1957.

POPMA, A. M.: Carcinoma of the eyelids. Acta. Un. Int. Cancr. *12*:384, 1956.

REESE, A. B.: Tumors of the Eye. New York, Paul B. Hoeber, 1953, p. 8.

RUBIN, P., and CASARETT, G. W.: Clinical Radiation Pathology, vol. 2. W. B. Saunders Co., Philadelphia, p. 662–702.

SCHULZ, M. D., and STETSON, C. G.: Radiation therapy of malignant lesions about the eye. Radiology *61*:786–795, 1953.

CHAPTER 26

Chemosurgery—Electrodessication

CHEMOSURGERY

By Perry Robins, M.D.

MALIGNANT TUMORS OF THE SKIN may be effectively treated by a number of methods which include excision, radiation therapy, cryotherapy, and electrodessication and curettage. Another modality for the management of skin cancer in use and uniquely suited for these lesions is chemosurgery.

Chemosurgery was introduced by Frederic Mohs more than 30 years ago and is currently being performed in many leading medical centers around the country.

With the chemosurgery technic, as the name implies, the tissue is first treated with a chemical agent and then surgically excised. The most important aspect of this procedure is the systematic microscopic examination of all surgically excised specimens at each stage of its removal. This allows the physician to identify precisely the extent of the tumor, which permits the total removal of the neoplasm under microscopic control. It provides the highest cure rate and at the same time sacrifices the minimum amount of normal tissue.

The following diagram is presented to show the steps in the Mohs technic (fig. 303):

A. The extent of the tumor is outlined and measured.

B. Frequently it is necessary to increase the percutaneous absorption of the zinc chloride fixative by the use of a keratolytic agent such as dichloracetic acid. The white discoloration shown is caused by the coagulation of epidermal proteins.

C. Zinc chloride paste, a 40 per cent solution of zinc chloride paste in stibinite, is applied in a thin layer. The thickness of the layer of paste applied will determine the depth of fixation. A thin layer of paste is all that is necessary to fix to a depth of 2 mm. in a twenty-four hour period.

Chief, Section Chemosurgery; Assistant Professor of Clinical Dermatology, New York University School of Medicine.

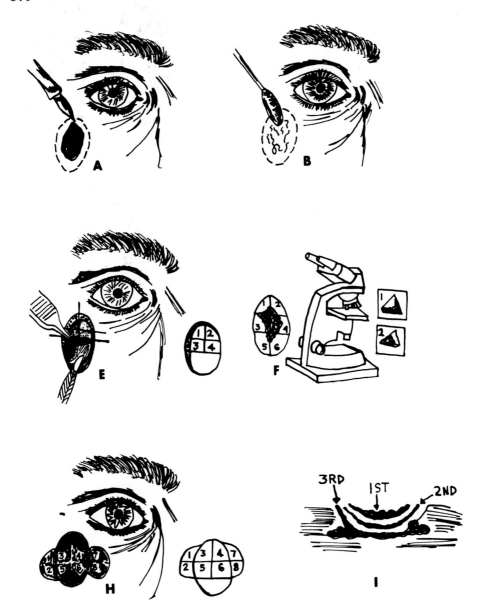

FIG. 303. Steps in the Mohs Technic of Chemosurgery.
A. Estimation of extent of tumor.
B. Dichloracetic acid applied.
C. Zinc chloride fixative paste applied.
D. Occlusive dressing.
E. Excision and mapping one day later.
F. Frozen section and examination.
G. Reapplication of paste to positive areas.
H. Second extension and mapping.
 I. Cross section of extension and depth.
J. Extent of lesion.
K. Healing one month later.

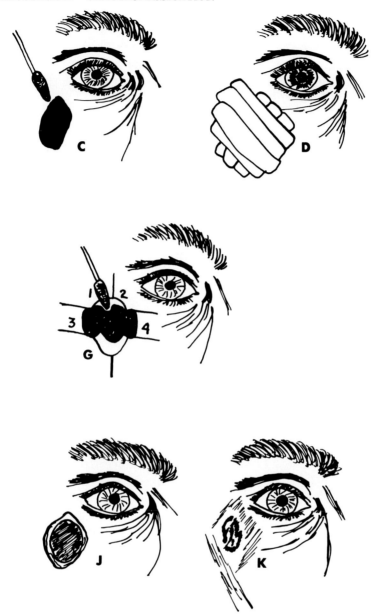

FIG. 303 (Continued)

D. Occlusive dressings are then used to cover the paste. This is necessary to avoid the effects of humidity which will cause the paste to liquify and reduce the rate of penetration of the zinc chloride. Often no analgesic is required during the period in which the fixative is penetrating the tissue.

E. After the fixative has been allowed to act for a few hours, the first layer of fixed tissue is surgically excised with a scalpel. The tissue is preferably removed in a saucer-like shape. There is minimal pain and little bleeding since the incision is made through fixed tissue.

Specimens of 1 to 2 mm. in thickness are cut into small pieces of approximately 1 cm. square which is a convenient size for the technician to section and for the physician to examine.

Dyes are applied to the edge of the specimen to indicate medial from lateral, superior from inferior. The location of the colored edges are indicated on a map. The red dye is mercurochrome. The blue dye is ordinary washing blue or Prussian blue. Marking two edges is usually sufficient. The origin and size of each specimen is indicated on a map. Each piece of tissue is assigned a consecutive number on the map and this order is maintained as more specimens are removed.

F.   After specimens have been removed and the map of the lesion is drawn, the patient waits until the frozen sections have been prepared by the technician and histologically examined. In producing frozen sections, the tissue is placed upside down on the microtome stage so that the undersurface of the flat specimen can be cut. If the microscopic section of the specimen reveals cancer, it is presumed that the next layer of adjacent tissue contains cancer. Where areas of cancer are found, their locations are marked in red pencil on the map.

G.   Fixative is then reapplied only to that area in which cancer has been located microscopically. This limitation to the treatment of the cancerous area is the important feature which allows for essentially selective destruction of the neoplasm and sacrifices the minimum amount of normal tissue.

H.   The procedure is repeated until the cancer-free level is reached.

I. and J.   There remains a layer of fixed tissue which sloughs off in several days. The granulation tissue is then exposed. It is remarkably vascular and highly resistant to infection.

K.   The lesion granulates in surprisingly rapidly, often with good cosmetic effects.

Dr. Mohs (1956) reported 129 consecutive cases of histologically proven basal cell carcinomas with a five-year cure rate of 93.4 per cent. These cases included both early and advanced cancers, many previously treated by other modalities which failed to completely destroy the neoplasms. Of this group, thirty patients were previously treated by other modalities and showed a cure rate of 83.3 per cent. This compares with 98.4 per cent in sixty-one cases having no prior treatment. With lesions measuring up to 3 cm. the cure rate was 98.5 per cent. Only eight lesions were reported to be larger than 3 cm. with a cure rate of 50 per cent. Deeply invasive tumors had a greater per cent of recurrence with a cure rate of 89.7 per cent (49 cases) as compared to the less invasive type with a cure rate of 100 per cent (42 cases).

The site of origin of basal cell epitheliomas plays an important part

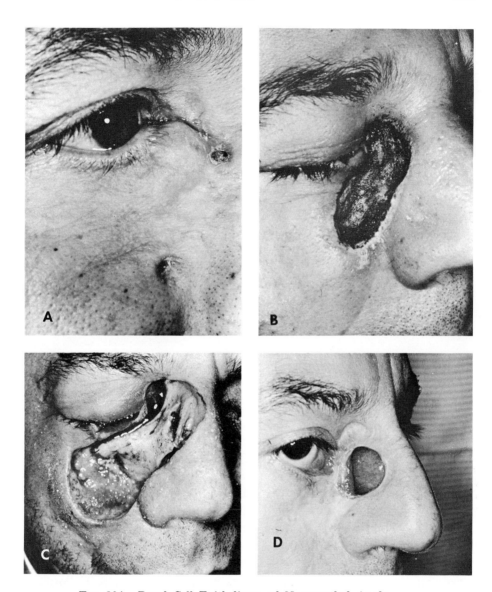

FIG. 304.   Basal Cell Epithelioma of Nasocanthal Angle.
A.   Recurrence after five resections.
B.   Application of zinc chloride paste after resection of tumor mass.
C.   Extent of upper and lower lid involvement.
D.   Healing one year later; prior to reconstruction.

in prognosis. Deeply invasive lesions of the canthal regions are more likely to produce serious complications than less invasive lesions (fig. 304). The latter are commonly found on the upper and lower lids.

In the treatment of squamous-cell carcinoma of the eyelids, a recent report showed a cure rate of 92.4 per cent. This included large and small lesions. The smaller sized lesions showed even a higher cure rate.

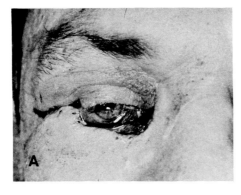

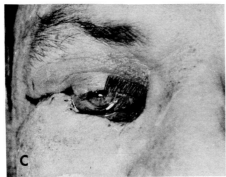

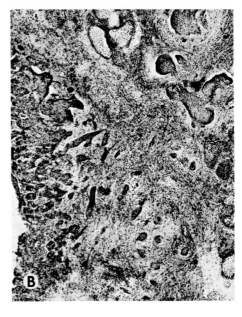

FIG. 305.   Recurrence of Basal Cell after Three Surgical Excisions.
A.   Recurred tumor of lower lid.
B.   Frozen section showing basal cell epithelioma in center and conjunctival
area.
C.   Shaded area shows upper lid involvement.

Tumors on the lid and the periorbital area can be surgically excised
by the chemosurgical method with minimal complications. Tumors situated at the eyelid margin can present some problems if the chemical
fixative should come in contact with the cornea. This can be eliminated by
excising a layer of unfixed tissue and having frozen sections of it prepared. The sources of the specimen are recorded on a map. Following
the removal of cancer on the lid margin, the defect site usually heals
spontaneously often leaving a remarkably small defect.

Cancers of medial and lateral canthi can be removed chemosurgi-
cally or by removing fresh tissue. In either event, it is possible to follow
the tumor a considerable distance into the orbit and still leave a functioning eye.

In the preparation of the histologic slides the architectural structures of the cells are not significantly altered. Thus, it is possible for the
physician to detect malignancies where present.

It is often difficult to determine the borders of a tumor, especially when the lesion site has been treated previously. However, with the chemosurgical technic, tumor tissue is readily identified and extensions can be followed out to their terminations. It is frequently difficult to judge on clinical examination if adjacent scar tissue is involved. Should tumor cells be present they can be easily detected by the chemosurgical technic. There is no delay in examining the histologic material in comparison with routine paraffin sections. The frozen tissue is cut immediately, stained for microscopic examination and is ready to be interpreted within a few minutes after the excision.

Extensions of tumors from the eyelids deep into the inner and outer canthus is not a rare occurrence, especially in cases which have been previously treated by surgery or radiation (fig. 305). Bizarre extensions must be considered each time a lesion in this area is encountered. Clinical judgment by palpation and approximation is insufficient for the total extirpation of these more difficult tumors. With the chemosurgical procedure, as previously stated, these tumors can be traced to their termination.

COMMENTS

Conservatism is the most important advantage of the chemosurgical procedure in removing tumors of the periorbital and eyelid areas. It is unnecessary to sacrifice more than 1 to 2 mm. of normal tissue beyond the extent of the tumor. There have been no deaths reported with this procedure. It is safe, and can be used on patients in poor health. Most frequently tumors are limited to the older age group. The Mohs technic allows such patients to undergo the procedure without serious complications. With a cellular response that is produced in the tissue there is a reduction in the incidence of infection and lastly, healing is surprisingly rapid; often a good cosmetic result is achieved without plastic reconstruction.

Where extensive tumor has left a large defect (fig. 306), the surgeon, because of the reliability of the procedure, can consider earlier repair than otherwise would be considered safe. He can feel free to go ahead knowing that the area is free of malignancy.

There is always the tendency—however subconscious—for a surgeon to save as much healthy appearing tissue as possible in order to make subsequent repair easier. (A recent report by Einaugler and Henkind showed 50 per cent inadequate resection in lid tumor excisions.) This helps swell the surgical recurrence rate and helps reduce it with a modality such as chemosurgery. The eye is a vital organ and the chemosurgical type of careful conservative treatment is best adapted to keep it safe, especially where other methods have failed.

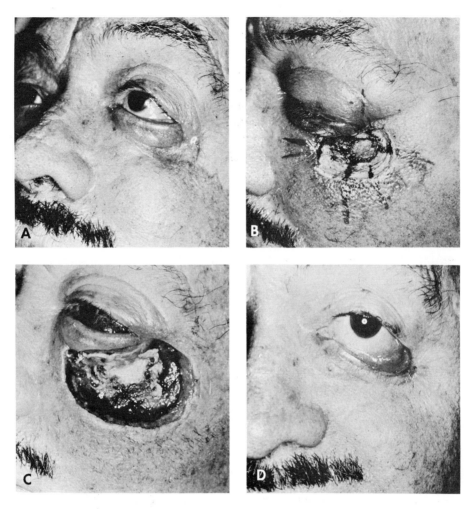

FIG. 306. Basal Cell Epithelioma of Fifteen Years' Duration.
A. Recurrence following three excisions and skin grafts.
B. Stage three level at which tumor was detected. (See figure 303*I*.)
C. Extent of lesion.
D. Healing after six months' duration. Ectropion was repaired at a later date.

CONCLUSION

The advantages of the chemosurgical procedure are unprecedented reliability, conservatism, low operative mortality, good healing without adverse sequelae and the feasibility of the operation to many patients in poor health. Lastly, where other standard modalities have been unsuccessful, chemosurgery offers a chance for cure. Physicians are now being trained in this procedure in many leading medical centers and facilities should be available to most patients in the not too distant future.

COMMENT: A SURGICAL VIEWPOINT

BY SIDNEY A. FOX, M.D.

Chemotherapy has probably been with us longer than history records and the use of cytostatic and escharotic chemicals in liquids, unguents and pastes has been sporadically recorded over the centuries. This, of course, is a modality of destruction. It acts—like irradiation—by necrotizing tissue.

A number of years ago Bayer E 39 (ethyleneimine quinone), a cytostatic and mitotic poison, was introduced by Domogk and used both intravenously and locally for malignancies. Pillat was the first to use it on eyelid tumors. He reported 31 successful cases in 1958 in which there were no adverse bone marrow or vascular changes. Others who have used it also reported good results with no side effects. In some cases, however, despite obvious clinical cures, tumor cells were still demonstrable. Hence long periods of observation are recommended or microscopic examination of scar tissue is suggested.

In 1941 Mohs reported his method of microscopically controlled serial cancer excision in which tissues are examined repeatedly by frozen section after chemical fixation. The method is beautifully described above by Dr. Robins. He has pointed out its advantages: conservation of healthy tissue, safety of important structures especially around the eye, reduction of infection and rapid healing. Obviously Dr. Robins, an expert in this particular modality, sees advantages in its use in all types, sizes and positions of tumors.

As in radiotherapy, much is made of the fact that the patient need not always be hospitalized. But chemosurgery, like irradiation, treats malignancies by tissue destruction and it may be accompanied by considerable local pain. Hence the patient cannot always carry on his normal gainful activities after application of the escharotic paste.

While small lesions may heal without subsequent corrective surgery, lid margin lesions should never be left unrepaired, as Dr. Robins suggests, unless they are of minimal depth. Every ophthalmologist knows how easily lid notching can occur after marginal resections. Larger lesions, with rare exceptions, all require surgical repair (figs. 304, 305 and 306). This, of course, means hospitalization and loss of time by the patient.

For the ophthalmic surgeon this chemosurgical technic would seem to be of most value in cases of deep infiltrating lesions especially in the nasocanthal angle where the medial canthal ligament and even the deeper lacrimal sac may show involvement. There is usually no line of demarcation and the lesion often has to be removed in bits and pieces. Here Mohs' technic of serial frozen sections of the area after surgery can be of significant assistance in assuring complete removal. I have found it so. (Incidentally, a recent report by Gooding, White and Yatsuhashi shows that only one-third of tumors reported as incompletely removed show recurrence.)

In lid areas other than the medial canthus, clean primary surgical removal, with frozen section examinations if deemed necessary, and immediate plastic repair would seem to be a less time consuming and more logical procedure. Healing is at least as good following surgery and immediate repair as following chemosurgery.

ELECTRODESSICATION

Electrodessication and electrocoagulation are of some value in cases of small, obviously benign lesions such as lid margin warts, keratoses, etc. This modality spares the cilia and does not impair the integrity of the lid margin. Another advantage is that the eye rarely has to be patched after its use. It is also valuable in minor cases of trichiasis where only a few cilia need be epilated (fig. 203).

One or two precautions should be observed. If the coagulation needle is buried too deeply, scarring may occur. Also in dark pigmented individuals unpigmented areas may appear (as in the removal of xanthelasma) which may be a more conspicuous blemish than the original lesion. Usually these light patches disappear after some months, however.

When the lesion is benign beyond peradventure of a doubt electrodessication is permissible. Figure 307A shows a fibrotic wart of the right lower lid involving the ciliary margin.

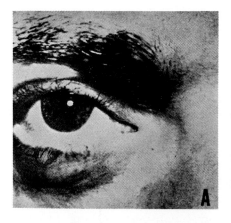 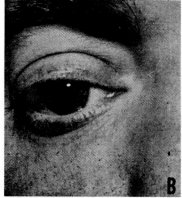

FIG. 307.   Use of Electrodessication—Ciliary Margin.
A.   Wart of right lower lid ciliary margin.
B.   Result after electrodessication.

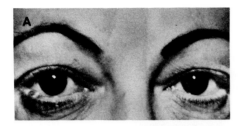
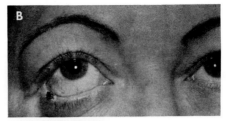
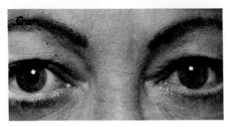

FIG. 308. Electrodessication of Flat Marginal Papilloma.
A. Papilloma of right lower lid.
B. Appearance after dessication.
C. Final result.

Procedure (fig. 307): The area is infiltrated with anesthesia. (Despite what has been claimed, electrodessication is not a painless procedure and anesthesia is advised.) A current just strong enough to cause a moderate spark is used and applied in an interrupted fashion (i.e., on and off) until the eschar created is even with the normal skin surface. No dressing is necessary. The area is examined in about two weeks for any residue (fig. 307B). If necessary, a little more dessication is done to eradicate lesion remnants.

A similar procedure was followed with the marginal lesion shown in figure 308A. The appearance after treatment (fig. 308B) shows the flat brown eschar on the surface of the lid margin. The eschar is lost in approximately two weeks leaving no residual scarring (fig. 308C).

Comment: The advantages of this modality are ease of application and simplicity of postoperative care. The faults are uncertainty as to whether the whole lesion has been removed and absence of a specimen for pathologic study. Hence it must be emphasized again that benignancy of the lesion must be assured before this method is used. Few such lesions exist (there are a few) before a pathology report is obtained.

REFERENCES

EINAUGLER, R. B., and HENKIND, P.: Basal cell epithelioma of the eyelid. Apparent incomplete removal. Am. J. Ophth. 67:413, 1969.

GOODING, C. A., WHITE, G., and YATSUHASHI, M.: Significance of marginal extension in excised basal cell carcinoma. New England J. of Med. 273:923, 1965.

MARX, J., and WILLOMITZER, H.: Zur chemotherapie des Lidkarzinomas mit "Bayer E 39." Klin. Monatsbl. Augenh. *133*:535, 1958.

MOHS, F. E.: Chemosurgery in Cancer, Gangrene and Infections. Springfield, Ill., Charles C Thomas, 1956.

————: Microscopically guided excision of cancer of the skin by means of chemosurgery. J. Ark. Med. Soc., November, 1968.

PILLAT, A.: Die Virkung des Cytostaticum Bayer E 39 bei malignen Geschwilsten der lider. Wien, Klin. Wchnschr. 383, 1958.

SZUJEWSKI, H. A.: Definitive treatment for tumors of the eyelids. Western Med., July, 1966.

Index